Clinical Exercise Testing

Progress in Respiratory Research

Vol. 32

Series Editor *Chris T. Bolliger,* Cape Town

KARGER

Basel · Freiburg · Paris · London · New York ·
New Delhi · Bangkok · Singapore · Tokyo · Sydney

Clinical Exercise Testing

Volume Editors *Idelle M. Weisman,* El Paso, Tex.
R. Jorge Zeballos, El Paso, Tex.

83 figures, 10 in color, and 97 tables, 2002

KARGER

Basel · Freiburg · Paris · London · New York ·
New Delhi · Bangkok · Singapore · Tokyo · Sydney

Idelle M. Weisman, MD

Human Performance Laboratory
Department of Clinical Investigation
Pulmonary-Critical Care Service
William Beaumont Army Medical Center
El Paso, Tex.
and
Department of Medicine
Pulmonary-Critical Care Division
University of Texas Health Science Center at San Antonio
San Antonio, Tex., USA

R. Jorge Zeballos, MD, DMSc

Department of Anesthesia
Texas Tech Regional Health Science Center
and
Human Performance Laboratory
Department of Clinical Investigation
William Beaumont Army Medical Center
El Paso, Tex., USA

Library of Congress Cataloging-in-Publication Data

Clinical exercise testing / volume editors, Idelle M. Weisman, R. Jorge Zeballos.
p. ; cm. – (Progress in respiratory research, ISSN 1422-2140 ; v. 32)
Includes bibliographical references and index.
ISBN 3805572980 (hardcover : alk. paper)
1. Exercise tests. 2. Lungs – Diseases – Diagnosis. 3. Cardiopulmonary system – Diseases – Diagnosis.
I. Weisman, Idelle M. II. Zeballos, R. Jorge. III. Series.
[DNLM: 1. Exercise Test. WG 141.5.F9 C641 2002]
RC734.E87.C554 2002
616.1′075–dc21 2002016243

Bibliographic Indices. This publication is listed in bibliographic services, including Current Contents® and Index Medicus.

Drug Dosage. The authors and the publisher have exerted every effort to ensure that drug selection and dosage set forth in this text are in accord with current recommendations and practice at the time of publication. However, in view of ongoing research, changes in government regulations, and the constant flow of information relating to drug therapy and drug reactions, the reader is urged to check the package insert for each drug for any change in indications and dosage and for added warnings and precautions. This is particularly important when the recommended agent is a new and/or infrequently employed drug.

P.O. Box, CH–4009 Basel (Switzerland)
www.karger.com
Printed in Switzerland on acid-free paper by
Reinhardt Druck, Basel
ISBN 3–8055–7298–0, ISSN 1422–2140

Contents

Foreword

Clinical exercise testing has been an area of personal interest for me for many years. It could therefore only have been a matter of time until I would have liked to see a volume in the book series *Progress in Respiratory Research* dedicated to this topic. Volume 32 is the result of this desire. The most important thing in the initial planning phase was, as always, to find the ideal volume editor(s), respected scientists in the field who can deliver the goods in time. Until now we have always been lucky in this respect. For this 32nd volume I did not have to think a long time who I was going to ask. Idelle Weisman, one of the outstanding experts in Cardiopulmonary Exercise Testing (CPET), came to my mind almost immediately. I have known her for some years now and have always admired her knowledge but at least as much her continued enthusiasm for both research in and teaching of CPET. When I approached her she immediately accepted the task, but asked me to do it together with her long-time colleague, Jorge Zeballos, a further name which does not need introduction. Their choice of chapter authors united a team of recognized specialists in their respective field.

The set was almost a guarantee for success. From there to the finished book, however, it took a lot of staying power by everyone to get everything done on time.

Dear Reader, when you look at the final product you will easily see what a high-powered book you are holding in your hands. In 25 well-written chapters all the relevant information about CPET is covered, from the physiologic responses to exercise, the set-up of an exercise lab, the methodology of clinical exercise testing, the varying patterns of response to exercise in different disease states, and very importantly to the clinical applications, everything you might want to know has been covered. As you read the book you will easily understand why CPET is becoming increasingly more important to help in clinical decision-making in the management of patients. The book is a must for anyone interested in clinical exercise testing.

Again, the publisher, S. Karger AG, Basel, Switzerland, has done a great job in bringing out a very attractive book with excellent quality of print. The appealing appearance of each single volume of *Progress in Respiratory Research* continues to be another key factor for the ever increasing success of the 'blue' book series. I would like to express a sincere thank you to Idelle and Jorge, to all chapter contributors, as well as to the staff at Karger.

C.T. Bolliger, Series Editor

Preface

Clinical Exercise Testing is increasingly being used in clinical medicine, as functional assessment has become an integral component of patient evaluation; this reflects in part a growing awareness of the limitations of traditional resting cardiopulmonary measurements in reliably estimating functional performance and outcome. A spectrum of clinical exercise testing modalities is available; which test to use depends on the question(s) being asked and the available resources. In turn, Cardiopulmonary Exercise Testing (CPET) has gained increasing popularity with a wide spectrum of clinical application over the last 25 years because of the valuable information it provides in patient diagnosis and management. This issue of *Progress in Respiratory Research* is testimony to the expanding list of clinical applications.

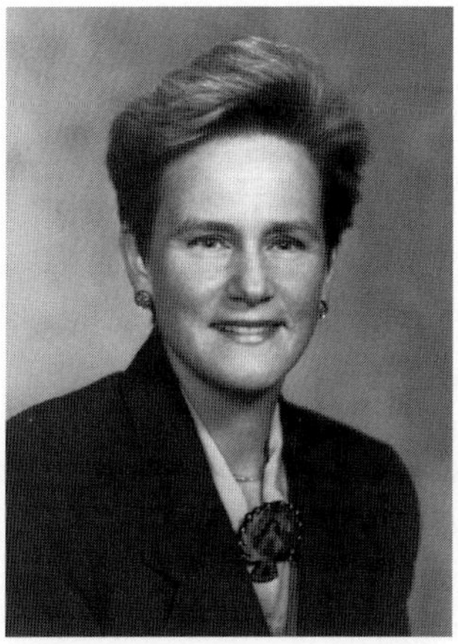

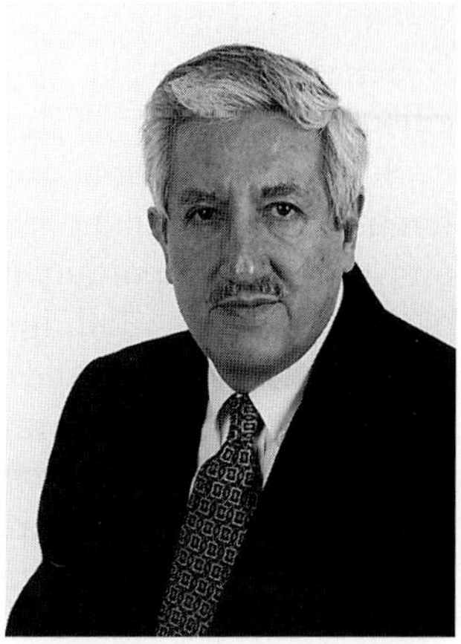

We were very excited about the *Progress in Respiratory Research* issue on Clinical Exercise Testing, as it would provide an opportunity for presentation of a comprehensive interdisciplinary update by well-respected experts that would focus on clinical application and highlight recent developments/practices based on current scientific knowledge and technologic advances. For CPET this would also reinforce the importance/value of the integrative exercise response in clinical assessment; that is, the ability to quantitate the patient's whole exercise response as well as contributions and interactions of individual components and thereby provide answers to questions not possible from other clinical exercise testing modalities. This issue explores the most widely used clinical exercise testing modalities with an emphasis on CPET. Furthermore, these comprehensive albeit succinct and cogent updates will be particularly useful to clinical readers challenged with keeping up with the remarkable information expansion in this area and the on-going need to assess clinical relevancy.

The expert contributors to this issue have provided timely, clinically oriented, and practical updates/reviews, which together represent a well-balanced perspective of clinical exercise testing for the new millennium. In that regard, we believe that this issue will be helpful to a wide audience – pulmonologists, cardiologists, pediatricians, exercise physiologists, rehabilitation specialists, respiratory therapists, etc. This issue begins with a state-of-the-art review of exercise physiology and limitation to exercise in normal subjects and is followed by a chapter on skeletal muscle function and energy metabolism during exercise which is currently a very 'hot' investigational topic. Modalities of clinical exercise testing provides a low-tech to high-tech functional assessment overview which concentrates on the 6-minute walk test, the shuttle test, and stair climbing, and addresses when these and more high-tech tests including graded exercise testing and CPET would be appropriately used. This is followed by a chapter providing basic and practical information related to equipment, methodology, protocols, conduct of the test, and also addresses important quality control issues for CPET. An article on deconditioning and training highlights the physiologic response to training and relates current knowledge to practical considerations for clinical application.

Since exertional dyspnea is a common reason for referral for exercise testing, mechanisms and measurement of dyspnea are also discussed. Another chapter addresses the patient with unexplained dyspnea after initial non-diagnostic work-up and emphasizes the role of CPET used as part of a step approach in the assessment of these challenging cases. A chapter on the aging pulmonary system and exercise provides insight and information that is extremely relevant as increasing numbers of senior citizens exercise.

Subsequent discussions evaluate exercise testing in different patient populations. A trio of complimentary chapters addresses important cardiovascular topics – the role of CPET in heart failure and transplantation discusses physiologic responses and current drug therapies, the role of cardiac rehabilitation in heart failure and cardiac transplantation discusses exercise prescription and monitoring and to complete the picture, non-invasive exercise testing modalities for ischemia discusses the most current technologies and clinical decision analysis for their use. A trio of chapters comprehensively evaluates important COPD topics including the role of CPET in evaluating exercise intolerance, exercise response patterns, exercise limitation, exercise training, and functional evaluation in lung volume reduction surgery. The next two chapters address the role of CPET in Interstitial Lung Disease and in Pulmonary Vascular Disease and a third discusses asthma and exercise.

This is followed by articles evaluating the use of exercise testing in specific clinical settings: in the evaluation of Impairment-Disability; in the Preoperative Evaluation for lung resection; in the evaluation of patients with metabolic myopathy and other neuromuscular disorders; in the evaluation of patients with Lung and Heart-Lung Transplantation, and in the evaluation of patients with other systemic diseases including obesity, diabetes, hyperthyroidism and chronic fatigue syndrome.

Previous monographs on clinical exercise testing have not included chapters on important population cohorts including pregnant/post-partum women and children, which have been included in this issue. Importantly, the chapter on exercise in children will appeal not only to pediatricians and pediatric sub-specialists, but also to adult pulmonologists and cardiologists who will provide care for the increasing number of children surviving into adulthood.

The subject of the last chapter is interpretation of cardiopulmonary exercise testing, which uses illustrative case studies to highlight the integrative approach to cardiopulmonary exercise testing and its role in the clinical decision-making process. Finally, it should be noted that most of these articles were written within the last 6 months of 2001 and includes 'hot-off-the-press' information that will remain clinically relevant for some time.

Our vision for this issue was to demonstrate how the information obtained from cardiopulmonary exercise testing impacts and enhances the clinical decision-making process including diagnosis, prognosis, severity, progression, and response to treatment in different clinical settings. Furthermore, we wanted to demonstrate how CPET complements and enhances other diagnostic modalities and can be an integral component in the clinical decision-making process. Enormous progress has been made but CPET still remains underutilized. Hopefully, the contents of this issue will stimulate more widespread use and discussion so that the full potential and limitations of cardiopulmonary exercise testing in the clinical decision-making process will be realized.

Acknowledgements

We are grateful to S. Karger AG, Switzerland and to Chris Bolliger, Editor of the *Progress in Respiratory Research* series, for allowing us the opportunity to assemble this outstanding group of articles. We believe that they will be a valuable resource and will appeal to a broad spectrum of readers interested in clinical exercise testing – from those who order exercise tests to answer important clinical questions to those who perform the testing. We would also like to express our appreciation to the expert contributors for their efforts to make this an updated 'state-of-the-art' book in Clinical Exercise Testing.

Special thanks are extended to Raul Hernandez, David Lopez and Luz Torres at William Beaumont Army Medical Center, El Paso, Texas, for their diligence and dedication in helping me complete this project. We would like to thank the command at William Beaumont Army Medical Center for their support in completing this project, and all colleagues who over the years have referred patients to the Human Performance Laboratory so that we might contribute to the clinical decision-making process. Finally, this issue is dedicated to our families for their patience, tolerance and ongoing support.

Idelle M. Weisman, R. Jorge Zeballos, Volume Editors

Weisman IM, Zeballos RJ (eds): Clinical Exercise Testing.
Prog Respir Res. Basel, Karger, 2002, vol 32, pp 1–17

Cardiovascular and Respiratory System Responses and Limitations to Exercise

Joshua R. Rodman Hans C. Haverkamp Sinéad M. Gordon Jerome A. Dempsey

The John Rankin Laboratory of Pulmonary Medicine, Department of Preventive Medicine, University of Wisconsin at Madison., Wisc., USA

Summary

The design and dimensions of the healthy pulmonary system are nearly perfect to meet the considerable demands on O_2 transport and CO_2 elimination imposed by physical exercise. In our chapter, we briefly describe the features of the nervous system pathways and the structure of the airways, lung surface area and respiratory muscles which ensure both the completeness of gas exchange at the level of alveolar gas, pulmonary capillaries and arterial blood and the high level of mechanical efficiency with which the respiratory muscle pump operates. We also discuss the absence of a physical training effect on pulmonary vs. systemic structures which determine O_2 delivery and the implications of a relatively underbuilt lung and chest wall to exercise-induced arterial hypoxemia, diaphragm fatigue and the distribution of systemic vascular conductance and blood flow.

Introduction

Muscular exercise presents multiple challenges to the cardiorespiratory system's goals of maintaining adequate O_2 and CO_2 transport to meet increased metabolic demands while minimizing the increase in work performed by the heart and respiratory muscles. Despite marked O_2 desaturation (<10% $S\bar{v}O_2$) and CO_2 retention ($P\bar{v}CO_2$ >80 mm Hg) in mixed venous blood as $\dot{V}O_2$ and $\dot{V}CO_2$ reach maximum levels, PO_2 and PCO_2 in blood leaving the lung remains near resting levels and we rarely become consciously aware of our breathing. These near perfect responses are universal in health and even small increases in arterial PCO_2 above resting levels or sensations of dyspnea during exercise should be treated with great suspicion of impending or underlying pathophysiology. This chapter describes the essential cardiovascular and respiratory responses to exercise in health, discusses their underlying mechanisms and also deals briefly with circumstances where the healthy respiratory system may fail regarding its homeostatic missions, thereby presenting a potential limitation to exercise performance.

Neurochemical Control of Exercise Hyperpnea

The precision with which alveolar ventilation is increased during exercise can be appreciated by examining the near constancy of alveolar (and arterial) carbon dioxide pressure ($PACO_2$ (and $PaCO_2$)) during steady-state exercise of mild-to-moderate intensity (fig. 1). The alveolar ventilation equation states that

$$PACO_2 = \frac{\dot{V}CO_2}{\dot{V}} \cdot K$$

The fact that $PaCO_2$ (and arterial oxygen pressure (PaO_2)) is maintained near constant during exercise means that alveolar ventilation ($\dot{V}_A$) increases in proportion to

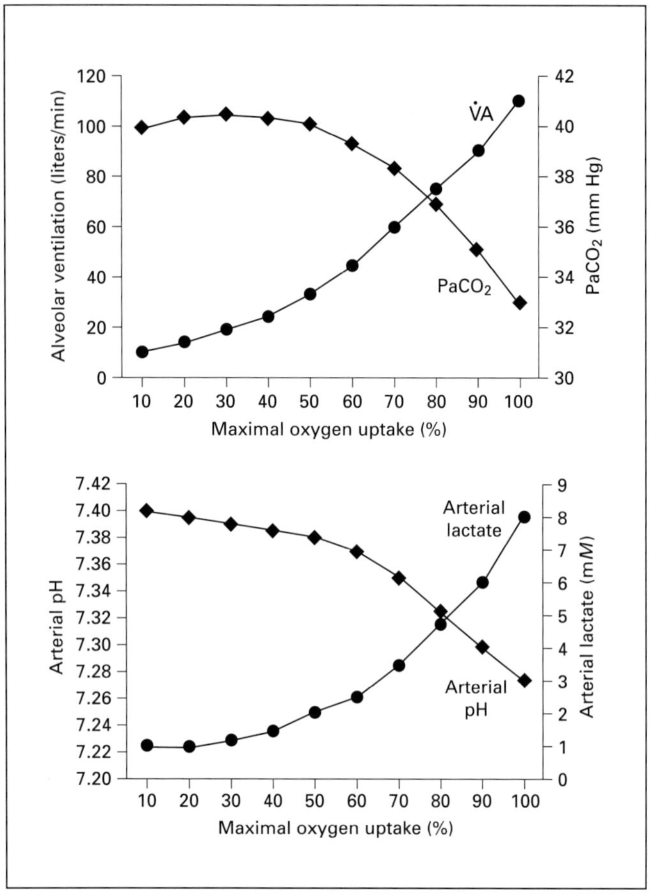

Fig. 1. Alveolar ventilation, arterial PCO_2, arterial lactate, and arterial pH during progressive exercise to maximum in a healthy young adult. As exercise intensity increases, a progressive lactic acidosis occurs which causes a decrease in arterial pH despite the concomitant hyperventilation (fall in $PaCO_2$). Data compiled from the authors' laboratory.

tissue CO_2 production ($\dot{V}CO_2$) (fig. 1). The complex question is: 'What powerful drives to breathe also change with exercise so precisely and quickly in concert with the increase in muscle CO_2 production?' Despite 120+ years of debate and often ingenious experimentation of this question, the exact mechanism(s) remain unresolved and intensely debated [see ref. 12 for recent review]. We have chosen to summarize this vast literature with the following generalizations, which we believe are supported by most experiments in both humans and animals. As with the control of heart rate and cardiac output (CO) in exercise, both feedback and feed-forward mechanisms operate in concert to mediate the hyperpneic response.

The feed-forward or 'central command' mechanism likely underlies the fast ventilatory response at exercise onset and remains the dominant stimulus to increase respiratory motor output at each level of exercise. This feed-forward ventilatory stimulation originates from higher locomotor centers (diencephalon, mesencephalon, and/or hypothalamic regions) and rises in parallel with central command to locomotor spinal motor neurons thus stimulating phrenic, intercostal, and lumbar respiratory motor neurons via descending neural pathways through the dorsal and ventral medullary areas responsible for generating respiratory motor output. There is no direct experimental evidence supporting ventilatory stimulation via the normally occurring increase in central locomotor command. Rather, support for this hypothesis comes primarily from electrical and pharmacological stimulation of motor areas in the supramedullary CNS to produce locomotion in decorticate cats. This stimulation increases ventilation (and cardiac output) even when the locomotor muscles are paralyzed [46].

Attempts have been made to increase central locomotor command (i.e., effort) in humans independently of muscle force output by using spinal blockade, partial muscle paralysis, studying patients with selected spinal cord lesions, or using hypnotic suggestion of exercise in normal intact subjects [78, 89, 91]. Inferences are then made about the role of central command during actual exercise based on the substantial hyperpnea and tachycardia observed under these conditions. However, we cannot be sure how closely, if at all, these changes in so-called 'central locomotor command' mimic those normally occurring during exercise. Does the increased locomotor 'effort' under these nonphysiologic conditions originate from the same motor areas of the higher CNS and travel the same descending neural pathways as normally occurs during whole body exercise?

In summary, the available evidence in animal models and the descriptive evidence in humans points toward a feed-forward stimulus from higher locomotor centers that is sufficiently powerful and precisely in tune with locomotor needs to explain much of the immediate and perhaps even steady-state hyperpnea achieved during exercise. However, final proof of this hypothesis requires that we be capable of mimicking, in isolation, all of the important characteristics of a truly physiological central locomotor command. Certainly, this is not an easy requirement and will not be met with current experimental approaches.

There is also a great deal of evidence supporting the view that feedback from unmyelinated metaboreceptors (type IV) and thinly myelinated mechanoreceptors (type

Fig. 2. Schema of two sets of influences (locomotor and respiratory) over autonomic control of cardiac output and blood flow distribution during exercise. Traditional central locomotor command effects parasympathetic outflow to the SA node for control of heart rate and sympathetic constrictor outflow to heart, skeletal muscle, and inactive vasculature. Feedback effects from working limb locomotor muscle effect sympathetic outflow. Aortic and carotid sinus baroreceptors undergo 'resetting' during exercise which permit heart rate and blood pressure to rise concomitantly. Newer data on respiratory system influences is included depicting excitatory metaboreceptor reflex effects from the diaphragm and expiratory muscles on vasoconstrictor sympathetic outflow (SNA), and an inhibitory feedback effect of lung inflation on SNA. Two additional respiratory-related sympathetic vasoconstrictor effects may include the influence of an increasing central respiratory motor output (which is strong in debuffered animals but may be masked by inhibitory feedback in intact humans) and the influence of carotid chemoreceptor stimulation, which likely occurs during heavy exercise.

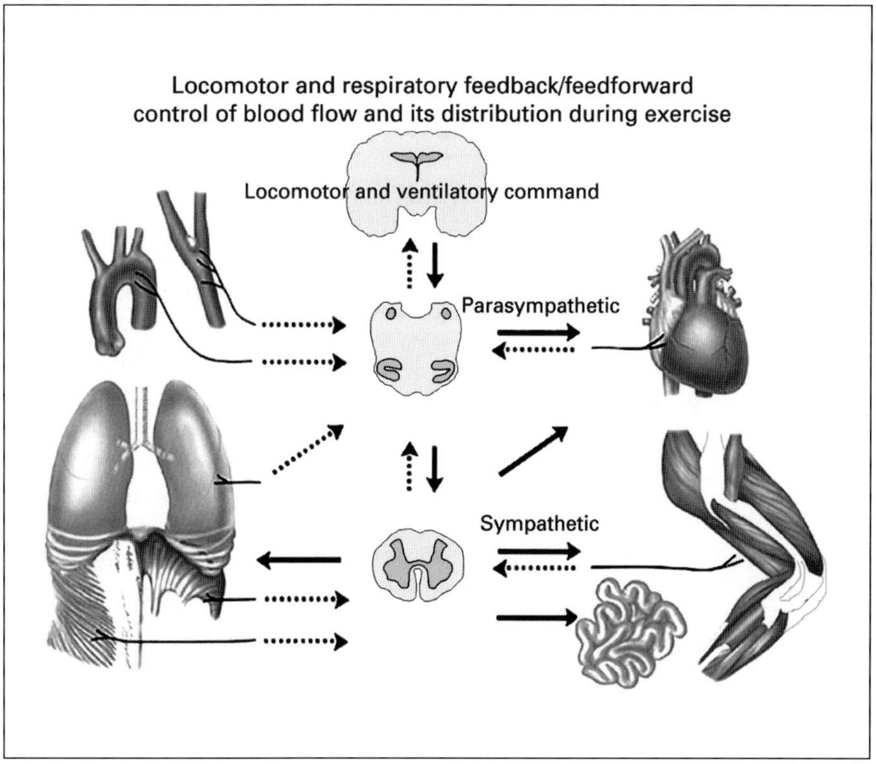

III) from contracting skeletal muscle contribute to regulation of the cardiorespiratory responses to exercise (fig. 2). Until recently, these muscle receptors were only thought to increase their activity in response to experimental perturbations such as ischemia, vessel distention, or electrical stimulation of motor nerves [46]. However, Kaufman and Forster [46] have shown that locomotion induced by electrical stimulation of locomotor centers in the higher CNS increases type III and IV afferent nerve activity in response to the 'exercise stimulus,' per se. Presence of this feedback effect is much more difficult to demonstrate in humans although increases in ventilation can be produced by local muscle ischemia, lower body positive pressure, vascular distention, or electrical stimulation of muscle. Evidence suggests a synergistic effect on the ventilatory response between feed-forward and feedback effects, especially as exercise intensity increases [91].

'CO_2 flow' back to the lung has logically been proposed as a regulating mechanism of hyperpnea primarily because of the tight correspondence between $\dot{V}_A$ and $\dot{V}CO_2$ during exercise. Receptors in the heart (mechanoreceptors) or lung (chemoreceptors) and magnified oscillations of arterial pH and PCO_2 stimulating carotid chemoreceptors have all been suggested as the 'missing stimulus' which changes in proportion to CO_2 flow with exercise [46]. However, these stimuli are not obligatory for the exercise hyperpnea to occur as shown by the normal ventilatory response to moderate exercise in humans with denervated lungs or carotid bodies, or in animal models where cardiac output and/or venous CO_2 concentrations can be controlled.

The hyperventilation of heavy exercise occurs at work rates requiring >70% $\dot{V}O_2$max reducing $PaCO_2$ as an arterial lactic acidosis develops. Three types of 'extra' stimuli to breathe appear to play a role here including: (a) curvilinear increases in the feedback stimulus as lactic acid and heat accumulate in working limb and respiratory muscles; (b) curvilinear increases in the feed-forward central command stimulus as more and more motor units are recruited in an attempt to maintain force output as limb and respiratory muscles fatigue [12], and (c) the added influence of carotid chemoreceptor stimulation in heavy work due to the addition of large quantities of hydrogen ions, norepinephrine, and potassium to arterial blood [12, 46]. Controversy exists, however, as denervation of the carotid bodies shows opposite effects on the hyperventilatory response to heavy exercise when tested in asthmatic humans (who exhibit a markedly blunted ventilatory

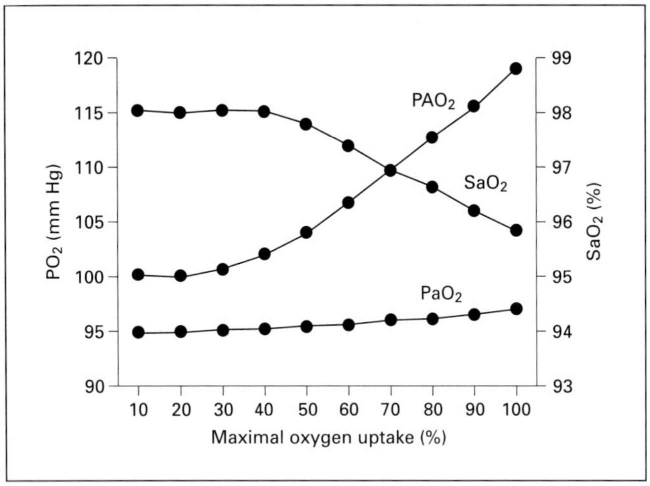

Fig. 3. Alveolar PO_2, arterial PO_2, and saturation of hemoglobin with oxygen during progressive exercise to maximum in a healthy, young adult. In spite of the progressively widened A-aDO_2, arterial PO_2 is maintained at resting levels during all exercise intensities. SaO_2 falls primarily because of a temperature and pH-mediated effect on the oxyhemoglobin dissociation curve. Data compiled from the authors' laboratory.

response following denervation) compared to animal models (who show an enhanced ventilatory response following denervation) [46]. We favor a combination of the aforementioned three mechanisms to explain the hyperventilatory response to heavy exercise.

Mechanics of Breathing during Exercise

During exercise, the respiratory control system functions to increase ventilation of the alveoli sufficient to maintain alveolar O_2 and CO_2 at or near resting levels while minimizing the mechanical work performed by the respiratory muscles [54, 57]. Minimizing the mechanical work, and therefore the metabolic cost of breathing will allow for: (1) a greater amount of cardiac output to be available for delivery to working limb muscle [28]; (2) a reduction in respiratory muscle energy store depletion [17], and (3) minimize sensory input and discomfort from the chest wall and lung reducing the potential for development of dyspnea or sensations of increased respiratory effort. These effects will delay limb and respiratory muscle fatigue thereby maximizing exercise performance [32].

During submaximal exercise, the increase in $\dot{V}_A$ is proportional to the increase in metabolic rate so that arterial O_2 and CO_2 remain constant (fig. 1, 3). As exercise progresses from mild through moderate intensity, $\dot{V}_A$ is increased primarily through increases in tidal volume (V_T) which: (1) reduces the dead space to tidal volume ratio (V_D/V_T), and therefore the 'wasted' portion of each inspiration, and (2) minimizes the flow-resistive work of breathing which is more closely related to breathing frequency (fb). The exercise-induced increases in V_T are achieved by encroaching into both the inspiratory and expiratory reserve lung volumes [33]. Encroachment into the expiratory reserve volume (i.e. reducing end-expiratory lung volume (EELV) below relaxation functional residual capacity (FRC)) is accomplished by recruitment of expiratory muscles [2] and is beneficial as it: (1) provides a passive contribution to the subsequent inspiration due to outward recoil of the rib cage upon termination of expiration; (2) lengthens the inspiratory muscles thereby placing them at a more optimal position for generating force during the subsequent inspiration, and (3) keeps the operating lung volumes on the linear (high compliance) portion of the pressure-volume curve over a greater range (fig. 4). As exercise intensity progresses from moderate to higher levels, V_T begins to impinge upon the flatter (stiffer) portion of the pressure-volume curve ($V_T > 75\%$ TLC; fig. 4). At this point of reduced lung compliance, V_T plateaus and further increases in $\dot{V}_A$ are accomplished solely through increases in fb [34].

An implicit consequence of increasing fb is a reduction in both inspiratory (TI) and expiratory (TE) time, which means flow must increase if a given lung volume change is to be maintained. Figure 5 illustrates the maximal flow volume loop generated by subjects at rest and is indicative of the capacity of the airways and respiratory muscles to produce flow and volume. In the healthy untrained adult, it can be seen that the capacities of both the airways and respiratory muscles to produce flow and volume are well in excess of those achieved during maximal exercise. A portion of the system's large capability to generate flow can be attributed to the coordinated efforts of numerous muscles that are recruited as exercise intensity increases including the diaphragm, scalenes, sternocleidomastoids, intercostals, abdominals, and pectorals. The metabolic capacities of these muscles are large and their biochemical properties quite heterogeneous [59], which provides for great functional versatility. Although most of the respiratory muscles are highly fatigue-resistant compared to limb muscles [24], they are susceptible to fatigue (especially during prolonged exercise at intensities $>80\%$ $\dot{V}O_2$max), which can effect sympathetic discharge, limb blood flow, and exercise performance (see 'Cardiorespiratory Interac-

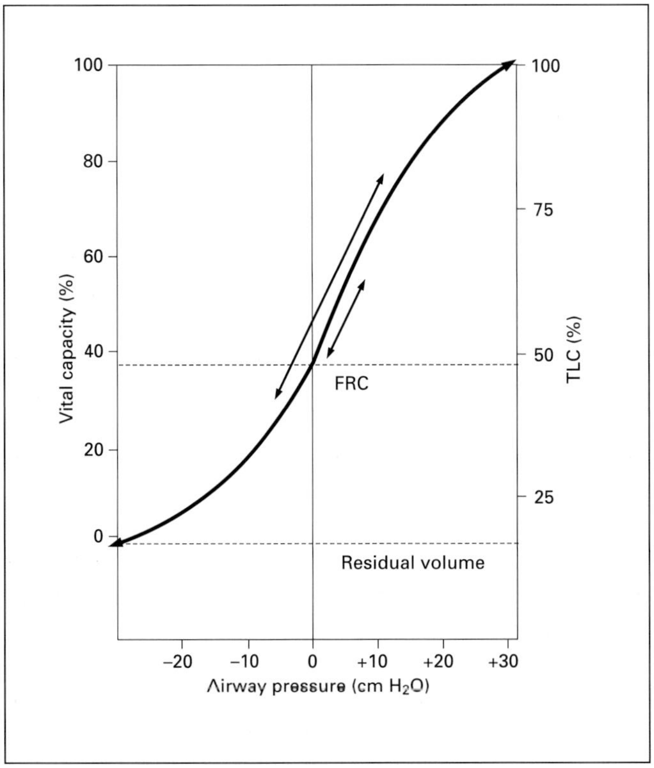

Fig. 4. Relaxation pressure-volume curve of the lung and chest wall. The subject inspires (or expires) to a certain volume from the spirometer, the tap is closed, he then relaxes his respiratory muscles. Modified from Powers et al. [59]. Less of a volume change is achieved for a given change in pressure generation at lower and higher lung volumes than compared to the mid-range volumes (decreased efficiency, i.e. compliance, at low and high lung volumes). Operating lung volumes at rest and during exercise are indicated by the short and long arrows, respectively. These volumes lie on the linear portion of the curve. Note the reduction in FRC during exercise due to abdominal expiratory muscle recruitment.

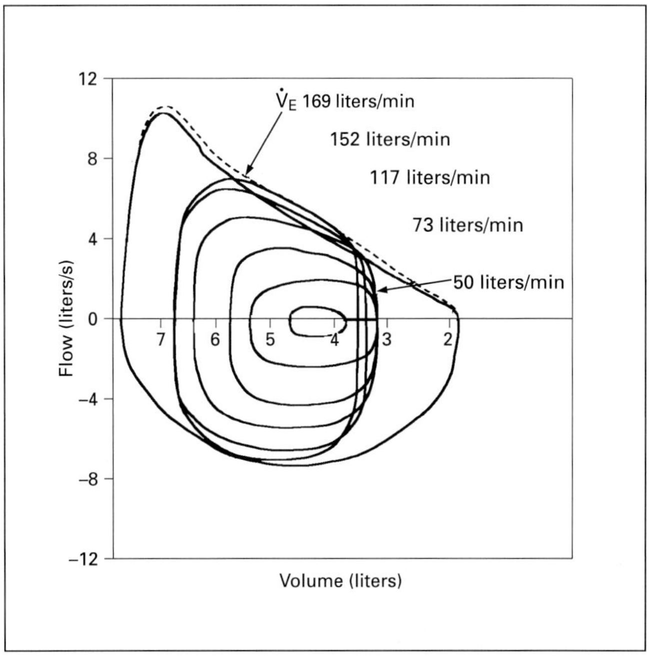

Fig. 5. Flow-volume relationship before, during, and after exercise in young adult males. The largest solid lined envelope is the mean maximal volitional effort for all subjects before exercise. The smallest loop is that obtained at rest. Note that all subjects show a reduced FRC during mild-to-moderate exercise (middle loops). Untrained subjects ($\dot{V}O_2$max = 35–50 ml/kg/min) with a mean V_E of 117 liters/min at maximal exercise show no significant flow limitation (i.e. impingement onto the maximal volitional loop), while highly trained subjects ($\dot{V}O_2$max = 60–83 ml/kg/min) with a mean maximal V_E of 150–190 liters/min but normal maximal flow-volume envelopes show significant expiratory flow limitation during strenuous and maximal exercise. The largest envelope (dotted line) represents the mean postexercise loop of all subjects and exceeds the maximal pre-exercise loop due to exercise-induced bronchodilation. Data compiled from Inbar et al. [42].

tions during Exercise and Respiratory Limitations to Exercise Performance').

Despite the large increases in both inspiratory and expiratory flows during exercise, flow resistance remains at or near resting levels due to a variety of precisely controlled mechanisms including: (1) a shift from predominantly nasal to oro-nasal breathing routes (normally occurs at levels of $\dot{V}_A$ equal to 20–40 liters/min [7]); (2) enhanced recruitment of laryngeal [14], tongue [88], and nasal [88] inspiratory muscles which serves to stiffen the airway and prevent negative pressure-induced airway narrowing; (3) coordinated activation of thoracic and abdominal respiratory muscles preventing paradoxical movement of the thorax [3]; (4) decreased expiratory 'braking' due to reductions in laryngeal adductor [14] and postinspiratory diaphragm muscle activity, and (5) sympathetic nervous system-mediated constriction of the vasculature in pulmonary and nasal mucosa which increases airway diameter [64].

The capabilities of the lung and respiratory muscles in the healthy, untrained adult are well in excess of the demands placed on them during exercise. As mentioned above, the flow rates and volume changes seen during maximal exercise are well within the maximal volitional flow-volume loops obtained at rest (fig. 5). Similarly, the amount of force generation required of the inspiratory muscles, as well as their velocity of shortening are only 40–60% of capacity at maximal exercise in the untrained individual. However, these numbers approach 90% of the system's capacity in the endurance-trained athlete [11] (see 'Respiratory Limitations to Exercise Performance').

Dyspnea

A critical aspect of the feedback control of breathing during exercise is its influence on suprapontine brain structures including the cortex, which are manifested as an 'awareness' of ventilatory effort and possibly even unpleasant sensations known as 'dyspnea'. Afferent fibers originating in the chest wall musculature and vagal afferents from the lung project all the way to the cerebellum and cerebral cortex. Furthermore, medullary inspiratory and expiratory pattern generator neurons project to the mid-brain and higher CNS. These neural connections may provide the sensory information that allows mechano- and chemostimuli to be perceived consciously.

Under what conditions does this cortical awareness of breathing and dyspnea occur during exercise? An increased drive to breathe by itself does not cause dyspnea, at least under conditions of mild to moderate exercise despite 10-fold increases in ventilation. Only in heavy exercise is the increased sensory input sufficient to engage the higher CNS and produce awareness of ventilatory effort. However, an increased drive to breathe combined with some form of mechanical impedance to flow or volume (i.e. an imbalance between neuromuscular effort and lung volume change) results in dyspneic sensations. Diseases which increase airway resistance, reduced lung/chest wall compliance, or cause respiratory muscle weakness create discrepancies between neuromuscular effort and ventilatory output, even during moderate intensity exercise. Hyperinflation of the lung secondary to expiratory flow limitation during exercise gives rise to extreme dyspnea because above a certain threshold lung volume, inspiratory efforts are opposed by inward recoil of the chest wall plus a stiffened lung (see fig. 4).

Pulmonary Gas Exchange

The alveolar to arterial PO_2 difference (A-aDO_2) is a measure of gas exchange efficiency from the alveoli to the pulmonary capillaries. At rest in the healthy human, the A-aDO_2 is ~ 5 mm Hg [11] and progressively widens during exercise of increasing intensity to values of ~ 20 mm Hg during maximal exercise [80] (fig. 3). Potential mechanisms causing the increased A-aDO_2 during exercise include a worsening maldistribution of ventilation to perfusion ($\dot{V}_A/\dot{Q}$), increased contributions from a fixed anatomical shunt, and/or a limitation for the diffusion of oxygen from alveoli to pulmonary capillary.

The ratio of $\dot{V}_A$ to $\dot{Q}$ can be partitioned into inter- (among regions) and intraregional (within a region) distributions for $\dot{V}_A$ and $\dot{Q}$. With respect to the interregional differences, both $\dot{V}_A$ and $\dot{Q}$ are greater at the base and less at the apex of the lung, a difference that has traditionally been thought to be primarily a function of gravity. However, recent evidence in primates and horses suggests only a small role for gravity effects on the pulmonary blood flow distribution during resting [21, 22] and exercising conditions [15]. Rather, it is suggested that the geometry of the pulmonary vascular tree is the principle determinant of interregional pulmonary perfusion heterogeneity and, thus, both structural heterogeneity and gravity effects result in the variability of resistances to blood flow that cause unequal distributions of $\dot{Q}$ vertically within the lung. Additionally, the rate of decline in $\dot{Q}$ from base to apex is greater than for $\dot{V}_A$ so that overall $\dot{V}_A/\dot{Q}$ is greater than 1 at the top, and less than 1 at the base of the lung at rest. Thus, an unequal distribution between ventilation and perfusion along the vertical plane of the lung also contributes to the interregional differences in $\dot{V}_A/\dot{Q}$ and some of the A-aDO_2 at rest and during exercise.

Intraregional differences in $\dot{V}_A$ distribution refer to the differences within a horizontal plane of the lung and arise due to variations in resistance of the airways within a region. Similarly, intraregional heterogeneity in $\dot{Q}$ is a function of the complex nature of the pulmonary vessels, which have random structural differences in diameter, length, and branching angles.

At rest, the A-aDO_2 is due almost entirely to a mismatch between $\dot{V}_A$ and $\dot{Q}$ within the lung. During exercise of increasing intensity [20, 80] and duration [38], the overall distribution of ventilation and perfusion throughout the lung likely becomes progressively slightly more nonuniform. This increase in overall $\dot{V}_A/\dot{Q}$ nonuniformity (as measured by the multiple inert gas technique (MIGET)) likely reflects the net effect of a more uniform topographical distribution (interregional) of $\dot{V}_A/\dot{Q}$ [5] and a less uniform intraregional $\dot{V}_A/\dot{Q}$ distribution. Despite this increase in nonuniformity of $\dot{V}_A/\dot{Q}$, the overall mean $\dot{V}_A$ increases out of proportion to $\dot{Q}$ with increasing exercise intensity. The resultant 3- to 4-fold higher overall $\dot{V}_A/\dot{Q}$ for the lung in heavy exercise vs. rest means that elevated alveolar PO_2s are present across all $\dot{V}_A/\dot{Q}$ units; thus, end-pulmonary-capillary PO_2 is maintained despite the marked reduction in mixed venous O_2 content and increased nonuniformity of $\dot{V}_A/\dot{Q}$ distribution.

The mechanisms accounting for the greater maldistribution of $\dot{V}_A/\dot{Q}$ during exercise remain largely unknown although possibilities include: (a) minor structural variations in airway and/or lung blood vessels could become further manifested during exercise as ventilatory and circulatory flows increase; (b) high flow rates could potentially irritate the airways resulting in airway secretions that effect the distribution of ventilation; (c) vascular tone could be altered during exercise, and/or (d) mild interstitial edema could develop during exercise if the lymphatic system does not adequately drain fluid leaking across the pulmonary capillary membrane into the interstitial space. Interstitial edema might be expected to effect the distributions of $\dot{V}_A$ and $\dot{Q}$ by increasing resistance to air and blood flow in affected areas. Additionally, if the fluid flux were to overwhelm the system so that it accumulated in the alveoli, gas exchange would be severely compromised. An increased transvascular fluid movement does occur during exercise [10], and several mechanisms exist to explain this including: (1) increased recruitment and distension of the pulmonary vasculature during exercise results in an increased total vascular surface area; (2) high pulmonary capillary transmural pressures during intense exercise may cause capillary stress failure and subsequent fluid leakage, and/or (3) the release of inflammatory mediators during exercise elicited by high flow rates and/or mechanical stress may increase vascular permeability resulting in fluid exudation/transudation. In healthy individuals however, the increased transcapillary flux does not result in appreciable accumulation of fluid within the interstitial space, primarily because of the lungs tremendous capacity to increase lymph flow and thus fluid drainage during exercise [10]. Also, the decrease in pulmonary vascular resistance that occurs during exercise attenuates the rise in pulmonary artery pressure minimizing the outward driving pressure for transcapillary fluid flux during exercise.

The second contributing factor to the A-aDO_2 is a right-to-left shunt of mixed venous blood (refers to blood that enters the arterial system without passing through the lungs). A fixed 1–2% extrapulmonary shunt exists in the normal human lung of which the thebesian veins are most important. Deoxygenated blood from these vessels empties directly into the left heart and mixes with oxygenated blood leaving the lungs, thus lowering PaO_2. The extrapulmonary shunt becomes progressively more important in determining the A-aDO_2 during exercise of increasing intensity as $C\bar{v}O_2$ falls.

A third potential contributing factor to the increased A-aDO_2 during exercise is failure of mixed venous blood in the pulmonary capillaries to equilibrate with alveolar oxygen pressure. Diffusion disequilibrium may occur between alveolar PO_2 and blood leaving the pulmonary capillaries if the time required for equilibration is greater than the time a red blood cell spends in a gas exchanging portion of the lung. The average time a red blood cell (RBC) spends in a pulmonary capillary is known as transit time and is determined by the ratio of pulmonary capillary blood volume to pulmonary blood flow. At rest, transit time is approximately 0.75 s while only ~0.40 s is required for the RBC to equilibrate with alveolar PO_2. During high-intensity exercise, however, transit time may be reduced to ~0.40 s or less which may result in incomplete oxygenation of hemoglobin (see 'Respiratory Limitations to Exercise Performance').

The rate of diffusion for O_2 across the alveolar-capillary membrane is determined by several factors that are quantitatively expressed in Fick's law of diffusion,

$$\text{Volume of gas} = \frac{D \times A \times (P_1 - P_2)}{T}$$

where D is a diffusion constant for the gas of interest, A is the surface area of the alveolar-capillary membrane, $P_1 - P_2$ is the partial pressure difference between gas in the alveoli and red blood cell, and T is the thickness of the blood-gas barrier membrane. The thickness and surface area depend on the structure of the blood-gas barrier, which is well designed to maximize diffusion across the membrane. While it is extremely thin (0.2–0.3 μm) [19] which is extremely important (see Fick's law of diffusion above), its design maintains the strength necessary to withstand the high transmural pressures developed during exercise. The interface consists of three primary components including the capillary endothelium, alveolar epithelium, and extracellular matrix (which is further comprised of the alveolar and capillary basement membranes). Situated in the middle of the extracellular matrix is an ultrathin layer of type IV collagen, which probably provides most of the strength to the blood-gas barrier [84]. The arrangement of type IV collagen is well designed to withstand the large transmural pressures generated during exercise. Additionally, the tremendous total surface area of the alveolar-capillary interface (approximately 50–100 m^2) [19] maximizes diffusion potential (see Fick's law of diffusion above). Thus, the extreme thinness and large surface area of the blood-gas barrier provide an optimal environment for diffusion of oxygen from the alveoli to pulmonary capillary during exercise. The only suggestion

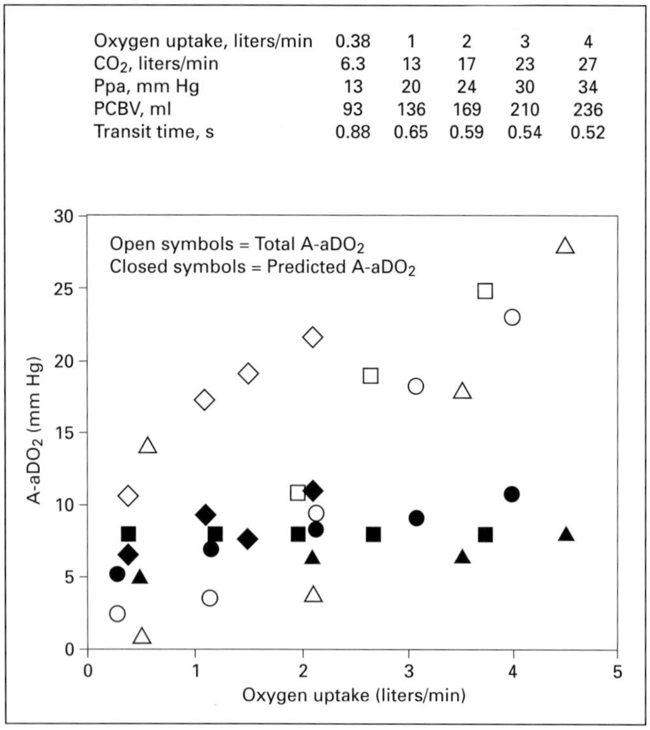

Fig. 6. Total A-aDO_2 (open symbols) and A-aDO_2 due to $\dot{V}_A/\dot{Q}$ mismatch predicted by MIGET (closed symbols) during exercise of increasing intensity in four separate studies [20, 26, 62, 77]. Data from each study are represented by separate symbols. Also included are average values of oxygen uptake ($\dot{V}O_2$), cardiac output (CO), pulmonary artery pressure (Ppa), pulmonary capillary blood volume (PCBV), and pulmonary capillary transit time. Ppa was calculated from the regression equation of [60] and PCBV from [39]. To illustrate, at a $\dot{V}O_2$ of ~ 3 liters/min, results from Hammond et al. [26] (represented by circles) measured a total A-aDO_2 of 18 mm Hg, while the A-aDO_2 attributable to $\dot{V}_A/\dot{Q}$ mismatch was 9 mm Hg. This $\dot{V}O_2$ corresponds to a CO of ~ 23 liters/min which brings Ppa, PCBV, and transit time to 30 mm Hg, 210 ml, and 0.54 s, respectively.

for a loss of blood-gas barrier integrity in humans comes from highly trained cyclists working at maximal intensity [37]; concentrations of red blood cells, total protein, and leukotriene B_4 measured in their broncho-alveolar lavage (BAL) fluid were significantly higher after a maximal 7-min uphill bike ride compared to a group of untrained subjects who did not perform an exercise bout. Unfortunately, the more appropriate test would have been to compare BAL fluid in the athletes before and after a maximal exercise bout as these results could have been due solely to subject selection bias.

The lung is further protected from significant diffusion disequilibrium by virtue of its low resistance pulmonary vasculature, which possesses a great capacity to dilate. During exercise, pulmonary artery pressure rises, pulmonary vascular resistance falls, and a passive expansion of the pulmonary capillary bed occurs mainly in lung regions that were under-perfused at rest with respect to $\dot{V}_A$. This expansion acts to maintain RBC transit time in the face of an increased cardiac output. Thus, only when cardiac output rises out of proportion to the pulmonary capillary blood volume does the possibility exist for a diffusion limitation to occur. Given the maximal cardiac output of a healthy, untrained person (~ 20 liters/min) and the great capacity for expansion of the pulmonary capillary bed, a limitation for diffusion is unlikely. Thus, if diffusion disequilibrium is involved in the increased A-aDO_2, it will likely only contribute during near-maximal to maximal exercise in the trained individual with a high cardiac output and rarely be involved in the increased A-aDO_2 during submaximal exercise [38].

The MIGET (multiple inert gas elimination technique) can be used to indirectly assess the contributions from diffusion limitation and extra-pulmonary shunt to the widened A-aDO_2 during exercise. Since the MIGET quantifies $\dot{V}_A/\dot{Q}$ inequality, a predicted value for the A-aDO_2 (assuming complete diffusion equilibration and no extra-pulmonary shunt) can be calculated and compared to the measured A-aDO_2. If the measured A-aDO_2 is greater than that predicted from the MIGET, a diffusion disequilibrium and/or extrapulmonary shunt must account for the difference although it is difficult to discern the relative contributions from each of the two. Using this technique, several authors have shown a significant difference between predicted and measured A-aDO_2 during exercise [26, 63, 80] and attribute this difference solely to diffusion disequilibrium. However, these studies found that the A-aDO_2 due to ventilation-perfusion mismatch (predicted) was less than the total A-aDO_2 during sub-maximal levels of exercise ($\dot{V}O_2$ ~ 2 liters/min) when cardiac output and pulmonary capillary blood volume are well below maximal levels, transit time is ~ 0.6 s, and pulmonary vascular pressures are well below those required for interstitial fluid accumulation due to capillary stress failure (fig. 6). Thus, it seems highly unlikely that alveolar-capillary diffusion disequilibrium actually occurs at these moderate exercise intensities. Alternatively, the extrapulmonary shunt may be responsible for a significant portion of the uncoupling between measured and predicted A-aDO_2 that occurs during submaximal exercise. Indeed, it was determined that during moderate exercise, an extrapulmonary shunt of 1% of cardiac output could explain all of the A-aDO_2 that remained after accounting for that due to $\dot{V}_A/\dot{Q}$ maldistribution [20]. It is important to emphasize that the MIGET technique is not free from error as shown in studies which have predicted the A-aDO_2 attributable to ventilation-perfusion inequality and found this value to be (impossibly) in excess of the actual total A-aDO_2 [38, 77].

In summary, the increased A-aDO_2 during exercise results from a maldistribution of $\dot{V}_A/\dot{Q}$ as well as contributions from diffusion disequilibrium and/or extrapulmonary shunt as exercise intensity increases. The combined effects of the latter two may comprise greater than 50% of the A-aDO_2 during heavy exercise in trained individuals [38, 63] and may account for the occurrences of exercise-induced arterial hypoxemia (see 'Respiratory Limitations to Exercise Performance').

Cardiovascular System Responses to Exercise

At rest, skeletal muscle receives less than 20% of total cardiac output. The fraction of cardiac output delivered to muscle increases during exercise, so that at maximal intensity, skeletal muscle receives approximately 80% of total cardiac output. Although cardiac output increases roughly in proportion to $\dot{V}O_2$, redistribution of flow from 'inactive' areas of the circulation (mainly the visceral organs) is necessary to supply the flow requirements of active muscle. Thus, blood flow to working muscle during exercise depends on appropriate: (1) increases in cardiac output; (2) increases in vascular resistance to skin, viscera, and other inactive tissues (including nonworking skeletal muscle), and (3) decreases in vascular resistance to working muscle. The underlying mechanisms are shown in figure 2.

During exercise, cardiac output must increase to meet the contracting muscle's requirement for flow. The increase in cardiac output occurs through increases in both heart rate and stroke volume and is thought to be mediated via feed-forward mechanisms. The concept of 'central command' states that medullary cardiovascular centers are activated in parallel with α-motoneurons at the onset of and throughout exercise. Evidence for this mechanism comes from experiments in which attempted muscle contraction raised cardiac output to nearly the same extent in subjects with temporary neuromuscular blockade as did actual contractions observed in control conditions. Additionally, cardiac output often increases in an anticipatory fashion (i.e. before exercise even begins).

The increase in heart rate that begins prior to and during mild and moderate intensity exercise is caused primarily by withdrawal of parasympathetic outflow to the SA node. As exercise intensity increases, further increases in heart rate are caused by sympathetic stimulation of the SA node. The SA node is further stimulated by circulating catecholamines, which are secreted into the plasma by the adrenal glands in response to sympathetic activation. Stroke volume increases during the early stages of upright exercise and reaches a plateau at submaximal workloads equal to approximately 40% of $\dot{V}O_2$max in healthy, untrained adults. The increase in stroke volume is due to the combined effects of increased venous return and the positive ionotropic effects of sympathetic stimulation on heart muscle.

Skeletal muscle contraction elicits a reflex increase in sympathetic outflow to several key vascular beds, which in turn causes widespread vasoconstriction contributing to the exercise-induced rise in blood pressure. This reflex is triggered by stimulation of mechano- and chemoreceptors located within working muscle. Although the precise nature of the stimulus is not known, exercise-induced blood pressure increases are closely correlated with increases in muscle venous lactate concentration and decreases in pH. Reflex sympathetic activation is the primary mechanism causing redistribution of cardiac output away from nonworking muscle and inactive tissue to provide more blood flow to working muscle. It is important to note that reflex increases in sympathetic outflow occur to active, as well as inactive skeletal muscle. Although sympathetic tone probably constrains the increase in limb muscle blood flow during exercise, local mechanical and chemical factors provide strong vasodilator influences opposing the constrictor influence and are probably the most important regulators of flow during exercise. During contraction, the blood vessels within skeletal muscle are mechanically compressed to the extent that flow is impeded; subsequent relaxation of the muscle allows flow to increase. Thus, rhythmic contraction and relaxation of skeletal muscle (as occurs during activities such as walking or running) imparts energy onto the blood vessels propelling blood out of the muscle vascular bed thereby facilitating venous return. The 'muscle pump' is thought to be almost entirely responsible for the immediate increase in blood flow that occurs at the onset of exercise. The mechanical effects of rhythmic contraction also play an important role in exercise vasodilation. Specifically, the muscle pump intermittently increases and decreases extravascular pressure (i.e. within the muscle) resulting in hyperemia.

The search for specific chemical mediators of exercise vasodilation has been partially successful. Many by-products of muscle contraction (e.g. potassium, adenosine,

CO_2, lactate, nitric oxide) are capable of producing vasodilation although none are obligatory for exercise hyperemia to occur [46].

In summary, the cardiovascular system response to exercise is regulated by interplay between neural, chemical, and mechanical factors. Increases in sympathetic nervous system activity triggered by feedback and feed-forward mechanisms are responsible for the exercise-induced increase in cardiac output and redistribution of blood flow from inactive to active tissue. In exercising muscle (including the heart), metabolic vasodilation is the predominant hemodynamic influence. Cerebral blood flow remains constant during exercise, even in the face of a small rise in systemic blood pressure; however, in heavy exercise, hypocapnia (secondary to the hyperventilatory response) will cause local cerebral vasoconstriction.

Cardiorespiratory Interactions during Exercise

The heart of the healthy individual is very sensitive to changes in preload which means the mechanical effects of inspiration and expiration impact cardiac output and blood flow distribution during exercise, especially that of high intensity. These influences are complex and include the following: (1) a more negative intrathoracic pressure during inspiration increases venous return and stroke volume (unless the negative pressure is too great and/or sustained too long during inspiration which could collapse the inferior vena cava, or unless an increased right atrial and ventricular volumes compromised left-ventricular expansion due to interventricular dependence) [65]; (2) active expiration during exercise causes large positive intra-thoracic and intra-abdominal pressures which may counterbalance the potential positive influences of negative intrathoracic pressure during inspiration on venous return and stroke volume, and (3) if inspiration is accomplished primarily with the diaphragm, diaphragmatic descent will increase intra-abdominal pressure during inspiration reducing the pressure gradient from the limbs to the abdomen thus impeding venous return [91].

Available evidence in the exercising human demonstrates that the negative intrathoracic pressure normally generated during inspiration exerts enough of a preload effect on the heart to account for a significant fraction of the increase in stroke volume and cardiac output during exercise. Wexler et al. [87] measured blood flow velocity in the inferior vena cava of humans during mild supine exercise and found cyclical increases in venous return during inspiration and reductions during expiration. Harms et al. [30] used proportional assist mechanical ventilation to unload the respiratory muscles and decrease the negativity of intrathoracic pressure during inspiration. They observed a reduction in stroke volume and cardiac output at all exercise intensities up to maximum, although a portion of the reduction was related to concomitant reductions in $\dot{V}O_2$.

In addition to the aforementioned mechanical effects of intra-thoracic and abdominal pressure swings on cardiac function, respiratory muscle work leading to diaphragm fatigue (which does occur during heavy exercise) exerts significant effects on sympathetic nervous system outflow to skeletal muscle (MSNA) and limb muscle blood flow. Using microneurographic recordings from the peroneal nerve of the resting limb, St. Croix et al. [71] demonstrated that repeated voluntary inspiratory efforts leading to diaphragm fatigue in otherwise resting subjects caused a time-dependent increase in MSNA (despite a coincident increase in MAP). Sheel et al. [68] subsequently demonstrated that this increased MSNA coincided with an increase in limb vascular resistance (LVR) and a 20–40% reduction in limb blood flow ($\dot{Q}_L$). This sympathetically-mediated limb vasoconstriction was not induced by voluntary increases in central respiratory motor output per se as voluntary increases in central respiratory motor output without fatigue actually reduced MSNA and LVR and increased $\dot{Q}_L$. The time-dependent effects of diaphragm fatigue on sympathetically-mediated limb vasoconstriction parallel those caused by fatiguing rhythmic handgrip or expiratory muscle contractions. These data in humans support a physiological role for the type III and IV receptors in respiratory muscle [13] and are consistent with the activation of these receptors during fatiguing diaphragmatic contractions induced by phrenic nerve stimulation in the anesthetized rat [35]. Furthermore, electrical or pharmacological stimulation of thin fiber phrenic nerve afferents in anesthetized animals causes constriction of coronary arterioles [74] and several other systemic vascular beds [41].

How these isolated findings apply to normal whole body exercise in humans is not clear. We do know that in humans performing heavy cycling exercise, unloading the normal work of breathing with a mechanical ventilator causes vasodilation and increased blood flow to the exercising limb [28]. These cardiovascular effects do not occur if respiratory muscle unloading is applied during moderate intensity exercise during which diaphragm fatigue does not occur [85]. Considering all available data together, it is likely that an accumulation of metabolites in fatiguing respiratory muscle during exercise triggers an increased sympathetic outflow increasing the total constrictor outflow to systemic vascular beds. We do not know, however, if this specific metaboreflex from respiratory muscle, by itself, is sufficiently powerful to override local vasodilator metabolites and impede blood flow to the exercising limb. We can only view these data as indicative of a respiratory-cardiovascular link during exercise that deserves serious consideration along with the more traditional feed-forward and feedback locomotor influences within the grand scheme of autonomic control of the circulation during exercise (fig. 2).

Respiratory Limitations to Exercise Performance

The combined aerobic capacity of all the organ systems involved in O_2 transport and utilization is $\dot{V}O_2max$. $\dot{V}O_2max$ is the plateau in $\dot{V}O_2$ eventually achieved as work rate increases during a progressive exercise test. The Fick equation defines the determinants of $\dot{V}O_2max$.

$$\dot{V}O_2max = CO_{max} \times [\text{arterial } O_2 \text{ content} - \text{mixed venous } O_2 \text{ content}]_{max}$$

Thus, $\dot{V}O_2max$ can be thought of as being limited by the capacity to transport O_2 to working muscle ($CaO_2 \times CO_{max}$) or by the capacity of working muscle to extract and utilize the available O_2.

The majority of evidence indicates that exercise capacity in the healthy, untrained human at sea-level is limited by the supply of O_2 delivered to working muscles rather than by their capacity to oxidize it [81]. Specifically, $\dot{V}O_2max$ is increased: (a) in proportion to arterial O_2 content when either O_2 carrying capacity is augmented via added red cells (i.e. blood 'doping') or inspiring very high concentrations of O_2 [79], or (b) when CO_{max} is increased by adding total circulating blood volume [82] or surgically removing the constraint of the pericardium [72]. In turn, maximal stroke volume and cardiac output are believed to be the major limiting factors to systemic O_2 transport and therefore $\dot{V}O_2max$ in most healthy subjects exercising at sea level. Extremely sedentary humans ($\dot{V}O_2max$ <35 ml/kg/min) do not show this dependency of $\dot{V}O_2max$ on O_2 transport and may be limited by the oxidative capacity of skeletal muscle [66].

The healthy pulmonary system is so well designed that it has traditionally been thought of as being 'overbuilt' and able to provide adequate gas exchange during all types and intensities of exercise. However, this once prevailing view is no longer widely accepted. Evidence has accumulated that indicates the respiratory system may limit exercise performance by two different mechanisms including: (1) the development of exercise-induced arterial hypoxemia, and (2) fatiguing levels of respiratory muscle work.

Pulmonary gas exchange in the healthy, untrained person is usually adequate at all levels of exercise intensity as arterial PO_2 is maintained at resting levels (fig. 3). However, significant decreases (3–13%) in the saturation of hemoglobin with oxygen (SaO_2) have been shown to occur during exercise at sea level in healthy, habitually active humans [11, 31, 58]. These findings provide evidence that the normal respiratory system is not always able to adequately accomplish its primary task of gas exchange. This phenomenon is known as exercise-induced arterial hypoxemia (EIAH) and results from a fall in arterial PO_2 and a pH or temperature-induced rightward shift of the oxyhemoglobin dissociation curve. Individuals with greater aerobic capacity are far more likely to develop EIAH although there is marked variation within groups of similar fitness levels [31].

The causes of EIAH are multifactorial and may originate from the observation that exercise training elicits adaptations in the cardiovascular and muscular systems without changing the gas exchange surface of the lung (see 'Effects of Endurance Training on the Respiratory System'). The two primary variables with which EIAH most often correlate are: (1) an excessively widened $A\text{-}aDO_2$, and (2) an insufficient hyperventilatory response to the exercise stimulus. In a well-trained athlete with a high maximal oxygen uptake, the $A\text{-}aDO_2$ may reach values of 40 mm Hg or greater at maximal exercise intensities compared with a maximal value of ~25 mm Hg in a healthy but untrained person. However, an excessively widened $A\text{-}aDO_2$ does not necessarily predispose one to develop EIAH as PaO_2 will be maintained if alveolar ventilation is increased in proportion to the widened $A\text{-}aDO_2$. Thus, individuals who have an excessively widened $A\text{-}aDO_2$ in conjunction with a blunted hyperventilatory response to exercise are the most susceptible to EIAH.

The mechanisms responsible for the widened $A\text{-}aDO_2$ during exercise were discussed in detail above (see 'Pulmonary Gas Exchange') and will not be rediscussed here except to mention that an excessively widened $A\text{-}aDO_2$ (>30 mm Hg) during exercise is likely due to a severe maldistribution of $\dot{V}_A/\dot{Q}$, diffusion limitation for O_2, and/or a greater contribution from extrapulmonary shunt than is normally seen. In trained athletes at high exercise intensities, the possibility for a significant limitation for diffusion cannot be discounted as their high CO_{max} (25–30 liters/min) combined with a normal (untrained) maximal

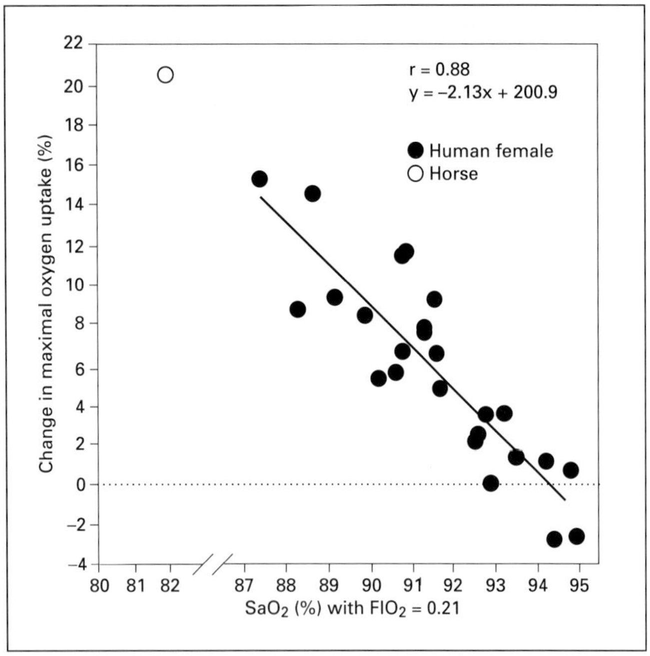

Fig. 7. Relationship between percent change in $\dot{V}O_2max$ when EIAH was prevented (with supplemental O_2) and SaO_2 during maximal exercise in normoxia. The intercept of the regression line at zero change in maximal oxygen consumption indicates that preventing EIAH began to have a significant effect on $\dot{V}O_2max$ when SaO_2 was between 93 and 95% (i.e. a 3% reduction below resting levels). Data compiled from Harms et al. [31].

pulmonary capillary blood volume of ~220 ml [62] places their estimated average red blood cell transit time at 0.35–0.40 s [36]. This puts these individuals at the limit needed for O_2 equilibration between alveoli and red blood cell during maximal exercise. Indeed, total pulmonary transit time (right to left ventricle) is significantly correlated with the magnitude of the A-aDO_2 in trained athletes [36].

The degree of hyperventilation, as reflected by the decrease in $PaCO_2$ from rest, is significantly correlated with EIAH [11, 29] as women who hyperventilated more were less likely to develop EIAH at a given work rate compared to women who hyperventilated less [29]. The mechanisms proposed to explain an inadequate hyperventilatory response to exercise include: (1) a low hypoxic and/or hypercapnic drive related to blunted chemoreceptor sensitivity [27], and/or (2) a mechanical constraint to the exercise hyperpnea [43, 53]. Although the development of EIAH has been shown to correlate with a reduced hypoxic and hypercapnic ventilatory response at rest and reduced ventilatory equivalent for CO_2 during exercise [23, 27], it is important to remember that CO_2 retention does not occur during high-intensity exercise indicating that alveolar ventilation is always adequate with regard to $\dot{V}CO_2$. Mechanical limitations to breathing during high-intensity exercise may also prevent an increase in minute ventilation irrespective of respiratory motor output. Indeed, ventilation increased and $PaCO_2$ decreased when subjects who exhibited expiratory flow limitation during exercise breathing room air subsequently performed the same exercise bout while breathing heliox [53].

It is important to note that a substantial portion of the decreased SaO_2 during exercise can be attributed to a pH and/or temperature-induced rightward shift of the hemoglobin dissociation curve. This was recently demonstrated in a group of runners during constant load high intensity treadmill exercise in which PaO_2 rose progressively over time while SaO_2 fell progressively because of increasing temperature and acidosis [86].

Evidence that EIAH limits exercise performance comes from studies where $\dot{V}O_2max$ increased in subjects when small amounts of supplemental inspired O_2 were given just sufficient to prevent the decreases in arterial oxygen content that occurred during normoxic exercise [31, 58]. The magnitude of the increase in maximal oxygen consumption correlated with the severity of EIAH achieved during normoxic exercise (fig. 7). The likely mechanism for the increased $\dot{V}O_2max$ is a widened a-$\bar{v}O_2$ difference in proportion to the increased CaO_2 [47]. Further, it has been demonstrated that hypoxemia begins to have a significant effect on $\dot{V}O_2max$ when SaO_2 drops 3–4% below resting levels [31]. SaO_2 during maximal exercise in most healthy, untrained individuals is approximately 94–95% [23, 27] placing them at a level of desaturation that would not be expected to compromise performance. However, many trained athletes commonly reach SaO_2 levels of 87–92% during maximal exercise [11, 31], which would cause a 5–15% reduction in $\dot{V}O_2max$.

The second major cause of a respiratory limitation to exercise performance involves fatiguing levels of respiratory muscle work. Fatiguing levels of respiratory muscle work are normally achieved during exercise in trained and untrained healthy people (>80% $\dot{V}O_2max$) and presumably during lighter intensity work in patients with chronic pulmonary and/or heart disease. The degree of respiratory muscle work needed to sustain the hyperpnea of strenuous exercise in a trained athlete can account for up to 16% of maximal $\dot{V}O_2$ [1] and cardiac output [30]. This significant demand for blood flow by the respiratory muscles does not influence the adequacy of ventilation, but may compromise perfusion of limb muscle thereby limiting its ability to perform work. Evidence of a competition for blood flow between the respiratory and limb muscles originates from data obtained in highly fit cyclists exercising at 90% $\dot{V}O_2$max who demonstrated decreases in limb blood flow commensurate with respiratory muscle loading, and even more physiologically relevant, increases in limb blood flow when the normal work of breathing was unloaded using a proportional assist ventilator [28].

In subsequent work, Harms et al. [32] studied highly fit cyclists, each of whom completed 11 randomized trials on a cycle ergometer at a workload requiring 90% $\dot{V}O_2$max under conditions of increased (loading), decreased (unloading), or normal (control) respiratory muscle work. They found that time to exhaustion was significantly increased with unloading the normal work of breathing in 76% of trials by an average of 1.3 min (14%) and significantly decreased with loading in 83% of the trials by an average of 1 min (15%) compared with control. Additionally, respiratory muscle unloading during exercise reduced $\dot{V}O_2$ and the rate of rise in dyspnea and limb discomfort (fig. 8). It was postulated that unloading the normal work of breathing during heavy exercise improved performance due to a redistribution of blood flow to the working limb, which could delay fatigue and reduce the perception of limb muscle discomfort. Other studies have used assisted mechanical ventilation to reduce the normal work of breathing at lower exercise intensities in healthy subjects and found no effect on ventilation or endurance time [18, 48, 85], suggesting that respiratory muscle fatigue must occur for unloading to improve performance. On the other hand, respiratory muscle unloading during exercise in patients with chronic heart failure had marked effects on improving exercise performance, even during moderate intensity exercise [55]. This effect may reflect the enhanced ventilatory response to exercise and limited cardiac output available in these patients.

Recent evidence has shown that fatiguing contractions of respiratory muscle in otherwise resting subjects increase efferent sympathetic nerve activity [71] and decrease limb blood flow [68]. These findings suggest that respiratory muscle fatigue, which has been shown to occur in healthy humans during heavy exercise [44, 50] could negatively impact limb work capacity due to blood flow redistribution even when cardiac output is not near maximal levels. It has thus been postulated that specific respiratory muscle training (either breathing against resistive loads or voluntary hyperpnea at rest) might improve exercise performance by: (1) delaying respiratory muscle fatigue and its subsequent effects on blood flow distribution, and/or (2) reducing subjective perception of muscular effort (both limb and respiratory). Results on the topic have been varied [4, 42, 70] and are likely due to differences in training paradigms, subject populations, performance testing protocols, and/or placebo effects on tests of maximum volitional performance.

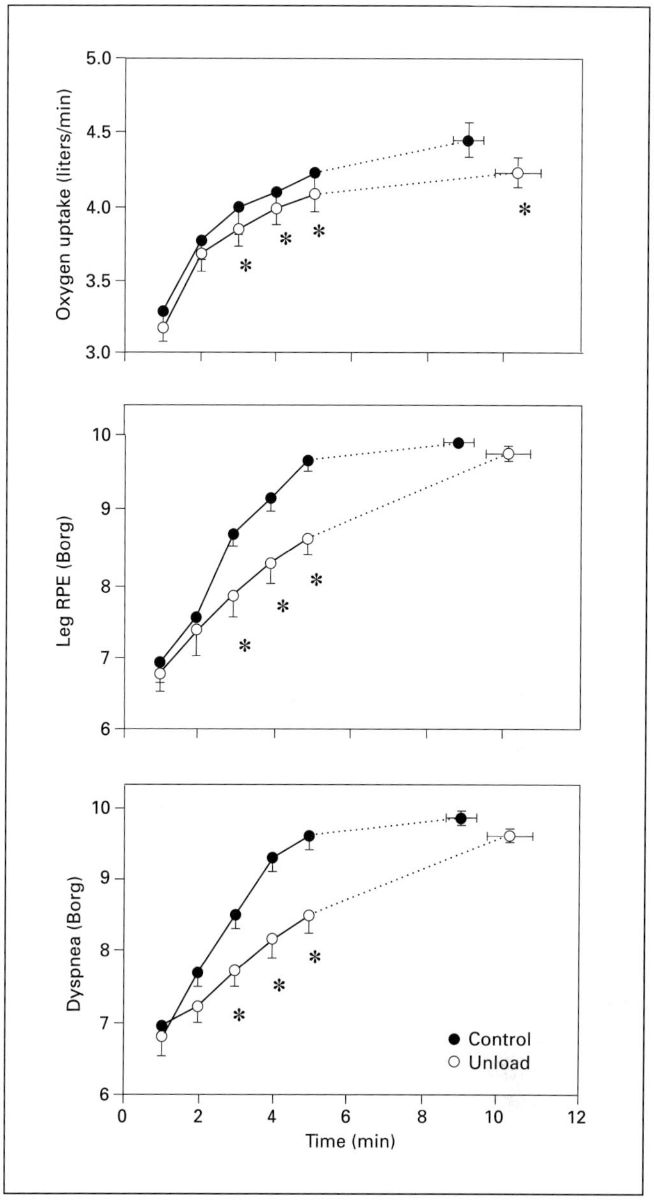

Fig. 8. Effects of respiratory muscle unloading on endurance exercise performance. Group mean data (n = 7) are shown for minutes 1–5 of exercise and at exhaustion. * Significant difference from control, $p < 0.05$. Data compiled from Harms et al. [32].

In summary, EIAH and the cardiovascular consequences of respiratory muscle fatigue are two mechanisms through which exercise performance and $\dot{V}O_2max$ are limited. However, these limitations do not generalize equally to all humans or all conditions. Specifically, EIAH occurs during sub-maximal exercise (short or long duration) only in the habitually active, while an increase in sympathetic outflow due to diaphragm fatigue can occur in anyone.

Aging alters the way in which the respiratory system limits exercise. With normal healthy aging, the lung loses elastic recoil, the chest wall and pulmonary arterioles increase in stiffness, and the gas exchange surface diminishes. This results in greater dead-space ventilation, expiratory flow limitation, and hyperinflation during exercise leading to dyspnea. EIAH occurs in many aged fit humans with $\dot{V}O_2max$ in the 40- to 45-ml/kg/min range (which is 50+% greater than normal at age 70 years) and pulmonary vascular resistance during exercise is higher in older vs. young healthy subjects at any given $\dot{V}O_2$.

Hypoxia of high altitude makes the respiratory system the primary limiting factor to exercise because: (a) diffusion limitation is enhanced and EIAH occurs much more readily (even at <1,000 m altitude if the absolute work load is sufficiently high); (b) local hypoxic vasoconstriction causes increased pulmonary vascular resistance which often precipitates edema formation during exercise, and (c) carotid chemoreceptor stimulation causes a marked hyperventilatory response to exercise along with increases in inspiratory and expiratory muscle work which enhance diaphragm fatigue and dyspnea.

Effects of Endurance Training on the Respiratory System

Endurance training-induced structural adaptations within the cardiovascular and muscular systems have been well documented [51, 83]. Whether training-induced changes in lung structure occur (i.e., lung diffusion surface area or parenchymal structure) is more controversial. Although exercise has been suggested to have an effect on lung development since the early 1900s, more recent data comparing habitually active vs. sedentary animals of the same body size but 3-fold differences in $\dot{V}O_2max$ (e.g. horse vs. cow) reported little difference in the alveolar-capillary interface despite significant differences in heart and limb muscle mitochondrial volume and capillary density [83]. Absence of an activity-induced effect on lung structure is further supported by data showing that daily exercise training is without effect on pulmonary diffusion surface area in the maturing lung of newborn guinea pigs [67]. Also, highly trained human athletes show no difference in diffusion capacity of the lung for carbon monoxide or pulmonary capillary blood volume at rest or any given exercise level compared to healthy, untrained subjects [62]. Exceptional cases have been found in competitive female swimmers who demonstrated significant increases in vital capacity (~9%) and total lung capacity (~7%) following 12 weeks of intense endurance training [9]. Larger than average vital and total lung capacities have also been shown in long distance swimmers compared to sprint trained and noncompetitive swimmers [69] although the differences noted in this cross-sectional study could have been solely due to subject selection bias. Longitudinal findings in elderly subjects demonstrated that habitual physical activity and high aerobic capacity do not prevent the normal deterioration in resting lung function (primarily reduced elastic recoil) or the high levels of expiratory flow limitation which occur during exercise in the healthy pulmonary system over the sixth and seventh decades of life [52].

It is possible that exercise training is not an intense or specific enough stimulus to cause adaptation, as there are only a few chronic stimuli to which the structure and function of the healthy lung are known to adapt. One of these stimuli is chronic hypoxia, which has been shown to increase alveolar and capillary number (expansion of the gas exchange surface area) in rats and dogs born and trained in hypoxia. Similarly, high-altitude residents of mountains (such as the Peruvian Andes and North American Rockies) show marked increases (30–50%) in pulmonary diffusion capacity at rest and during exercise [6]. A second stimulus to which the lung is adaptable is pneumonectomy where compensatory growth of the remaining lung occurs [40, 75]. Daily stretching of the adult lung and respiratory muscles over a 5-week period as occurs during programs of specific respiratory muscle training have been shown to elicit small but significant increases in vital capacity and peak flow [49].

In contrast to the lung, the respiratory muscles undergo changes in histochemical [24, 73] and biochemical [24, 25, 59, 73] properties in response to whole-body training or a chronic overload stimulus [16, 76]. Whole body exercise training has been shown to promote a shift from glycolytic to oxidative myosin heavy chain (MHC) isoforms [73] and significant increases (20–30%) in mitochondrial enzyme activity within the costal diaphragm of rodents [24, 59, 73]. Interestingly, these training protocols did not elicit changes in the crural diaphragm unless 90-min training sessions of moderate-to-high intensity exercise were used, indicating that these two regions of the diaphragm have different patterns of recruitment. Studies of the expiratory muscles also indicate significant increases (10–26%) in their oxidative capacity highlighting their recruitment during exercise [25, 59]. When training-induced changes in the metabolic capacity of the respiratory muscles are compared to those in locomotor muscles of similar fiber type, locomotor muscles display a notably higher increase (40–80%) [24, 25, 73]. These between-muscle differences are probably related to differences in the metabolic demand placed on these muscles during exercise and/or differences in the pre-training levels of oxidative enzymes across limb and respiratory muscle. Voluntary wheel running has shown that a volitional training stimulus can induce significantly greater adaptations in the oxidative capacity of inspiratory and expiratory rat muscle than the aforementioned fixed-load treadmill training protocols [25], possibly because the animals can either: (1) perform intermittent high intensity bouts of exercise for many weeks, and/or (2) reach daily running distances that are more than those of treadmill exercise models. It appears that the more intense the training regime the greater the adaptations, although there appears to be a threshold beyond which adaptation fails to occur as demonstrated by severe endurance training [56].

To date there are no published reports regarding the effects of whole-body endurance training upon cellular alterations in human respiratory muscle as biopsies are extremely difficult to obtain. However, costal diaphragm samples from chronic heart failure patients, who exhibit persistently elevated levels of minute ventilation at rest and during exercise in the face of reduced cardiac outputs, have shown significantly elevated oxidative (64%) and lipolytic (41%) capacities [76]. This illustrates the ability of the human diaphragm to change its metabolic properties in response to chronic overload.

A more recent question regarding possible training effects on the lung involves pulmonary vascular reactivity, or more specifically, enhanced vasodilation of pulmonary arteries in response to acetylcholine (ACh). Augmented pulmonary vasorelaxation could allow for a greater drop in pulmonary vascular resistance at any given cardiac output during exercise, which would presumably represent a favorable adaptation as the decreased pulmonary arterial pressure would reduce the chance of developing pulmonary edema during heavy intensity exercise. A recent study in this area demonstrated that short-term training (7 days) increased endothelial nitric oxide synthase (eNOS) protein and endothelium-dependent relaxation in porcine conduit pulmonary arteries [45]. These findings on pulmonary vascular reactivity are consistent with studies reporting training-induced effects on limb vascular reactivity [51]. These data from pigs confirm in part a previous training study in male rabbits that reported enhanced endothelium-dependent relaxation in pulmonary arteries following 8 weeks of training [8]. The exact mechanisms leading to these changes have not yet been determined but it has been suggested in the porcine model that acute exercise increases the shear stress imposed upon the endothelial lining of blood vessels leading to increased upregulation of eNOS protein. Surprisingly, much longer training periods (16 weeks) in pigs failed to change endothelium-dependent relaxation in pulmonary or systemic arteries [45] and no satisfactory explanation is forthcoming to explain the apparent discrepancy between short- and long-term training. We know of no human data that speaks for this proposed training effect and, as discussed previously, there is no evidence that pulmonary capillaries respond to physical training. In short, these findings point to a previously unappreciated and potentially beneficial effect of physical training on the pulmonary circulation.

References

1 Aaron EA, Seow KC, Johnson BD: Oxygen cost of exercise hyperpnea: Implications for performance. J Appl Physiol 1992;72:1818–1825.
2 Ainsworth DM, Smith CA, Eiker SW, Henderson KS, Dempsey JA: The effects of chemical versus locomotory stimuli on respiratory muscle activity in the awake dog. Respir Physiol 1989;78:163–176.
3 Aliverti A, Cala SJ, Duranti R, Ferrigno G, Kenyon CM, Pedotti A, Scano G, Sliwinski P, Macklem PT, Yan S: Human respiratory muscle actions and control during exercise. J Appl Physiol 1997;83:1256–1269.
4 Boutellier U: Respiratory muscle fitness and exercise endurance in healthy humans. Med Sci Sports Exer 1998;30:1169–1172.
5 Bryan AC, Bentivoglio LG, Beerel F, MacLeish H, Zidulka A, Bates DV: Factors affecting regional distribution of ventilation and perfusion in the lung. J Appl Physiol 1964;19:395–402.
6 Cerny FJ, Dempsey JA, Reddan WG: Pulmonary gas exchange in non-native residents of high altitude. J Clin Invest 1973;52:2993–2999.
7 Chadha TS, Birch S, Sackner MA: Oro-nasal distribution of ventilation during exercise in normal subjects and patients with asthma and rhinitis. Chest 1987;92:1037–1041.
8 Chen HI, Li HT: Physical conditioning can modulate endothelium-dependent vasorelaxation in rabbits. Arterioscler Thromb 1993;13:852–856.
9 Clanton TL, Dixon GF, Drake J, Gadek JE: Effects of swim training on lung volumes and inspiratory muscle conditioning. J Appl Physiol 1987;62:39–46.

10 Coates G, O'Brodovich H, Jeffries AL, Gray GW: Effects of exercise on lung lymph flow in sheep and goats during normoxia and hypoxia. J Clin Invest 1984;74:133–141.
11 Dempsey JA, Hanson PG, Henderson KS: Exercise-induced arterial hypoxemia in healthy human subjects at sea level. J Physiol 1984; 355:161–175.
12 Dempsey JA, Forster HV, Ainsworth DM: Regulation of hyperpnea, hyperventilation, and respiratory muscle recruitment during exercise; in Dempsey JA, Pack AI (eds): Regulation of Breathing. New York, Marcel Dekker, 1995, pp 1065–1133.
13 Duron B: Intercostal and diaphragmatic muscle endings and afferents; in Hornbein TF (ed): Regulation of Breathing, Part I. New York, Marcel Dekker, 1981, pp 473–540.
14 England SJ, Bartlett D Jr: Changes in respiratory movements of the human vocal cords during hyperpnea. J Appl Physiol 1982;52:780–785.
15 Erickson HH, Bernard SL, Glenny RW, Fedde RM, Polissar NL, Basaraba RJ, Walther SM, Gaughan EM, McMurphy R, Hlastala MP: Effect of furosemide on pulmonary blood flow distribution in resting and exercising horses. J Appl Physiol 1999;86:2034–2043.
16 Farkas GA, Roussos C: Adaptability of the hamster diaphragm to exercise and/or emphysema. J Appl Physiol 1982;53:1263–1272.
17 Fregosi RF, Dempsey JA: The effect of exercise in normoxia and acute hypoxia on respiratory muscle metabolites. J Appl Physiol 1986;60: 1274–1283.
18 Gallagher CG, Younes M: Effect of pressure support on ventilation and respiratory muscle mechanics in heavy exercise. J Appl Physiol 1989;66:1824–1837.
19 Gehr P, Bachofen M, Weibel ER: The normal lung: Ultrastructure and morphometric estimation of diffusion capacity. Respir Physiol 1978; 32:121–140.
20 Gledhill N, Froese AB, Dempsey JA: Ventilation to perfusion distribution during exercise in health; in Dempsey JA, Reed CE (eds): Muscular Exercise and the Lung. Wisconsin, University of Wisconsin Press, 1977, pp 325–344.
21 Glenny RW, Bernard S, Robertson TH, Hlastala MP: Gravity is an important but secondary determinant of regional pulmonary blood flow in upright primates. J Appl Physiol 1999;86: 623–632.
22 Glenny RW, Lamm WJE, Bernard SL, An D, Chornuk M, Pool SL, Wagner WW, Hlastala MP, Robertson HT: Physiology of a microgravity environment: Redistribution of pulmonary perfusion during weightlessness and increased gravity. J Appl Physiol 2000;89:1239–1248.
23 Gore CJ, Hahn AG, Scroop GC, Watson DB, Norton KI, Wood RJ, Campbell DP, Emonson DL: Increased arterial desaturation in trained cyclists during maximal exercise at 580 m altitude. J Appl Physiol 1996;80:2204–2210.
24 Gosselin LE, Betlach M, Vailas AC, Thomas DP: Training-induced alterations in young and senescent rat diaphragm muscle. J Appl Physiol 1992;72:1506–1511.
25 Halseth AE, Fogt DL, Fregosi RF, Henriksen EJ: Metabolic responses of rat respiratory muscles to voluntary exercise training. J Appl Physiol 1995;79:902–907.
26 Hammond MD, Gale GE, Kapitan KS, Ries A, Wagner PD: Pulmonary gas exchange in humans during exercise at sea level. J Appl Physiol 1986;60:1590–1598.
27 Harms CA, Stager JM: Low chemoresponsiveness and inadequate hyperventilation contribute to exercise-induced hypoxemia. J Appl Physiol 1995;79:575–580.
28 Harms CA, Babcock MA, McClaran SR, Pegelow DF, Nickele GA, Nelson WB, Dempsey JA: Respiratory muscle work compromises leg blood flow during maximal exercise. J Appl Physiol 1997;82:1573–1583.
29 Harms CA, McClaran SR, Nickele GA, Pegelow DF, Nelson WB, Dempsey JA: Exercise-induced arterial hypoxemia in healthy young women. J Physiol 1998;507:619–628.
30 Harms CA, Wetter TJ, McClaran SR, Pegelow DF, Nickele G, Nelson W, Dempsey JA: Effect of respiratory muscle work on cardiac output and its distribution during maximal exercise. J Appl Physiol 1998;85:609–618.
31 Harms CA, McClaran SR, Nickele GA, Pegelow DF, Nelson WB, Dempsey JA: Effect of exercise-induced arterial O_2 desaturation on $\dot{V}O_2$max in women. Med Sci Sports Exer 2000; 32:1101–1108.
32 Harms CA, Wetter TJ, St. Croix CM, Pegelow DF, Dempsey JA: Effects of respiratory muscle work on exercise performance. J Appl Physiol 2000;89:131–138.
33 Henke KG, Sharratt M, Pegelow D, Dempsey JA: Regulation of end-expiratory lung volume during exercise. J Appl Physiol 1988;64:135–146.
34 Hey EN, Lloyd BB, Cunningham DJC, Jukes MGM, Bolton DPG: Effects of various respiratory stimuli on the depth and frequency of breathing. Respir Physiol 1966;1:193–205.
35 Hill J: Discharge of group IV phrenic afferent fibers increases during diaphragmatic fatigue. Brain Res 2000;856:240–244.
36 Hopkins SR, Belzberg AS, Wiggs BR, McKenzie DC: Pulmonary transit time and diffusion limitation during heavy exercise in athletes. Respir Physiol 1996;103:67–73.
37 Hopkins SR, Schoene RB, Henderson WR, Spragg RG, Martin TR, West JB: Intense exercise impairs the integrity of the pulmonary blood-gas barrier in elite athletes. Am J Respir Crit Care Med 1997;155:1090–1094.
38 Hopkins SR, Gavin TP, Siafakas NM, Haseler LJ, Olfert IM, Wagner H, Wagner PD: Effect of prolonged, heavy exercise on pulmonary gas exchange in athletes. J Appl Physiol 1998;85: 1523–1532.
39 Hsia CCW, McBrayer DG, Ramanathan M: Reference values of pulmonary diffusing capacity during exercise by a rebreathing technique. Am J Respir Crit Care Med 1995;152: 658–665.
40 Hsia CC, Herazo LF, Ramanathan M, Johnson RL, Wagner PD: Cardiopulmonary adaptations to pneumonectomy in dogs. II. $\dot{V}_A/\dot{Q}$ relationships and microvascular recruitment. J Appl Physiol 1993;74:1299–1309.
41 Hussain S, Chatillon A, Comtois A, Roussos C, Magder S: Chemical activation of thin fiber phrenic afferents. II. Cardiovascular responses. J Appl Physiol 1991;70:77–86.
42 Inbar O, Weiner P, Azgad Y, Rotstein A, Weinstein Y: Specific inspiratory muscle training in well-trained endurance athletes. Med Sci Sports Exer 2000;32:1233–1237.
43 Johnson BD, Saupe KW, Dempsey JA: Mechanical constraints on exercise hyperpnea in endurance athletes. J Appl Physiol 1992;73: 874–886.
44 Johnson BD, Babcock MA, Suman OE, Dempsey JA: Exercise-induced diaphragmatic fatigue in healthy humans. J Physiol (London) 1993;460:385–405.
45 Johnson LR, Rush JW, Turk JR, Price EM, Laughlin MH: Short-term exercise training increases ACh-induced relaxation and eNOS protein in porcine pulmonary arteries. J Appl Physiol 2001;90:1102–1110.
46 Kaufman MP, Forster HV: Reflexes controlling circulatory, ventilatory, and airway responses to exercise; in Rowell L, Sheperd J (eds): APS Handbook of Physiology: Exercise. New York, Oxford Press,1996, pp 381–447.
47 Knight DR, Schaffartzik W, Poole DC, Hogan MC, Bebout DE, Wagner PD: Effects of hyperoxia on maximal leg O_2 supply and utilization in men. J Appl Physiol 1993;75:2586–2594.
48 Krishnan B, Zintel T, McParland C, Gallagher CG: Lack of importance of respiratory muscle load in ventilatory regulation during heavy exercise in humans. J Physiol (Lond) 1996;490: 537–550.
49 Leith DE, Bradley M: Ventilatory muscle strength and endurance training. J Appl Physiol 1976;41:508–516.
50 Loke J, Mahler DA, Virgulto JA: Respiratory muscle fatigue after marathon running. J Appl Physiol 1982;52:821–824.
51 McAllister RM, Laughlin MH: Short-term exercise training alters responses of porcine femoral and brachial arteries. J Appl Physiol 1997; 82:1438–1444.
52 McClaran SR, Babcock MA, Pegelow DF, Reddan WG, Dempsey JA: Longitudinal effects of aging on lung function at rest and exercise in healthy active fit elderly adults. J Appl Physiol 1995;78:1957–1968.
53 McClaran SR, Wetter TJ, Pegelow DF, Dempsey JA: Role of expiratory flow limitation in determining lung volumes and ventilation during exercise. J Appl Physiol 1999;86:1357–1366.
54 Mead J: Control of respiratory frequency. J Appl Physiol 1980;49:528–532.
55 O'Donnell DE, D'Arsigny C, Raj S, Abdollah H, Webb KA: Ventilatory assistance improves exercise endurance in stable congestive heart failure. Am J Respir Crit Care Med 1999;160: 1804–1811.

56 Okumoto T, Imoto T, Katsuta S, Wada M: Severe endurance training fails to change myosin heavy-chain distribution of diaphragm. Respir Physiol 1996;104:39–43.
57 Otis AB, Fenn WO, Rahn H: Mechanics of breathing in man. J Appl Physiol 1950;2:592–607.
58 Powers SK, Lawler J, Dempsey JA, Dodd S, Landry G: Effects of incomplete pulmonary gas exchange on $\dot{V}O_2$max. J Appl Physiol 1989;66: 2491–2495.
59 Powers SK, Farkas GA, Criswell D, Herb RA, Zambito K, Dodd S: Metabolic characteristics of primary inspiratory and expiratory muscles in the dog. J Appl Physiol 1994;77:2188–2193.
60 Rahn H, Otis AB, Chadwick LE, Fenn WO: The pressure-volume diagram of the thorax and lung. Am J Physiol 1946;146:161–178.
61 Reeves JT, Dempsey JA, Grover RF: Pulmonary circulation during exercise; in Weir EK, Reeves JT (eds): Pulmonary Vascular Physiology and Pathophysiology. New York, Marcel Dekker,1989, pp 107–133.
62 Reuschlein PS, Reddan WG, Burpee J, Gee JB, Rankin J: Effect of physical training on the pulmonary diffusing capacity during sub-maximal work. J Appl Physiol 1968;24:152–158.
63 Rice AJ, Thornton AT, Gore CJ, Scroop GC, Greville HW, Wagner H, Wagner PD, Hopkins SR: Pulmonary gas exchange during exercise in highly trained cyclists with arterial hypoxemia. J Appl Physiol 1999;87:1802–1812.
64 Richerson HB, Seebohm PM: Nasal airway response to exercise. J Allergy 1968;41:269–284.
65 Robotham JL, Rabson J, Permutt S, Sagawa K, Shoukas AA, Bromberger-Barnea B: Left ventricular hemodynamics during respiration. J Appl Physiol 1979;47:1295–1303.
66 Roca J, Agusti AGN, Alonso A, Poole DC, Viegas C, Barbera JA, Rodriguez-Roisin R, Ferrer A, Wagner PD: Effects of physical training on muscle O_2 transport at $\dot{V}O_2$max. J Appl Physiol 1992;73:1067–1976.
67 Ross KA, Thurlbeck WM: Lung growth in newborn guinea pigs: Effects of endurance exercise. Respir Physiol 1992;89:353–364.
68 Sheel AW, Derchak PA, Morgan B, Pegelow D, Jacques AJ, Dempsey JA: Fatiguing inspiratory muscle work causes reflex reductions in resting leg blood flow. J Physiol 2001;537:277–289.
69 Shephard RJ, Godin G, Campbell R: Characteristics of sprint, medium, and long-distance swimmers. Eur J Appl Physiol 1974;32:99–116.
70 Sonetti DA, Wetter TJ, Pegelow DF, Dempsey JA: Effects of respiratory muscle training vs. placebo on endurance exercise performance. Respir Physiol 2001;127:185–199.
71 St. Croix CM, Morgan BJ, Wetter TJ, Dempsey JA: Reflex effects from a fatiguing diaphragm increase sympathetic efferent activity (MSNA) to limb muscle in humans. J Physiol (Lond) 2000;529:493–504.
72 Stray-Gunderson J, Musch TI, Haidet GC, Swain DP, Ordway GA, Mitchell JH: The effect of pericardectomy on maximal oxygen consumption and maximal cardiac output in untrained dogs. Circ Res 1986;58:523–530.
73 Sugiura T, Morimoto A, Murakami N: Effects of endurance training on myosin heavy-chain isoforms and enzyme activity in the rat diaphragm. Pflügers Arch 1992;421:77–81.
74 Szulczyk A, Szulczyk P, Zywuszko B: Analysis of reflex activity in cardiac sympathetic nerve induced by myelinated phrenic nerve afferents. Brain Res 1988;447:109–115.
75 Thet LA, Law DJ: Changes in cell number and lung morphology during early post-pneumonectomy lung growth. J Appl Physiol 1984;56: 975–978.
76 Tikunov B, Levine S, Mancini D: Chronic congestive heart failure elicits adaptations of endurance exercise in diaphragmatic muscle. Circulation 1997;95:910–916.
77 Torre-Bueno JR, Wagner PD, Saltzman HA, Gale GE, Moon RE: Diffusion limitation in normal humans during exercise at sea level and simulated altitude. J Appl Physiol 1985;58: 989–995.
78 Victor RG, Secher NH, Lyson T, Mitchell JH: Central command increases muscle sympathetic nerve activity during intense intermittent isometric exercise in humans. Circ Res 1995; 76:1710–1717.
79 Wagner PD: New ideas on limitations to $\dot{V}O_2$max. Exer Sport Sci Rev 2000;28:10–14.
80 Wagner PD, Gale GE, Moon RE, Torre-Bueno JR, Stolp BW, Saltzman HA: Pulmonary gas exchange in humans exercising at sea level and simulated altitude. J Appl Physiol 1986;61: 260–270.
81 Wagner PD: Determinants of maximal oxygen transport and utilization. Annu Rev Physiol 1996;58:21–50.
82 Warburton DE, Gledhill N, Quinney HA: Blood volume, aerobic power, and endurance performance: Potential ergogenic effect of volume loading. Clin J Sport Med 2000;10:59–66.
83 Weibel ER, Taylor CR, Hoppeler H: Variations in function and design: Testing symmorphosis in the respiratory system. Respir Physiol 1992;87:325–348.
84 West JB: Cellular responses to mechanical stress: Pulmonary capillary stress failure. J Appl Physiol 2000;89:2483–2489.
85 Wetter TJ, Harms CA, Nelson WB, Pegelow DF, Dempsey JA: Influence of respiratory muscle work on $\dot{V}O_2$ and leg blood flow during submaximal exercise. J Appl Physiol 1999;87: 643–651.
86 Wetter TJ, St. Croix C, Pegelow DF, Sonetti DA, Dempsey JA: Effects of exhaustive exercise on pulmonary gas exchange and airway function in females. J Appl Physiol 2001;91: 847–858.
87 Wexler LD, Bergel DH, Gae IT, Makin CS, Mills CJ: Velocity of blood flow in normal human vena cava. Circ Res 1968;23:349–359.
88 Williams JS, Janssen PL, Fuller DD, Fregosi RF: Influence of posture and breathing route on neural drive to upper airway dilator muscles during exercise. J Appl Physiol 2000;89:590–598.
89 Williamson JW, McColl R, Mathews D, Mitchell JH, Raven PB, Morgan WP: Hypnotic manipulation of effort sense during dynamic exercise: Cardiovascular responses and brain activation. J Appl Physiol 2001;90:1392–1399.
90 Williput R, Rondeux C, DeTroyer A: Breathing affects venous return from legs in humans. J Appl Physiol 1984;57:971–976.
91 Winchester PK, Williamson JW, Mitchell JH: Cardiovascular responses to static exercise in patients with Brown-Séquard syndrome. J Physiol 2000;527.1:193–202.

Joshua Rodman
John Rankin Laboratory of
Pulmonary Medicine
Department of Preventive Medicine
504 North Walnut Street
University of Wisconsin at Madison
Madison WI 53705 (USA)
Tel. +1 608 262 9499, Fax +1 608 262 8235
E-Mail jrrodman@students.wisc.edu

Weisman IM, Zeballos RJ (eds): Clinical Exercise Testing.
Prog Respir Res. Basel, Karger, 2002, vol 32, pp 18–29

Muscular Alterations in Chronic Obstructive Pulmonary Disease and Chronic Heart Failure at Rest and during Exercise

Harry R. Gosker[a] Nicole H.M.K. Uszko-Lencer[b] Emiel F.M. Wouters[a]
Ger J. van der Vusse[c] Annemie M.W.J. Schols[a]

Departments of [a]Pulmonology, [b]Cardiology and [c]Physiology, Maastricht University, Maastricht, The Netherlands

Summary

Reduced skeletal muscle performance contributes to exercise intolerance in COPD and CHF patients, independent of the severity of local organ dysfunction. Striking similarities are observed in morphological and metabolic abnormalities in peripheral skeletal muscle between these two disorders, pointing towards a decreased oxidative capacity. Both diseases also share striking differences between peripheral muscles and the diaphragm, which may therefore require a different therapeutical approach. The following possible underlying factors of muscular alterations in COPD and CHF are discussed: hypoxia, oxidative stress, disuse, weight loss and altered substrate metabolism.

According to the definitions of the World Health Organization chronic diseases are not only characterized by their primary impairments, but also by the resulting disabilities or even handicaps [1]. Although the primary impairments in chronic obstructive pulmonary disease (COPD) and chronic heart faulure (CHF) clearly differ, there is a striking resemblance in the systemic consequences of these diseases and their effect on exercise capacity and health status. Skeletal muscle function in COPD and CHF has long been ignored as potential contributor by focusing on the ventilatory and cardiac limitations of exercise performance, respectively; but recent research has shown that skeletal muscle function is impaired in moderate to severe COPD and CHF and also is an important predictor of exercise limitation in both diseases [2–4]. Muscle function depends, among others, on perfusion, muscle mass, fibre composition and energy metabolism [5]. It can be inferred that alterations in one or more of these determinants play a role in reduced muscle performance. Indeed, both in COPD and in CHF such changes have been found and striking similarities between the two etiologically distinct disorders appear to be present.

In this paper we will first present an overview of clinical studies that have investigated impaired muscle function with special emphasis on muscle morphology and energy metabolism in COPD and CHF. In the second part of the paper, potential causes will be discussed including hypoxia, oxidative stress, disuse, weight loss and altered substrate metabolism.

Muscular Alterations in COPD and CHF

Muscle Performance

Muscle performance is largely characterized by strength and endurance. Strength is defined as the capacity of the muscle to develop maximal force and endurance as the capacity of the muscle to maintain a certain force in time, thus to resist fatigue. Loss of either one of these aspects results in muscle weakness and, hence, in impaired muscle performance. Numerous studies have now convincingly demonstrated that COPD and CHF are commonly associated with muscle weakness [6–8]. Hamilton et al. [3] found significantly reduced strengths of both peripheral and respiratory muscles in patients suffering from respiratory failure, heart failure, or a combination of both as compared to healthy subjects. However, strength and endurance seem not to be affected in the same way in respiratory and peripheral muscles. This is illustrated by the poor correlation between the strengths of both muscle groups in both disorders [7, 8], compared to a much stronger correlation in healthy subjects [9]. It implies that the strength component of muscle weakness is affected differently in peripheral and respiratory muscles. In healthy subjects, as well as in patients, exercise limiting symptoms are the sense of leg effort (exertional discomfort) and/or breathlessness (exertional dyspnoea) [10, 11]. Despite correlations between peripheral muscle strength and performance in COPD and CHF [7, 10], reduced *endurance* (~ fatigue) seems to be the dominating limiting factor in peripheral muscles in these patients, since the sense of leg effort was one of the main reasons to stop exercise [3, 11–13]. Recently, it has been shown that early lactic acidosis occurs in COPD during exercise [14] and that this is largely the result of lactate release from the lower exercising limb [15]. In CHF reports lactate release is thought to be a result of decreased blood flow to the peripheral muscles. Muscle acidosis is a contributing factor to muscle fatigue [16].

Fatigue probably is *not* the main limiting factor in respiratory muscle function. Morrison et al. [17] found that COPD subjects have decreased respiratory muscle strength and endurance. Fatigue of the respiratory muscle may indeed occur during exercise, but it is not certain whether this is an independent determinant of exercise capacity [12, 18, 19]. In addition, it is unlikely that the respiratory muscles from exercising COPD patients contribute to the lactate response mentioned earlier [20]. It also should be emphasized that the respiratory muscles must operate against the mechanical airway impedances in this specific disorder [21], for which the force component of respiratory muscle function is most likely of great importance. For CHF it was found that respiratory muscle strength and not respiratory muscle fatigability correlated with the degree of dyspnoea [22]. It thus seems that strength is the limiting aspect of muscle performance in the respiratory muscle, whereas endurance limitation dominates in peripheral muscles. However, more detailed studies are required to clarify the individual roles of strength and endurance limitation in peripheral and respiratory muscles in COPD and CHF.

Muscle Morphology

In both CHF [10, 23] and COPD [2, 24–27] marked loss of muscle mass or decline in cross-sectional area is observed. This muscle wasting plays an important role in the loss of exercise tolerance in these patients. Morphological alterations may also be related to muscle function impairment, although direct relationship with exercise performance have not (yet) been shown. Some histological information is available on abnormalities in skeletal muscle in CHF but hardly any on COPD. Recently, reduced fibre cross-sectional area has been demonstrated in the vastus lateralis of COPD [28] and CHF [29]. Gertz et al. [30] found no sings of increased fibrosis or other alterations in intercostal muscles from patients with respiratory failure, whereas endomyosal fibrosis has been found in skeletal muscle of a limited number of CHF patients [31]. Increased acid phosphatase activity, a lysosomal enzyme contributing to protein degradation, has been found in the quadriceps of some patients with CHF [32] or respiratory failure [27]. Increased lipid deposits have been found in the quadriceps, biceps and deltoids of some patients with CHF [27, 32]. Very contradicting results have been obtained with respect to capillary density in peripheral skeletal muscle in CHF. A normal capillary density has been found [27], which is in confirmation with other studies where both a reduced capillary/fibre ratio and atrophy resulted in an unchanged capillary density [32]. An unaltered capillary/fibre ratio has also been reported; however, capillary density increased due to fibre atrophy [34]. In contrast, reduced capillary density in combination with a reduced capillary/fibre ratio has been shown in CHF patients [35] and even in heart transplantation recipients [36]. Thus, there is an overall tendency for a reduced capillary/fibre ratio, but depending on the degree of atrophy the capillary density may even be increased. This has recently been confirmed for COPD [25]. In a few studies morphometry of mitochondria has been performed using electron microscopy, showing that mitochondrial volume densities in skeletal muscle are lower in CHF patients compared to control subjects [35, 37], which was still the case 10 months after heart transplantation [36]. Histochemical alterations reflecting mitochondrial abnormalities have also been reported in biceps muscle biopsies of COPD patients [27]. These results suggest that oxidative capacity in peripheral skeletal muscles may be altered.

Muscle Fibre Type Distribution

The most remarkable muscle alteration in COPD and CHF is a relative shift in fibre composition which seems to occur in opposite direction in peripheral and respiratory muscle. Fibre typing is mainly performed histochemically, based on the differences in myosin ATPase activities, or immunocytochemically [38]. Adult mammalian skeletal muscle contains four myosin heavy chain (MyHC) isoforms, namely type I, IIa, IIb and IIx [39]. In most older studies fibre typing is limited to determining fibre types I, IIa and IIb. Furthermore, human fibres formerly identified as being IIb with myosin ATPase staining are probably IIx fibres [40]. Therefore the notation IIb/x will be used in the subsequent text. Fibre type I has a slow-twitch and develops a relative small tension, but since it depends mainly on aerobic metabolism it is fatigue resistant. In contrast, fibre type IIb/x has a fast-twitch and develops large tensions, but it is susceptible for fatigue, since in type IIb/x fibres energy conversion is based on anaerobic, glycolytic metabolism. Fibre type II has intermediate properties in that it also has a fast twitch, develops a moderate tension, is relatively resistant to fatigue and is apt to work under both aerobic and anaerobic conditions [5, 38]. A decrease of the percentage of type I fibres and a corresponding increase in type II (mainly type IIb/x) fibres compared to normal subjects has been reported for COPD [25, 41, 42] and for CHF [32–35, 43] in limb muscles. In addition, recently we demonstrated increased proportions of I/IIa and IIa/IIx hybrid fibres in COPD [44]. These fibres may represent transformation intermediates in the I→IIx shift. In contrast to peripheral muscles, a shift from type IIb/x to type I fibres has been reported in the diaphragm in both COPD and CHF patients. Despite some variation in the results obtained till now, there is most likely a I→IIb/x shift in peripheral muscles and a IIb/x→I shift in the respiratory muscle. It is feasible that these shifts have functional consequences in the affected muscles, since the distinct fibre types have different contractile properties with respect to twitch and fatigue resistance. Therefore, in COPD and CHF, a I→IIb/x shift accompanied by more glycolytic and less oxidative capacity in peripheral muscles implies loss of fatigue resistance. This change might contribute to the observed loss of exercise tolerance, since peripheral muscle fatigue is the main limiting factor in these patients. This is confirmed by a study in which a faster twitch response in combination with less resistance to fatigue was observed in leg muscles of CHF patients [45]. Accordingly, a IIb/x→I shift towards more oxidative metabolism in the respiratory muscle implies a shift towards a more fatique-resistant, but less strength adapted muscle. This too is in line with our notion that strength and not fatigue seems to be the main limiting factor for respiratory muscle function.

Muscle Energy Metabolism

Considerable amounts of data are available on skeletal muscle metabolism in CHF and COPD, partly because of the applicability of ^{31}P-nuclear magnetic resonance (^{31}P-NMR) which has enabled a direct and non-invasive assessment of tissue levels of high-energy phosphates and pH. High levels of adenosine triphosphate (ATP), creatine phosphate (CrP) and nicotinamide adenine dinucleotide in the reduced form (NADH) reflect a high energy state, whereas elevated levels of adenosine diphosphate (ADP), adenosine monophosphate (AMP), inorganic phosphate (Pi) and oxidized nicotinamide adenine dinucleotide (NAD^+) commonly reflect a low energy state. Lactate and glycogen levels are often measured, but it must be noted that low levels may reflect either increased clearance or reduced formation and vice versa for high levels. Although activities of enzymes involved in muscle energy metabolism do not reflect the physiological situation since only maximal activities are obtained under the optimal circumstances of in vitro measurements, they do provide an indication for adaptations in expressions of proteins involved in metabolic pathways. Typical oxidative enzymes are citrate synthase (CS), succinate dehydrogenase (SDH) and β-hydroxyacyl-CoA dehydrogenase (HAD). Typical glycolytic enzymes are hexokinase (HK), phosphofructokinase (PFK) and lactate dehydrogenase (LDH), the latter catalysing the last step of anaerobic glycolysis. Measurements of substrate and cofactor levels in peripheral skeletal muscle of COPD and CHF patients indicate impaired energy metabolism (see table 3). Most striking are the observed reduced levels of the high-energy phosphates in rest. Pouw et al. [46] observed higher Pi/Crp and ADP/ATP ratios associated with slightly, but statistically significantly elevated inosine monophosphate (IMP) levels. The latter may be due to increased degradation of accumulating AMP by deamination, which probably reflects reduced aerobic capacity [47]. The situation becomes even worse during exercise: greater increase of the Pi/CrP ratio and a faster drop in pH were found in the calf muscle of COPD patients [48, 49] and of CHF patients [34, 50, 51] performing exercise. Similar results have been obtained for the forearm muscle [51, 52] (table 1). In addition, a slower recovery of CrP was observed

Table 1. Changes in muscle energy metabolism during exercise

Disorder	Ref.	Muscle	Variables of NMR spectroscopy					
			PCr	Pi/PCr	PCr/(PCr+Pi)	ATP	relATP	pH
COPD	54	calf	↓					↓
	53	calf		↑		=		↓
	55	calf		↑			↓	↓
	56	quadriceps		=				=
	57	forearm			↓ NS			=
	58	forearm		↑	↓		↑	↓
CHF	60	calf*	=	=	=	=	=	=
	60	calf**		↑		=	↑	↓
	59	calf			=			↓
	34	calf						↓
	61	calf						↓
	57	forearm		↓ NS				=

Pi = Inorganic phosphate; PCr = phosphocreatine; ATP = adenosime triphosphate; relATP = ATP corrected for Pi/PCr; ↑ significantly increased compared to controls; ↓ significantly decreased compared to controls; = means in patients not significantly different from controls; * compared to sedentary controls; ** compared to trained controls.

Table 2. Muscle energy metabolism in the recovery phase after exercise

Disorder	Ref.	Muscle	Variables of NMR spectroscopy					
			PCr/RT$^1/_2$	PCr/(PCr+Pi)/RT$^1/_2$	Pi/PCr	RT$^1/_2$	pH	pH/RT$^1/_2$
COPD	53	calf	↑					
	54	calf	=					
	55	calf	↑					
	58	forearm		↑				↑
	57	forearm			↑		↓	↑
CHF	60	calf*				=		
	60	calf**				=		
	61	calf	↑					
	57	forearm	↑		↓	↑	↓ NS	

Pi = Inorganic phosphate; PCr = phosphocreatine; RT$^1/_2$ = recovery halftime; ↑ significantly increased compared to controls; ↓ significantly decreased compared to controls; = means in patients not significantly different from controls; * compared to sedentary controls; ** compared to trained controls.

after exercise [34, 49–52]. COPD patients also show a prolonged half-time (RT½) for pH [53–55, 57, 58] (table 2). These results suggest that rephosphorylation of high-energy phosphates is less efficient in these patients both during and after muscular exercise. In CHF patients, Chati et al. [60] compared NMR spectra of calf muscles during exercise with sedentary and trained controls. They found no difference between patients and sedentary controls and concluded deconditioning being an important factor for the abnormalities. In addition, glycogen contents in patients tend to be lower, whereas lactate levels are higher (table 3). It thus seems that anaerobic energy metabolism is enhanced and since this process yields far less ATP compared to complete oxidative degradation of

Table 3. Muscle metabolite concentrations in COPD and CHF

Metabolite	Muscle	Disorder	Direction	References
CrP	QF	COPD	↓	30, 124, 125, 126*
	QF	CHF	↓	127, 128*
ATP	QF	COPD	↓	30, 124, 125, 126*
	QF	CHF	↓	127, 128*
IMP	TA	COPD	↑	46
Glycogen	QF	CHF	↓	32, 127, 128
	QF	COPD	↓	124, 125*
Lactate	QF	COPD	↑	30, 126
	QF	CHF	↑	129
Pyruvate	QF	CHF	↑	32
	QF	COPD	↑	14

ATP = Adenosine triphosphate; CrP = creatine phosphate; IMP = inosine monophosphate; QF = quadriceps femoris; TA = tibialis anterior; * nearly reached significance.

Table 4. Muscle enzyme activities

Enzyme	Muscle	Disorder	Direction	References
CS	QF	COPD	↓	130, 131
	QF	CHF	↓	32, 34, 129, 132
	DIA	CHF	↑	133
HAD	QF	COPD	↓	130, 131
	QF	CHF	↓	32, 34, 129, 132
	DIA	CHF	↑	133
SDH	QF	COPD	↓	131
	QF	CHF	↓	32, 132
LDH	QF	COPD	↑	131
	QF	CHF	↑	129*
	DIA	CHF	↓	133
	DIA	COPD	↓	134
HK	QF	CHF	↓	132
	DIA	COPD	↓	134
PFK	QF	COPD	↑	131

CS = Citrate synthase; HAD = β-hydroxyacyl-CoA dehydrogenase; SDH = succinate dehydrogenase; HK = hexokinase; PFK = phosphofructokinase; LDH = lactate dehydrogenase; QF = quadriceps femoris; DIA = diaphragm.

glucose this could explain the reduced high-energy phosphate levels.

Analysis of enzyme activities too suggest an overall increase of glycolytic and an overall decrease of oxidative activities in peripheral muscles of both COPD and CHF patients (table 4). Since these enzyme activities depend largely on the fibre type [62], it is likely that this shift in activities is related to the shift in fibre distribution mentioned above. Whether enzyme activities adapt to the fibre type redistribution or the other way around remains unclear. Due to technical difficulties with ^{31}P-NMR and muscle biopsies of the diaphragm and accessory respiratory muscles, very little is known about energy metabolism in these muscles. However, the observed alterations for enzyme activities (table 4) are in confirmation with the morphological data, in that oxidative enzyme activities are reduced and glycolytic enzyme activities are increased. As in peripheral muscles, this shift probably results from the shift in fibre type distribution.

Possible Underlying Factors

Hypoxia

In COPD and CHF oxygen delivery to peripheral and respiratory muscles may be insufficient, caused by either hypoxemia and/or reduced blood supply. In both cases muscle tissue may become hypoxic and this could lead to the adaptive changes in skeletal muscle as those described above. In this respect relevant information is now available from mountaineering expeditions (lasting at least 6 weeks above 5,000 m), since oxygen is limited at this altitude. Under these conditions reductions in mitochondrial volume densities, in oxidative enzyme activities and in cross sectional areas of muscle fibers were found in the quadriceps [63, 64]. But such expeditions are accompanied by strenuous physical activity, which also causes muscular adaptations other than those caused by hypoxia. In fact, the effect of training in combination with hypoxia may even cause a shift towards more oxidative metabolism [65].

More information about the effect of hypoxia on muscle has been obtained from animal studies. Several of these studies have shown that hypoxia can indeed lead to the muscular alterations as described for limb muscles in COPD and CHF: (1) Reduced fibre diameters in combination with unaffected numbers of capillaries, resulting in increased capillary densities, have been reported in rats exposed to hypoxia [66, 67]. (2) Some studies revealed that hypoxia depresses protein synthesis [68, 69], including in muscle tissue [68]. Chronic hypoxia inhibits the normal conversion of type IIa to type I fibres in growing rats, resulting in a predominating proportion of type IIa fibres compared to control rats [70]. So hypoxia does not directly cause a type I → II fibre shift, but causes an abnormal fibre type distribution from alterations in muscular development. It is feasible that in COPD and CHF a similar mechanism underlies the abnormal fibre type distribution in the regeneration of damaged muscle or the adaptation of muscles to consequences of the disease. (3) There is evidence that hypoxia causes a shift towards glycolytic metabolism, resulting in an increased lactate-to-pyruvate ratio [71, 72] and reduced malate dehydrogenase, a citric acid enzyme [73]. (4) Hypoxia causes stimulation of glucose transport [74] and increased levels of membrane-associated glucose transporters (GLUT1 and GLUT4) in rat muscle [75].

It should be noted, however, that in COPD and CHF this reduction of oxidative capacity does not occur in the diaphragm. It is feasible that hypoxia causes an endurance training effect in the diaphragm due to increased ventilation, which overrides its direct effect ultimately resulting in a shift towards more aerobic metabolism.

Oxidative Stress

Oxidative stress may be another factor contributing via reactive oxygen species to muscle damage. In both COPD and CHF increased plasma levels of lipid peroxidation products have been found [76, 77]. Sources of free oxygen radicals are: (1) Mitochondria, since 2–5% of the total oxygen consumed is not fully reduced in the electron transport chain and may leak away as superoxide radicals [78, 79]. (2) Immune cells activated during inflammation [80]. Monocytes and macrophages produce cytokine tumor necrosis factor-α (TNFα) which may in turn induce oxidative stress in myocytes [81]. Elevated TNFα blood levels have indeed been found in both COPD [82, 83] and CHF [84, 85], in particular in those patients characterized by weight loss and/or muscle wasting. (3) Xanthine oxidase, in case of a low energy state, is involved in the degradation of AMP [79]. The above-mentioned elevated IMP levels in COPD [46] indeed suggest enhanced AMP breakdown. Susceptibility to these free radicals largely depends on the antioxidant status of tissue [79]. The main antioxidant scavengers and enzymes are, amongst others, reduced glutathione, vitamin E (in cell membranes), superoxide dismutase (SOD), glutathione peroxidase and catalase [79, 86]. Long-term training stimulates the defense system against oxygen free radicals [78, 79, 86] and the disuse of muscles thus may lack this antioxidant stimulating trigger resulting in a reduced antioxidant status. Chronic hypoxia probably acts in the same way, since limitations of oxygen supply are indeed found to be associated with reductions in SOD activity in mammalian tissues like brain, lungs and heart, although this change was not found in skeletal muscle tissue [87, 88]. In addition, in myocytes (obtained from chronic hypoxic human myocardium) cultured at low oxygen tension, antioxidant enzyme activities were lower than in myocytes cultured at a higher oxygen tension, illustrating the direct modulatory effect of oxygen [89]. In vivo and in vitro hypoxia-reoxygenation studies revealed that oxygen oversupply following a period of oxygen shortage may give rise to free radical formation in myocytes [87, 90]. Accordingly, in COPD and CHF chronic hypoxia may result in a reduced antioxidant status and occasional bouts of exercise may cause a boost of free radicals exceeding the capacity of the defence system [78]. It is also feasible that the reduced oxidative capacity in the patients itself leads to enhanced oxidative stress, since the sudden oversupply of oxygen during exercise is inefficiently metabolised.

Reactive oxygen species are well capable of damaging lipids and proteins [78, 79, 86, 91]. Radicals that react with fatty acyl moieties in membrane phospholipids cause a chain reaction of peroxidations increasing the membrane permeability [91]. Maintenance of membrane integrity is crucial for: (1) Adequate functioning of the respiratory chain, since the driving force for oxidative ATP synthesis is the electrochemical proton gradient over the inner membrane of the mitochondrion, which is generated during the electron transfer from NADH to oxygen [92]. (2) To prevent intracellular calcium overload, caused by damaged sarcoplasmatic reticulum membrane, in combination with impaired activity of calcium ATPases, which accompanies oxidative stress in animal myocytes [78, 87, 90, 93], and may further uncouple respiration from ATP production through extensive depolarisation of the inner membrane [94].

Protein oxidation by oxygen free radicals leads to formation of carbonyl groups on amino acid residues, which may modify the structure and/or chemical properties of the proteins affected [95]. These alterations may cause decline in function or even complete protein unfolding. The latter gives rise to enhanced susceptibility to proteinases. These modified proteins may also be recognized as foreign substances and, hence, be attacked by the immune system. Whether radical induced protein damage plays a role in the abnormalities in muscles of COPD and CHF patients is unclear. It has been shown in animal studies that in vivo induced oxidative stress caused myofibrillar muscle protein modification and that these proteins were rapidly degraded by proteases [96]. Thus theoretically, muscle atrophy can be enhanced by radical induced protein damage. Indeed, it has been shown that a calcium overload is involved in muscle atrophy [97] and that vitamin E deficiency facilitates muscle wasting and necrosis [98], both probably mediated by oxidative damage to proteins. Also, in human skeletal muscle it has been shown that mitochondria and mitochondrial proteins were more susceptible to oxidative damage compared to other subcellular components [99], which suggests that protein damage may cause impaired oxidative metabolism.

As opposed to necrosis, which is the result of exogenous damage as described above, apoptosis of muscle cells is an active process of cell death, which recently also has been associated with oxidative stress [100]. In this study the exposure of rat myoblasts to nitric oxide or hydrogen peroxidase led to apoptotic cell death. Since these chemical stimuli are also released by immune cells, it cannot be excluded that apoptosis underlies muscle wasting during inflammation.

Disuse

Disuse (low level of physical exercise because of their disease) of skeletal muscle is also a factor that most likely contributes to the observed muscle alterations in COPD and CHF. This results in: (1) Muscle weakness, due to reduced motor neuron activity and muscle wasting [38, 101]. (2) Relative reduction in the percentage of type I fibres and an increase in the percentage of type IIb/x fibres [38, 102]. (3) A decline in activity of enzymes involved in oxidative energy conversion, which occurs both in type I and type II fibres [102], suggesting that it can occur even without any change in fibre composition. (4) A negative effect on the antioxidant status enhances the risk of oxidative damage. As mentioned above, the diaphragm is probably not disused and a kind of endurance training effect may even occur. This may not only be true for COPD, but for CHF as well, since especially in severe CHF dyspnoea and elevated ventilation occur already at rest [13, 103].

Weight Loss and Altered Substrate Metabolism

Weight loss commonly occurs in COPD [104, 105] and in CHF [23, 106] and is an independent determinant of mortality [107, 108]. In both disorders in particular loss of FFM is an important determinant for exercise capacity [2, 24, 109]. Determination of body composition, and not only weight, with respect to nutritional depletion is very important since at least in COPD different patterns of weight loss can be distinguished: predominant loss of fat mass, predominant loss of fat-free mass or a combination of both. Predominant loss of fat mass involves an impaired balance between energy requirement and energy intake. Although limited information is available in CHF patients, a negative energy balance commonly occurs in COPD as a result of either a decreased dietary intake, elevated energy requirements or a combination of both. Total daily energy metabolism (TDE) can be divided in 3 components: resting energy expenditure (REE), measured under fasting conditions in the early morning, diet induced thermogenesis (DIT) and physical activity induced (PAI) thermogenesis. REE comprises the major part of TDE, DIT on average only 10–15% and PAI can be highly variable. While in many chronic wasting diseases, REE is increased, probably related to an enhanced systemic inflammation, TDE is not different from healthy control subjects due to a compensatory decrease in daily activities. In contrast, TDE in COPD was found to be increased as a result of an increased PAI [110]. It is yet unclear to what extent an increased PAI is related to a decreased mechanical or a decreased metabolic efficiency and what the contributing role is of peripheral skeletal muscles versus the diaphragm.

In a situation of semistarvation, either primarily due to increased energy requirements or due to decreased dietary intake, loss of both fat mass and fat-free mass occurs, but the loss of fat-free mass is relatively preserved. Therefore, intrinsic muscle abnormalities besides loss of muscle mass must account for impaired muscle performance. Studies on muscle function and histology in anorexia nervosa patients provide strong data on the effect of undernutrition per se on muscles. Muscle performance is markedly impaired in these patients [111–113] and is associated with weight loss, loss of muscle mass and fibre atrophy (particularly of type II fibres) [114, 115]. We recently demonstrated selective fibre type IIx atrophy in COPD patients associated with a reduced fat-free mass, suggesting a role for undernutrition in this disease too [44]. Data from animal studies confirm these effects of undernutrition. Decreased activities of enzymes involved in glycolytic and mitochondrial pathways have been reported from muscle biopsies of patients with anorexia nervosa [99, 111], with glycolytic capacity being affected the most [111]. The contribution of nutritional depletion to a shift from oxidative to glycolytic metabolism in COPD and CHF patients needs further investigation.

Disproportionate loss of fat-free mass often referred as cachexia, involves an impaired balance between protein anabolism and catabolism. Protein depletion itself may impair skeletal muscle performance as reflected by reduced maximum voluntary handgrip strength, reduced respiratory muscle strength and an increased fatigability of in vivo electrically stimulated adductor pollicis muscle [116]. Predominant loss of fat-free mass with relative preservation of fat mass also points towards alterations in substrate metabolism. Partly independent of pulmonary or cardiac cachexia, other disease characteristics like hypoxia or hypercapnia may alter substrate metabolism. Insulin has a central role in substrate metabolism. Hyperinsulinemia has been described in COPD and insulin resistance commonly occurs in CHF. While nearly no data are available regarding carbohydrate and fat metabolism in fasting, fed or stressed states, protein metabolism has been subject of recent investigations in COPD. In nondepleted COPD patients, an increased whole-body protein turnover was observed at rest and specifically in emphysema a suppressed whole body protein turnover was observed during and immediately after exercise [118, 119]. Whole-body protein turnover, however, does not necessarily reflect muscle protein turnover. A study in underweight patients with emphysema reported a reduced muscle protein synthesis [117], while protein degradation was not increased [119, 120]. It is feasible that amino acids are required in other processes than muscular protein synthesis, such as gluconeogenesis. Besides, recent data also showed intrinsic alterations in the amino acid profile of peripheral skeletal muscles. Most consistent results were found with respect to the amino acid glutamate (GLU). Intracellular GLU has various important functions, as it plays an important role in preserving high-energy phosphates in muscle through different metabolic mechanisms. GLU concentration is high in the free amino acid pool of human skeletal muscle. Intracellular GLU is known as an important precursor for the antioxidant glutathione (GSH) and glutamine synthesis in the muscle. Muscle GLU is indeed highly associated with muscle GSH, and patients with emphysema suffer from decreased muscular GLU and GSH levels [122]. Studies have shown that in healthy human muscle, the GLU pool functions to generate tricarboxylic acid (TCA) intermediates during the first minutes of exercise, which is achieved via the alanine aminotransferase reaction (pyruvate + GLU $\rightarrow$ alanine + α-ketoglutarate) at the cost of GLU. Moreover, this reaction can shunt the pyruvate accumulated during exercise towards alanine instead of lactate, suggesting a possible role of the intracellular GLU level in the lactate response to exercise. In line with this hypothesis early lactic acidosis during exercise in patients with COPD was indeed associated with a reduction in muscle GLU [14]. Not only at rest, but also during 20 min of submaximal constant cycle exercise a different response in amino acid status was found in skeletal muscle and plasma of COPD patients as compared with healthy age-matched controls [123]. A significant reduction of most muscle amino acids was present postexercise, whereas several plasma amino acids were increased, suggesting an enhanced amino acid release from muscle in COPD during exercise. The increase in plasma alanine and glutamine was even higher postexercise, suggesting enhanced nitrogen efflux. Although investigation of substrate metabolism in COPD and CHF is still in its infancy, the available studies clearly point towards therapeutic perspective, not only in cachectic patients, but also as anabolic stimulus to enhance muscle and exercise performance. In frail elderly it has indeed been observed that oral amino acid intake stimulates the transport of amino acids into muscle, and that there is a direct link between amino acid transport and protein synthesis when ingested before exercise or some time after exercise.

Conclusions

This review underscores that reduced skeletal muscle performance markedly contributes to exercise intolerance in COPD and CHF patients. Morphologic and metabolic abnormalities occur in the skeletal muscles of these patients which, in both disorders, probably are determined by the same set of contributing factors. Both diseases also share striking differences between peripheral muscles and the diaphragm which, therefore, may require a different therapeutical approach.

References

1 Wood PH: Appreciating the consequences of disease: The international classification of impairments, disabilities, and handicaps. WHO Chron 1980;34:376–380.

2 Schols AM, Mostert R, Soeters PB, Wouters EF: Body composition and exercise performance in patients with chronic obstructive pulmonary disease. Thorax 1991;46:695–699.

3 Hamilton AL, Killian KJ, Summers E, Jones NL: Muscle strength, symptom intensity, and exercise capacity in patients with cardiorespiratory disorders. Am J Respir Crit Care Med 1995;152:2021–2031.

4 Steele IC, Moore A, Nugent AM, Riley MS, Campbell NPS, Nicholls DP: Non-invasive measurement of cardiac output and ventricular ejection fractions in chronic cardiac failure: Relationship to impaired exercise tolerance. Clin Sci 1997;93:195–203.

5 Armstrong RB: Muscle fiber recruitment patterns and their metabolic correlates; in Horton HS, Terjung RL (eds): Exercise, Nutrition, and Energy Metabolism. New York, Macmillan, 1988, pp 9–26.

6 Bernard S, LeBlanc P, Whittom F, Carrier G, Jobin J, Belleau R, Maltais F: Peripheral muscle weakness in patients with chronic obstructive pulmonary disease. Am J Respir Crit Care Med 1998;158:629–634.

7 Gosselink R, Troosters T, Decramer M: Peripheral muscle weakness contributes to exercise limitation in COPD. Am J Respir Crit Care Med 1996;153:976–980.

8 Chua TP, Anker SD, Harrington D, Coats AJ: Inspiratory muscle strength is a determinant of maximum oxygen consumption in chronic heart failure. Br Heart J 1995;74:381–385.

9 Lands LC, Heigenhauser GJ, Jones NL: Respiratory and peripheral muscle function in cystic fibrosis. Am Rev Respir Dis 1993;147:865–869.

10 Harrington D, Anker SD, Chua TP, Webb Peploe KM, Ponikowski PP, Poole Wilson PA, Coats AJ: Skeletal muscle function and its relation to exercise tolerance in chronic heart failure. J Am Coll Cardiol 1997;30:1758–1764.

11 Killian KJ, Leblanc P, Martin DH, Summers E, Jones NL, Campbell EJ: Exercise capacity and ventilatory, circulatory, and symptom limitation in patients with chronic airflow limitation. Am Rev Respir Dis 1992;146:935–940.

12 Belman MJ: Exercise in patients with chronic obstructive pulmonary disease. Thorax 1993;48:936–946.

13 Myers J, Salleh A, Buchanan N, Smith D, Neutel J, Bowes E, Froelicher VF: Ventilatory mechanisms of exercise intolerance in chronic heart failure. Am Heart J 1992;124:710–719.

14 Engelen MPKJ, Schols AMWJ, Does JD, Wouters EFM: Exercise induced lactate increase in relation to physical activity level and peripheral muscle substrates in COPD. Am J Respir Crit Care Med 1999;159:A475.

15 Maltais F, Jobin J, Sullivan MJ, Bernard S, Whittom F, Killian KJ, Desmeules M, Bélanger M, LeBlanc P: Metabolic and hemodynamic responses of lower limb during exercise in patients with COPD. J Appl Physiol 1999;84:1573–1580.

16 Mainwood GW, Renaud JM: The effect of acid-base balance on fatigue of skeletal muscle. Can J Physiol Pharmacol 1985;63:403–416.

17 Morrison NJ, Richardson J, Dunn L, Pardy RL: Respiratory muscle performance in normal elderly subjects and patients with COPD. Chest 1989;95:90–94.

18 Decramer M, Aubier M: The respiratory muscles: Cellular and molecular physiology. Eur Respir J 1997;10:1943–1945.

19 Fitting JW: Respiratory muscle fatigue limiting physical exercise? Eur Respir J 1991;4:103–108.

20 Engelen MP, Casaburi R, Rucker R, Carithers E: Contribution of the respiratory muscles to the lactic acidosis of heavy exercise in COPD. Chest 1995;108:1246–1251.

21 O'Donnell DE, Webb KA: Exertional breathlessness in patients with chronic airflow limitation: The role of lung hyperinflation. Am Rev Respir Dis 1993;148:1351–1357.

22 Mancini DM, Henson D, LaManca J, Levine S: Respiratory muscle function and dyspnea in patients with chronic congestive heart failure. Circulation 1992;86:909–918.

23 Wilson JR, Mancini DM: The mechanism of extertional fatigue in heart failure. Cardioscience 1990;1:13–17.

24 Engelen MP, Schols AM, Wouters EF: Nutritional depletion in relation to respiratory and peripheral skeletal muscle function in out-patients with COPD. Eur Respir J 1994;7:1793–1797.

25 Whittom F, Jobin J, Simard PM, Leblanc P, Simard C, Bernard S, Belleau R, Maltais F: Histochemical and morphological characteristics of the vastus lateralis muscle in patients with chronic obstructive pulmonary disease. Med Sci Sports Exerc 1998;30:1467–1474.

26 Rochester DF: Body weight and respiratory muscle function in chronic obstructive pulmonary disease. Am Rev Respir Dis 1986;134:646–648.

27 Sato Y, Asoh T, Honda Y, Fujimatsu Y, Higuchi I, Oizumi K: Morphologic and histochemical evaluation of muscle in patients with chronic pulmonary emphysema manifesting generalized emaciation. Eur Neurol 1997;37:116–121.

28 Gosker HR, Engelen MPKJ, Mameren van H, Dijk van PJ, Vusse van der GJ, Wouters EFM, Schols AMWJ: Muscle fibre type IIX atrophy is involved in the loss of fat-free mass in chronic obstructive pulmonary disease. Am J Clin Nutr 2001;in press.

29 Vescovo G, Volterrani M, Zennaro R, Sandri M, Ceconi C, Lorusso R, Ferrari R, Ambrosio GB, Dalla Libera L: Apoptosis in skeletal muscle of patients with heart failure: Investigation of clinical and biochemical changes. Heart 2000;84:431–437.

30 Gertz I, Hedenstierna G, Hellers G, Wahren J: Muscle metabolism in patients with chronic obstructive lung disease and acute respiratory failure. Clin Sci Mol Med 1977;52:395–403.

31 Dunnigan A, Staley NA, Smith SA, Pierpont ME, Judd D, Benditt DG, Benson DW Jr: Cardiac and skeletal muscle abnormalities in cardiomyopathy: Comparison of patients with ventricular tachycardia or congestive heart failure. J Am Coll Cardiol 1987;10:608–618.

32 Lipkin DP, Jones DA, Roud JM, Poole Wilson PA: Abnormalities of skeletal muscle in patients with chronic heart failure. Int J Cardiol 1988;18:187–195.

33 Sullivan MJ, Green HJ, Cobb FR: Skeletal muscle biochemistry and histology in ambulatory patients with long-term heart failure. Circulation 1990;81:518–527.

34 Mancini DM, Coyle E, Coggan A, Beltz J, Ferraro N, Montain S, Wilson JR: Contribution of intrinsic skeletal muscle changes to ^{31}P NMR skeletal muscle metabolic abnormalities in patients with chronic heart failure. Circulation 1989;80:1338–1346.

35 Drexler H, Riede U, Münzel T, König H, Funke E, Just H: Alterations of skeletal muscle in chronic heart failure. Circulation 1992;85:1751–1759.

36 Lampert E, Mettauer B, Hoppeler H, Charloux A, Charpentier A, Lonsdorfer J: Structure of skeletal muscle in heart transplant recipients. J Am Coll Cardiol 1996;28:980–984.

37 Hambrecht R, Fiehn E, Yu J, Niebauer J, Weigl C, Hilbrich L, Adams V, Riede U, Schuler G: Effects of endurance training on mitochondrial ultrastructure and fiber type distribution in skeletal muscle of patients with stable chronic heart failure. J Am Coll Cardiol 1997;29:1067–1073.

38 McComas AJ: Skeletal Muscle: Form and Function. Champaign, Human Kinetics, 1996.

39 Schiaffino S, Reggiani C: Molecular diversity of myofibrillar proteins: Gene regulation and functional significance. Physiol Rev 1996;76:371–423.

40 Pereira Sant'Ana JA, Ennion S, Sargeant AJ, Moorman AF, Goldspink G, Sant'ana Pereira J, Young A: Comparison of the molecular, antigenic and ATPase determinants of fast myosin heavy chains in rat and human: A single-fibre study. Pflügers Arch 1997;435:151–163.

41 Satta A, Migliori GB, Spanevello A, Neri M, Bottinelli R, Canepari M, Pellegrino MA, Reggiani C: Fibre types in skeletal muscles of chronic obstructive pulmonary disease patients related to respiratory function and exercise tolerance. Eur Respir J 1997;10:2853–2860.

42 Hildebrand IL, Sylvén C, Esbjörnsson M, Hellström K, Jansson E: Does chronic hypoxaemia induce transformations of fibre types? Acta Physiol Scand 1991;141:435–439.

43 Sullivan MJ, Duscha BD, Klitgaard H, Kraus WE, Cobb FR, Saltin B: Altered expression of myosin heavy chain in human skeletal muscle in chronic heart failure. Med Sci Sports Exerc 1997;29:860–866.

44 Gosker HR, Mameren H, Schols, AMWJ: Fiber type redistribution in limb muscle in COPD occurs through gradual changes in myosin isoform content. Eur Respir J 2000; 16(suppl 31):p559s.

45 Harridge SD, Magnusson G, Gordon A: Skeletal muscle contractile characteristics and fatigue resistance in patients with chronic heart failure. Eur Heart J 1996;17:896–901.

46 Pouw EM, Schold AMWJ, Wouters EFM: Elevated inosine monophosphate levels in resting muscle of patients with stable COPD. Am J Respir Crit Care Med 1998;157:453–457.

47 Dudley GA, Terjung RL: Influence of aerobic metabolism on IMP accumulation in fast-twitch muscle. Am J Physiol 1985;248:C37–42.

48 Thompson CH, Davies RJ, Kemp GJ, Taylor DJ, Radda GK, Rajagopalan B: Skeletal muscle metabolism during exercise and recovery in patients with respiratory failure. Thorax 1993; 48:486–490.

49 Payen JF, Wuyam B, Levy P, Reutenauer H, Stieglitz P, Paramelle B, Le Baw JF: Muscular metabolism during oxygen supplementation in patients with chronic hypoxemia. Am Rev Respir Dis 1993;147:592–598.

50 Mancini DM, Walter G, Reichek N, Lenkinski R, McCully KK, Mullen JL, Wilson JR: Contribution of skeletal muscle atrophy to exercise intolerance and altered muscle metabolism in heart failure. Circulation 1992;85:1364–1373.

51 Kemp GJ, Thompson CH, Stratton JR, Brunotte F, Conway M, Adamopoulos S, Arnolda L, Radda GK, Rajagopalan B: Abnormalities in exercising skeletal muscle in congestive heart failure can be explained in terms of decreased mitochondrial ATP synthesis, reduced metabolic efficiency, and increased glycogenolysis. Heart 1996;76:35–41.

52 Stratton JR, Kemp GJ, Daly RC, Yacoub M, Rajagopalan B: Effects of cardiac transplantation on bioenergetic abnormalities of skeletal muscle in congestive heart failure. Circulation 1994;89:1624–1631.

53 Wuyam B, Payen JF, Levy P, Bensaidane H, Reutenauer H, Le Bas JF, Benabid AL: Metabolism and aerobic capacity of skeletal muscle in chronic respiratory failure related to chronic obstructive pulmonary disease. Eur Respir J 1992;5:157–162.

54 Thompson CH, Davies RJ, Kemp GJ, Taylor DJ, Radda GK, Rajagopalan B: Skeletal muscle metabolism during exercise and recovery in patients with respiratory failure. Thorax 1993; 48:486–490.

55 Payen JF, Wuyam B, Levy P, Reutenauer H, Stieglitz P, Paramelle B, Le Bas JF: Muscular metabolism during oxygen supplementation in patients with chronic hypoxemia. Am Rev Respir Dis 1993;147:592–598.

56 Evans AB, al-Himyary AJ, Hrovat MI, Pappagianopoulos P, Wain JC, Ginns LC, Systrom DM: Abnormal skeletal muscle oxidative capacity after lung transplantation by ^{31}P-MRS. Am J Respir Crit Care Med 1997;155:615–621.

57 Tata H, Kato H, Misawa T, Sasaki F, Hayashi S, Takahashi H, Kutsumi Y, Ishizaki T, Nakai T, Miyabo S: ^{31}P-nuclear magnetic resonance evidence of abnormal skeletal muscle metabolism in patients with chronic lung disease and congestive heart failure. Eur Respir J 1992;5: 163–169.

58 Kutsuzawa T, Shioya S, Kurita D, Haida M, Ohta Y, Yamabayashi H: ^{31}P-NMR study of skeletal muscle metabolism in patients with chronic respiratory impairment. Am Rev Respir Dis 1992;146:1019–1024.

59 Okita K, Yonezawa K, Nishijima H, Hanada A, Ohtsubo M, Kohya T, Murakami T, Kitabatake A: Skeletal muscle metabolism limits exercise capacity in patients with chronic heart failure. Circulation 1998;98:1886–1891.

60 Chati Z, Zannad F, Jeandel C, Lherbier B, Escanye JM, Robert J, Aliot E: Physical deconditioning may be a mechanism for the skeletal muscle energy phosphate metabolism abnormalities in chronic heart failure. Am Heart J 1996;13:560–566.

61 Mancini DM, Ferraro N, Tuchler M, Chance B, Wilson JR: Detection of abnormal calf muscle metabolism in patients with heart failure using phosphorus-31 nuclear magnetic resonance. Am J Cardiol 1988;62:1234–1240.

62 Essén-Gustavsson B, Henriksson J: Enzyme levels in pools of microdissected human muscle fibres of identified type: Adaptive response to exercise. Acta Physiol Scand 1984;120:505–515.

63 Hoppeler H, Desplanches D: Muscle structural modifications in hypoxia. Int J Sports Med 1992;13:S166–S168.

64 Howald H, Pette D, Simoneau JA, Uber A, Hoppeler H, Cerretelli P: Effects of chronic hypoxia on muscle enzyme activities. Int J Sports Med 1990;11:S10–S14.

65 Melissa L, MacDougall JD, Tarnopolsky MA, Cipriano N, Green HJ: Skeletal muscle adaptations to training under normobaric hypoxic versus normoxic conditions. Med Sci Sports Exerc 1997;29:238–243.

66 Bigard AX, Brunet A, Guezennec CY, Monod H: Effects of chronic hypoxia and endurance training on muscle capillarity in rats. Pflügers Arch 1991;419:225–229.

67 Snyder G, Farrelly C, Coelho J: Adaptations in skeletal muscle capillarity following changes in oxygen supply and changes in oxygen demands. Eur J Appl Physiol 1992;65:158–163.

68 Preedy VR, Smith DM, Sugden PH: The effects of 6 hours of hypoxia on protein synthesis in rat tissues in vivo and in vitro. Biochem J 1985;228:179–185.

69 Kwast KE, Hand SC: Acute depression of mitochondrial protein synthesis during anoxia: Contributions of oxygen sensing, matrix acidification, and redox state. J Biol Chem 1996;271: 7313–7319.

70 Ishihara A, Itoh K, Oishi Y, Itoh M, Hirofuji C, Hayashi H: Effects of hypobaric hypoxia on histochemical fibre-type composition and myosin heavy chain isoform component in the rat soleus muscle. Pflügers Arch 1995;429:601–606.

71 Pastoris O, Dossena M, Foppa P, Arnaboldi R, Giorini A, Villa RF, Benzi G: Modifications by chronic intermittent hypoxia and drug treatment on skeletal muscle metabolism. Neurochem Res 1995;20:143–150.

72 Pastoris O, Gorini A, Vercesi L, Taglietti M, Dossena M: Modification of the skeletal muscle energy metabolism induced by intermittent normobaric hypoxia and treatment with biological pyrimidines. Farmaco Sci 1985;40:442–453.

73 Takahashi H, Kikuchi K, Nakayama H: Effect of chronic hypoxia on oxidative enzyme activity in rat skeletal muscle. Ann Physiol Anthropol 1993;12:363–369.

74 Cartee GD, Douen AG, Ramlal T, Klip A, Holloszy JO: Stimulation of glucose transport in skeletal muscle by hypoxia. J Appl Physiol 1991;70:1593–1600.

75 Xia Y, Warshaw JB, Haddad GG: Effect of chronic hypoxia on glucose transporters in heart and skeletal muscle of immature and adult rats. Am J Physiol 1997;273:R1734–1741.

76 Rahman I, Morrison D, Donaldson K, MacNee W: Systemic oxidative stress in asthma, COPD, and smokers. Am J Respir Crit Care Med 1996;154:1055–1060.

77 Keith M, Geranmayegan A, Sole MJ, Kurian R, Robinson A, Omran AS, Jeejeebhoy KN: Increased oxidative stress in patients with congestive heart failure. J Am Coll Cardiol 1998; 31:1352–1358.

78 Giuliani A, Cestaro B: Exercise, free radical generation and vitamins. Eur J Cancer Prevention 1997;6:S55–67.

79 Ji LL: Exercise, oxidative stress, and antioxidants. Am J Sports Med 1996;24:S20–24.

80 Reid MB: Reactive oxygen and nitric oxide in skeletal muscle. News Physiol Sci 1996;11: 114–119.

81 Buck M, Chojkier M: Muscle wasting and dedifferentiation induced by oxidative stress in a murine model of cachexia is prevented by inhibitors of nitric oxide synthesis and antioxidants. EMBO J 1996;15:1753–1765.

82 de Godoy I, Donahoe M, Calhoun WJ, Mancino J, Rogers RM: Elevated TNF-alpha production by peripheral blood monocytes of weight-losing COPD patients. Am J Respir Crit Care Med 1996;153:633–637.

83 Schols AM, Buurman WA, Staal van den Brekel AJ, Dentener MA, Wouters EF: Evidence for a relation between metabolic derangements and increased levels of inflammatory mediators in a subgroup of patients with chronic obstructive pulmonary disease. Thorax 1996; 51:819–824.

84 Levine B, Kalman J, Mayer L, Fillit HM, Packer M: Elevated circulating levels of tumor necrosis factor in severe chronic heart failure. N Engl J Med 1990;323:236–241.

85 Anker SD, Clark AL, Kemp M, Salsbury C, Teixeira MM, Hellewell PG, Coats AJ: Tumor necrosis factor and steroid metabolism in chronic heart failure: Possible relation to muscle wasting. J Am Coll Cardiol 1997;30:907–1001.
86 Clarkson P: Antioxidants and physical performance. Crit Rev Food Sci Nutr 1995;35:131–141.
87 Ferrari R, Ceconi C, Curello S, Alfieri O, Visioli O: Myocardial damage during ischaemia and reperfusion. Eur Heart J 1993;14:25–30.
88 Liu J, Simon LM, Phillips JR, Robin ED: Superoxide dismutase (SOD) activity in hypoxic mammalian systems. J Appl Physiol 1977; 42:107–110.
89 Li RK, Mickle DA, Weisel RD, Kemp M, Salsbury C, Teixeira MM, Hellewell PG, Coats AJ: Effect of oxygen tension on the anti-oxidant enzyme activities of tetralogy of Fallot ventricular myocytes. J Mol Cell Cardiol 1989;21: 567–575.
90 Smith DR, Stone D, Darley-Usmar VM: Stimulation of mitochondrial oxygen consumption in isolated cardiomyocytes after hypoxia-reoxygenation. Free Radic Res 1996;24:159–166.
91 Haramaki N, Packer L: Oxidative stress indices in exercise; in Sen KC, Packer L, Hänninen O (eds): Exercise and Oxygen Toxicity. Amsterdam, Elsevier Science, 1994, pp 77–87.
92 Stryer L: Biochemistry. New York, Freeman, 1988.
93 Xu KY, Zweier JL, Becker LC: Hydroxyl radical inhibits sarcoplasmic reticulum Ca^{2+}-ATPase function by direct attack on the ATP binding site. Circ Res 1997;80:76–81.
94 Minezaki K, Suleiman M, Chapman R: Changes in mitochondrial function induced in isolated guinea-pig ventricular myocytes by calcium overload. J Physiol Lond 1994;476: 459–471.
95 Dean RT, Fu SL, Stocker R, Davies MJ: Biochemistry and pathology of radical-mediated protein oxidation. Biochem J 1997;324:1–18.
96 Nagasawa T, Hatayama T, Watanabe Y, Tanaka M, Niisato Y, Kitts DD: Free radical mediated effects on skeletal muscle protein in rats treated with fe nitrilotriacetate. Biochem Biophys Res Commun 1997;231:37–41.
97 Soares JM, Duarte JA, Carvalho J: The possible role of intracellular Ca^{2+} accumulation for the development of immobilization atrophy. Int J Sports Med 1993;14:437–439.
98 Thomas PK, Cooper JM, King RH, Workman JM, Schapira AH, Goss Sampson MA, Muller DP: Myopathy in vitamin E deficient rats: muscle fibre necrosis associated with disturbances of mitochondrial function. J Anat 1993; 183:451–461.
99 Haycock JW, Jones P, Harris JB: Differential susceptibility of human skeletal muscle proteins to free radical induced oxidative damage: A histochemical, immunocytochemical and electron microscopical study in vitro. Acta Neuropathol Berl 1996;92:331–340.
100 Stangel M, Zettl UK, Mix E, Zielasek J, Toyka KV, Hartung HP, Gold R: H_2O_2 and nitric oxide-mediated oxidative stress induce apoptosis in rat skeletal muscle myoblasts. J Neuropathol Exp Neurol 1996;55:36–43.
101 Berg HE, Tesch PA: Changes in muscle function in response to 10 days of lower limb unloading in humans. Acta Physiol Scand 1996;157:63–70.
102 Terjung RL, Dudley GA, Meyer RA: Metabolic and circulatory limitations to muscular performance at the organ level. J Exp Biol 1985;115:307–318.
103 Messner-Pellenc P, Brasileiro C, Ahmaidi S, Mercier J, Ximenes C, Grolleau R, Prefaut C: Exercise intolerance in patients with chronic heart failure: Role of pulmonary diffusing limitation. Eur Heart J 1995;16:201–209.
104 Gray-Donald K, Gibbons L, Martin JG: Effect of nutritional status on exercise performance in patients with chronic obstructive pulmonary disease. Am Rev Respir Dis 1989; 140:1544–1548.
105 Efthimiou J, Fleming J, Gomes C, Spiro SG: The effect of supplementary oral nutrition in poorly nourished patients with chronic obstructive pulmonary disease. Am Rev Respir Dis 1988;137:1075–1082.
106 Carr JG, Stevenson LW, Walden JA, Heber D: Prevalence and hemodynamic correlates of malnutrition in severe congestive heart failure secondary to ischemic or idiopathic dilated cardiomyopathy. Am J Cardiol 1989; 63:709–713.
107 Schols AMWJ, Slangen J, Volovics L, Wouters EMF: Weight loss is a reversible factor in the prognosis of chronic obstructive pulmonary disease. Am J Respir Crit Care Med 1998;157:1791–1797.
108 Anker SD, Ponikowski P, Varney S, Chua TP, Clark AL, Webb-People KM, Harrington D, Kox WJ, Poole-Wilson PA, Coats AJS: Wasting as independent risk factor for mortality in chronic heart failure. Lancet 1997;349:1050–1053.
109 Schols AM, Soeters PB, Dingemans AM, Mostert R, Frantzen PJ, Wouters EF: Prevalence and characteristics of nutritional depletion in patients with stable COPD eligible for pulmonary rehabilitation. Am Rev Respir Dis 1993;147:1151–1156.
110 Baarends EM, Schols AM, Pannemans DL, Westerterp KR, Wouters EF: Total free living energy expenditure in patients with severe chronic obstructive pulmonary disease. Am J Respir Crit Care Med 1997;155:549–554.
111 McLoughlin DM, Spargo E, Wassif WS, Newham DJ, Peters TJ, Lantos PL, Russell GF: Structural and functional changes in skeletal muscle in anorexia nervosa. Acta Neuropathol Berl 1998;95:632–640.
112 Russel DM, Prendergast PJ, Darby PL, Garfinkel PE, Whitwell J, Jeejeebhoy KN: A comparison between muscle function and body composition in anorexia nervosa: The effect of refeeding. Am J Clin Nutr 1983;38:229–237.
113 Rigaud D, Moukaddem M, Cohen B, Malon D, Reveillard V, Mignon M: Refeeding improves muscle performance without normalization of muscle mass and oxygen consumption in anorexia nervosa patients. Am J Clin Nutr 1997;65:1845–1851.
114 Lindboe CF, Askevold F, Slettebo M: Changes in skeletal muscles of young women with anorexia nervosa: An enzyme histochemical study. Acta Neuropathol Berl 1982; 56:299–302.
115 Essen B, Fohlin L, Thoren C, Saltin B: Skeletal muscle fibre types and sizes in anorexia nervosa patients. Clin Physiol 1981;1:395–403.
116 Hill GL: Body composition research: Implications for the practice of clinical nutrition. J Parenter Enteral Nutr 1992;16:197–218.
117 Morrison WL, Gibson JN, Scrimgeour C, Rennie MJ: Muscle wasting in emphysema. Clin Sci 1988;75:415–420.
118 Engelen MPKJ, Deutz NEP, Wouters EFM, Schols AMWJ: Enhanced whole body protein turnover in patients with chronic obstructive pulmonary disease. Am J Respir Crit Care Med 2000;162:1488–1492.
119 Aguilani B, Goldstein Shapses S, Pajon A, Levy P, Sarrot F, Leverve X, Page E, Askanazi J: Muscle protein degradation in severely malnourished patients with chronic obstructive pulmonary disease subject to short-term total parenteral nutrition. J Parenter Enteral Nutr 1992;16:248–254.
120 Goldstein SA, Thomashow BM, Kvetan V, Askanazi J, Kinney JM, Elwyn DH: Nitrogen and energy relationships in malnourished patients with emphysema. Am Rev Respir Dis 1988;138:636–644.
121 Engelen MPKJ, Deutz NEP, Wouters EFM, Mosterd R, Schols AMWJ: Suppressed response in whole body protein turnover to exercise in patients with emphysema; thesis, 2000.
122 Engelen MPKJ, Schols AMWJ, Does JD, Deutz NEP, Wouters EFM: Altered glutamate metabolism is associated with reduced muscle glutathione levels in patients with emphysema. Am J Respir Crit Care Med 2000; 161:98–103.
123 Engelen MPKJ, Wouters EFM, Deutz NEP, Does JD, Schols AMWJ: Effects of exercise on amino acid metabolism in patients with chronic obstructive pulmonary disease. Am J Respir Crit Care Med 2000;163:859–864.
124 Jakobsson P, Jorfeldt L, Brundin A: Skeletal muscle metabolites and fibre types in patients with advanced chronic obstructive pulmonary disease (COPD), with and without chronic respiratory failure. Eur Respir J 1990; 3:192–196.
125 Hughes RL, Katz H, Sahgal V, Campbell JA, Hartz R, Shields TW: Fiber size and energy metabolites in five separate muscles from patients with chronic obstructive lung diseases. Respiration 1983;44:321–328.

126 Fiaccadori E, Del Canale S, Vitali P, Coffrini E, Ronda N, Guariglia A: Skeletal muscle energetics, acid-base equilibrium and lactate metabolism in patients with severe hypercapnia and hypoxemia. Chest 1987;92:883–887.
127 Broqvist M, Arnqvist H, Dahlström U, Larsson J, Nylander E, Permert J: Nutritional assessment and muscle energy metabolism in severe chronic congestive heart failure – effects of long-term dietary supplementation. Eur Heart J 1994;15:1641–1650.
128 Opasich C, Aquilani R, Dossena M, et al: Biochemical analysis of muscle biopsy in overnight fasting patients with severe chronic heart failure. Eur Heart J 1996;17:1686–1693.
129 Schaufelberger M, Eriksson BO, Held P, Swedberg K: Skeletal muscle metabolism during exercise in patients with chronic heart failure. Heart 1996;76:29–34.
130 Maltais F, Simard AA, Simard C, Jobin J, Desgagnes P, LeBlanc P: Oxidative capacity of the skeletal muscle and lactic acid kinetics during exercise in normal subjects and in patients with COPD. Am J Respir Crit Care Med 1996;153:288–293.
131 Jakobsson P, Jorfeldt L, Henriksson J: Metabolic enzyme activity in the quadriceps femoris muscle in patients with severe chronic obstructive pulmonary disease. Am J Respir Crit Care Med 1995;151:374–377.
132 Sullivan MJ, Green HJ, Cobb FR: Altered skeletal muscle metabolic response to exercise in chronic heart failure: Relation to skeletal muscle aerobic enzyme activity. Circulation 1991;84:1597–1607.
133 Tikunov B, Levine S, Mancini D: Chronic congestive heart failure elicits adaptations of endurance exercise in diaphragmatic muscle. Circulation 1997;95:910–916.
134 Sánchez J, Bastien C, Medrano G, Riquet M, Derenne JP: Metabolic enzymatic activities in the diaphragm of normal men and patients with moderate chronic obstructive pulmonary disease. Bull Eur Physiopathol Respir 1984;20:535–540.

A.M.W.J. Schols
Department of Pulmonology
University Hospital Maastricht
PO Box 5800
NL–6202 AZ Maastricht (The Netherlands)
Tel. +31 43 3875046, Fax +31 43 3875051
E-Mail a.schols@pul.unimaas.nl

Weisman IM, Zeballos RJ (eds): Clinical Exercise Testing.
Prog Respir Res. Basel, Karger, 2002, vol 32, pp 30–42

Modalities of Clinical Exercise Testing

R. Jorge Zeballos[a] Idelle M. Weisman[b]

[a]Department of Internal Medicine, Texas Tech University Health Sciences Center and Department of Clinical Investigation, Human Performance Laboratory, William Beaumont Army Medical Center, El Paso, Tex.; [b] Human Performance Laboratory, Department of Clinical Investigation, Pulmonary-Critical Care Service, William Beaumont Army Medical Center, El Paso, Tex., and Department of Medicine, Pulmonary-Critical Care Division, University of Texas Health Science Center at San Antonio, San Antonio, Tex., USA

Summary

Currently, clinical exercise testing is increasingly utilized in clinical practice in order to optimize patient management and provide answers to questions not available from resting cardiopulmonary tests. There are several modalities of clinical exercise testing designed to evaluate and to answer different clinical question(s). The selection of clinical exercise testing modality should be based on the clinical question, facilities and expertise available including consideration of the cost effectiveness of the different tests. The most popular clinical exercise tests are the 6-minute walk test, exercise-induced bronchospasm test, cardiac stress test and cardiopulmonary exercise test. The main applications of clinical exercise testing include the evaluation of exercise intolerance and unexplained dyspnea; early diagnosis of cardiopulmonary diseases; evaluation of coronary artery disease and exercise-induced asthma; assessment of functional capacity; preoperative surgical evaluation; prognosis of cardiopulmonary diseases; evaluation of therapeutic interventions; oxygen prescription, and prescription for pulmonary rehabilitation.

Clinical exercise tests are utilized in a variety of clinical situations [1]. They provide functional information useful for patient management which cannot be obtained from resting pulmonary and/or cardiac measurements [2–5]. Furthermore, exertional symptoms correlate poorly with resting cardiopulmonary measurements [4, 6].

There are several modalities of clinical exercise testing used in clinical practice. Some provide basic information, are low tech, and simple to perform, while others provide a more complete assessment of all the physiological systems involved in exercise and require more complex technology. Table 1 shows the most popular clinical exercise tests in order of increasing complexity.

Modality selection should be based on the clinical question(s) to be addressed and on the available equipment and facilities. Some examples of clinical scenarios that can be encountered and the appropriate clinical exercise modality to be used follow. A test for exercise-induced bronchospasm would be appropriate for a patient who is young and complains of breathing difficulties post-exercise. However, asthma has a bimodal distribution and exercise-induced bronchoconstriction as a cause of unexplained dyspnea occurs commonly in older patients [7]. For a patient over 40 years old with chest tightness and/or chest pain triggered by exercise, a cardiac stress test on a treadmill would be the first choice, although the use of a cycle ergometer would also be acceptable. If these modalities were not available, a Master two-step test could be another less frequently used alternative. If the reason for testing is the diagnosis of unexplained dyspnea or exercise intolerance, early cardiopulmonary exercise testing (CPET) would be most beneficial in clinical decision-making [8]. CPET is also most appropriate in situations in which it is important to differentiate between cardiac and pulmonary etiologies for exercise limitation; to answer questions related to underlying mechanisms of

The opinions or assertions contained herein are the private views of the authors and are not to be construed as official or as reflecting the views of the Department of the Army or the Department of Defense.

Table 1. Modalities of clinical exercise testing

Modalities	Technical requirement	Intensity	Evaluation	Standardization	Reproducibility	Cost
Stair climbing	0	Near max/max	Postoperative risk Functional capacity	0	0	0
Master two-step test	+	Near max	Ischemia Functional capacity	+	++	$
6MWT	+	Submax/near max	Functional capacity	++	++	$
Shuttle test	++	Max	Functional capacity	+++	++	$
EIB	+++	Submax	Airway hyperreactivity	++	++	$$
GXT	+++	Submax	Ischemia Arrhythmias	+++	+++	$$$
CPET	++++	Max	Functional capacity Global/individual system function	++	+++	$$$$

6MWT = 6-min walk test; EIB = exercise-induced bronchospasm; GXT = cardiac stress test; CPET = cardiopulmonary exercise test.

exercise limitation, and when it is necessary to objectively determine aerobic capacity ($\dot{V}O_2$ peak) as in patients being evaluated for cardiac transplantation. When the reason for the test is to evaluate the functional response to a medical intervention, the six-minute walk test (6MWT) would probably be the more cost effective; alternatively, a shuttle test could also be used, but is technically more demanding. Recent work, however, has demonstrated that a constant work CPET is more sensitive than 6MWT in detecting responses to treatment [9]. For evaluation of heart and/or lung transplantation, either the cardiopulmonary (preferable) or the 6MWT can be used. Often they are used together as they provide complementary information. Interpretation of CPET results may be more complex, but in turn provide more insight into the different etiologies for exercise intolerance [10]. In hospitals that do not have facilities or equipment to perform sophisticated exercise tests, stair climbing could be used in the preoperative evaluation of patients for lung resection.

Stair Climbing

This is the simplest and most basic of all clinical exercise testing modalities, which does not require costly or sophisticated equipment. Historically, surgeons have used stair climbing to assess postoperative risk before more advanced techniques like CPET were available. Stair climbing is still used in some clinical centers for its practicality in the evaluation of postoperative complications. This test imposes a progressive stress on the cardiopulmonary system and skeletal muscles, providing a basic assessment of functional capacity.

Methodology

There is no standardized procedure or consensus on how to perform the test. Variations in methodology and in the reporting of results among different authors make comparisons of results difficult.

In essence, the test consists of asking the patients to climb as many stairs as possible until they are limited by symptoms including dyspnea, exhaustion, leg fatigue, chest pain and dizziness [11]. Some authors instruct the patients to climb at their own pace [12] and others at a brisk pace [11]. Also, some authors ask the patients to use the railing for balance [13] while others ask them to climb without rail holding [11]. To improve reproducibility and safety it would be better to let the patients choose their own pace (as in the 6MWT) and to use the railing for balance.

Optional measurements include the timing of the test and the use of pulse oximetry [12]. In addition, heart rate and dyspnea index have been reported at rest and at the end of the test in some studies [14]. However, these values were not used in the interpretation of the tests.

Another source of variability is the form in which the results are reported. The majority of studies report the results by the number of flights of stairs climbed. However, there is no uniformity of the basic definition of one 'flight of stairs'. Some papers include all the stairs between floors as one flight and in others they describe two flights of stairs with a landing on the middle between floors. Since the number of stairs per flight and the height of the stairs is not the same in all the health centers, it would be advisable to report the number of stairs climbed and also the height of the stairs. This information would allow a better comparison of results among different studies. Another practical approach would be to report the results as the number of floors climbed instead of flights of stairs.

For safety reasons, it would be advisable to have a technician trained in cardiopulmonary resuscitation conducting the test. Also, a physician and a resuscitation cart should be available in the proximity were the test is being performed.

There are several studies that have measured the energy cost of stair climbing (expressed in kcal and $\dot{V}O_2$) which are discussed in the paper of Bassett et al. [15] However, some studies cited for measurement of $\dot{V}O_2$ during stair climbing in reality were performed during bench stepping or during exercise on the Stair Master. Limited data exist in measurement of $\dot{V}O_2$ during actual stair climbing. In the study of Pollock et al. [11], $\dot{V}O_2$ was measured during stair climbing and during a maximal incremental cardiopulmonary exercise test on a cycle ergometer in 31 patients with chronic obstructive pulmonary disease (COPD). The authors reported a good correlation ($r = 0.7$) between the number of steps climbed and $\dot{V}O_2$. Also, the investigators reported that the $\dot{V}O_2$, heart rate and blood pressure were higher at stair climbing peak than during peak cycle ergometry.

Several studies have reported calculated $\dot{V}O_2$ during stair climbing [12, 16], but as has been discussed previously the calculations have a significant margin of error and also they complicate unnecessarily the test.

Applications of the Stair Climbing Test

The main application of stair climbing is in the preoperative evaluation of postoperative complications of patients undergoing thoracic or upper abdominal surgery. It is unclear when stair climbing began to be utilized in the evaluation of surgical patients. Van Nostrand et al. [17] in a retrospective study in patients undergoing pneumonectomy demonstrated a mortality of 50% in patients who were unable to climb two flights of stairs and that the mortality rate decreased to 11% in patients who were able to climb two flights of stairs. In another retrospective study in patients who had undergone lung resection, the authors observed that patients unable to climb three flight of stairs had a higher number of complications compared to patients who were able to climb three flights of stairs [16]. In a study of 16 patients at high risk for pulmonary resection, the authors reported that the patients who were unable to climb 44 steps had a higher risk of medical complications [12]. Girish et al. [13] in a prospective study in patients undergoing thoracotomy or upper abdominal laparotomy demonstrated that the inability to climb two flights of stairs was associated with a positive predicted value of 82% for the development of postoperative complications. The results of the cited studies appear to support the concept that the inability to climb two flights of stairs may be associated with a higher risk of postoperative complications.

Most recently, stair climbing has been used in other clinical settings including evaluation of functional capacity in patients with COPD [11, 14].

Master Two-Step Test

The stress step tests consist of the subject walking up and down on a stool or bench at an established rate. This is one of the oldest, most basic and simplest exercise tests. Several variations of the original concept have been done in regard to the step height, rate of step-ups per minute and number of steps. These different protocols were called the Harvard step test, the Master step test, progressive step test, the graded step test, etc. [18]. The Master two-step test is the one that has become the most popular [19].

This test had been widely accepted and used in the past for the diagnosis of ischemic heart diseases. Its popularity began to decline in the 1970s, although it continues to be used sporadically [20]. The advantages of the test are its simplicity, low-tech equipment, and that it is fairly inexpensive. The disadvantages include difficulty in measuring work rate, safety issues related to the risk of stumbling, and difficulty in cardiac monitoring, and in performing cardiopulmonary measurements. This step test is suitable for office and field studies. With the step tests it is possible to reach $\dot{V}O_2max$ or near $\dot{V}O_2max$ [21].

Methodology

The equipment consists of three steps (benches) in a row: the first one is 9 in high, the middle is 18 in, and the last is 9 in. The subject walks up and down the three steps. After going up and over, the patient then turns and repeats the procedure for a determined number of times to be completed in 1.5 min [19]. The number of ascents is chosen from tables established for men and women based on age and weight [22]. ECG is monitored before and immediately after the test or continuously during the test.

Six-Minute Walk Test

The 6MWT is gaining popularity because it is a practical, simple test to perform that does not require high-tech equipment or advanced technical training and because it provides an objective assessment of exercise tolerance/functional status (capacity). Also, walking is an activity familiar to almost everyone [23].

Traditionally, the qualitative evaluation of functional capacity has been done by clinicians questioning their patients about the amount of physical activity performed. Based on this concept, Balke [24] developed a simple test to evaluate functional capacity measuring the distance run in a 15-min best effort. Cooper [25] used a 12-minute walk test (12MWT) for evaluation of the level of physical fitness of healthy individuals. This test was subsequently adapted to assess disability in patients with chronic bronchitis [26]. In order to accommodate patients with respiratory disease for whom walking 12 min was too exhausting, Butland et al. [27] shortened the time to 2 and 6 min. They compared the results of these two tests with the standard 12MWT and concluded that: (1) 12 min is an unnecessarily long duration, (2) that the 2-min walk is less powerful in discriminating between subjects, and (3) that the 6MWT appeared to be the best option for patients with respiratory disease.

This test consists of measuring the maximal distance that a patient can walk on a flat hard surface in a period of 6 min. It is a self-paced walk in a measured corridor [28]. It evaluates the global and integrated responses of all the systems involved during exercise, which includes the pulmonary and cardiovascular systems, systemic circulation, peripheral circulation, blood, neuromuscular units, muscle metabolism, etc. However, this test does not provide specific information on the function of each one of the different organs and systems involved in exercise and of the mechanism of exercise limitation as is possible with CPET. Also, contrary to CPET in which the maximal exercise capacity is determined, the 6MWT assesses the submaximal level of functional capacity.

Table 2. Applications of the 6MWT

Evaluation of medical interventions
Pharmacological
Patients with heart disease [76]
Patients with pulmonary disease [9]
Surgical
Lung transplantation [77]
Lung resection [12]
Lung volume reduction surgery [78, 79]
Pulmonary rehabilitation [80]
Prediction of morbidity and mortality
Patients with heart failure [77, 81]
Patients with COPD [82]
Primary pulmonary hypertension [83]
Evaluation of functional capacity
Patients with heart disease [56, 84]
Patients with pulmonary disease
COPD [85]
ILD [86]
Patients with peripheral vascular disease [87]
Patients with cystic fibrosis [37]
Normal subjects [46]
As predictor of $\dot{V}O_2$ peak [30, 81]

Indications

The 6MWT has been used successfully as an outcome measure of different types of interventions, including pharmacological, surgical and pulmonary rehabilitation. Also, it is often used for functional assessment in a wide spectrum of clinical entities. In addition, it had been used with promising results to predict morbidity and mortality in patients with cardiopulmonary diseases. A detailed list of the indications of the 6MWT appears in table 2.

Solway et al. [29] have published a very complete and comprehensive review of the applications of the walking tests, including the 6MWT.

Important Factors That Impact the Results of the 6MWT

Length and Shape of the Course. Although most studies have used courses of approximately 30 m, there are others that have used 20 m [30] and 50 m [31]. It is possible that in a shorter corridor, the distance walked could be less because more turns are involved. However, in a recent study, Wiese [32] did not find significant differences in

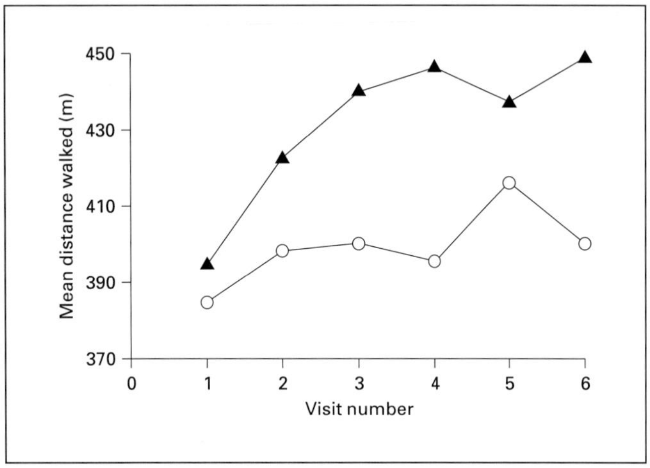

Fig. 1. Mean distance walked in the 6MWT by encouraged (▲) and nonencouraged (○) groups of patients. From Guyatt et al. [26], with permission.

the distance walked in straight tracks ranging from 50 to 64 ft. Also, it appears that in a continuous track (round) the patients walk longer than in a straight track.

Training Effect. Walking distance in patients with pulmonary and heart disease can increase significantly with repeated tests; however, no significant changes were demonstrated after the third test (fig. 1) [27, 28, 33–36]. In a study in which 24 patients with chronic bronchitis performed a 5-minute walk test three times in a day and repeated it every week for 4 weeks, the distance walked increased continuously from the first test of the first day to the last test of the fourth week, even though the mean increase in distance was of 21 m only [34]. Nevertheless, in a study in children with cystic fibrosis, no differences were reported between two 6MWTs performed 1 week apart [37]. The observed training effect appears to be related to coordination, stride length, overcoming of anxiety, etc. As such, it is recommended that two practice tests be performed before baseline measurements are obtained (third test). In many clinical situations, it is difficult and impractical to perform two practice tests before the valid one (third test). Since at this time the clinical relevance of the practice tests is not clear, it appears that a reasonable approach would be to perform two 6MWTs with at least 1 h of rest between them and to report the highest 6MWT.

Encouragement. Guyatt et al. [28, 33] have clearly demonstrated that encouragement significantly increases the distance walked by patients (fig. 1). Since the reproducibility for tests with and without encouragement was similar, it would be advisable to perform the 6MWT with encouragement to obtain better results. The encouragement should be consistent for all patients.

Supplemental Oxygen. The beneficial effect of O_2 supplementation on walking distance has clearly been shown [36, 38]. If during the first practice test, SpO_2 drops below 85%, supplemental O_2 should be prescribed for subsequent 6MWT. If O_2 supplementation is indicated, all the 6MWT should be performed using the same modality of delivery and the same O_2 flow.

Medications. A significant improvement in the distance walked after administration of bronchodilators in COPD patients has been demonstrated [39]. Therefore, it is important to be consistent in the administration of medication(s) before the 6MWT. The administration of medication will be determined by the objective of the test.

Recommended Methodology for the 6MWT

One of the shortcomings of the 6MWT is the lack of a widely accepted standardized protocol [40]. This represents a potential source of intra- and inter-subject variability of an important functional outcome variable. A well-performed 6MWT requires attention to several methodological issues as recommended by Guyatt et al. [28]. Since the main use of the 6MWT is to follow up medical interventions, it is critical that the 6MWT protocol be applied consistently in all the subjects. The American Thoracic Society (ATS) is in the process of publishing a statement with guidelines for the 6MWT [41]. The methodology presented in this chapter will incorporate the most popular techniques and procedures actually in use and the recommendations obtained from the draft of the ATS document on the 6MWT [41].

Track for 6MWT. The 6MWT should be performed indoors, preferably along a long, flat, straight, enclosed corridor (environmental conditions are more comfortable and consistent). The walking course should be 30 m (100-foot corridor) [28]. The extremes of the course should be marked on the floor with colored tape or with traffic cones and the length of the track should be marked every 3 m with pieces of tape stuck to the lower part of the wall.

Patient Preparation. Patient instructions for the 6MWT should include wearing comfortable clothing and shoes (sneakers) and avoid vigorous exercise 2 h before the test. In order to minimize intra-individual variability, the 6MWT should be performed at the same time each testing day. A light breakfast is permitted before morning tests. The usual medication regimen should be maintained the day of the walking test.

Monitor. The monitor must have a stopwatch or a countdown timer, a tape measure, a sphygmomanometer, a worksheet on a clipboard to annotate the results of the test, and a chair. Optionally, and only when additional information is requested, a Borg dyspnea scale and a portable pulse oximeter would be required. The monitor should be standing near the starting line (do not walk with the patient) keeping track of the time, counting the number of laps walked and telling the patient the time and words of encouragement. The monitor should stop the test if the patient presents one of the medical complications described in the 'Safety Considerations' section.

6MWT Protocol. Before beginning the test and prior to taking the resting measurements, the patient should be at rest, sitting on a chair, for at least 10 min. Heart rate (HR) and blood pressure should be measured to check for contraindications. Optionally, the patient's rate of perceived dyspnea and overall fatigue using the Borg scale [42] and/or SpO_2 could be assessed. Measurements should be performed (standing) before and immediately after the test.

The instructions must be literally the same for all patients tested and for each test: 'The object of this test is to walk as far as possible for six minutes. You will walk back and forth between the marks of the course. Six minutes is a long time to walk, so you will be exerting yourself. You will probably get out of breath or become exhausted. You are permitted to slow down, to stop, and to rest as necessary. You may lean against the wall while resting, but resume walking as soon as you are able to do so in order to complete the 6MWT. During the test, you will be regularly informed of the elapsed time and you will be encouraged to do your best. Remember that your goal is to walk as far as possible in 6 min' [23, 41].

The words of encouragement and notification of time should be also consistent for all the patients. Each minute of the test, the monitor will provide the same encouragement telling the patient 'You are doing well' or 'keep up the good work' (do not use other words of encouragement) and will also tell the patient the minutes left to the end of the test, in order to help adjust and maintain a good pace [33, 41]. For example, 'you are doing well, you have four minutes to go'.

At the end of the 6 min, the monitor must instruct the patient to stop and mark the place with a tape. He/she must immediately perform the pertinent measurements (HR, blood pressure, Borg scale, SpO_2). The distance walked is measured using the number of completed laps (60 m) plus the distance to the start point, using as a guide the markers placed on the wall and a tape measure. The distance should be reported in meters.

Measurements. The main outcome of the 6MWT is the maximal distance walked by the patient in 6 min. Other measurements including HR, blood pressure, SpO_2 and perceived dyspnea have been shown not to be useful indices of functional capacity; however, they are usually measured for safety reasons as well as for providing a more complete characterization of patient performance. During serial evaluations of medical interventions, it is possible that improvement may be manifested by reduced symptoms despite no change in the distance walked. Recently, a new approach to the interpretation of the 6MWT in the assessment of functional exercise tolerance, using a multivariable assessment that includes HR, oxygen desaturation, perceived dyspnea and effort has been proposed [43].

Practice Test. As discussed previously, the need of a practice tests to evaluate the functional status of the patient will be determined for the reason of the test. If it is a one time evaluation or the repeated tests are more than 1 month apart, 6MWT evaluation with only one test may be acceptable, but if the medical intervention requires more frequent evaluations, at least two tests would be required with at least 1 h between them. The highest 6MWT should be used as the baseline for the post-intervention tests.

Safety Considerations

Contraindications for the 6MWT are similar to those described elsewhere for CPET [44]. However, it is unknown if medical complications would occur if such patients would perform the 6MWT, therefore the suggested contraindications are dictated by the experience of the investigators and by the need of being prudent. The reasons for stopping the 6MWT are similar to the ones recommended for CPET [44]; the most important are [23]: chest pain, intolerable dyspnea, mental confusion or lack of coordination, leg cramps, sudden onset of pallor, sweating, evolving lightheadedness and SpO_2 <85% (if monitored).

It appears that the exercise risks are less than for CPET, since in the 6MWT, the patients determine the intensity of exercise that 'they know they can tolerate safely'. The 6MWT has been used safely in 800 patients with cardiomyopathy or primary pulmonary hypertension [45]. Enright and Sherrill [46] performed this test in thousands of elderly persons without untoward events.

The technician performing the test must have training in cardiopulmonary resuscitation. The presence of a physician is not necessary, however it would be advisable if he/she is available in the same building where the test is being performed in case of an emergency. A resuscitation cart must be available in close proximity to the area where the 6MWT is being administered.

Reference Values and Clinical Significance

Scarce literature is available on normal reference values for the 6MWT. Recently, Enright and Sherrill [46] published a set of reference equations for the 6MWT in healthy adults (aged 40–80 years). In this study, the median distance walked was 576 m for healthy men and 494 m for healthy women. Trooster et al. [31] evaluated 51 healthy 50- to 85-year-old subjects and reported a mean of 631 m. The average distance walked by males was 84 m greater than females. As a ball park reference of 6MWT results to be expected, Redelmeier et al. [47] reported that for patients with COPD, the average distance achieved during the 6MWT was 371 m (range 119–705 m). In that study, the authors estimate that the smallest difference in 6MWT distances associated with a noticeable clinical difference in patients' perception of exercise performance was 54 m [47]. However, in the same paper, the authors reported that in 68% of the reviewed literature on statistical significant differences due to medical interventions, the differences in the 6MWT were less than 54 m. In addition, a meta-analysis demonstrated that the best estimate of the beneficial effect of pulmonary rehabilitation for COPD patients on the 6MWT was 56 m [48]. It appears that differences between 6MWT of approximately 55 m may have clinical significance. However, more studies are needed to validate this number; additionally, it would probably be better if clinical significant changes were expressed in percentage change from baseline.

Reproducibility

The 6MWT has good reproducibility, which is comparable or better to other lung function and exercise tests. Noseda et al. [49] studied the reproducibility of lung function and exercise testing over a long interval in 20 COPD patients. They showed that the coefficient of variation of patients tested on four occasions at 1-month intervals was (mean and range) 5% (1.0–8.9) for HRmax; 9.0% (2.4–19.5) for $\dot{V}O_2max$; 9.0% (1.5–21.4) for 12 MWT; 10.2% (2.3–26.4) for FEV_1. Although in this study the 12 MWT was used, the results can be extrapolated to the 6MWT because of the high correlation that has been shown between both walking tests. Other authors have reported similar results [27, 34]. Also, it has been reported that the questionnaires for the subjective evaluation of functional status have larger variability (22–33%) than the 6MWT (8–9%) [50].

Comparison with Other Clinical Evaluators of Functional Capacity

A 6MWT is often used in lieu of CPET when the latter is either unavailable or impractical. Compared to CPET, the 6MWT represents more of a submaximal and motivational test. A good correlation, however, has been reported between the 6MWT and maximal oxygen consumption ($\dot{V}O_2max$) in patients with end-stage lung disease ($r = 0.73$) [51]. In some clinical situations, the 6MWT provides physiologic information that may be more realistic than $\dot{V}O_2max$ in the evaluation of daily activities. The information provided by a 6MWT is complimentary to CPET, but does not replace it.

In almost all clinical exercise tests, the work rate intensity is imposed on subjects. Considering that in the 6MWT, patients choose their own intensity of exercise (self-paced) and also that most activities of daily living are performed at submaximum levels of exertion, the 6MWT appears to better reflect the functional exercise level for daily physical activities.

Some have suggested that endurance testing (constant work exercise) on the treadmill or cycle ergometer may be more helpful in the evaluation of functional capacity in COPD patients compared to maximal incremental exercise testing; however, the constant work test requires an initial maximal incremental exercise test to determine the level of constant work rate. This may be time consuming and appear to be more motivationally dependent and less reproducible than the 6MWT [49]. However, in more recent work comparing different exercise modalities, a cycle endurance constant work exercise protocol was more sensitive than conventional 6MWT in detecting the effects of therapeutic interventions (inhaled anticholinergic agents) on exercise performance in patients with COPD [9].

The shuttle-walking test (discussed in detail below) requires the patient to walk at speeds which increase every minute until the patient cannot maintain the required walking speed. This test would be more comparable to a maximal symptom-limited incremental treadmill test. Not surprisingly, the 'shuttle test' has been reported to have a better correlation with $\dot{V}O_2max$ compared to the standard 6MWT. However, the shuttle test is more complicated and more difficult to perform. The potential for cardiovascular problems may be greater, especially in elderly COPD, since patients are pushed to exercise more intensely without ECG monitoring.

A better correlation has been reported between the 6MWT with several questionnaires on quality of life than with $\dot{V}O_2max$ [50]. It has been also shown that the 6MWT correlates well with subjective evaluation after different interventions [52, 53].

6MWT on the Treadmill

The 6MWT can be performed on a treadmill and has been proposed in situations in which a long (30-meter) hallway or corridor may not be available. During this test, the patient walks on the treadmill for 6 min continuously self-adjusting the speed of the treadmill in order to set the pace [54]. The advantages of a treadmill 6MWT include the availability of continuous cardiovascular and oximetry monitoring, the ease of supplemental O_2 device carriage, and the avoidance/inconvenience of performing the test outside the laboratory. However, a treadmill 6MWT may undermine the basic principles of the 6MWT, which are low tech and self-paced. Furthermore, a treadmill 6MWT may be difficult for the elderly because of coordination problems of walking on the treadmill while simultaneously controlling the speed.

In a recent study in lung disease patients, which compared treadmill 6MWT vs. conventional 6MWT, the distance walked on the treadmill was, not surprisingly, 14% less than corridor walking. This most probably reflects less familiarity with treadmill walking. The authors concluded that both test results were not interchangeable [54]. Similarly, Swerts et al. [55] reported longer distances for the corridor as compared to the treadmill 6MWT in 11 patients with severe COPD. In contrast, other authors have reported similar distances walked on the treadmill as compared to the corridor 6MWT in controls, patients with chronic heart failure [56], and in severe COPD [57]. However, it is interesting to note that in the study in chronic heart failure patients [56], 22% participants were unable to perform the treadmill test and 17% covered very short distances on the treadmill as compared to the corridor. More studies are needed to clarify if the 6MWT on the treadmill is comparable to the corridor 6MWT. Alternatively, if treadmill testing were available/desired, an endurance constant work protocol at 0% elevation and at a steady speed comfortable for the patient might be preferable. This approach is practical, simple and has been extensively used in the past, but requires more rigorous prospective comparative investigation.

Shuttle-Walking Test

A newer modality of walking tests is the 'shuttle-walking test' which uses an audio signal from a cassette tape to direct the walking pace of the patient [58]. The protocol requires the patient to walk at speeds, which increase every minute, up and down a 10-meter course. The test ends when the patient cannot maintain the required walking speed. This test would be more comparable to a maximal symptom-limited incremental treadmill test. Although a good correlation with 6MWT has been reported [58], the shuttle-walking test, not surprisingly, correlates better with $\dot{V}O_2$max than the 6MWT [59, 60]. However, the shuttle test is more complicated and more difficult to perform. The shuttle-walking test probably does not reflect daily activities, as does the 6MWT, which is a submaximal test. The shuttle-walk test can have a potentially greater risk of medical complications than the CPET because an ECG is not monitored. Presently, this test is less popular than the 6MWT, with its main use reported in the UK.

Constant Work Shuttle-Walking Test

Recently, an externally controlled, constant-paced, walking test has been developed to evaluate the endurance capacity of patients [61]. This test was designed to complement the incremental shuttle-walk test. The rationale for this test is that most activities of everyday living represent sustained submaximal levels of exercise. The advantage of this test over the 6MWT is that, since this is an externally controlled constant walking test, the variability would be less than for the 6MWT (which is a self-paced test). The disadvantage would be that it is more complicated and technically demanding than the 6MWT and that this test would require an incremental shuttle-walk test to determine the walking speed.

The methodology is the same as for the incremental shuttle test, that is a 10-meter course and an audio signal to control the pace. The walking speed is selected based on the percentage (75–95%) of the maximal speed reached during the incremental shuttle test. Several cassette tapes with speeds that range between 1.80 and 6.00 km/h are available. The patients are instructed to walk for as long as possible until reaching exhaustion following the audio signal from the cassette tape with the walking speed selected.

It appears that very few studies using this methodology have been published, one of them by the same authors who developed this field test [62]; it was used to evaluate the effect of ambulatory oxygen and an ambulatory ventilator on endurance exercise in COPD. At the present time, it is too premature to comment about the clinical significance of this constant walking test.

Exercise-Induced Bronchospasm Testing

Exercise-induced bronchospasm (EIB) is defined as a bronchospastic event that occurs after vigorous exercise. It is usually self-limited and remits spontaneously. It generally reaches its peak about 5–10 min after cessation of exercise and usually resolves in another 20–30 min. It is seldom life-threatening. Common symptoms of EIB are wheezing, shortness of breath, chest pain or tightness, cough and deterioration in exercise performance [63, 64]. It is generally established that EIB is caused by a loss of heat, water, or both from the lung during exercise caused by the hyperventilation that accompanies exercise [64]. Exercise is one of the most common precipitants of acute asthma encountered in clinical practice [65].

EIB testing is primarily useful in the diagnosis of airway hyperreactivity, particularly in patients who complain of exercise intolerance and unexplained dyspnea.

Bronchodilators and other inhaled agents should be withheld prior to testing. Spirometry (FVC and FEV_1) is measured before (baseline) and at 5, 15 and 30 min post-exercise. A positive test is reflected as a reduction of FEV_1 or FVC of 15% after exercise [64, 66]. A widely used protocol involves constant work exercise on the treadmill or on the cycle ergometer for 6–8 min at an intensity necessary to elicit a HR of ≈80% of the maximum predicted, so that $\dot{V}_E$ will increase sufficiently to trigger bronchoconstriction in those with hyperreactive airways [67]. Exercise-induced bronchoconstriction is observed in 70–80% of patients with clinically recognized asthma. However, this test is less sensitive than a methacholine challenge test for the evaluation of airway hyperreactivity [68], especially in patients with unexplained dyspnea [69]. For a more comprehensive explanation of exercise-induced asthma the reader is referred to the corresponding chapter of this book ('Asthma and Exercise').

Cardiac Stress Test or Graded Exercise Test

This test is used primarily for the diagnosis of coronary artery disease (myocardial ischemia), arrhythmias, and to assess therapeutic interventions (medications, interventional techniques, surgery). It is the most widely used clinical exercise testing modality in the United States with extensive literature documenting its efficacy [70]. This test is performed on a treadmill. During the test, ECG and blood pressure are monitored. The Bruce protocol is the most popular and consists of five progressive stages, each 3 min in duration. Stage I: 1.7 mph and 10% grade, stage II: 2.5 mph and 12% grade, stage III: 3.4 mph and 14% grade, stage IV: 4.2 mph and 16% grade, and stage V: 5.0 mph and 18% grade. The single most reliable indicator of exercise-induced ischemia is ST-segment depression [70]. Other ECG abnormalities are also used as supplementary indicators of ischemia. In general, however, and ischemia notwithstanding, the Bruce protocol cannot define underlying pathophysiology. For more complete information about the topic of this section, please see the chapter on 'Ischemic Heart Disease'.

Cardiopulmonary Exercise Testing

CPET is the most complete of all the clinical exercise tests. CPET involves the measurement of oxygen uptake ($\dot{V}O_2$), carbon dioxide output ($\dot{V}CO_2$), minute ventilation ($\dot{V}_E$), and other variables, in addition to the monitoring of 12-lead ECG, blood pressure, and pulse oximetry (SpO_2) during a maximal symptom-limited incremental exercise test on the cycle ergometer or on the treadmill. When appropriate, the additional measurement of arterial blood gases provides important information on pulmonary gas exchange. An evaluation, using the Borg scale, of the symptoms limiting exercise is also necessary [42].

Maximal exercise testing can be safely performed in the vast majority of patients with respiratory disease with careful monitoring of the ECG and arterial oxygen saturation (SaO_2) [71, 72].

Why Perform CPET?

CPET provides information not available from the previously described clinical exercise testing modalities. CPET permits: objective determination of functional capacity ($\dot{V}O_2max$) and impairment; evaluation of the mechanisms of exercise limitation, such as the contribution of different organ systems involved in exercise (i.e., heart, lungs, blood and/or skeletal muscles); differentiation between heart and lung disease; diagnosis of the causes of exercise intolerance/dyspnea on exertion; monitoring of disease progression and response to treatment; early diagnosis of several clinical disorders, and determination of the appropriate intensity and duration of exercise for cardiopulmonary rehabilitation (prescription) [5, 18].

In addition, resting cardiopulmonary measurements do not provide an adequate prediction of functional capacity. Spirometry only estimates a patient's ventilatory capacity and not the ventilatory requirements for exercise. Although many studies have demonstrated a correlation between FEV_1 and $\dot{V}O_2max$ in patients, with COPD, the variability of the prediction would limit its applicability for the individual patient [2, 73]. Similarly, for patients with interstitial lung disease, spirometry and total lung capacity have been inconsistent predictors of $\dot{V}O_2max$. However, patients with significantly low resting DLco are likely to experience abnormal gas exchange response during exercise [74]. The predictive value of less severe resting DLco is less certain [3]. Finally, resting ECG and systolic performance variables (i.e., left ventricular ejection fraction) cannot reliably predict exercise performance and functional capacity [75].

Clinical Applications

The spectrum of clinical applications for CPET has broadened and increased significantly during the last few years. Comprehensive CPET is useful in a wide variety of clinical settings (table 3). Its impact can be appreciated in all phases of clinical decision-making including diagnosis, assessment of severity, disease progression, prognosis, and response to treatment. In practice, CPET is considered when specific questions persist following consideration of basic clinical data including history, physical examination, CXR, PFTs and resting ECG. Please see other chapters in the present issue which provide a more comprehensive explanation of methodology, normal exercise response and CPET results interpretation, as well as the application of CPET in different clinical entities.

Table 3. Clinical applications of cardiopulmonary exercise testing

Evaluation of exercise intolerance [5, 70, 88]
Assessment of functional capacity ($\dot{V}O_2$ peak)
Determination of exercise limitation
Evaluation of unexplained dyspnea [8, 89]
Assessing contribution of cardiac and pulmonary etiology in coexisting disease
Symptoms disproportionate to resting pulmonary and cardiac tests
When initial resting cardiopulmonary testing is nondiagnostic
Evaluation of patients with cardiovascular disease
Heart failure [90]
Prognosis of morbidity and mortality [91, 92]
Evaluation of therapeutic interventions [93]
Evaluation of patients with respiratory diseases
Assessment of functional impairment
COPD [94, 95], ILD [96], PVD [83], cystic fibrosis [97]
Detection of gas exchange abnormalities [10, 74]
Determination of magnitude of hypoxemia for O_2 prescription [98]
Evaluation of therapeutic interventions [99]
Surgical evaluation
Lung resectional surgery, [100, 101] lung volume reduction surgery [102]
Evaluation for heart [103], lung, heart-lung transplantation [104, 105]
Exercise prescription and monitoring response
Pulmonary rehabilitation [106, 107]
Cardiac rehabilitation [108]
Health promotion (wellness) [71]
Evaluation for impairment-disability [109]

References

1 Weisman IM, Zeballos RJ: Clinical exercise testing. Clin Chest Med 2001;22:679–701.
2 Carlson DJ, Ries AL, Kaplan RM: Prediction of maximum exercise tolerance in patients with COPD. Chest 1991;100:307–311.
3 Sue DY, Oren A, Hansen JE, Wasserman K: Diffusing capacity for carbon monoxide as a predictor of gas exchange during exercise. N Engl J Med 1987;316:1301–1306.
4 Szlachcic J, Massie BM, Kramer BL, Topic N, Tubau J: Correlates and prognostic implication of exercise capacity in chronic congestive heart failure. Am J Cardiol 1985;55:1037–1042.
5 Wasserman K, Hansen JE, Sue DY, Casaburi R, Whipp BJ: Principles of Exercise Testing and Interpretation, ed 3. Philadelphia, Lippincott-Williams & Wilkins, 1999.
6 Killian KJ, Leblanc P, Martin DH, Summers E, Jones NL, Campbell EJ: Exercise capacity and ventilatory, circulatory and symptom limitation in patients with chronic airflow limitation. Am Rev Respir Dis 1992;146:935–940.
7 Martinez FJ, Stanopoulos I, Acero R, Becker FS, Pickering R, Beamis JF: Graded comprehensive cardiopulmonary exercise testing in the evaluation of dyspnea unexplained by routine evaluation. Chest 1994;105:168–174.
8 Weisman IM, Zeballos RJ: Clinical evaluation of unexplained dyspnea. Cardiologia 1996;41: 621–634.
9 Oga T, Nishimura K, Tsukino M, Hajiro T, Ikeda A, Izumi T: The effects of oxitropium bromide on exercise performance in patients with stable chronic obstructive pulmonary disease. A comparison of three different exercise tests. Am J Respir Crit Care Med 2000;161: 1897–1901.
10 Weisman IM, Zeballos RJ: An integrated approach to the interpretation of cardiopulmonary exercise testing. Clin Chest Med 1994;15: 421–445.
11 Pollock M, Roa J, Benditt J, Celli B: Estimation of ventilatory reserve by stair climbing. A study in patients with chronic airflow obstruction. Chest 1993;104:1378–1383.
12 Holden DA, Rice TW, Stelmach K, Meeker DP: Exercise testing, 6-min walk, and stair climb in the evaluation of patients at high risk for pulmonary resection. Chest 1992;102: 1774–1779.
13 Girish M, Trayner E Jr, Dammann O, Pinto-Plata V, Celli B: Symptom-limited stair climbing as a predictor of postoperative cardiopulmonary complications after high-risk surgery. Chest 2001;120:1147–1151.
14 Montes de Oca M, Ortega Balza M, Lezama J, Lopez JM: Chronic obstructive pulmonary disease: Evaluation of exercise tolerance using three different exercise tests. Arch Bronconeumol 2001;37:69–74.

15 Bassett DR, Vachon JA, Kirkland AO, Howley ET, Duncan GE, Johnson KR: Energy cost of stair climbing and descending on the college alumnus questionnaire. Med Sci Sports Exerc 1997;29:1250–1254.

16 Olsen GN, Bolton JW, Weiman DS, Hornung CA: Stair climbing as an exercise test to predict the postoperative complications of lung resection. Two years' experience. Chest 1991;99: 587–590.

17 Van Nostrand D, Kjelsberg MO, Humphrey EW: Preresectional evaluation of risk from pneumonectomy. Surg Gynecol Obstet 1968; 127:306–312.

18 Jones NL: Clinical Exercise Testing, ed 4. Philadelphia, Saunders, 1997.

19 Master AM, Rosenfeld I: 'Two-step' exercise test brought up to date. NY State J Med 1961; 61:1850–1857.

20 Yoshida K, Utsunomiya T, Morooka T, Yazawa M, Kido K, Ogawa T, Ryu T, Ogata T, Tsuji S, Tokushima T, Matsuo S: Mental stress test is an effective inducer of vasospastic angina pectoris: Comparison with cold pressor, hyperventilation and master two-step exercise test. Int J Cardiol 1999;70:155–163.

21 Shephard RJ: Tests of maximum oxygen intake. A critical review. Sports Med 1984;1:99–124.

22 Master AM: The two-step exercise electrocardiogram: A test for coronary insufficiency. Ann Intern Med 1950;32:842–863.

23 Sciurba FC, Slivka WA: Six-minute walk testing. Semin Respir Crit Care Med 1998;19:383–392.

24 Balke B: A simple field test for the assessment of physical fitness. CARI Report 1963;63:18.

25 Cooper KH: A means of assessing maximal oxygen intake. Correlation between field and treadmill testing. JAMA 1968;203:201–204.

26 McGavin CR, Gupta SP, McHardy GJ: Twelve-minute walking test for assessing disability in chronic bronchitis. Br Med J 1976; 1:822–823.

27 Butland RJA, Pang J, Gross ER, Woodcock AA, Geddes DM: Two-, 6-, and 12-minute walking tests in respiratory disease. Br Med J 1982;284:1607–1608.

28 Guyatt GH, Sullivan MJ, Thompson PJ, Fallen EL, Pugsley SO, Taylor DW, Berman LB: The 6-minute walk: A new measure of exercise capacity in patients with chronic heart failure. Can Med Assoc J 1985;132:919–923.

29 Solway S, Brooks D, Lacasse Y, Thomas S: A qualitative systematic overview of the measurement properties of functional walk tests used in the cardiorespiratory domain. Chest 2001;119:256–270.

30 Lipkin DP, Scriven AJ, Crake T, Poole-Wilson PA: Six-minute walking test for assessing exercise capacity in chronic heart failure. Br Med J 1986;292:653–655.

31 Troosters T, Gosselink R, Decramer M: Six-minute walking distance in healthy elderly subjects. Eur Respir J 1999;14:270–274.

32 National Emphysema Treatment Trial: Six-minute walk distance in severe COPD; reliability and effect of walking course layout and length. Annual Meeting of the American College of Chest Physicians, San Francisco, Oct 25, 2000.

33 Guyatt GH, Pugsley SO, Sullivan MJ, Thompson PJ, Berman L, Jones NL, Fallen EL, Taylor DW: Effect of encouragement on walking test performance. Thorax 1984;39:818–822.

34 Knox AJ, Morrison JF, Muers MF: Reproducibility of walking test results in chronic obstructive airways disease. Thorax 1988;43:388–392.

35 Riley M, McParland J, Stanford CF, Nicholls DP: Oxygen consumption during corridor walk testing in chronic cardiac failure. Eur Heart J 1992;13:789–793.

36 Leach RM, Davidson AC, Chinn S, Twort CH, Cameron IR, Bateman NT: Portable liquid oxygen and exercise ability in severe respiratory disability. Thorax 1992;47:781–789.

37 Gulmans VA, van Veldhoven NH, de Meer K, Helders PJ: The six-minute walking test in children with cystic fibrosis: Reliability and validity. Pediatr Pulmonol 1996;22:85–89.

38 Roberts CM, Bell J, Wedzicha JA: Comparison of the efficacy of a demand oxygen delivery system with continuous low flow oxygen in subjects with stable COPD and severe oxygen desaturation on walking. Thorax 1996;51:831–834.

39 Grove A, Lipworth BJ, Reid P, Smith RP, Ramage L, Ingram CG, Jenkins RJ, Winter JH, Dhillon DP: Effects of regular salmeterol on lung function and exercise capacity in patients with chronic obstructive airways disease. Thorax 1996;51:689–693.

40 Elpern EH, Stevens D, Kesten S: Variability in performance of timed walk tests in pulmonary rehabilitation programs. Chest 2000;118:98–105.

41 American Thoracic Society: Guidelines for the six-minute walk test. Am J Respir Crit Care Med 2002 (in revision).

42 Borg GAV: Psychophysical bases of perceived exertion. Med Sci Sports Exerc 1982;14:377–381.

43 Van Stel HF, Bogaard JM, Rijssenbeek-Nouwens LH, Colland VT: Multivariable assessment of the 6-min walking test in patients with chronic obstructive pulmonary disease. Am J Respir Crit Care Med 2001;163:1567–1571.

44 Zeballos RJ, Weisman IM: Behind the scenes of cardiopulmonary exercise testing. Clin Chest Med 1994;15:193–213.

45 Barst RJ, Rubin LJ, McGoon MD, Caldwell EJ, Long WA, Levy PS: Survival in primary pulmonary hypertension with long-term continuous intravenous prostacyclin. Ann Intern Med 1994;121:409–415.

46 Enright PL, Sherrill DL: Reference equations for the six-minute walk in healthy adults. Am J Respir Crit Care Med 1998;158:1384–1387.

47 Redelmeier DA, Bayoumi AM, Goldstein RS, Guyatt GH: Interpreting small differences in functional status: The six-minute walk test in chronic lung disease patients. Am J Respir Crit Care Med 1997;155:1278–1282.

48 Lacasse Y, Wong E, Guyatt GH, King D, Cook DJ, Goldstein RS: Meta-analysis of respiratory rehabilitation in chronic obstructive pulmonary disease. Lancet 1996;348:1115–1119.

49 Noseda A, Carpiaux JP, Prigogine T, Schmerber J: Lung function, maximum and submaximum exercise testing in COPD patients: Reproducibility over a long interval. Lung 1989; 167:247–257.

50 Guyatt GH, Thompson PJ, Berman LB, Sullivan MJ, Townsend M, Jones NL, Pugsley SO: How should we measure function in patients with chronic heart and lung disease? J Chronic Dis 1985;38:517–524.

51 Cahalin L, Pappagianopoulos P, Prevost S, Wain J, Ginns L: The relationship of the 6-min walk test to maximal oxygen consumption in transplant candidates with end-stage lung disease. Chest 1995;108:452–459.

52 Guyatt GH, Townsend M, Keller J, Singer J, Nogradi S: Measuring functional status in chronic lung disease: Conclusions from a randomized control trial. Respir Med 1991; 85(suppl B):17–21.

53 Niederman MS, Clemente PH, Fein AM, Feinsilver SH, Robinson DA, Ilowite JS, Bernstein MG: Benefits of a multidisciplinary pulmonary rehabilitation program. Improvements are independent of lung function. Chest 1991;99: 798–804.

54 Stevens D, Elpern E, Sharma K, Szidon P, Ankin M, Kesten S: Comparison of hallway and treadmill six-minute walk tests. Am J Respir Crit Care Med 1999;160:1540–1543.

55 Swerts PM, Mostert R, Wouters EF: Comparison of corridor and treadmill walking in patients with severe chronic obstructive pulmonary disease. Phys Ther 1990;70:439–442.

56 Peeters P, Mets T: The 6-minute walk as an appropriate exercise test in elderly patients with chronic heart failure. J Gerontol A Biol Sci Med Sci 1996;51:M147–M151.

57 Beaumont A, Cockcroft A, Guz A: A self-paced treadmill walking test for breathless patients. Thorax 1985;40:459–464.

58 Singh SJ, Morgan MD, Scott S, Walters D, Hardman AE: Development of a shuttle walking test of disability in patients with chronic airways obstruction. Thorax 1992;47:1019–1024.

59 Singh SJ, Morgan MD, Hardman AE, Rowe C, Bardsley PA: Comparison of oxygen uptake during a conventional treadmill test and the shuttle walking test in chronic airflow limitation. Eur Respir J 1994;7:2016–2020.

60 Morales FJ, Martinez A, Mendez M, Agarrado A, Ortega F, Fernandez-Guerra J, Montemayor T, Burgos J: A shuttle walk test for assessment of functional capacity in chronic heart failure. Am Heart J 1999;138:291–298.

61 Revill SM, Morgan MD, Singh SJ, Williams J, Hardman AE: The endurance shuttle walk: A new field test for the assessment of endurance capacity in chronic obstructive pulmonary disease. Thorax 1999;54:213–222.

62 Revill SM, Singh SJ, Morgan MD: Randomized controlled trial of ambulatory oxygen and an ambulatory ventilator on endurance exercise in COPD. Respir Med 2000;94:778–783.
63 National Heart, Lung and Blood Institute. National Asthma Education Program. Expert Panel Report: Guidelines for the Diagnosis and Management of Asthma. National Heart, Lung and Blood Institute. National Asthma Education Program. Expert Panel Report. J Allergy Clin Immunol 1991;88:425–534.
64 National Heart, Lung and Blood Institute. National Asthma Education and Prevention Program. Expert Panel Report 2: Guidelines for the Diagnosis and Management of Asthma. Bethesda, National Institutes of Health, 1997, Publ No 97-4051.
65 American Thoracic Society: Standards for the diagnosis and care of patients with chronic obstructive pulmonary disease and asthma. Am Rev Respir Dis 1987;136:225–244.
66 European Respiratory Society: Airway responsiveness. Standardized challenge testing with pharmacological, physical and sensitizing stimuli in adults. Eur Respir J Suppl 1993;16:53–83.
67 Cypcar D, Lemanske RF Jr: Asthma and exercise. Clin Chest Med 1994;15:351–368.
68 American Thoracic Society: Guidelines for methacholine and exercise challenge testing –1999. Am J Respir Crit Care Med 2000;161: 309–329.
69 Zeballos RJ, Weisam IM, Connery SM, Bradley JP: Standard treadmill vs. incremental cycle ergometry in the evaluation of airway hyperreactivity in unexplained dyspnea (abstract). Am J Respir Crit Care Med 1999;159: A419.
70 ACC/AHA/ACP-ASIM: Guidelines for the management of patients with chronic stable angina: Executive summary and recommendations. A Report of the American College of Cardiology/American Heart Association Task Force on Practice Guidelines (Committee on Management of Patients with Chronic Stable Angina). Circulation 1999;99:2829–2848.
71 American College of Sports Medicine: ACSM's Guidelines for Exercise Testing and Prescription, ed 5. Baltimore, Williams & Wilkins, 1995.
72 American Heart Association: Exercise standards. A statement for healthcare professionals from the American Heart Association. Writing Group. Circulation 1995;91:580–615.
73 LoRusso TJ, Belman MJ, Elashoff JD, Koerner SK: Prediction of maximal exercise capacity in obstructive and restrictive pulmonary disease. Chest 1993;104:1748–1754.
74 Risk C, Epler GR, Gaensler EA: Exercise alveolar-arterial oxygen pressure difference in interstitial lung disease. Chest 1984;85:69–74.
75 Myers J, Froelicher VF: Hemodynamic determinants of exercise capacity in chronic heart failure. Ann Intern Med 1991;115:377–386.
76 Sueta CA, Gheorghiade M, Adams KF Jr, Bourge RC, Murali S, Uretsky BF, Pritzker MR, McGoon MD, Butman SM, Grossman SH, et al: Safety and efficacy of epoprostenol in patients with severe congestive heart failure. Epoprostenol Multicenter Research Group. Am J Cardiol 1995;75:34A–43A.
77 Kadikar A, Maurer J, Kesten S: The six-minute walk test: A guide to assessment for lung transplantation. J Heart Lung Transplant 1997;16: 313–319.
78 Sciurba FC, Rogers RM, Keenan RJ, Slivka WA, Gorcsan J, 3rd, Ferson PF, Holbert JM, Brown ML, Landreneau RJ: Improvement in pulmonary function and elastic recoil after lung-reduction surgery for diffuse emphysema. N Engl J Med 1996;334:1095–1099.
79 Criner GJ, Cordova FC, Furukawa S, Kuzma AM, Travaline JM, Leyenson V, O'Brien GM: Prospective randomized trial comparing bilateral lung volume reduction surgery to pulmonary rehabilitation in severe chronic obstructive pulmonary disease. Am J Respir Crit Care Med 1999;160:2018–2027.
80 Roomi J, Johnson MM, Waters K, Yohannes A, Helm A, Connolly MJ: Respiratory rehabilitation, exercise capacity and quality of life in chronic airways disease in old age. Age Ageing 1996,25.12–16.
81 Cahalin LP, Mathier MA, Semigran MJ, Dec GW, DiSalvo TG: The six-minute walk test predicts peak oxygen uptake and survival in patients with advanced heart failure. Chest 1996;110:325–332.
82 Kessler R, Faller M, Fourgaut G, Mennecier B, Weitzenblum E: Predictive factors of hospitalization for acute exacerbation in a series of 64 patients with chronic obstructive pulmonary disease. Am J Respir Crit Care Med 1999;159: 158–164.
83 Miyamoto S, Nagaya N, Satoh T, Kyotani S, Sakamaki F, Fujita M, Nakanishi N, Miyatake K: Clinical correlates and prognostic significance of six-minute walk test in patients with primary pulmonary hypertension. Comparison with cardiopulmonary exercise testing. Am J Respir Crit Care Med 2000;161:487–492.
84 O'Keeffe ST, Lye M, Donnellan C, Carmichael DN: Reproducibility and responsiveness of quality of life assessment and six-minute walk test in elderly heart failure patients. Heart 1998;80:377–382.
85 Bernstein ML, Despars JA, Singh NP, Avalos K, Stansbury DW, Light RW: Reanalysis of the 12-minute walk in patients with chronic obstructive pulmonary disease. Chest 1994;105: 163–167.
86 Chang JA, Curtis JR, Patrick DL, Raghu G: Assessment of health-related quality of life in patients with interstitial lung disease. Chest 1999;116:1175–1182.
87 Montgomery PS, Gardner AW: The clinical utility of a six-minute walk test in peripheral arterial occlusive disease patients. J Am Geriatr Soc 1998;46:706–711.
88 Jones NL, Killian KJ: Exercise limitation in health and disease. N Engl J Med 2000;343: 632–641.
89 Flaherty KR, Wald J, Weisman IM, Zeballos RJ, Schork MA, Blaivas M, Rubenfire M, Martinez FJ: Unexplained exertional limitation. Characterization of patients with a mitochondrial myopathy. Am J Respir Crit Care Med 2001;164:425–432.
90 Wasserman K, Zhang YY, Gitt A, Belardinelli R, Koike A, Lubarsky L, Agostoni PG: Lung function and exercise gas exchange in chronic heart failure. Circulation 1997;96:2221–2227.
91 Robbins M, Francis G, Pashkow FJ, Snader CE, Hoercher K, Young JB, Lauer MS: Ventilatory and heart rate responses to exercise: Better predictors of heart failure mortality than peak oxygen consumption. Circulation 1999;100:2411–2417.
92 Stelken AM, Younis LT, Jennison SH, Miller DD, Miller LW, Shaw LJ, Kargl D, Chaitman BR: Prognostic value of cardiopulmonary exercise testing using percent achieved of predicted peak oxygen uptake for patients with ischemic and dilated cardiomyopathy. J Am Coll Cardiol 1996;27:345–352.
93 Ziesche S, Cobb FR, Cohn JN, Johnson G, Tristani F: Hydralazine and isosorbide dinitrate combination improves exercise tolerance in heart failure. Results from V-HeFT I and V-HeFT II. The V-HeFT VA Cooperative Studies Group. Circulation 1993;87: VI56–VI64.
94 Richardson RS, Sheldon J, Poole DC, Hopkins SR, Ries AL, Wagner PD: Evidence of skeletal muscle metabolic reserve during whole body exercise in patients with chronic obstructive pulmonary disease. Am J Respir Crit Care Med 1999;159:881–885.
95 O'Donnell DE, Lam M, Webb KA: Spirometric correlates of improvement in exercise performance after anticholinergic therapy in chronic obstructive pulmonary disease. Am J Respir Crit Care Med 1999;160:542–549.
96 Marciniuk DD, Gallagher CG: Clinical exercise testing in interstitial lung disease. Clin Chest Med 1994;15:287–303.
97 Nixon PA, Orenstein DM, Kelsey SF, Doershuk CF: The prognostic value of exercise testing in patients with cystic fibrosis. N Engl J Med 1992;327:1785–1788.
98 Harris-Eze AO, Sridhar G, Clemens RE, Gallagher CG, Marciniuk DD: Oxygen improves maximal exercise performance in interstitial lung disease. Am J Respir Crit Care Med 1994;150:1616–1622.
99 Belman MJ, Botnick WC, Shin JW: Inhaled bronchodilators reduce dynamic hyperinflation during exercise in patients with chronic obstructive pulmonary disease. Am J Respir Crit Care Med 1996;153:967–975.
100 Bolliger CT, Perruchoud AP: Functional evaluation of the lung resection candidate. Eur Respir J 1998;11:198–212.
101 Weisman IM: Cardiopulmonary exercise testing in the preoperative assessment for lung resection surgery. Semin Thorac Cardiovasc Surg 2001;13:116–125.

102 Sciurba FC: Early and long-term functional outcomes following lung volume reduction surgery. Clin Chest Med 1997;18:259–276.
103 Ramos-Barbon D, Fitchett D, Gibbons WJ, Latter DA, Levy RD: Maximal exercise testing for the selection of heart transplantation candidates: Limitation of peak oxygen consumption. Chest 1999;115:410–417.
104 Williams TJ, Patterson GA, McClean PA, Zamel N, Maurer JR: Maximal exercise testing in single and double lung transplant recipients. Am Rev Respir Dis 1992;145:101–105.
105 Howard DK, Iademarco EJ, Trulock EP: The role of cardiopulmonary exercise testing in lung and heart-lung transplantation. Clin Chest Med 1994;15:405–420.
106 American Thoracic Society: Pulmonary rehabilitation – 1999. American Thoracic Society. Am J Respir Crit Care Med 1999;159:1666–1682.
107 Maltais F, LeBlanc P, Jobin J, Berube C, Bruneau J, Carrier L, Breton MJ, Falardeau G, Belleau R: Intensity of training and physiologic adaptation in patients with chronic obstructive pulmonary disease. Am J Respir Crit Care Med 1997;155:555–561.
108 Strzelczyk TA, Quigg RJ, Pfeifer PB, Parker MA, Greenland P: Accuracy of estimating exercise prescription intensity in patients with left ventricular systolic dysfunction. J Cardiopulm Rehabil 2001;21:158–163.
109 Ortega F, Montemayor T, Sanchez A, Cabello F, Castillo J: Role of cardiopulmonary exercise testing and the criteria used to determine disability in patients with severe chronic obstructive pulmonary disease. Am J Respir Crit Care Med 1994;150:747–751.

R. Jorge Zeballos, MD
Department of Internal Medicine
Texas Tech University Health Sciences Center
4800 Alberta Avenue
El Paso, TX 79905 (USA)
Tel. +1 915 833 3350, Fax +1 775 243 1377
E-Mail rjzeballos@yahoo.com

Weisman IM, Zeballos RJ (eds): Clinical Exercise Testing.
Prog Respir Res. Basel, Karger, 2002, vol 32, pp 43–59

Methods for Cardiopulmonary Exercise Testing

Kenneth C. Beck[a] Idelle M. Weisman[b]

[a]Physiological Imaging Laboratory, Department of Radiology, University of Iowa, Iowa City, Iowa;
[b]Human Performance Laboratory, Department of Clinical Investigation, Pulmonary-Critical Care Service, William Beaumont Army Medical Center, El Paso, Tex., and Department of Medicine, Pulmonary-Critical Care Division, University of Texas Health Science Center at San Antonio, San Antonio, Tex., USA

Summary

Over the last 20 years, CPET has expanded to include a wide spectrum of clinical applications. This has challenged clinical exercise testing laboratories to provide flexible, yet standardized methodological approaches relevant to clinical decision-making. Standardization of important methodological practices/processes is necessary to optimize clinical application [1]. This chapter will review the practical aspects of setting up a clinical exercise-testing laboratory for the evaluation of both healthy subjets and patients and will utilize the most widely accepted/applied criteria, as standardization is an evolving process. The following topics will be included: equipment, methodology for the determination of metabolic responses to exercise and for quantifying external work, protocols, monitoring, conduct of the test, patient safety, and emerging methodology for the evaluation of ventilatory limitation.

Exercise Testing Equipment

Layout of a typical clinical exercise testing laboratory is shown in figure 1. During a cardiopulmonary exercise test (CPET), an external work load is imposed on the patient while physiological monitoring documents changes in external work intensity, metabolic gas exchange, oxygen saturation of arterial blood using pulse oximetry (SpO_2), electrocardiograph (ECG), blood pressure, and possibly arterial blood gases or additional specialized tests such as spirometry and exercise tidal flow volume loops.

The opinions or assertions contained herein are the private views of the authors and are not to be construed as official or as reflecting the views of the Department of the Army or the Department of Defense.

Measuring Exercise Intensity: Ergometry

Exercise uses the body's internal energy stores to perform useful external work. Work is equal to the force times the distance over which it acts; the rate of performance of the external work is defined as power. The unit of work is the joule (equal to 1 Newton·meter) and power is measured in joules·s^{-1} or watts. Power output is also commonly expressed in kilopond meters per minute, where 100 W = 612 kp·m·min^{-1} [2]. The external power output should be quantifiable by measuring force (on pedals, or on the tread), distance (crank length, tread length) and time.

The quantitative assessment of power output is made using either a cycle ergometer or a treadmill. With cycle ergometers, the power output is measured directly by measuring the resistance required to turn the pedals (torque, usually with an internal force transducer) and crank revolutions per minute (RPM). Power output is torque times RPM. With the treadmill, determining the precise power output is more difficult. External energy consumed while walking or running on a flat motorized treadmill is essentially zero, although clearly the metabolic energy requirement increases with walking speed. The metabolic requirement for walking is derived entirely from work

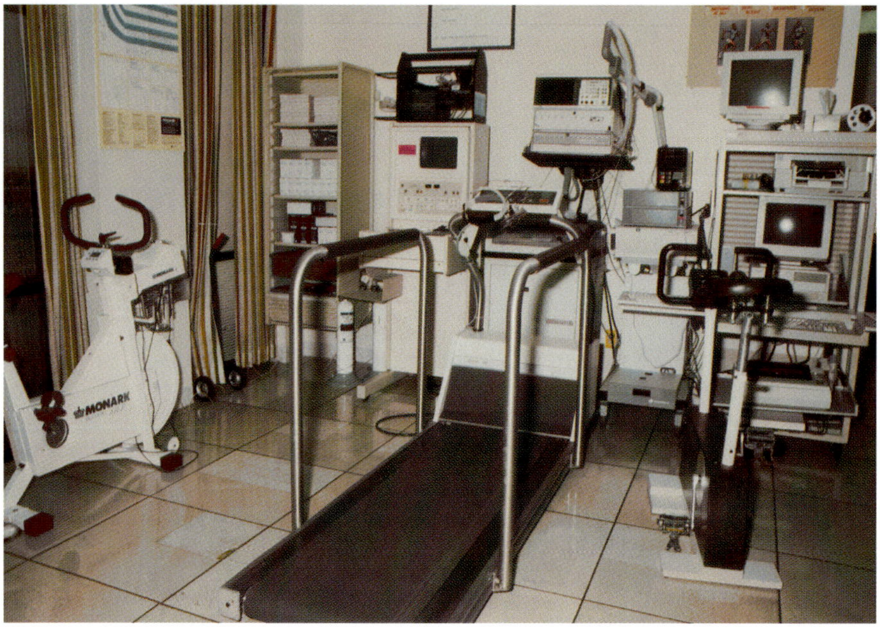

Fig. 1. Cardiopulmonary exercise testing (CPET) laboratory. Shown are a treadmill, electrically braked cycle ergometer (right) and a mechanically braked cycle ergometer ('Monarch', left). At rear is the collection of monitoring equipment including computer for acquisition of breath-by-breath metabolic data, and ECG machine. Photograph courtesy of the Human Performance Laboratory, William Beaumont Army Medical Center, El Paso, Tex.

Table 1. Comparison of ergometers used in CPET

	Cycle ergometer	Treadmill
$\dot{V}_{O_2}$max	lower	higher
Leg muscle fatigue	often limits performance	less often limits performance
Work rate quantification	yes	estimation only
Blood gas collection	easier	more difficult
Instrumentation noise and artifacts	less	more
Safety	safer	less safe (?)
Weight bearing in obese	less	more
More appropriate for	patients	active normals

required to move the limbs, and from the up and down motion against gravity. When the treadmill is inclined, power output increases due to the work against gravity needed to prevent downward motion. Thus, power output is related to body weight in addition to treadmill speed and elevation [3, 4]. The treadmill can impose noise on instrumentation signals such as ECG, blood pressure, and gas exchange measurements. $\dot{V}_{O_2}$max is often 5–10% lower on the cycle as only the leg muscles are used during exercise; consequently, leg fatigue is often the limiting factor to exercise performance. For quantitative assessment of exercise response in the clinical laboratory, electronically braked cycle ergometry is preferable to treadmill testing for several reasons summarized in table 1: direct quantitation of work rate, less noise (artifact) on ECG, easier to collect blood samples during exercise, less expensive, and safer across a wide spectrum of clinical patient populations.

Metabolic and Ventilatory Responses

There are four basic measurements that are essential in quantitating the response to exercise: Oxygen consumption ($\dot{V}_{O_2}$), carbon dioxide production ($\dot{V}_{CO_2}$), heart rate (HR), and expired minute ventilation ($\dot{V}_E$). In turn, an impressive number of derived variables can be measured during CPET; their impact on the interpretative process and clinical decision-making has been noted previously [5–7] and reviewed in the chapter on Interpretation. Historically $\dot{V}_{O_2}$ and $\dot{V}_{CO_2}$ measurements were made by timed collection of expired gas into large collection bags [8]. Today, the two most common methods for providing rapid on-line analysis are the mixing chamber technique [6, 9] and breath-by-breath technique [10], both of which require continuous measurement of expiratory flow (or occasionally volume) and continuous gas concentration.

Expiratory Flow and Volume Measurement. Most equipment measures instantaneous flow using a pneumotachograph and integrates that signal to obtain volume. Pneumotachographs operate on a number of different principles, the most common of which are listed in table 2. Note that each type exploits different properties

Table 2. Methods for continuous measurement of flow and volume (types of pneumotachographs)

	Principle of operation	Advantages	Disadvantages
Screen-type	Differential pressure across screen element Proportional to gas density and viscosity	Linear response	Seriously affected by moisture or sputum impaction Not disposable
Bernoulli or Pitot tube	Differential pressure within gas stream Proportional to gas density	Not seriously affected by moisture or sputum Lightweight Disposable	Highly nonlinear response requires computerized compensation
Hot wire anemometer	Current maintains temperature of resistance wires Exploits heat capacity of gas	Not seriously affected by mosture buildup Linear response	May be affected by sputum impaction Not disposable
Turbine	Registers volume, not flow Counts revolutions of lightweight spinning fan blade	Least sensitive to changes in gas species (may be affected slightly by gas density or viscosity change) Not seriously affected by moisture Constant calibration (one revolution = fixed volume)	May be affected by sputum impaction 'Over spin' due to intertia requires computerized compensation Not disposable

of the gas (density for screens and Pitot tubes, heat capacity for the hot wire). If a study is being undertaken with an inspired gas other than room air (e.g. high O_2, or He/O_2 breathing), the manufacturer of the equipment must be consulted and validation should be performed.

The calibration curve of any pneumotachograph can be affected by its mounting location in the system because of entrance and exit effects of flowing gases. Thus, care must be taken to ensure proper attachment to the exercise equipment prior to daily calibration. A common means for daily calibration is with a 3L gas syringe. The calibration procedure should include pumping the syringe at various rates to confirm that output of the pneumotachograph is independent of flow over the range expected during exercise [11, 11A]. The internal resistance and dead space volume of the pneumotachograph and associated valves must be taken into consideration. Although good data regarding the effect of breathing resistance on exercise response are not available, a resistance of more than 1–2 cm $H_2O \cdot l^{-1} \cdot s^{-1}$ will likely be sensed by subjects at high levels of exercise. Added dead space of equipment will manifest itself as an increase in ventilatory requirement, particularly at rest and lower levels of exercise.

Gas Concentration. Measurement of $\dot{V}_{O_2}$ and $\dot{V}_{CO_2}$ requires determination of concentrations of O_2 and CO_2 in the expired and inspired air in addition to flow or volume. If the classic bag collection technique is being used, the time taken to analyze the gas is not a critical issue, and chemical gas absorption methods are often used (Haldane and Scholander techniques). Real time data analysis requires more rapid analyzers. Essential requirements for a gas analyzer include speed of response, linearity, stability of calibration, and independence of output (i.e. presence of CO_2 does not affect O_2 measurement). Validation of these properties can be accomplished with a set of 3–4 precision grade gas tanks. Testing at least one of these gases both dry and humidified will identify how the analyzer is affected by water vapor.

Basic Concepts of Metabolic Measurements

Bag collection, mixing chamber, and breath-by-breath methods all use the same set of basic equations to calculate $\dot{V}_{O_2}$ and $\dot{V}_{CO_2}$. These equations express the mass balance of O_2 and CO_2 by quantifying the amount of the gas taken in during inspiration less the amount given off during expiration. The following basic equations are used [2, 6]:

$$\dot{V}_{O_2} = \dot{V}_I \cdot F_{IO_2} - \dot{V}_E \cdot F_{\bar{E}O_2},$$

where over-dotted V's indicate timed collections of gas volumes and the subscript $\bar{E}$ indicates mixed expired gas, as in a well mixed bag of expired gas. This equation has both inspired and expired gas volumes, but only one of these volumes needs to be measured, usually expired volume:

$$\dot{V}_I(STPD) = \dot{V}_E(STPD) \cdot F_{\bar{E}N_2}/F_{IN_2} = \dot{V}_E(STPD) \cdot (1.0 - F_{\bar{E}O_2} - F_{\bar{E}CO_2})/F_{IN_2},$$

where F_{IN_2} is inspired N_2 concentration (0.79 for room air) and $F_{\bar{E}N_2}$ is the mixed expired N_2 (in a bag).

The equation for $\dot{V}_{CO_2}$ is the reverse of the one for $\dot{V}_{O_2}$ (expired CO_2 volume minus inspired CO_2 volume), but the CO_2 concentration is near zero in room air, so the inspired volume is often omitted:

$\dot{V}_{CO_2} = \dot{V}_E \cdot F_{\bar{E}CO_2} - \dot{V}_I \cdot F_{ICO_2}$, but since $F_{ICO_2} \approx 0$,

$\dot{V}_{CO_2} = \dot{V}_E \cdot F_{\bar{E}CO_2}$

The metabolic measurements $\dot{V}_{O_2}$ and $\dot{V}_{CO_2}$ are expressed in standard temperature and pressure conditions (STPD). The conversion from ATPS (ambient temperature and pressure, saturated), to STPD is performed using:

$$\text{ATPS to STPD} = \frac{P_{bar} - P_{H_2O}(t)}{760} \cdot \frac{273}{273 + t},$$

where P_{bar} is barometric pressure (mm Hg), t is room temperature in °C and $P_{H_2O}(t)$ is determined from lookup tables of water vapor pressure against temperature.

The minute ventilation of the lungs is usually reported in body temperature pressure saturated conditions. The conversion from SPTD to BTPS is straightforward, since it involves three numbers that do not vary:

$$\text{STPD to BTPS} = \frac{760}{P_{bar} - P_{H_2O}(37\,°C)} \cdot \frac{310}{273} = \frac{863}{P_{bar} - 47}$$

Example: In a laboratory at about 700 feet altitude above sea level (P_{bar} = 740 mm Hg) and typical room temperature of 22 °C, a one minute collection of expired gas, or measurements obtained from a mixing chamber system, might be as follows: $\dot{V}_E$ = 50 liters/min, $F_{\bar{E}O_2}$ = 16.7%, $F_{\bar{E}CO_2}$ = 4.0%.

- The $\dot{V}_E$ in STPD conditions is found from the conversion of ATPS to STPD: (740 – 20)/760 × 273/295 = 0.8767, so $\dot{V}_E$(STPD) is 43.84 liters.
- The inspired volume is obtained from 43.84 × (1.0 – 0.167 – 0 .04)/0.79 = 43.98 liters/min.
- $\dot{V}_{CO_2}$ = 43.84 × 0.040 = 1.75 liters/min.
- $\dot{V}_{O_2}$ = 43.98 × 0.2095 – 43.84 × 0.167 = 1.89 liters/min.
- Reported $\dot{V}_E$(BTPS) = 43.84 × 863/(740 – 47) = 54.6 liters/min.

Effects of Water Vapor. Expired gas is warmed and humidified compared to inspired gas. Water vapor represents about the same fractional concentration as CO_2 in expired air, but is a much lower concentration in inspired air of most laboratory environments. Water vapor is never measured directly, and rapid gas analyzers used in most commercial systems (with the exception of the few that rely on mass spectrometry) require the gas sample to be dried before analysis because the analyzers are either damaged or their output affected by water vapor. It is common for manufacturers to use drying gas sample lines, in which water vapor is absorbed in transport from the mouth to the gas analyzers. Drying sample lines are prone to failure, and this failure to correct adequately for water vapor in the expired gas can be a surprisingly large (20–25%) source of error in either breath-by-breath or mixing chamber systems [12].

Breath-by-Breath and Effects of Gas Analyzer Time Delay. The breath-by-breath method samples gas flow and concentration over the breath to obtain inspired and expired volumes of CO_2 and O_2 per breath. These quantities are then used in mass balance equations combined with breath timing information to determine $\dot{V}_{O_2}$ and $\dot{V}_{CO_2}$ extrapolated to 1 min. A technical hurdle is the fact that flow measurement occurs nearly instantaneously, but gas concentration signals are delayed by the transit time of the gas along the sampling tubing into the instrument. When performing breath by breath integration, it is important to temporally realign the gas concentration and flow signals [13, 14]. Most automated commercial systems have computer software that accomplishes this realignment with a built-in calibration routine that determines the delay time that is used.

Mixing Chamber. The mixing chamber technique directs expiratory gas into a 5- to 10-liter chamber with internal baffles to facilitate mixing. Mixed gas concentration and expiratory flow are measured continuously near the outlet of the box. In addition to the delay time for gas concentration measurement mentioned above, the gas concentration signal of a mixing chamber system is delayed relative to the flow signal by the time to transport exhaled gas from the breathing valve to the mixing chamber. Because of changing $\dot{V}_E$ during exercise, the latter delay is not a fixed time period, but is determined from the ratio of (tubing volume + box volume)/$\dot{V}_E$. Computerized systems can make real time adjustments for this varying delay.

Comparing Metabolic Measurement Techniques

Of the three methods for assessing $\dot{V}_{O_2}$, $\dot{V}_{CO_2}$ and $\dot{V}_E$, the breath-by-breath technique has become the most common, although there are still many mixing chamber systems in use (table 3). Both are acceptable for clinical exercise testing. Direct bag collection is usually reserved for validation studies. The breath-by-breath method requires a digital computer to carry out the calculations in real time but has the advantages of flexibility and high time resolution for changes in metabolic rate or ventilation.

Table 3. Comparison of techniques for measuring $\dot{V}_{O_2}$, $\dot{V}CO_2$ and $\dot{V}_E$

Feature	Breath-by breath	Mixing chamber	Bag collections
Accuracy	variable, depends on calibration of flow meter, gas analyzer and handling of water vapor	variable, depends on calibration of flow meter, gas analyzer and handling of water vapor	high for steady state conditions
Laboratory space	low, needs computer, compact gas analyzers, calibration tanks	low, needs computer or strip chart recorder, compact gas analyzers, calibration tanks	high, needs means to collect gas volumes in large bags, measurement of large gas volumes (Tissot spirometer) and high precision gas analysis equipment
Patient interface	lightweight pneumotachograph and gas sampling lines allow freedom of movement	requires expired gas tubing to mixing chamber, restricting movement	requires expired gas tubing to expired bag, restricting movement
Technical ease of use	equipment is usually portable, and requires daily calibration	equipment is usually portable, requires daily calibration	requires setup of bulky equipment; gas analysis methods (Haldane, Scholander) are usually laborious
Time resolution	may be breath-by breath	variable, may be 30–60 s at low ventilation rates, but nearly breath-by-breath at high ventilations	usually 60 s bag collection, can do 30 s collections at high intensities
Immediacy of results	computerized real time computations and displays	computerized real time computations and displays	data are usually calculated after exercise testing

However, there is also a high degree of breath-to-breath variability in the data. Some of the breath-to-breath variability is caused by variations in mismatch between inspired and expired volume of each breath, leading to variation in gas stores in the lung [14, 15]. For practical purposes, most laboratories use averaging techniques to smooth the noise. There are two broad choices for averaging methods: average over time or average over fixed number of breaths. For both, the longer the averaging interval and the more breaths in the average, the more the data are smoothed [16–18]. However, there is a trade-off: as data are smoothed, rapid changes may be obscured. As peak $\dot{V}_{O_2}$ usually occurs during a period of non-steady state metabolic response, it could be underestimated. When averaging by fixed number of breaths, the time interval of the average decreases as breathing rate increases late in exercise. A 20- to 30-second moving average is probably a good choice for routine testing, though up to 60 s averaging may be appropriate to mimic traditional bag collections [2]. Additional studies are required to determine the clinical significance of these different interval-averaging techniques.

The $\dot{V}_{O_2}$ and $\dot{V}_{CO_2}$ data coming from mixing chamber systems are smoother than unaveraged breath-by-breath data simply because the mixing chamber provides a physical averaging mechanism. In addition to the inability to measure P_{ETO_2} and P_{ETO_2}, the only real disadvantage of mixing chamber systems over breath-by-breath systems is the lack of time resolution. However, modern mixing chamber systems have improved time resolution, while true breath-by-breath time resolution is generally not necessary in clinical testing situations.

Quality Control and Validation of Equipment

The equipment manufacturer should provide data sheets indicating results of validation testing. It is the responsibility of the laboratory to insure continuous accuracy over time as the equipment ages. Periodic quality control (QC) testing often makes the assumption that either the ergometer or the metabolic measuring equipment is operating properly. For instance, it is common to validate metabolic measurement systems by having a normal subject exercise at a given intensity while measuring their $\dot{V}_{O_2}$, $\dot{V}_{CO_2}$, and $\dot{V}_E$ and comparing the values obtained with those expected at the work intensity setting [3, 6, 11A]. If the ergometer is not properly calibrated, an 'error' would be detected in metabolic data.

Reproducibility of Measurements

As with all laboratory measurements, there is some inherent 'noise' or uncertainty in the measurement of responses to exercise. Consideration of the uncertainty of CPET variables is important because of its impact on the interpretation of CPET results. Numerous studies have shown the test-retest variability of both metabolic measurements ($\dot{V}_{O_2}$, $\dot{V}_{CO_2}$, and $\dot{V}_E$) and external work intensi-

Table 4. Reproducibility of maximal exercise capacity in normals and selected patient populations

Ref. No.	Sample size	* V_{O_2}max	* $V_E$max	AT	Maximal power	Disease
20	6	8.4%	4.4%	12.1%	5.5%	normal
88	10	5.0%	7.0%	13.0%	7.0%	normal
89	11	3.0%	5.0%	–	3.7%	COPD
90	20	9.0%	8.1%	–	9.7%	COPD
91	13	6.6%	6.3%	–	13.8%	COPD
19	6	5.3%	5.5%	–	5.6%	ILD
92	11	4.1%	6.3%	–	3.6%	CHF

* Table adapted from Marciniuk et al. [19]. Table entries are coefficient of variation (SD/mean) of the indicated variable. AT = The $\dot{V}_{O_2}$ at the anaerobic threshold; COPD = chronic obstructive pulmonary disease; ILD = interstitial lung disease; CHF = chronic heart failure.

ties is quite low in both normal and patient populations when individuals are retested in the same laboratory [19] (table 4). Because exercise testing is strongly dependent on patient motivation, which in turn can be affected by motivational skills of testing personnel, there may be some variability within a laboratory among testing personnel. In addition, variability between laboratories is affected by adequacy of equipment calibration and maintenance. The variability among testing personnel and among laboratories has not been extensively studied. Finally, time of day [20] and laboratory environment (temperature, humidity) may affect test results. To achieve good comparable data for comparison purposes, laboratories should strive to standardize as many of these variables as possible within the testing laboratory.

Ergometer Validations

Treadmill validation is relatively easy, requiring checking of the accuracy of the % elevation and speed of the belt. This evaluation should be performed with a subject running on the treadmill, because the weight of the subject can alter treadmill speed. Validation of belt speed is easily performed by counting the number of times a mark or piece of tape affixed to the tread cycles around per minute.

Cycle ergometers (arm or leg) are more difficult to validate. Timed counting of pedal revolutions validates the tachometer. Some manufacturers provide a 'static' calibration device that allows the user to perform checks of the internal force transducer. Static calibration does not check the internal resistance of the cycle, nor does it check the accuracy of the controller mechanism. Dynamic calibration is more difficult to perform and requires an external means of turning the cycle's crank while measuring the torque. Such calibrators are commercially available through independent vendors who will provide on-site validation or manufacturers who will loan or rent these devices for validation studies [21, 22].

Quality Control of Metabolic Measurements: The Physiologic QC

Optimizing quality control of metabolic measurements is best accomplished by establishing a program of regular 'physiologic calibration' tests in one or more individuals (usually healthy, willing, and available hospital employees) at a fixed number of exercise intensities. Because the effect of small errors in the time delay adjustment between the pneumotachograph and gas analyzer is amplified at high breathing rates [13], it is relatively easy (and preferable) to test at both normal and high breathing rates for a more complete accuracy check. Gas exchange simulators have become available that can be used for periodic validation [23]. However, use of these simulators is not a replacement for adequate physiologic validation. The gas from the simulator is usually at room temperature, with normal humidity, so errors that can occur with defective gas drying mechanism might not be picked up with the devices.

A reasonable algorithm for a physiologic QC program would proceed as follows. First, ensure that the ergometer is functioning properly and registering accurate power output. Select a subject who is likely to remain available for periodic testing and determine his/her $\dot{V}_E$, $\dot{V}_{O_2}$, and $\dot{V}_{CO_2}$ while exercising at either a fixed intensity or preferably at several intensities (e.g. 50, 100, 150 W on a cycle) at least 4 times. The data are then entered into a QC database to obtain an average for each intensity level including range (95% confidence interval = 1.96 × SD). At regular intervals, the same person should perform the same exercise, and the results of $\dot{V}_E$, $\dot{V}_{O_2}$, and $\dot{V}_{CO_2}$ are compared with the established 95% confidence interval. If data are outside this interval, repeat the test either in the same person or in another subject with established data. If both measures are outside the limits, then an equipment check is in order (pneumotachograph, gas analyzer, drying gas sampling line, etc.). If one or both measurements are within tolerance, add them to the QC database. When six or more data points have thus been added to the database, recalculate the 95% confidence interval [11A].

The most frequent causes for error in the metabolic measurements in our experience are failure of the gas analyzer or failure of the mechanism for drying the gas sample. Other errors that can occur are in the alignment of flow and gas concentration signals, in gas flow measurement, or in ergometer calibration (rare).

Exercise Protocols

The choice of testing protocol is guided largely by the goals of the exercise evaluation; either treadmill or cycle ergometry can be used. Several protocols for clinical exercise testing are available and include: (1) a progressive incremental exercise test in which workload is increased (usually every 1–2 min) or continuously in a ramp fashion; (2) a multi-stage (usually every 3 min or 'pseudo steady-state' exercise protocol, and (3) a constant work rate protocol in which the work rate is maintained constant for a variable period of time (5–30 min).

Incremental testing protocols change the exercise intensity in regular time intervals so that intensity increases slowly until volitional exhaustion. Design of an incremental protocol has two major elements: the size of the increment in work intensity and the time period for each stage. In cycle ergometry, the size of the increment can be changed by altering either the resistance on the pedals or, in case of simple devices with frictional bands, the pedal cadence. Modern feedback controlled cycles control the power output in watts by adjusting resistance on the pedals to keep power output constant within a range of pedal cadences. With treadmills, speed and elevation of the treadmill determine the increment, which is usually expressed in METS, or metabolic equivalents compared to rest. The time period for each increment is usually 1–3 min. Because the cardiac and metabolic responses to a sudden change in work intensity have a nearly exponential time course with a time constant (time to attain 63% of the total response) of about 30 s in normal subjects (shorter in trained subjects, longer in disease [24]) 2- to 3-min stages will result in nearly complete adaptation to changes in intensity at the end of the test interval.

It has become popular to impose 'ramp' increases in external power output, especially when using cycle ergometers. Ramp protocols increase power output nearly continuously, so true steady state is never attained. It can be shown, however, that cardiac and metabolic responses during ramp protocols represent steady state values with a time lag that is determined by the time constant of the response to step change in power output [25]. Similar metabolic and cardiopulmonary values have been obtained using the 1-min incremental or ramp protocols and therefore, either is acceptable for clinical purposes [25–28]. Maximal exercise capacity determined by ramp protocols has been shown to be reasonably accurate when compared with incremental protocols in both elderly subjects [29] and patients with COPD [30].

After attaining the maximal or peak exercise intensity, the patient should be allowed to 'cool down' by performing unloaded pedaling or slow walking on the level treadmill while monitoring ECG, SpO_2 and heart rate. Importantly, the heart rate recovery may provide important independent prognostic information for mortality and morbidity [31, 32]. Heart rate recovery has been defined as peak HR – HR at 1 min [31] or peak HR – HR at 2 min [32]. Furthermore, current available data has come from treadmill testing; although it is likely valid heart rate recovery still requires further testing for application in cycle ergometry.

Cycle Ergometry

Incremental or Ramp Protocols. Cycle ergometry is the preferable mode of exercise testing in patients with respiratory diseases (table 1). Exercise protocols designed to determine $\dot{V}_{O_2}$max as one end point should be designed to last approximately 10 min [33]. Patients will exercise until volitional exhaustion is achieved or the test is terminated based on the judgment of the monitor. A predaling frequency of 60 rpm appears optimal although this can vary between 40 and 70 rpm. A popular protocol for obtaining cardiopulmonary measurement using cycle ergometry is outlined in table 5. The patient sits for 3 min on the cycle with the nose clip and mouthpiece in place for baseline measurements. A warm-up period of usually 3 min follows; some prefer unloaded cycling for this warm-up whereas others prefer low-intensity exercise (5–20 W). However, patients with advanced lung disease are often unable to warm-up for 3 min even at unloaded cycling and therefore, this must be individualized. An

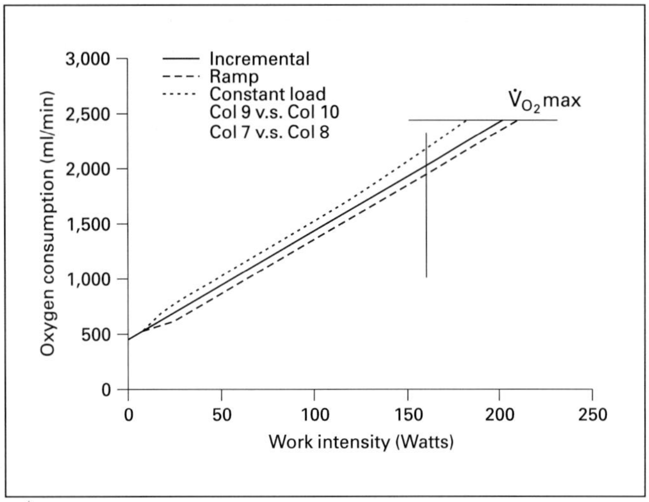

Fig. 2. Comparison of $\dot{V}_{O_2}$ during ramp, incremental and constant work exercise. Schematic graph which demonstrates that at any submaximal work rate, $\dot{V}_{O_2}$ will be higher during constant work compared to incremental or ramp exercise testing (vertical line). Though $\dot{V}_{O_2}$max may be comparable among the three protocols, the maximal power output will be lowest with the constant load protocol (horizontal line).

Table 5. Incremental exercise protocol (cycle ergometry)

	Familiarization ↓ Patient preparation (ECG, pulse oximetry, blood pressure, ? arterial line) ↓
Cardiopulmonary measurements ($\dot{V}_{O_2}$, $\dot{V}_{CO_2}$, $\dot{V}_E$)	1–3 min resting data ↓ 1–3 min unloaded pedaling ↓ ≈10 min incremental exercise (5–30 W/min)
	↓ 10 min recovery (3 min unloaded cycling) (ECG, blood pressure, oximetry)

automated flywheel apparatus may be helpful to overcome the inertia of the pedals under these circumstances. Subsequently, the rate of increase in intensity depends on the pre-test estimation of the subject's capacity. Most patients with respiratory disease will exercise at work rate increments of 5 W (very debilitated disease) to 25–30 W/min (mild disease and/or very fit).

Pre-test estimations of maximal exercise capacity can be made by starting with predicted $\dot{V}_{O_2}$max then adjusting the prediction based on clinical assessment of the subject's capabilities. For instance, a young fit subject should be able to attain a $\dot{V}_{O_2}$max of about 40 $ml \cdot min^{-1} \cdot kg^{-1}$. A subject weighing 75 kg would have an estimated $\dot{V}_{O_2}$max of 3,000 $ml \cdot min^{-1}$. Using a rough rule of thumb that $\dot{V}_{O_2}$ increases about 9–11 $ml \cdot min^{-1}$ per watt of external power output, the estimated maximal power would be (3,000 – 500)/10 = 250 W. A $\dot{V}_{O_2}$ of 500 $ml \cdot min^{-1}$ is subtracted from the estimated $\dot{V}_{O_2}$max to correct for $\dot{V}_{O_2}$ during warm-up cycling (10–20 W). Thus, a 20–25 W/min protocol would bring the subject to near maximal within the 10–12 min guideline. A very fit subject might require 30 to as high as 50 W/min protocols, whereas less fit, smaller, or older subjects might require lesser increments. The increase in power output can be a steady ramp or incrementing intensity at the end of each 1- or 2-min period. Finally, recovery is monitored for at least 10 min during which the patient performs unloaded cycling for at least 3 min to prevent blood pooling in the legs.

Constant Work Protocols. Increasingly, constant work exercise at a standardized submaximal work load (based on an initial incremental exercise test) is being uilized to evaluate the impact of therapeutic interventions including exercise training, oxygen therapy, and lung volume reduction surgery. The relationship between $\dot{V}_{O_2}$ and work rate for a ramp protocol, a 1-min incremental exercise protocol and a constant work rate exercise protocol are shown in figure 2. At any submaximal external power output, $\dot{V}_{O_2}$ will be higher during a constant work protocol compared to either ramp or 1-min incremental protocols. The difference between constant work and the ramp or incremental protocols will likely be larger above compared to below the anaerobic threshold [34]. Constant work protocols can be performed on either a cycle ergometer or treadmill. Recent work has suggested that Borg dyspnea ratings, measurements of inspiratory capacity (as a reflection of dynamic hyperinflation) and endurance times during submaximal exercise were highly reproducible and sensitive in patients with severe COPD [35, 36]; furthermore, constant work endurance times were more sensitive than 6-min walk times in determining therapeutic effectiveness of pharmacological intervention [36].

A constant work protocol is also useful for corroboration of pulmonary gas exchange and as a possible alternative approach to obtain PaO_2, $P(A\text{-}a)O_2$, and VD/VT in lieu of arterial line placement during incremental exercise testing [37]. A work rate of 70% of the maximum work rate achieved during the incremental exercise test is used for the constant work test, which results in $\dot{V}_{O_2}$peak > 90% of the value obtained in the maximal exercise evaluation. An arterial blood gas obtained at rest is used for the rest-exercise comparison (see chapter on Interpretation – case studies). Additional validation of this approach is warranted.

Treadmill Protocols

Treadmill protocols are more complex because there are two variables that affect work intensity: speed and elevation. In the extreme, speed or elevation can be left constant while altering only the other variable (e.g. Balke protocol). The most common treadmill protocol is that designed by Bruce [3, 38]. However, there are other alternatives, listed in the guidelines published by the American College of Sports Medicine [3]. A comparison study of treadmill protocols found a slightly higher $\dot{V}_{O_2}$max using the Taylor vs. Bruce and Balke protocols [39]. The Taylor protocol is a discontinuous protocol involving 3-min stages of exercise separated by 5-min rest periods [39]. Consequently, it takes much longer to complete than continuous protocols and is, therefore, used less often in clinical exercise labs.

The Bruce and Balke protocols are the two most widely used treadmill protocols. The Bruce protocol is the standard for cardiac ischemia testing with the increment increase per stage approximately 50 W, too great for most respiratory patients [40]. In turn, protocols which approximate a constant rate of increase in work rate are better suited for cardiopulmonary exercise testing. The Balke protocol [41] maintains a constant speed at 3.3 mph as elevation is increased 1% every minute. This protocol can be modified to accommodate different levels of fitness, selecting an appropriate speed level (walking or running) as elevation is increased 1% every minute [5, 42].

Invasive vs. Noninvasive CPET

An important decision is whether a clinical exercise test requires the placement of an indwelling arterial catheter for blood gas analysis in order to answer relevant clinical question(s) [2, 7] (see chapter on 'Interpretation'). Clinically, this is usually not necessary. However, there are some clinical situations in which the additional information provided by arterial line placement may be helpful and, therefore, should be considered. These include: patients with pulmonary disease and suspicion of pulmonary gas exchange abnormalities like pulmonary vascular disease, COPD with low DLCO, interstitial lung disease; patients in whom documentation of psychogenic hyperventilation is necessary; patients in whom a non-invasive exercise test suggests the presence of a pulmonary gas exchange abnormality and the need for invasive measurements; patients in whom pulse oximetry may not be reliable (blacks, smokers, patients with poor perfusion) and in whom a more accurate SaO_2 assessment is required for O_2 prescription [43, 44] (see case studies in chapter on 'Interpretation').

A helpful blood sampling strategy includes samples at rest, during unloaded cycling, and then every other minute during incremental exercise and after 2 min of recovery. Arterial catheter placement into the radial artery is preferable as collateral circulation to the hand through the ulnar artery mitigates complications due to rare occurrences of arterial occlusion. The catheter is inserted after performing an Allen's test, which evaluates for the presence of such collateral circulation.

Valuable pulmonary gas exchange information may also be provided by a single radial arterial stick, which is usually attempted near peak exercise. However, assessing exercise gas exchange from a sample obtained from a single arterial stick at peak exercise when the patient is struggling to finish the test or immediately post exercise when the gas exchange milieu is already different from peak exercise conditions is problematic and should be discouraged. Misleading information may result as PaO_2 changes occur rapidly following the end of exercise and clinically significant abnormalities present at peak exercise can be missed [45]. An alternative strategy utilizing a single stick during minute 5 of constant work may be preferable as breathing pattern alterations are minimal compared to peak exercise using this approach (see constant work and chapter on 'Interpretation', case 2).

Monitoring

Blood Pressure and ECG

Heart rate is most accurately obtained from the R-R interval on the 12-lead electrocardiogram. Movement artifacts must be minimized by adequate skin preparation and use of electrodes designed for exercise testing [11A]. For optimal detection of myocardial ischemia and cardiac arrhythmias, serial 12-lead ECG tracings should be obtained during the exercise test. Care should be exercised when using averaged signals, and the raw tracings should always be consulted for final ECG interpretation.

Arterial blood pressure can be measured using either cuff (noninvasive) or indwelling arterial cannula and pressure transducer. Modern transducers are pre-calibrated, but they always need to be positioned at the mid-heart level for accurate readings. Care should also be exercised to exclude air bubbles from tubing and the transducer housing to optimize the frequency response of the signal. Because of peripheral amplification of the pulse pressure, direct readings from indwelling catheters may register higher (≈8–10 mm Hg) systolic and diastolic values compared to cuff [46, 47]. Cuff pressure measurement may also be problematic; motion associated with exercise can make auscultation difficult. Use of a miniature microphone attached to the arm and systems that filter out noise and amplify the pulses sometimes help, but these and automated blood pressure systems should be validated against standard cuff measurements before use. Exercise blood pressure criteria (see tables 7, 9) are based mostly on cuff measurements.

Pulse Oximetry

The pulse oximeter provides valuable real-time readout of changes in oxygen saturation (SpO_2) during exercise. As a result of the shape of the oxyhemoglobin dissociation curve, O_2 saturation is a relatively insensitive indicator of gas exchange abnormalities (see arterial blood gases). Oximeters operate by measuring light absorbance of tissues at several wavelengths, allowing differentiation between oxygenated and unoxygenated blood [48]. Pulse oximeters perform rapid analysis of the signals to allow differentiation between arterial and mixed venous blood during each pulse beat. Factors that will compromise their performance therefore include deficiencies in perfusion to the selected measuring site (usually finger or ear, but instruments are becoming available that attach to the forehead), interference from bright ambient lights, some types of finger nail polish, and skin pigmentation [11A, 43, 48, 49]. The accuracy of pulse oximetry compared to direct sampling of arterial blood is generally good (± 4%) as long as a good pulse signal is obtained, but the measurement is generally thought to be less accurate at saturations below about 88%; this is exacerbated in blacks [43]. Pulse oximeters measure both COHb and O_2Hb, unlike co-oximeters which can separate the two. Consequently, a patient with 5% COHb and 85% SaO_2 will have SpO_2 approximately 90%. Also, during exercise in some heart failure patients, the instrument may register a desaturation because of diminishing peripheral perfusion [44]. Thus, care should be exercised in interpreting any changes obtained by pulse oximetry alone. Significant desaturation, defined as $\Delta SpO_2 \geq 5$ mm Hg, should be confirmed with arterial blood gases [50].

In general, pulse oximeters are good for monitoring trending phenomena but not reliable for determining absolute magnitude of change. Quality assurance for pulse oximeters should include validation with arterial oxygen saturation and linear regression plots for each oximeter. This is important because some pulse oximeters underestimate while others overestimate arterial oxygen saturation especially at $SaO_2 < 88\%$. Pulse oximetry during exercise testing is considered standard of care: in the evaluation of patients with exertional dyspnea, in patients with resting hypoxemia, and patients with suspected exertional hypoxemia.

Arterial Blood Gases

As previously noted, it may be desirable to document the changes in pulmonary gas exchange during exercise in patients with heart or lung disease. Whereas most laboratories will use pulse oximetry (see above) to monitor arterial saturation, it is well appreciated that SpO_2 by itself provides a relatively crude index of changes in pulmonary gas exchange. P_{aO_2} and the alveolar to arterial oxygen tension difference ($P(A\text{-}a)O_2$ are much more sensitive indicators of gas exchange abnormalities. Arterial blood sampling including measurement of P_{aO_2}, P_{aCO_2}, pH, HCO_3, SaO_2 and calculation of $P(A\text{-}a)O_2$ and VD/VT is optimal. Suggested guidelines and caveats for arterial blood gas values during CPET appear in the chapter on 'Interpretation' [table 3 in ref. 7; also 5, 50, 51]. To calculate P_{AO_2}, use the alveolar air equation for O_2:

$$P_{AO_2} = P_{IO_2} - P_{aCO_2} \cdot \left[\frac{1}{R} - F_{IO_2} \cdot \frac{1-R}{R}\right],$$

where P_{IO_2} indicates the inspired partial pressure of O_2 ($F_{IO_2} \times (P_{bar} - 47)$,

$$R = \frac{\dot{V}_{CO_2}}{\dot{V}_{O_2}}$$

from metabolic measurements obtained at the same time as blood sampling, and F_{IO_2} is the inspired fraction of O_2 (usually 0.2095). A simpler form that is nearly as accurate especially when $R \approx 1.0$ is

$$P_{AO_2} = P_{IO_2} - \frac{P_{aCO_2}}{R}.$$

The $P(A\text{-}a)O_2$ is normally less than 10 mm Hg at rest, but may increase to about 20 even in normal subjects near maximal exercise. Widening of the $P(A\text{-}a)O_2$ more than this suggests significant gas exchange defects such as worsening $\dot{V}_A/Q$ inequalities, diffusion limitation, right-to-left shunt, or compounding of these factors by the inevitable fall in $P_{\bar{v}O_2}$ that occurs progressively with exercise.

If hypoxemia worsens without widening of the $P(A-a)O_2$, the hypoxemia is likely due to an inadequate ventilatory response and CO_2 retention rather than a primary gas exchange abnormality.

The VD/VT is also calculated using blood gases. To complete the calculation, an estimate of the mixed expired P_{CO_2} obtained at the same time as arterial blood sampling ($P\bar{E}_{CO_2}$) is necessary. Traditionally, this came from a bag collection of expired air. With mixing chamber systems, the number can be taken directly from the mixing chamber. Breath-by-breath systems will often provide that data, obtaining from the ratio of V_{CO_2}/V_T, where V_{CO_2} is expired volume of CO_2, averaged over a number of breaths, and both V_{CO_2} and V_T must be expressed in STPD conditions. The equation for VD/VT is

$$\frac{P_{aCO_2} - P\bar{E}_{CO_2}}{P_{aCO_2}}.$$

The VD/VT typically declines during exercise in healthy individuals, but it is higher in older subjects compared to younger subjects. VD/VT calculation should be based on P_{aCO_2} because P_{ETCO_2} is unreliable [52].

Table 6. Conduct of a cardiopulmonary exercise test

Pre-test patient check list
Reason(s) for CPET
Diagnosis, history, physical examination
ECG, PFTs, salient laboratory test results
Health questionnaire and physical activity profile
Compliant with pre-test instructions, especially medications
Consent form signed
Equipment and protocol selection
Incremental vs. constant work or both (1 h between tests)
Invasive vs. noninvasive test
Pre-test laboratory procedures
Quality control
Equipment calibration
Patient preparation
Familiarization
Monitoring devices – ECG, pulse oximetry, blood pressure
Arterial line placement (if warranted)
Cardiopulmonary exercise testing
Interpretation of integrative CPET results

Conduct of the Exercise Test

An overview for the conduct of a CPET appears in table 6. Reason(s) for CPET are usually given by the referring physician but is/are often obtained by consultation between the referring physician and the physician in charge of the exercise testing laboratory. A medical diagnosis and a summary of the salient features of the physical examination/medical history should accompany the exercise test request. The results of pulmonary function testing, EKG, chest X-ray and pertinent laboratory results should also be noted. The patient with the assistance of exercise lab personnel should respond to a short medical questionnaire. This should include questions related to cardiopulmonary and major systemic disease and current therapy, with special attention to medications that alter heart rate and blood pressure, those used for the treatment of cardiac insufficiency, and for treatment of pulmonary conditions such as asthma or COPD. Physical activity and symptom(s) levels, as well as risk factors for coronary artery disease should also be noted. A brief physical examination of the patient may be required to identify contraindications to performing CPET such as knee or other joint problems that can limit exercise performance. Patients may benefit from an exercise familiarization screening 'mini-session' which includes practicing cycling on the bike, or walking on the treadmill while wearing a noseclip, mouthpiece, pulse oximeter, etc. This is also a good opportunity to explain communication techniques during exercise including use of hand signs and symptoms scoring [53, 54]. The patient should be encouraged to ask questions and feel comfortable in the exercise-testing laboratory.

Absolute and relative contraindications to exercise testing are provided as a reference source and appear in table 7 [3, 6, 55–57]. Systemic hypertension is included, although there is disagreement about the level (systolic >200–250 mm Hg and diastolic >115–120 mm Hg measured at rest). Care should be exercised in testing pregnant women [3, 58] (see chapter on 'Exercise in Pregnancy'). The clinical judgment of the physician in charge of the test should prevail.

Preliminary Requirements for CPET

When the test is pre-scheduled, the subject should be issued some basic information about the conduct of the test and a list of instructions for preparation. Importantly, the patient is instructed on which medications should be taken or withheld prior to exercise testing. For cardiac transplantation or impairment-disability evaluation, patients should be tested on an optimized medication regimen. For evaluation of exercise-induced asthma, respiratory medications are usually withheld prior to exercise

Table 7. Contraindications to exercise testing

Absolute contraindications	
1	Recent myocardial infarction
2	Changes in the resting ECG that suggest acute or recent myocardial event
3	Unstable angina pectoris
4	Uncontrolled cardiac rhythm disturbances, either supraventricular or ventricular, particularly when compromising cardiac output
5	Severe aortic stenosis and known or suspected dissecting aortic aneurysm
6	Active or suspected acute pericarditis or myocarditis
7	Acute congestive heart failure
8	Recent systemic or pulmonary embolus
9	Acute febrile illness
10	Third degree a-v block without pacemaker control
11	Pulmonary edema or significant cor pulmonale
12	Physical disabilities or other inability to cooperate such as severe emotional or psychological distress
Relative contraindications	
1	Systemic hypertension
2	Resting tachycardia (>120 min^{-1})
3	Frequent ventricular or atrial ectopy
4	Moderate aortic stenosis
5	Moderate to severe pulmonary hypertension
6	Moderate valvular heart disease
7	Pregnancy
8	Known electrolyte abnormalities and severe anemia (Hb < 10 g/100 ml)

Additional absolute or relative contraindications can exist and clinical judgment should always be used to determine the appropriateness of performing an exercise test.

Table compiled from ref. 3, 6, 55, 56, 57.

Table 8. Borg perceived exertion scales

Category ratio scale		Linear scale	
numerical rating	descriptor	numerical rating	descriptor
0	nothing at all	6	
0.5	very, very slight (almost none)	7	very, very light
1	very slight	8	
2	slight	9	very light
3	moderate	10	
4	somewhat severe	11	fairly light
5	severe	12	
6		13	somewhat hard
7	very severe	14	
8		15	hard
9	very,very severe	16	
10	maximal	17	very hard
		18	
		19	very, very hard
		20	

Note: May substitute 'weak' for 'slight' and 'strong' for 'severe.' Table adapted from ref. 53, 54.

testing (see chapter on 'Exercise-Induced Asthma'). The patient should refrain from exercise the day of the test and to abstain from smoking for at least 8 h. The subject should avoid eating a heavy meal within 3 h of testing and should wear comfortable loose fitting clothing and shoes appropriate for exercise. If clinically warranted, PFTS including MVV and spirometry may be performed. Depending on the clinical question(s), lung volumes and DLCO should also be obtained. A resting arterial blood gas may be appropriate if hypoxemia is suspected.

Performing the Test

A consent document is signed, if required. Patient preparation includes the placement of ECG electrodes and if necessary, an arterial catheter. Skin preparation for the ECG lead placement is important to decrease the noise on the ECG tracing. The position of the 12-lead ECG electrodes proposed by Mason and Likar [59] is recommended. A supine resting 12-lead ECG should be obtained as the standard ECG for determination of resting abnormalities [60]. An upright baseline ECG is taken as resting baseline. The patient should be familiarized with the protocol including the incrementing work rate, monitoring devices, and the equipment.

If cycle ergometry is being used, the seat height should be carefully adjusted to optimum by having the patient slowly turn the pedals and look for slight angle of the knee when the pedal is at bottom of its swing, with little hip movement on the seat. Whether cycle ergometry or treadmill is the modality, the patient needs to be instructed in proper exercise technique: regular, constant revolution of pedals for cycle ergometry, and relaxed stride on a treadmill using the hands only for balance by touching the rails lightly with no tension in the arms.

Symptom scoring and blood pressure are usually obtained at the end of each stage, or every minute to 2 min in the case of continuous ramp protocols. Other measurements, such as arterial blood gases or flow-volume loop measurements can be obtained less frequently, such as every other minute. Symptoms can be assessed using a variety of instruments; the most popular are the original Borg perceived exertion scale or the modified category ratio scale

Table 9. Criteria for early termination of an exercise test

1	Clinical observation and judgement
2	Moderate to severe angina
3	>2 mm horizontal or downsloping ST segment depression or elevation
4	Serious arrhythmias
	Second or third degree atrioventricular block
	Sustained ventricular tachycardia
	Frequent premature ventricular contractions
	Atrial fibrillation with a rapid ventricular response
5	Severe hypertension (systolic pressure >260 mm Hg; diastolic pressure >115–120 mm Hg)
6	Drop in systolic blood pressure with increasing intensity accompanied by signs or symptoms, or drop below pre-exercise values
7	Severe wheezing in the chest or upper airways
8	Unusual or severe shortness of breath
9	Ataxia, vertigo, visual or gait problems, confusion or other signs of central nervous system disorder; and acute myocardial infarction
10	Physical or verbal manifestations of severe fatigue or shortness of breath
11	Signs of poor peripheral perfusion (pallor, cyanosis, cold clammy skin)
12	Leg cramps or extreme pain suggesting claudication

Modified from ref. 3, 68.

(table 8) [53, 54]. Increasingly, the modified category ratio scale is also being used for leg fatigue and chest pain. Alternatively, these symptoms can be assessed with simple 0–4 scales (0 = none, 4 = severe). Testing personnel should observe the patient for signs of fatigue or other symptoms, and monitoring ECG and gas exchange data.

When the patient stops exercise, it is important to determine the main causes for termination (shortness of breath, chest discomfort, leg fatigue or leg pain, etc.). The patient should be observed for signs of shortness of breath, faintness, unusual weakness or other symptoms. The subjective impression of the testing personnel of why exercise stopped should also be noted as this can differ from the patient's assessment. In some cases, auscultation can be performed to detect breath sounds either over the lung fields or the trachea and upper airway. As noted previously ('Exercise Protocols'), monitoring heart rate in the recovery period may provide valuable prognostic information [31, 32].

Criteria for terminating an exercise test appear in table 9 [2, 6, 61, 62]. If monitoring fails (e.g. ECG or blood pressure), consideration should be given to stopping, depending on the clinical circumstances. In the absence of terminating signs or symptoms, testing should be continued until volitional exhaustion. Verbal encouragement is often helpful in assuring a patient's maximal effort. A maximal exercise test is usually reflected by a patient achieving at least one of the following criteria: maximal predicted $\dot{V}_{O_2}$, heart rate, or $\dot{V}_E$ (relative to MVV), RER >1.15 or lactate >8 mEq/l [63]. A test may be discontinued because of serious ECG changes and/or significant symptoms. Despite a patient's best efforts, physiologic limitation due to symptom limitation is often not achieved; assessing patient effort under these circumstances is underscored. Finally, if medical complications arise, the medical monitor should terminate the test. In those situations, the patient should be observed until stable and physiologic variables have returned to baseline. Based on the judgment of the physician, admission to the hospital maybe warranted. Resuscitation equipment should always be available in the exercise laboratory.

Patient Safety

Extensive literature suggests that symptom-limited exercise testing in otherwise healthy individuals is a relatively safe procedure. In patients, a death rate of approximately 0.5 per 10,000 has been reported in a survey of 1,375 clinical exercise testing facilities [64]. In more than 70,000 maximal exercise tests performed in a preventive medicine clinic, no deaths were reported, with only 6 major medical complications [3]. In a very large study of cycle ergometry exercise testing involving >1 million sports persons and patients, 2 deaths per 100,000 tests were reported in patients with a chronic disease [65]. Sudden death during exercise testing was evaluated in eight studies analyzed by the American Heart Association revealing a rate of 0–5 per 100,000 exercise tests [66]. More recently, analysis of 75,828 exercise tests performed in the Veterans Affairs Health Care System revealed an event rate of 1.2 per 10,000 exercise tests performed (myocardial infarction, ventricular tachycardia) with no deaths [67]. It can be reasonably concluded therefore that exercise testing is safe, that the risk of medical complications during exercise testing is related to the underlying disease, and that the morbidity for patients resulting from exercise testing is 2–5 per 100,000 clinical exercise tests.

Evaluation of Ventilatory Limitations

Assessing the degree of ventilatory limitation has traditionally been based on the ventilatory reserve or on how close the maximal $\dot{V}_E$ achieved during exercise ap-

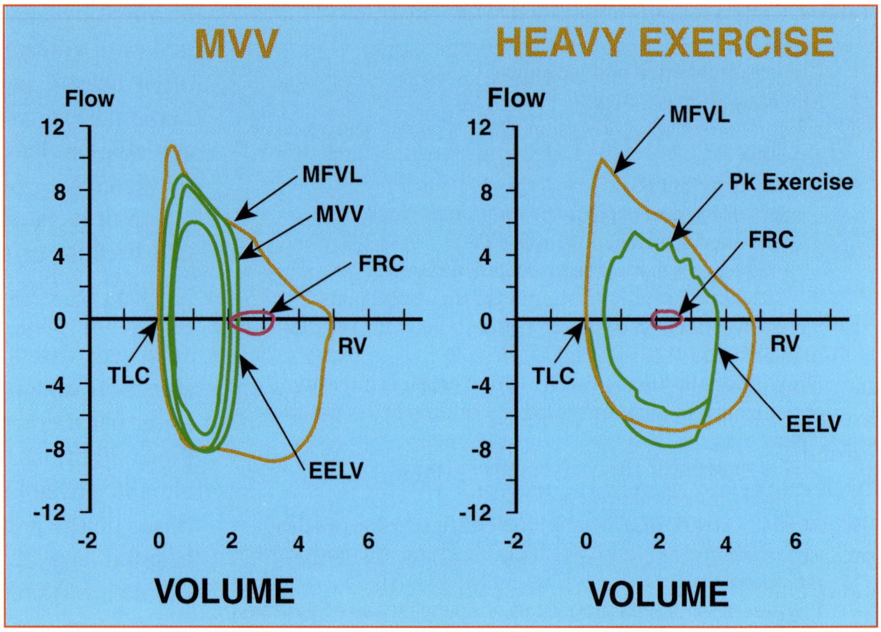

Fig. 3. Flow vs. volume loops obtained during a maximal voluntary ventilation (MVV) test and near maximal exercise in a healthy young adult. Note the encroachment on both the expiratory and inspiratory MFVL envelope, the higher lung volume and attendant increased elastic load which increases the work of breathing during the MVV maneuver compared with exercise. Figure adapted from Johnson et al. [86].

proaches the maximal voluntary ventilation (MVV) or some estimate of the MVV that is used as an index of ventilatory capacity. The standard maximal voluntary ventilation (MVV) test is obtained at rest by having a patient breathe in and out of a spirometer as hard as possible for 12–15 s [5, 6, 11]. A rough estimate of the MVV can be obtained from the FEV_1 obtained from spirometry multiplied by about 35–40 [68]. As there is considerable variability in the relationship of MVV to FEV_1 among subjects, especially those with lung disease [68], the 'calculated' MVV should be used only when directly measured MVV or other direct methods (see below) are not available.

Although the MVV is practical, simple, and widely applied, it most probably overestimates 'true' ventilatory capacity for two reasons: (1) the maneuver is a short high intensity effort that cannot be sustained [69], and (2) the breathing pattern adopted by most subjects is different from exercise ventilation in that breathing occurs at higher lung volumes and at higher respiratory rates (fig. 3) [70, 71], and involves a different pattern of muscle activation [72].

There has been a growing trend in both research and clinical laboratories to find alternative ways to evaluate ventilatory limitation during exercise [73]. This results from the appreciation that patients may discontinue exercise due to ventilatory constraints and dyspnea prior to achieving the classic indices associated with ventilatory limitation (i.e. minute ventilation ($\dot{V}_E$) that reached the maximum voluntary ventilation (MVV) or a rise in $PaCO_2$) and that ventilatory limitation is not an 'all or none' phenomenon. One approach that has gained popularity is the measurement of the exercise tidal flow volume loop (extFVL) and plotting it within the maximal flow volume loop (MFVL) [74–78]. This technique provides a good visual index of the degree of ventilatory constraint, allows a more detailed approach to defining ventilatory limitation (relative to the $\dot{V}_E$/MVV relationship), and has gained popularity due to the ease of measurement using many of the commercially available automated exercise systems. Figure 4 shows an example of the rest and peak exercise flow volume responses in a healthy, average fit adult plotted within the MFVL.

Table 10 lists indices of ventilatory constraint using extFVL plotted within the MFVL [73]. In addition, other parameters can be devised that provide more continuous information, such as the area between the extFVL and the MFVL. Further work must be done to determine which parameters in addition to visual inspection of the loops are useful diagnostic tools.

Another method for determining degree of flow limitation is the 'negative expiratory pressure' or NEP method [79–81]. This technique requires a negative pressure source to be connected at the mouth so that at randomly selected times during exercise, mouth pressure can be forced to be negative, usually about –10 cm H_2O, during expiration of one breath. An increase in expiratory flow during a breath where the NEP is applied compared with a normal breath is taken as evidence that flow limitation is *not* present.

Each of these techniques assesses ventilatory limitation in different ways. extFVL analysis is hampered by the fact that the MFVL determined by routine spirometry is affected by gas compression within the chest during the maximal expiratory effort [82–84], and that the MFVL curve itself can be affected by exercise [81, 84, 85]. In turn, the NEP technique is essentially an 'all or none phenomenon' unable to detect the approach to flow limitation, but rather only when flow limitation is present; furthermore, NEP by itself does not document changes in breathing strategy in response to actual or impending flow limitation [73]. Both techniques have their technical difficulties: the NEP requires additional instrumentation and means for measuring and generating the negative mouth pressures during expiration only, whereas the MFVL curve analysis requires drift-free volume and flow signals, and each measurement must be accompanied by a full inspiratory effort from the patient to determine inspiratory capacity [86]. The IC measurement, as a reflection of end-expiratory lung volume and overall operational lung volumes is becoming increasingly important in clinical decision-making [35, 75, 87]. A combination of the NEP technique and the use of extFVL/MFVL may provide the greatest amount of information on ventilatory constraints imposed by the lung and chest wall.

Acknowledgements

Supported by a General Clinical Research Center grant from the National Institutes of Health (MO1-RR00585) and NHLBI grants HL-52230 and HL064368.

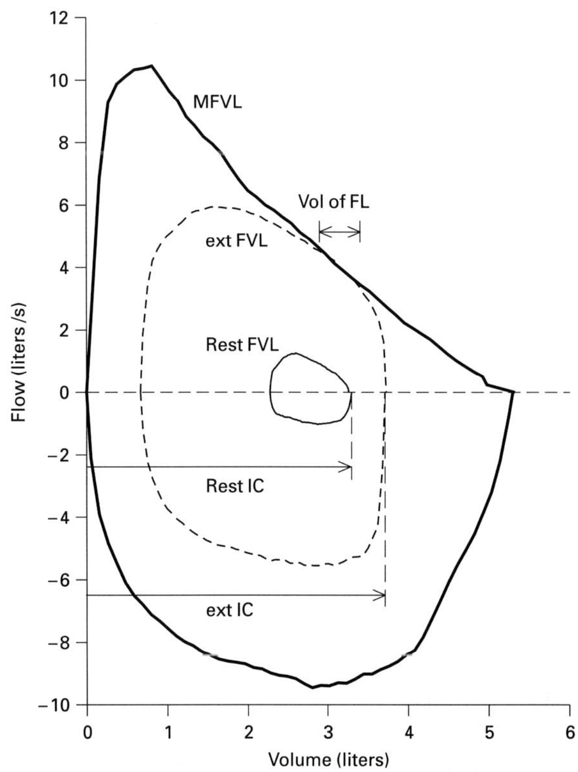

Fig. 4. Calculation of flow limitation (FL) and inspiratory capacity (IC) from exercise test flow-volume loops (ext FVL) and maximal flow-volume loops (MFVL). Flow limitation is quantified by measuring the volume over which the ext FVL flows meet or exceed the MFVL flows (Vol of FL) expressed as a % of the tidal volume. Another useful index of exercise adaptation is the change in inspiratory capacity (IC), here indicate for rest (rest IC) and exercise (ext IC). In this normal individual, the IC gets larger during exercise as end-expiratory lung volume (EELV) drops. In patients, EELV may rise as FL occurs earlier in exercise, causing IC to fall.

Table 10. Indices of ventilatory constraint using ext FVL plotted within the MFVL

Index	How it is assessed	Role in ventilatory contraints
Expiratory flow limitation (%FL)	% of ext FVL that meets or exceeds the MFVL	FL may indicate airway collapse, increasing WOB, and could trigger reflexes, increasing sensation of dyspnea
Elastic load	EILV/TLC ratio	high WOB, increased load on respiratory muscles
Dynamic rise in EELV	Fall in IC (EELV = TLC – IC)	reduces inspiratory muscle length, and increases elastic load
Inspiratory flow reserve	area between inspiratory limb of extFVL and MFVL	a measure of breathing reserve

EILV = End-inspiratory lung volume; TLC = total lung capacity; IC = inspiratory capacity; WOB = work of breathing.
Other terms defined in text or figure 4. Table adapted from Johnson et al. [73].

References

1 Weisman IM, Zeballos RJ: Cardiopulmonary exercise testing – the need for standardization: Pulmonary perspectives. Am Coll Chest Phys 1992;8:5–8.

2 Zeballos RJ, Weisman IM: Behind the scenes of cardiopulmonary exercise testing. Clin Chest Med 1994;15:193–213.

3 American College of Sports Medicine: Guidelines for Exercise Testing and Prescription, ed 6. Philadelphia, Lippincott Williams & Wilkins, 2000.

4 Astrand PO: Textbook of Work Physiology. New York, McGraw-Hill, 1977.

5 Wasserman K, Hansen JE, Sue DY, Casaburi R, Whipp BJ: Principles of Exercise Testing and Interpretation, ed 3. Philadelphia, Lippincott Williams & Wilkins, 1999.

6 Jones NL: Clinical Exercise Testing, ed 4. Philadelphia, Saunders, 1997.

7 Weisman IM, Zeballos RJ: An integrated approach to the interpretation of cardiopulmonary exercise testing. Clin Chest Med 1994;15:421–445.

8 Mitchell JH, Sproule BJ, Chapman CB: The physiological meaning of the maximal oxygen intake test. J Clin Invest 1958;37:538–547.

9 Hughson RL, Kowalchuk JM, Prime WM, Green HJ: Open-circuit gas exchange analysis in the non-steady-state. Can J Applied Sports Sci 1980;5:15–18.

10 Beaver WL, Wasserman K, Whipp BJ: On-line computer analysis and breath-by-breath graphical display of exercise function tests. J Appl Physiol 1973;34:128–132.

11 American Thoracic Society: Standardization of spirometry, 1994 update. Am J Respir Crit Care Med 1995;152:1107–1136.

11A Wanger J, Crapo RO, Irvin CG: Pulmonary function laboratory management and procedure manual: A project of the American Thoracic Society. American Thoracic Society, New York, NY, 1998/2001.

12 Beaver WL: Water vapor corrections in oxygen consumption calculations. J Appl Physiol 1973;35:928–931.

13 Proctor DN, Beck KC: Time delays adjustment to minimize errors in breath-by-breath measurement of $\dot{V}_{O_2}$ during exercise. J Appl Physiol 1996;81:2495–2499.

14 Hughson RL, Northey DR, Xing HC, Dietrich BH, Cochrane JE: Alignment of ventilation and gas fraction for breath-by-breath respiratory gas exchange calculations in exercise. Comp Biomed Res 1991;24:118–128.

15 Beaver WL, Lamarra N, Wasserman K: Breath-by-breath measurement of true alveolar gas exchange. J Appl Physiol 1981;51:1662–1675.

16 Sciurba FC, Owens GR, Ondriezek J: The effect of sample interval on maximal values obtained during incremental exercise. Am Rev Respir Dis 1991;143:A176.

17 Slivka WA: Sciurba FC: Parameters and power to measure a therapeutic effect (lung reduction surgery – LVRS) in advanced emphysema. Am J Respir Crit Care Med 1998;157:A92.

18 Myers J, Walsh D, Sullivan M, Froelicher V: Effect of sampling on variability and plateau in oxygen uptake. J Appl Physiol 1990;68:404–410.

19 Marciniuk DD, Watts R, Gallagher CG: Reproducibility of incremental maximal cycle ergometer testing in patients with restrictive lung disease. Thorax 1993;48:894–898.

20 Garrard CS, Emmons C: The reproducibility of the respiratory responses to maximum exercise. Respiration 1986;49:94–100.

21 Russell JC, Dale JD: Dynamic torquemeter calibration of bicycle ergometers. J Appl Physiol 1986;61:1217–1220.

22 Van Praagh E, Bedu M, Roddier P, Coudert J: A simple calibration method for mechanically breaked cycle ergometers. Int J Sports Med 1992;13:27–30.

23 Huszczuk A, Whipp BJ, Wasserman K: A respiratory gas exchange simulator for routine calibration in metabolic studies. Eur Respir J 1990;3:465–468.

24 Otsuka T, Kurihara N, Fujii T, Fujimoto S, Yoshikawa J: Effect of exercise training and detraining on gas exchange kinetics in patients with chronic obstructive pulmonary disease. Clin Physiol 1997;17:287–297.

25 Whipp BJ, Davis JA, Torres F, Wasserman K: A test to determine parameters of aerobic function during exercise. J Appl Physiol 1981;50:217–221.

26 Zhang YY, Johnson MC, Chow N, Wasserman K: Effect of exercise testing protocol on parameters of aerobic function. Med Sci Sports Exerc 1991;23:625–630.

27 Myers J, Buchanan N, Walsh D, Kraemer M, McAuley P, Hamilton-Wessler M, Froelicher VF: Comparison of the ramp versus standard exercise protocols. J Am Coll Cardiol 1991;17:1334–1342.

28 Tanner CS, Heise CT, Barber G: Correlations of the physiologic parameters of a continuous ramp versus an incremental James exercise protocol in normal children. Am J Cardiol 1991;67:309–312.

29 Bader DS, Maguire TE, Balady GJ: Comparison of ramp versus step protocols for exercise testing in patients > or = 60 years of age. Am J Cardiol 1999;83:11–14.

30 Miyahara N, Eda R, Takeyama H, Maeda T, Aoe K, Kunichika N, Kohara H, Harad M: Cardiorespiratory responses during cycle ergometer exercise with different ramp slope increments in patients with chronic obstructive pulmonary disease. Int Med 2000;39:15–19.

31 Nishime EO, Cole CR, Blackstone EH, Pashkow FJ, Lauer MS: Heart rate recovery and treadmill exercise score as predictors of mortality in patients referred for exercise ECG. JAMA 2000;284:1392–1398.

32 Cole CR, Foody JM, Blackstone EH, Lauer MS: Heart rate recovery after submaximal exercise testing as a predictor of mortality in a cardiovascularly healthy cohort. Ann Int Med 2000;132:552–555.

33 Buchfuhrer MJ, Hansen JE, Robinson TE, Sue DY, Wasserman K, Whipp BJ: Optimizing the exercise protocol for cardiopulmonary assessment. J Appl Physiol 1983;55:1558–1564.

34 Roston WL, Whipp BJ, Davis JA, Cunningham DA, Effors RM, Wasserman K: Oxygen uptake kinetics and lactate concentration during exercise in humans. Am Rev Respir Dis 1987;135:1080–1084.

35 O'Donnell DE, Lam M, Webb KA: Spirometric correlates of improvement in exercise performance after anticholinergic therapy in chronic obstructive pulmonary disease. Am J Respir Crit Care Med 1999;160:542–549.

36 Oga T, Nishimura K, Tsukino M, Hajiro T, Ikeda A, Izumi T: The effects of oxitropium bromide on exercise performance in patients with stable chronic obstructive pulmonary disease. A comparison of three different exercise tests. Am J Respir Crit Care Med 2000;161:1897–1901.

37 Zeballos RJ, Weisman IM, Connery SM: Comparison of pulmonary gas exchange measurements between incremental and constant work exercise above the anaerobic threshold. Chest 1998;113:602–611.

38 Bruce RA, Kusumi F, Hosmer D: Maximal oxygen intake and nomographic assessment of functional aerobic impairment in cardiovascular disease. Am Heart J 1973;85:546–562.

39 Froelicher VE Jr, Brammell H, Davis G, Noguera I, Stewart A, Lancaster MC: A comparison of the reproducibility and physiologic response to three maximal treadmill exercise protocols. Chest 1974;65:512–517.

40 Bruce RA, McDonough JR: Stress testing in screening for cardiovascular disease. Bull NY Acad Med 1969;45:1288–1305.

41 Nagle FS, Balke B, Naughton JP: Gradational step tests for assessing work capacity. J Appl Physiol 1965;20:745–748.

42 Pollock ML, Wilmore JH, Fox SM III: Exercise in Health and Disease. Philadelphia, Saunders, 1984.

43 Zeballos RJ, Weisman IM: Reliability of noninvasive oximetry in black subjects during exercise and hypoxia. Am Rev Resp Dis 1991;144:1240–1244.

44 Hansen JE, Cassaburi R: Validity of ear oximetry in clinical exercise testing. Chest 1987;91:333–337.

45 Ries AL, Fedullo PF, Clausen JL: Rapid changes in arterial blood gas levels after exercise in pulmonary patients. Chest 1983;83:454–456.

46 Rasmussen PH, Staats BA, Driscoll DJ, Beck KC, Bonekat HW, Wilcox WD: Direct and indirect blood pressure during exercise. Chest 1985;87:743–748.

47 Robinson TE, Sue DY, Huszczuk A, Weiler-Ravell D, Hansen JE: Intra-arterial and cuff blood pressure responses during incremental cycle ergometry. Med Sci Sports Exerc 1988;20:142–149.

48 Sinex JE: Pulse oximetry: Principles and limitations. Am J Emerg Med 1999;17:59–67.

49 Ralston AC, Webb RK, Runciman WB: Potential errors in pulse oximetry. III. Effects of interference, dyes, dyshaemoglobins and other pigments. Anaesthesia 1991;46:291–295.
50 Am Assoc Resp Care (AARC): Clinical practice guideline: Exercise testing for evaluation of hypoxemia and/or desaturation. Respir Care 1992;37:907–912.
51 Hansen JE, Sue DY, Wasserman K: Predicted values for clinical exercise testing. Am Rev Respir Dis 1984;129(suppl):S49–S55.
52 Lewis DA, Sietsema KE, Casaburi R, Wasserman K: Inaccuracy of non-invasive estimates of V_D/V_T in clinical exercise testing. Chest 1994;106:1476–1480.
53 Borg GAV: Psychophysical bases of perceived exertion. Med Sci Sports Exerc 1982;14:377–381.
54 Borg GAV: Perceived exertion as an indicator of somatic stress. Scan J Rehab Med 1970;2–3: 92–98.
55 Froelicher VF, Marcondes GD: Manual of Exercise Testing. St Louis, Mosby Year Book, 1989.
56 Zavala DC: Manual on Exercise Testing: A Training Handbook, ed 3. Iowa City, University of Iowa, 1993.
57 Pina IL, Balady GJ, Hanson P, Labovitz AJ, Madonna DW, Myers J: Guidelines for clinical exercise testing laboratories: A statement for healthcare professionals from the Committee on Exercise and Cardiac Rehabilitation, American Heart Association. Circulation 1995;91: 912–921.
58 American College of Obstetricians and Gynecologists Technical Bulletin: Exercise during pregnancy and the postpartum period. 1994; Number 189.
59 Mason RE, Likar I: Experimental and laboratory reports: A new system of multiple-lead exercise electrocardiography. Am Heart J 1966;71: 196–205.
60 Gamble P, McManus H, Jensen D, Froelicher V: A comparison of the standard 12-lead electrocardiogram to exercise electrode placements. Chest 1984;85:616–622.
61 Lollgen H, Ulmer H-V, Crean P (eds): Eur Heart Assoc Report of the Task Force Conference on Ergometry. Recommendations and standard guidelines for exercise testing. Eur Heart J 1988;9(suppl K):1–37.
62 Am College Card/Am Heart Assoc Guidelines for exercise testing: A report of the American College of Cardiology/American Heart Association Task Force on Practice Guidelines (Committee on Exercise Testing). J Am Coll Cardiol 1997;30:260–311.
63 Shephard RJ: Test of maximum oxygen intake: A critical review. Sports Med 1984;1:99–124.
64 Stuart RJ Jr, Ellestad MH: National Survey of exercise stress testing facilities. Chest 1980;77: 94–97.
65 Scherer D, Kaltenbach M: Frequency of life-threatening complications associated with stress testing. Dtsch Med Wochenschr 1979; 104:1161–1165.
66 American Heart Association: Exercise standards. A statement for healthcare professionals. Circulation 1995;91:580–615.
67 Myers J, Voodi L, Umann T, Froelicher VF: A survey of exercise testing: Methods, utilization, interpretation, and safety in the VAHCS. J Cardiopulm Rehab 2000;20:251–258.
68 Beck KC: Evaluating exercise capacity and airway function in the athlete; in Weiler JM (ed): Allergic and Respiratory Disease in Sports Medicine. New York, Marcel Dekker, 1997.
69 Freedman S: Sustained maximum voluntary ventilation. Resp Physiol 1970;8:230–244.
70 Hyatt RE: The interrelationships of pressure, flow and volume during various respiratory maneuvers in normal and emphysematous subjects. Am Rev Respir Dis 1961;83:676–683.
71 Olafsson S, Hyatt RE: Ventilatory mechanics and expiratory flow limitation during exercise in normal subjects. J Clin Invest 1969;48:564–573.
72 Klas JV, Dempsey JA: Voluntary versus reflex regulation of maximal exercise flow: Volume loops. Am Rev Respir Dis 1989;139:150–156.
73 Johnson BD, Beck KC, Zeballos RJ, Weisman IM: Advances in pulmonary laboratory testing. Chest 1999;116:1377–1387.
74 Johnson BD, Reddan WG, Seow KC, Dempsey JA: Mechanical constraints on exercise hyperpnea in a fit aging population. Am Rev Respir Dis 1991;143:968–977.
75 Babb TG: Ventilatory response to exercise in subjects breathing CO_2 or HeO_2. J Appl Physiol 1997;82:746–754.
76 Johnson BD, Saupe KW, Dempsey JA: Mechanical constraints on exercise hyperpnea in endurance athletes. J Appl Physiol 1992;73: 874–886.
77 Marciniuk DD, Watts R, Gallagher CG: Dead space loading and exercise limitation in patients with interstitial lung disease. Chest 1994; 105:183–189.
78 Marciniuk DD, Sridhar G, Clemens RE, Zintel TA, Gallagher CG: Lung volumes and expiratory flow limitation during exercise in interstitial lung disease. J Appl Physiol 1994;77:963–973.
79 Eltayara L, Becklake MR, Volta CA, Milic-Emili J: Relationship between chronic dyspnea and expiratory flow limitation in patients with chronic obstructive pulmonary disease. Am J Respir Crit Care Med 1996;154:1726–1734.
80 Mota S, Casn P, Drobnic F, Giner J, Ruiz O, Sanchis J, Milic-Emili J: Expiratory flow limitation during exercise in competition cyclists. J Appl Physiol 1999;86:611–616.
81 Koulouris NG, Dimopoulou I, Valta P, Finkelstein R, Cosio MG, Milic-Emili J: Detection of expiratory flow limitation during exercise in COPD patients. J Appl Physiol 1997;82:723–731.
82 Coates AL, Desmond KJ, Demizio D, Allen P, Beaudry PH: Sources of error in flow-volume curves: Effect of expired volume measured at the mouth vs. that measured in a body plethysmograph. Chest 1988;94:976–982.
83 Hyatt RE: Effort independence and forced expiratory flow. Chest 1980;77:246–248.
84 Rodarte JR: Detection of expiratory flow limitation during exercise in COPD patients (invited editorial). J Appl Physiol 1997;82:721–722.
85 Johnson BD, Scanlon PD, Beck KC: Regulation of ventilatory capacity during exercise in asthmatics. J Appl Physiol 1995;79:892–901.
86 Johnson BD, Weisman IM, Zeballos RJ, Beck KC: Emerging concepts in the evaluation of ventilatory limitation during exercise: The exercise tidal flow-volume loop. Chest 1999;116: 488–503.
87 Babb TG: Mechanical ventilatory constraints in aging, lung disease, and obesity: Perspective and brief review. Med Sci Sports Exerc 1999; 31(suppl):S12–S22.
88 Nordrehaug JE, Danielson R, Strangeland L, Rosland GA, Vik-Mo H: Respiratory gas exchange during treadmill exercise testing: Reproducibility and comparison of different exercise protocols: Technical notes. Scand J Clin Lab Invest 1991;51:655–658.
89 Cox NJM, Hendriks JCM, Binkhorst RA, Folgering HTM, van Herwaarden CLA: Reproducibility of incremental maximal cycle ergometer tests in patients with mild to moderate obstructive lung disease. Lung 1989;167:129–133.
90 Noseda A, Carpiaux JP, Prigogine T, Schmerber J: Lung function, maximum and submaximum exercise testing in COPD patients: Reproducibility over a long interval. Lung 1989; 167:247–257.
91 Owens MW, Kinasewitz GT, Strain DS: Evaluating the effects of chronic therapy in patients with irreversible air-flow obstruction. Am Rev Respir Dis 1986;134:935–937.
92 Meyer K, Westbrook S, Schwaibold M, Hajric R, Peters K, Roskamm H: Short-term reproducibility of cardiopulmonary measurements during exercise testing in patients with severe chronic heart failure. Am Heart J 1977;134: 20–26.

Kenneth C. Beck, PhD
Physiological Imaging Laboratory
Department of Radiology
University of Iowa Hospitals and Clinics
200 Hawkins Drive
Iowa City, IA 52242-1077 (USA)
Tel. +1 319 356 1381, Fax +1 319 356 1503
E-Mail kbeck@dpi.radiology.uiowa.edu

Weisman IM, Zeballos RJ (eds): Clinical Exercise Testing.
Prog Respir Res. Basel, Karger, 2002, vol 32, pp 60–71

Deconditioning, and Principles of Training

Thierry Troosters[a,b] Rik Gosselink[a,b] Marc Decramer[a,b]

[a]Respiratory Division and Respiratory Rehabilitation, University Hospital Gasthuisberg, Leuven,
[b]Faculty of Physical Education and Physiotherapy, Department of Rehabilitation Sciences,
Katholieke Universiteit Leuven, Belgium

Summary

Exercise capacity and muscle strength decline rapidly after onset of immobilization, bed rest or significant reduction in daily activities. The functional consequences of deconditioning are increased mortality and comorbidity risk. In patients with underlying chronic disease (like myocardial infarction, chronic obstructive pulmonary disease, congestive heart failure and renal failure), deconditioning has been associated with impaired prognosis, independently of the underlying primary disease process. Deconditioning is highly prevalent in elderly, where it is often catalyzed by sarcopenia, observed from the 6th to 7th decades on. The mechanisms of the rapid decline in skeletal muscle function with inactivity are yet not fully understood, but oxidative stress, suppression of insulin-like growth factor I and II and up-regulation of myostatin are currently suggested as key actors in the atrophy process. Because of the significant consequences of deconditioning, all efforts should be made to prevent and treat the onset, or further aggravation of the deconditioning process. Exercise training is a potent therapy for deconditioning. Training programs can consist of whole body exercise (endurance training) or resistance training, where isolated muscle groups are trained. It is widely accepted that exercise training is conducted at least 3 times weekly at high training intensity in order to improve exercise capacity and/or muscle strength. Special attention is needed for patients suffering from severe deconditioning or underlying illness. In these cases, more specific guidelines are proposed. The impact of both endurance and resistance training on the cardiovascular system and the skeletal muscle is impressive, and deconditioning is restored within weeks of adequate training. In order to prevent deconditioning, rather than to improve exercise performance, significantly less exercise is warranted. Once-weekly endurance training, or just few resistance exercises, may be sufficient to prevent deterioration of muscle function during periods of inactivity, or when formal training is ended. This is an important feature in the prevention of deconditioning and needs much more attention.

It is generally accepted that regular exercise improves functional capacity, prevents morbidity and positively influences survival [1]. Deconditioning results in significant morbidity and has been associated with compromised survival, and reduced quality of life. In a longitudinal study by Blair et al., who followed participants for 15 years [2], the least fit subjects had a threefold increased risk of dying compared to the most fit subjects. In a consecutive study the authors showed that subjects who improved their fitness over time reduced their relative risk for dying by approximately 50% [3]. The present chapter deals with both above-mentioned issues: deconditioning on the one hand, and exercise training as an important tool to treat deconditioning, and improve exercise performance on the other hand.

Reduction in exercise performance or skeletal muscle function may result from disease-specific processes, or may be the result of disuse, prolonged bed rest or sedentary lifestyle. For the purpose of this chapter we will refer to deconditioning as reduced exercise capacity and skeletal muscle function due to disuse (immobilization, bed rest,

Table 1. Summary of most important impacts of deconditioning, inactivity or bed rest on different organ systems (a list of review articles is added)

	Impact	Ref.
Cardiocirculatory system	Reduction in peak cardiac output, primarily through reduction of stroke volume Heart rate is increased at iso-work Plasma volume is reduced, as well as Hb content Orthostatic intolerance is present, probably as a consequence of cardiac atrophy and hypovolemia	129, 130, 5
Pulmonary system	Little impact on resting pulmonary function, reduced ventilatory efficiency	131, 132, 16
Endocrine system	Androgen levels decrease Insulin sensitivity decreases	133, 16
Skeletal	Bone loss, stiffness tendons	134
Central nervous system	Mental concentration impaired, sleep quality reduced	135

or sedentary lifestyle) in the absence of any underlying primary disease. The impact of specific diseases will be dealt with in other chapters. Skeletal muscle adaptations due to reduced activation (e.g. paralysis or motor neuron blockade) are beyond the scope of the present review. The focus of the present chapter will be on the skeletal muscles. However, the impact on different organ systems, and organ system responses, cannot be overlooked. Table 1 summarizes briefly the general impact of inactivity on the otherwise healthy body, along with a concise list of review papers dealing with the impact of inactivity on these specific organ systems.

Skeletal Muscle Abnormalities Associated with Deconditioning

In clinical practice, deconditioning is characterized by impaired functional status and reduced peak oxygen consumption [4]. In the classical study by Bengt Saltin et al. [4], the authors reported a reduction of 28% in VO_2peak after 20 days of bed rest. In a very recent follow-up study the authors suggest that 30 years of aging may have less impact on VO_2peak than 20 days of bed rest [5]. These data were later replicated by several other studies. The reduction in VO_2peak was reported to be related to the initial VO_2peak, and the duration of the bed rest [6]. Besides the reduction in peak exercise capacity, early onset of lactic acidosis [7–10] during incremental exercise testing has been reported. Typically the onset of lactate accumulation starts at a VO_2 less than 40% of the predicted maximal VO_2 [11]. After a period of deconditioning, the lactate threshold was reported to shift to lower workloads [12]. Muscle bioenergetics are impaired [13], due to significant reductions in β-hydroxyacyl-CoA dehydrogenase and citrate synthase, without changes in glycolytic enzyme activity. Conflicting data are reported on capillarization after relatively short-term (weeks to 3 months) immobilization or detraining [14, 15], but since exercise training increases capillarization, one may expect that long-term inactivity may reduce capillary density [16]. Although reduced peak exercise performance has been associated with reduced survival both in healthy subjects and patients with heart disease [17], consequences of deconditioning at submaximal exercise, and loss of skeletal muscle strength may be more relevant to the daily functioning.

Models of deconditioning using bed rest show rapid (within days to weeks) and impressive loss of skeletal muscle mass, a negative protein balance [18], accompanied by a disproportionately greater (≈30%) reduction in muscle strength [19, 20]. The latter has been attributed to the impaired maximal neural input (motor neuron recruitment) [20] resulting in a decreased ratio 'muscle strength to muscle cross-sectional area'. Reduction in specific tension of the muscle is evidenced by a significantly increased submaximal activation (EMG activity to elicit a torque of 100 nm) after bed rest. Even after a period as short as 10 days, these findings were observed (albeit less impressive) [21]. Occasionally, necrotic changes, cellular edema, extracellular mitochondria and disorganized myofibrils were reported after simulated microgravity, suggesting presence of myopathic changes besides atrophy [14].

After 42 days of bed rest, Ferretti et al. [22] observed a 16% reduction in peak oxygen consumption. These authors studied comprehensively all factors contributing to

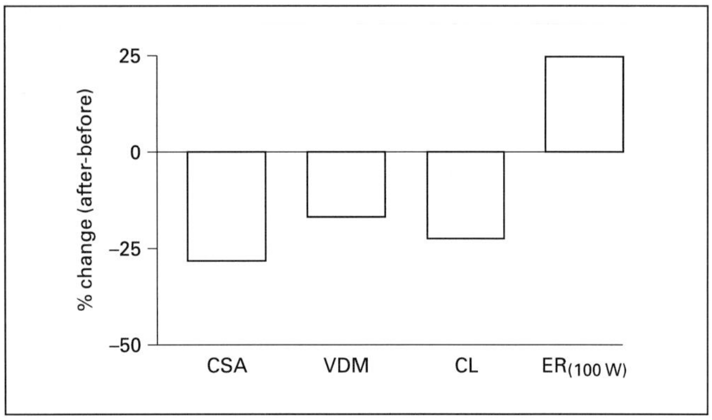

Fig. 1. Changes after 37 days of bed rest in healthy volunteers in (1) cross-sectional area of the thigh (CSA), (2) volume density of total mitochondria (VDM), (3) total capillary length (CL) in an identical muscle slice from [22] and (4) extraction ratio at iso (submaximal) work rate (100 W) ($ER_{(100\ W)}$) from the same study, published in Ferretti et al. [138].

the loss in peak VO_2. Figure 1 summarizes some of the important consequences of bed rest on the skeletal muscle, which contribute significantly to the reduced peak VO_2. Besides the important decrease in peak cardiac output, the authors found a reduced oxidative capacity of the limb muscles, and a reduced extraction of oxygen at isowork rate. It is noteworthy that in human muscle biopsies taken after bed rest, atrophy is consistently observed in all muscle fibers of the m. quadriceps [20], whereas in animal experiments atrophy is predominantly confined to type I (oxidative fibers). The changes seen in the muscle have been associated to the unloading of the muscle. Indeed, bed rest itself did not result in changes in the deltoid muscle [23], a muscle which remains functional during these experiments. It is generally accepted that the abnormalities observed after bed rest, are more most expressed in weight-bearing (antigravity) muscles [24].

Mechanisms of Deconditioning Induced Atrophy

The mechanisms that underlie the muscle atrophy are far from unraveled. Inactivity seems to be devastating to the muscle. Muscle wasting in humans starts almost immediately after application of bed rest [25]. It is important, however, that the alterations in the signaling process, detected at the mRNA levels, are often more impressive than the result at the protein level [26, 27]. Although decreased protein synthesis is probably the most important contributor to the negative protein balance [18, 28, 29], studies trying to stimulate protein synthesis by administrating anabolic hormone during hindlimb suspension [30] or bed rest [31] failed to show any effect on the atrophy. Protein balance, however, was better preserved by anabolic hormone administration, but there were no benefits in terms of muscle strength or function. These findings indicate that the impact of the mechanical stimulation of the muscle cannot be replaced by increasing protein synthesis alone. It has been suggested that increased oxidative stress induced by the inactivity may play a role [32], since administration of antioxidant vitamin E significantly counteracts the atrophy observed after immobilization of rat hindlimb [33]. Although appealing, oxidative stress alone cannot explain the processes related to muscle deconditioning and muscle wasting. Other mechanisms, such as up-regulation of myostatin, a promoter of muscle atrophy, and down-regulation of insulin-like growth factor II, have been suggested in recent literature to explain the atrophy seen after 17 days of space flight [34]. Elevated growth differentiation factor (GDF)-8 or myostatin levels have indeed been associated to sarcopenia in elderly subjects and during hindlimb unloading [35]. Insulin-like growth factor administration onto previously immobilized muscle showed in older rat to increase the proliferation potential of satellite cells and reduced the immobilization-induced atrophy [36]. Insulin-like growth factor I, on the other hand, may potentially suppress proteolysis (and thus atrophy) via its interaction with the ubiquitin pathways [37, 38]. A last family of factors which may play a role in the deconditioning observed after immobilization or bed rest may be the myogenic regulatory factors (MRFs). These regulatory factors bind to the regulatory regions of certain muscle genes and activate their transcription. Loughna and Brownson [39] showed that MRF4 was dramatically down-regulated in the soleus muscle (weight-bearing, oxidative muscle) after hindlimb immobilization. This, however, was not observed in other muscles. Other muscle-specific regulatory factors such as MyoD and myogenin, seem to play a less dominant role in the atrophy seen after hindlimb suspension in animal models [40]. In a recent report the serial analysis of gene expression (SAGE) technique was used to accurately measure the expression of genes to evaluate the effect of immobilization on gene expression in rat hindlimb (gastrocnemius) muscle [41]. Among other interesting findings, these authors report up-regulated genes involved in proteolysis after immobilization, whereas those involved in protein elongation were down-regulated. A threefold decrease in genes expression involved in energy metabolism was observed. Since most of the mechanisms remain far from elucidated, further research should focus on the mechanisms involved in the etiology of the muscle atrophy seen after short and longer periods of skeletal muscle unloading. Further insight in the mechanisms of deconditioning could yield a first approach to prevent muscle wasting during periods of inactivity. This may significantly reduce inactivity-related morbidity and/or mortality.

Deconditioning in Clinical Practice

Transition from clean animal models and clinical experiments to clinical practice is a complex step. Indeed, deconditioning is seldom an isolated process. Often it is associated with aging, cytotoxic drugs [42, 43], chronic undernutrition (insufficient protein uptake), or chronic disease inducing inactivity. Aging is in the context of the present chapter of particular interest, since subjects, as they get older, tend to decrease their accustomed level of activity [44], especially if they are institutionalized [45]. A recent analysis of the available literature revealed that in elderly (>65–70 years) only 30% of the total daily energy expenditure resulted from activities [46]. Aging itself has been associated with sarcopenia, defined as the age-specific, unintentional, loss of skeletal muscle mass [47], leading to reductions in muscle strength [48], functional exercise capacity [49] and peak oxygen consumption [50, 51]. Moreover, skeletal muscle of elderly showed to have less mitochondrial density, and decreased oxidative capacity per mitchondrial volume [52]. Unlike inactivity, aging has been associated, in cross-sectional studies, with predominantly fiber type II atrophy. In a recent longitudinal study, however, type I fiber proportion was significantly reduced after 10 years of follow-up [48], and a reduction of capillary to fiber ratio was observed. Aging is – as inactivity – associated with reduced satellite cell proliferation in humans [53], which has been suggested as an important step in the age-associated sarcopenia [36]. Interestingly, it was reported recently that aging is associated with increased amount of genetic point mutations, a phenomenon particularly present in the skeletal muscle [54]. Moreover, aging showed to be associated with significant denervation of muscle fibers [55, 56], which may be another potential pathway for the development of sarcopenia. The latter two observations may indicate that the reduction in muscle function frequently observed in elderly subjects is not only related to reduction in activity, but may be promoted by the aging process itself.

Impact of Deconditioning in Chronic Disease

Patients suffering from a chronic disease have impaired exercise performance, which can be at least partially attributed to deconditioning. Patients with chronic heart failure or chronic obstructive pulmonary disease (COPD) accumulate inactivity with aging, and disease-specific factors such as tissue hypoxia, inflammation, excessive oxidative stress, associated with excessive cytokine release, and deleterious effects of cytotoxic drugs such as corticosteroids [57]. This complex interaction of different factors makes it difficult to distinguish between the derangement in the skeletal muscle due to deconditioning alone, and these induced by disease-specific problems. The latter may result in myopathy rather than atrophy of the skeletal muscle [57]. The combination of systemic inflammation, increased oxidative stress, age-compromised genetically affected muscle, may make the muscle of patients with chronic diseases particularly vulnerable to even short bouts of inactivity. Disregarding its etiology, it has been convincingly shown that skeletal muscle weakness is an important contributor to exercise intolerance in COPD [58], congestive heart failure [59, 60] and renal failure [61].

The consistent finding that relatively short (8 weeks) exercise training in moderate COPD restores – to a large extent – skeletal muscle bioenergetics [62], lactic threshold [63] and oxidative enzymes [64], favors the hypothesis that muscle abnormalities in chronic diseases such as COPD are the net result of deconditioning only. It is however important to indicate that skeletal muscle strength and CSA did improve after rehabilitation, but did not return to normal values [65–67]. In healthy subjects, training studies after previous deconditioning almost unanimously report full recovery of skeletal muscle derangements after few weeks of exercise training [19, 68]. This observation, in combination with the description of myopathic changes [57], and the observation of patients in whom the relative muscle strength (strength/CSA) was clearly below normal, suggest that deconditioning alone cannot explain the abnormalities observed in the skeletal muscle function observed in patients suffering from chronic diseases [69]. Moreover, in animal models of heart failure, inactivity itself has formally been excluded as a contributing factor [70]. In the clinical setting however, we feel that both inactivity and intrinsic disease-induced changes contribute to the skeletal abnormalities and may strongly interact leading to clearly abnormal skeletal muscle function.

Treatment for Deconditioning

Exercise training has shown to be a potent therapy to reverse the muscular changes induced by deconditioning. Improved physical condition as a result of exercise training can be expected, and, as mentioned before, is related to improved survival. Reversal of deconditioning in patients after myocardial infarction showed to be directly related to reduced mortality [71] and subjects who improved their activity status had significantly lower risk of dying [3].

In the following section of this chapter, general principles of exercise training programs are discussed along with their recognized effects in healthy (deconditioned) subjects. Aerobic training (endurance and interval) and strength (resistance) training will be discussed. It is important to consider that the reported effects of exercise training show a large variability. A highly standardized training program in healthy subjects (age 17–65, n = 481) reported a 17% increase in VO_2 peak, with a range of –5 to +57% change in VO_2peak after training. It is important to mention that this study did not find any race, gender or age effect when the improvements of exercise training were expressed as relative gain, compared to baseline (% initial). From the same prestigious HERITAGE study, a genetic predisposition to VO_2peak responses after training was found [72], accounting for 47% of the variability in training response. The authors report 2.5 times more variability between families than within families. Hence, when effects of exercise training are appreciated in individual patients, the intrinsic predisposition of a subject to present a training effect on the outcome used in the assessment (e.g. VO_2peak) should be considered. Therefore, a large group of genetically unrelated subjects is needed to evaluate the general effects of a given exercise training program. Small studies possibly including genetically related subjects can potentially be misleading. A second comment refers to the impact of exercise training on daily life activities. Exercise training has shown to improve indices of physical function, and quality of life in virtually all patient groups in whom exercise training is applied as a therapeutic, or preventive approach. Transfer to actually increasing measured daily life activities is not always guaranteed [73–76]. If the aim of a training program is to increase daily activities, special attention should be paid to the implementation of the physiologic gains in the everyday life. This should be a point of attention for the persons supervising the training program.

General Principles of Exercise Training

Training can aim at improving general cardiovascular fitness, including improvement in peak oxygen uptake and muscle oxidative capacity, and may add to the prevention of chronic diseases such as cardiovascular disease [77], type II diabetes and colon cancer [78]. To achieve these effects, typically whole body endurance exercise training is applied. When the aim of the training program is to improve skeletal muscle force, or muscle cross-sectional area, resistance training can be applied, involving small muscle groups. These two training types are discussed consecutively in the section below.

Aerobic Exercise

The American College for Sports Medicine (ACSM) recently reviewed the available literature on aerobic exercise training in healthy subjects [79], and subsequently made guidelines for exercise training in elderly [80]. Table 2 summarizes the generally accepted features of exercise training sessions in order to result in significant physiological training effects.

The above-mentioned guidelines aim at improving physical fitness of unfit but otherwise healthy subjects. Applying these guidelines will result in improvements in peak oxygen consumption. The ACSM acknowledges that lower exercise intensity showed to be enough to reduce risk for chronic degenerative diseases, and result in both quantity and quality of life benefits. Exercise training programs aiming at treatment or prevention of chronic diseases often apply somewhat different training strategies. Although the general principles remain the basis of these training programs, the ACSM has introduced specific guidelines for training in patients with coronary heart disease [81], hypertension [82], osteoporosis [83] and obesity weight control. Training programs which can be used in the treatment of COPD are reviewed in this book in the chapter 'The Importance of Exercise Training in Pulmonary Rehabilitation', and in a recent European Respiratory Society document [84]. Training programs in different diseases and frail elderly may successfully deviate from the above-mentioned guidelines when the aim of the training program is to improve function, activities of daily living and general well-being, without improving VO_2peak. In this case, lower exercise intensities or shorter training time is allowed. From a meta-analysis summarizing 34 training studies, Londeree [85] concluded that physiological benefits from exercise training are only obtained when training intensity is at or above the ventilatory (and probably lactic) threshold in healthy sedentary subjects. A study investigating the effect of different exercise intensities on exercise capacity suggested that the intensity threshold should be approximately 40% of the VO_2peak. In the same study, exercise training at 80% of peak VO_2 resulted in more impressive benefits in exercise tolerance [86].

Table 2. Summary of American College of Sports Medicine Guidelines for developing and maintaining cardiorespiratory and muscular fitness [79]

	Minimal requirement exercise training (ACSM recommendations)
Intensity	55–90% of HR_{max}; 40–85% of oxygen uptake reserve or heart rate reserve (see footnote)
Duration/session	20–60 min, continuous or intermittent
Frequency	3–5 days per week
Mode	Whole body exercises (cycling, walking ...)

The heart rate reserve is calculated as $HR_{peak} - HR_{rest}$. The training intensity is calculated by adding a percentage of this value to the resting HR. Hence training pulse rate = resting pulse rate + [0.4 – 0.85 × (maximum HR – resting HR)]. Suppose that the resting heart rate and peak heart rate at the end of an incremental exercise test in a 55 year-old man would be respectively 71 and 166 min^{-1}. A reasonable training pulse would be 71 + [0.7 × (166 – 71)] = 136 min^{-1}. Training intensity according to VO_2 reserve is done using essentially the same strategy.

The guidelines on training intensity summarized in table 2 only apply for subjects in whom peak exercise performance is limited by reaching the boundaries of the cardiocirculatory system. In these subjects the peak heart rate reaches the predicted maximum heart rate, and cardiac output levels at peak exercise [87]. In subjects limited in their exercise performance for other reasons (heart failure, ventilatory limitation, gas exchange in the lung, or in the skeletal muscle, or plain skeletal muscle weakness, including myopathies), these guidelines should be applied with caution. Heart rate may be unreliable as the only variable in the appraisal of the training intensity. It is important to point out that high training intensity is warranted, and feasible, in most chronic diseases in order to achieve physiologic benefits of endurance exercise training. The intensity should be high relative to the performance capacity of the patients. Generally a training intensity at or around 70% of VO_2peak is considered adequate, both in health and chronic disease like COPD. Since peak work rate may considerably vary with different incremental exercise testing approaches, exercise training at 70% of the VO_2 reserve (VO_2rest + [0.7 × (VO_2rest – VO_2peak)] rather than at 70% of peak work rate should be achieved to be methodologically correct [88]. It has been suggested that lactate production is necessary to obtain physiological effects of exercise training [89]. However, more recent studies consistently showed that high relative workloads were a prerequisite to achieve training effects, independently of the achieved blood lactate accumulation [90–93]. Patients with chronic disease, including COPD [62], and chronic heart failure [94], show reduced intramuscular pH, suggestive of intramuscular acidosis at low work rates. This, however, is not necessarily accompanied by increased systemic blood lactate levels, since the total amount of working muscle mass may still be very small. Hence patients with chronic diseases, unlike deconditioned, but otherwise healthy subjects may achieve significant benefits from endurance training in the absence of whole body blood lactate accumulation during training, provided that the intensity is high, relative to the maximal workload patients can achieve.

Table 3. Alternative tools that can be used to assure high training intensity in the absence of maximal incremental exercise data

	Threshold for adequate training intensity
Blood lactate levels	4–5 mEq
Gas exchange threshold (GET)	At or around GET or ventilatory threshold [136]
Symptoms	Ability to talk while doing exercise
Symptom scores (e.g. Borg ratings)	5–6 on 10-point scale [137]

Measurements of VO_2 during all exercise modalities used in a training program is in most exercise training settings not feasible in the clinical routine. Since appropriate training intensity is critical to achieve physiological benefits, other means of estimating training intensity should be used. Table 3 summarizes other tools that may be used to successfully target training intensity.

The training time should be minimally 20–30 min. Typically, endurance training consists of 30 min continuous exercise training, but recent studies support that in sedentary subjects, this duration of exercise can be spread over the day (e.g. three bouts of 10 min), with similar effectiveness [95].

Practical Implementation of Endurance Training. Endurance training is preferably done on equipment which involves large muscle mass (whole body ergometers). Amongst them treadmills, rowing machines, steppers or stair climbing, and bicycles are the most popular. Cycle ergometers have the advantage that workload can be controlled and adjusted easily. On a treadmill and stepper, the workload imposed is highly dependent on the body weight of the subject. Rowing devices engage a large amount of skeletal muscle, which may result in difficulties in applying appropriate workload to each individual muscle in elderly and severely impaired patients with chronic diseases. Training effects will be specific to the exercise involved in the training, although some transfer to other activities may be achieved [96]. Hence, when training is performed on a bicycle, training effects will be much larger when evaluated during incremental bicycle exercise [97]. In this context, training programs for patients and frail elderly should preferably integrate activities relevant to their daily life. Hence training programs consisting solely of cycling in elderly and patients with chronic disease may result in important physiologic benefits, while benefits towards increased activities of daily living may be limited. Walking and stepping exercises may be more appropriate in gaining ADL benefits. Whatever exercise modality (or combination of different modalities) is decided to be appropriate, supervising physiotherapists, or physicians should reassure adequate (high) training intensity for each session (see table 3).

Endurance Training: Impact on the Muscle. Aerobic exercise training, as described above, has been studied extensively, both in humans and animal models. This training modality showed to improve both cardiovascular performance and general muscle oxidative capacity [98]. The latter is underscored by the larger peak arterial-venous oxygen content difference, and by the shift of the point at which lactate accumulates in the blood to higher exercise intensity [85]. This effect is the net result of intra-muscle fiber and extra-muscle fiber adaptations to endurance training. An increased oxygen supply to the muscle (through increased cardiac output, increased capillary vascular bed, and increased capillary to muscle fiber contacts) matches the increased peak oxygen demand. The increased capacity of the skeletal muscle to deal with the available oxygen is the net result of increased number of mitochondria, increased oxidative activity of the existing mitochondria, increased number (and CSA) of oxidative (fiber I, IIa) muscle fibers. Peak muscle oxygen extraction ratio only increases by approximately 10% in healthy sedentary subjects starting an endurance exercise program, while peak muscle VO_2 increases by approximately 40%. This illustrates that the increase in oxygen supply, and the increase in oxygen demand are both important factors to result in an appreciable effect of endurance training [99]. Hence in order to achieve large benefits in VO_2peak as seen in healthy young subjects, the peak oxygen supply should be increased. This is achieved by increasing peak cardiac output, and peak alveolar ventilation. In situations where the alveolar ventilation cannot be increased (e.g. obstructive lung disease), or cardiac output is limited by the disease (e.g. heart failure), improvement in VO_2peak is limited. Submaximal exercise capacity and skeletal muscle performance may virtually normalize after exercise training [62, 100]. In many chronic diseases VO_2peak can thus not be used as a unique measure of skeletal muscle adaptations to exercise training.

Within the skeletal muscle fiber, endurance training typically increases oxidative enzyme content. In younger subjects however the latter seems to be the result of an augmented mitochondrial density after training [101], whereas in elderly it may be the result of restoring mitochondrial function without apparent changes in mitochondrial density [102, 103]. A recent report by Starritt et al. [104] suggested that citrate synthase activity was increased after as few as 5 days of endurance training in healthy, young subjects. Although research has focussed on the local effects of endurance training on the muscle, or on whole body responses to exercise, systemic effects of endurance training should not be excluded, especially in selected patient groups. Indeed, Linke et al. [105] showed correction of radial artery endothelial dysfunction after lower limb exercise training. Other 'unexpected' secondary beneficial effects of exercise training may be improved immune system responses after training [106]. The clinical importance, of these systemic benefits of endurance exercise training, merits further research.

Although the changes in the skeletal muscles after endurance training are described extensively, the precise mechanisms which form the basis of the observed processes are not yet fully understood. It remains unclear which of the acute responses to a single exercise bout are carried forward to result in the final training effect after repeated bouts of endurance exercise over weeks.

Resistance/Strength Training

Resistance training targets isolated muscle groups. The training load is adjusted to the maximal performance of the muscle rather than to the whole exercising body. Three modalities of resistance training can be applied. These are classically subdivided based upon the speed of the movement, and the resistance applied over the range of motion, as indicated in table 4.

For concentric exercises the intensity of the training is mostly determined by the number of contractions and the number of sets of contractions (e.g. three sets of 10 contractions). The resistance is expressed relative to the maximal resistance (the maximal load that can be displaced once over the full range of motion, 1 repetition maximum, 1RM). Training programs using few repetitions are typical strength training programs, whereas lifting relatively low percentages of 1RM with a high number of repetitions result in more endurance training.

Practical Implementation of Resistance Training. Weightlifting training was introduced by Captain Delorme in 1945 in an attempt to increase muscle strength in injured soldiers. Resistance training can be done using free weights. Alternatively, a device can be used where the movement is limited to one specific muscle group, and the weight is applied through a system of pulleys. In the latter setup both movement and weights can be elegantly controlled and adjusted. Training programs generally apply a load of 60–80% of the weight that can be lifted once over the full range of motion (1RM). From a review of the literature, McDonagh and Davies [107] concluded that to improve strength, a load of at least 66% of the 1RM was required, and had to be lifted at least 10 times. Higher workloads however resulted in significantly more training effect. Empirically most training programs use 20–30 repetitions.

More sophisticated isokinetic (constant contraction velocity) equipment has been described to do resistance training, but these apparatus are very costly. This limits the application of isokinetic resistance training in general clinical practice. In healthy but frail elderly subjects, resistance training was successfully applied using 80% of 1RM applied through a cheap cable pulley system. Exercise days were alternated by days of rest. This program increased strength and improved functional capacity in frail institutionalized elderly. A secondary analysis of the data of the women in this trial by Nelson et al. [108] showed that the training program improved dynamic balance and was an effective means of preserving bone mineral density in postmenopausal women. Hence resistance training may be a cheap and cost-effective training strategy, especially in the elderly [109].

Table 4. Modalities for muscle strength measurements and training modalities

Isometric	Movement speed: zero; resistance variable*
Concentric	Movement in the direction of the muscle contraction: muscle shortening
Free weights and barbells	Movement speed: free; movement resistance: variable*
Isokinetic equipment	Movement speed: constant; movement resistance: variable*
CAM devices	Movement speed: variable; movement resistance: constant
Eccentric	Movement in the opposite direction of the muscle contraction

* Frequently used in resistance training in the clinical setting.

Impact on the Muscle. Resistance training is thought to improve neural activation both through well-matched pre- and postsynaptic adaptation in the neuromuscular junction [110], enhanced neural facilitation and increased maximal motor unit discharge rates [87, 111]. These changes account for approximately 90% of the increase in skeletal muscle strength in the first days or weeks of a resistance training program, especially in elderly subjects [111]. When training is continued, skeletal muscle strength increases further through increases in muscle hypertrophy. It is well accepted that after a single bout of high-intensity resistance exercise both protein breakdown and synthesis are increased. The net protein balance, however, is reported to be positive for 2 days following the acute exercise bout [112]. The effect of resistance training on the protein balance is unaffected by age. This suggests that both elderly and young subjects may benefit from this form of exercise [113]. Protein synthesis could result from increased mRNA transcriptional activity, or the acute exercise-induced increase in mixed muscle protein synthetic rate could be mediated through posttranscriptional events [114]. This is probably due to an improved efficiency of mRNA translation after resistance exercise [115].

The functional effect of resistance training has historically been characterized as increase in muscle strength, without large crossover effects to peak oxygen consumption, and tasks requiring predominantly oxidative (type I, IIa fiber) muscle work. This is probably due to the fact that most original observations were done in young subjects undergoing periods of heavy resistance training [116, 117]. In young, healthy persons, the impact of resistance training on whole body oxygen uptake is negligible [118].

Whether these observations hold in elderly subjects is currently debated. Literature supports clear oxidative capacity changes in skeletal muscles after resistance training in the elderly [102, 103]. In the last decade, resistance training gained interest in the treatment of sarcopenia in frail elderly. Fiattarone et al. [45] convincingly showed that resistance training improved strength, gait speed and mobility in frail subjects in their eight decade. An interesting recent observation by Greiwe et al. [119] may add to our understanding of the efficiency that resistance training showed in counteracting sarcopenia. The latter authors showed that TNFα expression in skeletal muscle of frail elderly was dramatically reduced after a resistance training program. Since the cytokine TNFα is a potent inductor of muscle wasting, the observation by Greiwe et al. may explain why resistance training showed to be successful, especially in the frail elderly. In patients with chronic diseases such as heart failure and COPD, resistance training has been applied as a way to increase the training stimulus to skeletal muscles, when whole body exercise capacity is limited by ventilatory and/or cardiocirculatory factors at relatively low workload. In patients with heart failure, resistance training showed to increase peak oxygen uptake [120]. In patients with COPD, strength training improved whole body endurance [121]. The addition of strength training to a regular endurance training program showed to restore muscle strength and muscle cross-sectional area more than endurance training alone in these patients [122].

Prevention of Deconditioning and Maintaining Training Effects

Abrupt ending of an exercise training period results in rapid loss of the benefits gained from it, even if the subject returns to normal sedentary daily life (and thus remains more active than during bed rest) [118]. It is accepted that the volume of exercise necessary to maintain physical condition is appreciably less than the amount of exercise necessary to improve exercise capacity. It has been generally accepted that healthy subjects lose less muscle mass as they remain more physically active [123, 124]. In the context of immobilization or bed rest, resistance training is an attractive tool since this form of training is adaptable to bedside situations. Among the many illustrations available in current literature is the one by Akima et al. [125] who showed that 30 isometric leg press contractions were sufficient to prevent the atrophy seen after 20 days of bed rest. Muscle protein synthesis was maintained during bed rest when resistance training was associated every other day during bed rest [28]. Alterations in fiber type composition and fiber atrophy were prevented in this setting. Whether muscle weakness can be completely prevented using this approach is debated [28, 126]. On completion of exercise training programs, adequate strategies should be applied to prevent the loss of exercise training-induced benefits. Studies by Hickson et al. [127, 128] showed that reducing training frequency, without reducing training intensity may be adequate to maintain training effect. Hence once a week training at high (see above) training intensity seems to be appropriate.

References

1 Blair SN: 1993 C.H. McCloy Research Lecture: Physical activity, physical fitness, and health. Res Q Exerc Sport 1993;64:365–376.

2 Blair SN, Kohl HW III, Paffenbarger RS Jr, Clark DG, Cooper KH, Gibbons LW: Physical fitness and all-cause mortality. A prospective study of healthy men and women. JAMA 1989; 262:2395–2401.

3 Blair SN, Kohl HW III, Barlow CE, Paffenbarger RS Jr, Gibbons LW, Macera CA: Changes in physical fitness and all-cause mortality. A prospective study of healthy and unhealthy men. JAMA 1995;273:1093–1098.

4 Saltin B, Blomqvist CG, Mitchell JH, Johnson RL, Wildenthal K, Chapman CB: Response to exercise after bed rest and after training. Circulation 1968;38:1–78.

5 McGuire DK, Levine BD, Williamson JW, Snell PG, Blomqvist CG, Saltin B, Mitchell JH: A 30-year follow-up of the Dallas bedrest and training study. Effect of age on cardiovascular response to exercise. Circulation 2001;104: 1350–1357.

6 Convertino VA: Cardiovascular consequences of bed rest: Effect on maximal oxygen uptake. Med Sci Sports Exerc 1997;29:191–196.

7 Wasserman K, Whipp BJ: Exercise physiology in health and disease. Am Rev Respir Dis 1975;112:219–249.

8 Weisman IM, Zeballos RJ: An integrated approach to the interpretation of cardiopulmonary exercise testing. Clin Chest Med 1994;15: 421–445.

9 Coyle EF, Martin WH III, Bloomfield SA, Lowry OH, Holloszy JO: Effects of detraining on responses to submaximal exercise. J Appl Physiol 1985;59:853–859.

10 Convertino VA, Karst GM, Kirby CR, Goldwater DJ: Effect of simulated weightlessness on exercise-induced anaerobic threshold. Aviat Space Environ Med 1986;57:325–331.

11 Wasserman K, Hansen JE, Sue DJ, Whipp BJ, Casaburi R: Principles of Exercise Testing and Interpretation, ed 2. Philadelphia, Williams & Wilkins, 1994, p 479.

12 Karvonen J, Rauhala E, Chwalbinska-Moneta J: The effects of three months slalom training on physical performance capacity. J Sports Med Phys Fit 1985;25:194–197.

13 Tartaglia MC, Chen JT, Caramanos Z, Taivassalo T, Arnold DL, Argov Z: Muscle phosphorus magnetic resonance spectroscopy oxidative indices correlate with physical activity. Muscle Nerve 2000;23:175–181.

14 Hikida RS, Gollnick PD, Dudley GA, Convertino VA, Buchanan P: Structural and metabolic characteristics of human skeletal muscle following 30 days of simulated microgravity. Aviat Space Environ Med 1989;60:664–670.
15 Coyle EF, Martin WH III, Sinacore DR, Joyner MJ, Hagberg JM, Holloszy JO: Time course of loss of adaptations after stopping prolonged intense endurance training. J Appl Physiol 1984;57:1857–1864.
16 Mujika I, Padilla S: Cardiorespiratory and metabolic characteristics of detraining in humans. Med Sci Sports Exerc 2001;33:413–421.
17 Vanhees L, Schepers D, Fagard R: Comparison of maximum versus submaximum exercise testing in providing prognostic information after acute myocardial infarction and/or coronary artery bypass grafting. Am J Cardiol 1997; 80:257–262.
18 Ferrando AA, Lane HW, Stuart CA, Davis-Street J, Wolfe RR: Prolonged bed rest decreases skeletal muscle and whole body protein synthesis. Am J Physiol 1996;270:E627–E633.
19 Vandenborne K, Elliott MA, Walter GA, Abdus S, Okereke E, Shaffer M, Tahernia D, Esterhai JL: Longitudinal study of skeletal muscle adaptations during immobilization and rehabilitation. Muscle Nerve 1998;21:1006–1012.
20 Berg HE, Larsson L, Tesch PA: Lower limb skeletal muscle function after 6 weeks of bed rest. J Appl Physiol 1997;82:182–188.
21 Berg HE, Tesch PA: Changes in muscle function in response to 10 days of lower limb unloading in humans. Acta Physiol Scand 1996;157:63–70.
22 Ferretti G, Antonutto G, Denis C, Hoppeler H, Minetti AE, Narici MV, Desplanches D: The interplay of central and peripheral factors in limiting maximal O_2 consumption in man after prolonged bed rest. J Physiol 1997;501:677–686.
23 Desplanches D, Hoppeler H, Mayet MH, Denis C, Claassen H, Ferretti G: Effects of bedrest on deltoideus muscle morphology and enzymes. Acta Physiol Scand 1998;162:135–140.
24 Portero P, Vanhoutte C, Goubel F: Surface electromyogram power spectrum changes in human leg muscles following 4 weeks of simulated microgravity. Eur J Appl Physiol Occup Physiol 1996;73:340–345.
25 Ferrando AA, Stuart CA, Brunder DG, Hillman GR: Magnetic resonance imaging quantitation of changes in muscle volume during 7 days of strict bed rest. Aviat Space Environ Med 1995;66:976–981.
26 Andersen JL, Schiaffino S: Mismatch between myosin heavy chain mRNA and protein distribution in human skeletal muscle fibers. Am J Physiol 1997;272:C1881–C1889.
27 Andersen JL, Gruschy-Knudsen T, Sandri C, Larsson L, Schiaffino S: Bed rest increases the amount of mismatched fibers in human skeletal muscle. J Appl Physiol 1999;86:455–460.
28 Ferrando AA, Tipton KD, Bamman MM, Wolfe RR: Resistance exercise maintains skeletal muscle protein synthesis during bed rest. J Appl Physiol 1997;82:807–810.
29 Goldspink DF: The influence of immobilization and stretch on protein turnover of rat skeletal muscle. J Physiol 1977;264:267–282.
30 Bricout VA, Serrurier BD, Bigard AX, Guezennec CY: Effects of hindlimb suspension and androgen treatment on testosterone receptors in rat skeletal muscles. Eur J Appl Physiol Occup Physiol 1999;79:443–448.
31 Zachwieja JJ, Smith SR, Lovejoy JC, Rood JC, Windhauser MM, Bray GA: Testosterone administration preserves protein balance but not muscle strength during 28 days of bed rest. J Clin Endocrinol Metab 1999;84:207–212.
32 Oishi K, Yokoi M, Maekawa S, Sodeyama C, Shiraishi T, Kondo R, Kuriyama T, Machida K: Oxidative stress and haematological changes in immobilized rats. Acta Physiol Scand 1999;165:65–69.
33 Appell HJ, Duarte JA, Soares JM: Supplementation of vitamin E may attenuate skeletal muscle immobilization atrophy. Int J Sports Med 1997;18:157–160.
34 Lalani R, Bhasin S, Byhower F, Tarnuzzer R, Grant M, Shen R, Asa S, Ezzat S, Gonzalez-Cadavid NF: Myostatin and insulin-like growth factor-I and -II expression in the muscle of rats exposed to the microgravity environment of the NeuroLab space shuttle flight. J Endocrinol 2000;167:417–428.
35 Baldwin KM: Effect of space flight on the functional, biochemical, and metabolic properties of skeletal muscle. Med Sci Sports Exerc 1996; 28:983–987.
36 Chakravarthy MV, Davis BS, Booth FW: IGF-I restores satellite cell proliferative potential in immobilized old skeletal muscle. J Appl Physiol 2000;89:1365–1379.
37 Wing SS, Bedard N: Insulin-like growth factor I stimulates degradation of an mRNA transcript encoding the 14 kDa ubiquitin-conjugating enzyme. Biochem J 1996;319:455–461.
38 Wing SS, Banville D: 14-kDa ubiquitin-conjugating enzyme: Structure of the rat gene and regulation upon fasting and by insulin. Am J Physiol 1994;267:E39–E48.
39 Loughna PT, Brownson C: Two myogenic regulatory factor transcripts exhibit muscle-specific responses to disuse and passive stretch in adult rats. FEBS Lett 1996;390:304–306.
40 Mozdziak PE, Greaser ML, Schultz E: Myogenin, MyoD, and myosin heavy chain isoform expression following hindlimb suspension. Aviat Space Environ Med 1999;70:511–516.
41 St Amand J, Okamura K, Matsumoto K, Shimizu S, Sogawa Y: Characterization of control and immobilized skeletal muscle: An overview from genetic engineering. FASEB J 2001;15: 684–692.
42 Gayan-Ramirez G, Vanderhoydonc F, Verhoeven G, Decramer M: Acute treatment with corticosteroids decreases IGF-1 and IGF-2 expression in the rat diaphragm and gastrocnemius. Am J Respir Crit Care Med 1999;159:283–289.
43 Ferrando AA, Stuart CA, Sheffield-Moore M, Wolfe RR: Inactivity amplifies the catabolic response of skeletal muscle to cortisol. J Clin Endocrinol Metab 1999;84:3515–3521.
44 Bortz WM, Bortz WM: How fast do we age? Exercise performance over time as a biomarker. J Gerontol A Biol Sci Med Sci 1996;51: M223–M225.
45 Fiatarone MA, O'Neill EF, Doyle Ryan N, Clements KM, Solares GR, Nelson ME, Roberts SB, Kehayias JJ, Lipsitz LA, Evans WJ: Exercise training and nutritional supplementation for physical frailty in very elderly people. N Engl J Med 1994;330:1769–1775.
46 Westerterp KR: Daily physical activity and ageing. Curr Opin Clin Nutr Metab Care 2000; 3:485–488.
47 Moulias R, Meaume S, Raynaud-Simon A: Sarcopenia, hypermetabolism and aging. Z Gerontol Geriatr 1999;32:425–432.
48 Frontera WR, Hughes VA, Fielding RA, Fiatarone MA, Evans WJ, Roubenoff R: Aging of skeletal muscle: A 12-year longitudinal study. J Appl Physiol 2000;88:1321–1326.
49 Troosters T, Gosselink R, Decramer M: Six-minute walking distance in healthy elderly subjects. Eur Respir J 1999;14:270–274.
50 McClaran SR, Babcock MA, Pegelow DF, Reddan WG, Dempsey JA: Longitudinal effects of aging on lung function at rest and exercise in healthy active fit elderly adults. J Appl Physiol 1995;78:1957–1968.
51 Fleg JL, Lakatta EG: Role of muscle loss in the age-associated reduction in VO_2 max. J Appl Physiol 1988;65:1147–1151.
52 Conley KE, Jubrias SA, Esselman PC: Oxidative capacity and ageing in human muscle. J Physiol 2000;526:203–210.
53 Decary S, Mouly V, Hamida CB, Sautet A, Barbet JP, Butler-Browne GS: Replicative potential and telomere length in human skeletal muscle: implications for satellite cell-mediated gene therapy. Hum Gene Ther 1997;8:1429–1438.
54 Wang Y, Michikawa Y, Mallidis C, Bai Y, Woodhouse L, Yarasheski KE, Miller CA, Askanas V, Engel WK, Bhasin S, Attardi G: Muscle-specific mutations accumulate with aging in critical human mtDNA control sites for replication. Proc Natl Acad Sci USA 2001;98:4022–4027.
55 Brooks SV, Faulkner JA: Skeletal muscle weakness in old age: Underlying mechanisms. Med Sci Sports Exerc 1993;26:432–439.
56 Luff AR: Age-associate changes in the innervation of muscle fibers and changes in the mechanical properties of motor units. Ann NY Acad Sci 1998;854:92–101.
57 Decramer M, de Bock V, Dom R: Functional and histologic picture of steroid-induced myopathy in chronic obstructive pulmonary disease. Am J Respir Crit Care Med 1996;153: 1958–1964.
58 Gosselink R, Troosters T, Decramer M: Peripheral muscle weakness contributes to exercise limitation in COPD. Am J Respir Crit Care Med 1996;153:976–980.
59 Drexler H, Riede U, Munzel T: Alterations of skeletal muscle in chronic heart failure. Circulation 1992;85:1751–1759.

60 Magnusson G, Kaijser L, Rong H: Exercise capacity in heart failure: Relative importance of heart and skeletal muscle. Clin Physiol 1996; 16:183–195.
61 Diesel W, Emms M, Knight BK, Noakes TD, Swanepoel CR, van Zyl SR, Kaschula RO, Sinclair-Smith CC: Morphologic features of the myopathy associated with chronic renal failure. Am J Kidney Dis 1993;22:677–684.
62 Sala E, Roca J, Marrades RM, Alonso J, Gonzalez De Suso JM, Moreno A, Barbera JA, Nadal J, de Jover L, Rodriguez-Roisin R, Wagner PD: Effects of endurance training on skeletal muscle bioenergetics in chronic obstructive pulmonary disease. Am J Respir Crit Care Med 1999;159:1726–1734.
63 Casaburi R, Patessio A, Ioli F, Zanaboni S, Donner CF, Wasserman K: Reductions in exercise lactic acidosis and ventilation as a result of exercise training in patients with obstructive lung disease. Am Rev Respir Dis 1991;143:9–18.
64 Maltais F, LeBlanc P, Simard C, Jobin J, Berube C, Bruneau J, Carrier L, Belleau R: Skeletal muscle adaptation to endurance training in patients with chronic obstructive pulmonary disease. Am J Respir Crit Care Med 1996;154: 442–447.
65 Troosters T, Gosselink R, Decramer M: Short- and long-term effects of outpatient rehabilitation in patients with chronic obstructive pulmonary disease: A randomized trial. Am J Med 2000;109:207–212.
66 Bernard S, Whittom F, LeBlanc P, Jobin J, Belleau R, Berube C, Carrier G, Maltais F: Aerobic and strength training in patients with chronic obstructive pulmonary disease. Am J Respir Crit Care Med 1999;159:896–901.
67 O'Donnell DE, McGuire M, Samis L, Webb KA: General exercise training improves ventilatory and peripheral muscle strength and endurance in chronic airflow limitation. Am J Respir Crit Care Med 1998;157:1489–1497.
68 Hakkinen K, Alen M, Kallinen M, Newton RU, Kraemer WJ: Neuromuscular adaptation during prolonged strength training, detraining and re-strength-training in middle-aged and elderly people. Eur J Appl Physiol 2000;83:51–62.
69 Bernard S, LeBlanc P, Whittom F, Carrier G, Jobin J, Belleau R, Maltais F: Peripheral muscle weakness in patients with chronic obstructive pulmonary disease. Am J Respir Crit Care Med 1998;158:629–634.
70 Simonini A, Long CS, Dudley GA: Heart failure in rats causes changes in skeletal muscle morphology and gene expression that are not caused by inactivity. Circ Res 1996;79:128–136.
71 Vanhees L, Fagard R, Thijs L, Amery A: Prognostic value of training-induced change in peak exercise capacity in patients with myocardial infarcts and patients with coronary bypass surgery. Am J Cardiol 1995;76:1014–1019.
72 Bouchard C, Leon AS, Rao DC, Skinner JS, Wilmore JH: Familial aggregation of VO_2max response to exercise training: Results from the HERITAGE family study. J Appl Physiol 1999;87:1003–1008.
73 Gottlieb SS, Fisher ML, Freudenberger R, Robinson S, Zietowski G, Alves L, Krichten C, Vaitkevicus P, McCarter R: Effects of exercise training on peak performance and quality of life in congestive heart failure patients. J Card Fail 1999;5:188–194.
74 Meijer EP, Westerterp KR, Verstappen FT: Effect of exercise training on total daily physical activity in elderly humans. Eur J Appl Physiol Occup Physiol 1999;80:16–21.
75 Morio B, Montaurier C, Pickering G, Ritz P, Fellmann N, Coudert J, Beaufrere B, Vermorel M: Effects of 14 weeks of progressive endurance training on energy expenditure in elderly people. Br J Nutr 1998;80:511–519.
76 Van Etten LM, Westerterp KR, Verstappen FT, Boon BJ, Saris WH: Effect of an 18-week weight-training program on energy expenditure and physical activity. J Appl Physiol 1997;82: 298–304.
77 Surgeon General's report on physical activity and health. From the Centers for Disease Control and Prevention. JAMA 1996;276:522.
78 Booth FW, Gordon SE, Carlson CJ, Hamilton MT: Waging war on modern chronic diseases: Primary prevention through exercise biology. J Appl Physiol 2000;88:774–787.
79 Pollock ML, Gaesser GA, Butcher JD, Després J, Dishman RK, Franklin BA, Garber CE: Position stand: The recommended quantity, and quality of exercise for developing and maintaining cardiorespiratory and muscular fitness, and flexibility in healthy adults. Med Sci Sports Exerc 1998;30.
80 Mazzeo RS, Cavanagh P, Evans WJ, Fiatarone MA, Hagberg J, McAuley E, Startzell J: Position stand ACSM: Exercise and physical activity for older adults. Med Sci Sports Exerc 1998; 30:992–1008.
81 American College of Sports Medicine position stand. Exercise for patients with coronary artery disease. Med Sci Sports Exerc 1994;26: i–v.
82 American College of Sports Medicine. Position Stand. Physical activity, physical fitness, and hypertension. Med Sci Sports Exerc 1993;25: i–x.
83 American College of Sports Medicine Position Stand. Exercise and physical activity for older adults. Med Sci Sports Exerc 1998;30:992–1008.
84 Donner CF, Decramer M: Pulmonary Rehabilitation. Eur Respir Monogr 2000;13:1–200.
85 Londeree BR: Effect of training on lactate/ventilatory thresholds: A meta-analysis. Med Sci Sports Exerc 1997;29:837–843.
86 Sady S, Katch V, Freedson P, Weltman A: Changes in metabolic acidosis: Evidence for an intensity threshold. J Sports Med Phys Fitness 1980;20:41–46.
87 McArdle WD, Katch FI, Katch VL: Exercise Physiology, Energy Nutrition and Human performance, ed 4. Baltimore, Williams & Wilkins, 1996, pp 1–849.
88 Debigare R, Maltais F, Mallet M, Casaburi R, LeBlanc P: Influence of work rate incremental rate on the exercise responses in patients with COPD. Med Sci Sports Exerc 2000;32:1365–1368.
89 Wasserman K, Sue DJ, Casaburi R, Moricca RB: Selection criteria for exercise training in pulmonary rehabilitation. Eur Respir J 1989; 7(suppl):604S–610S.
90 Punzal PA, Ries AL, Kaplan RW, Prewitt LM: Maximum intensity exercise training in patients with chronic obstructive pulmonary disease. Chest 1991;100:618–623.
91 Maltais F, LeBlanc P, Jobin J: Intensity of training and physiological adaptation in patients with chronic obstructive pulmonary disease. Am J Respir Crit Care Med 1997; 155:555–561.
92 Casaburi R, Porszasz J, Burns MR, Carithers ER, Chang RS, Cooper CB: Physiologic benefits of exercise training in rehabilitation of patients with severe chronic obstructive pulmonary disease. Am J Respir Crit Care Med 1997;155:1541–1551.
93 Troosters T, Gosselink R, Decramer M: Exercise training in COPD: How to distinguish responders from nonresponders. J Cardiopulm Rehabil 2001;21:10–17.
94 Van der Ent M, Jeneson JA, Remme WJ, Berger R, Ciampricotti R, Visser F: A noninvasive selective assessment of type I fibre mitochondrial function using ^{31}P-NMR spectroscopy. Evidence for impaired oxidative phosphorylation rate in skeletal muscle in patients with chronic heart failure. Eur Heart J 1998;19:124–131.
95 DeBusk RF, Stenestrand U, Sheehan M, Haskell WL: Training effects of long versus short bouts of exercise in healthy subjects. Am J Cardiol 1990;65:1010–1013.
96 Nieuwland W, Berkhuysen MA, Landsman ML, Lie KI, Rispens P: Training effects on peak VO_2, specific of the mode of movement, in rehabilitation of patients with coronary artery disease. Int J Sports Med 1998;19:358–363.
97 Pierce EF, Weltman A, Seip RL, Snead D: Effects of training specificity on the lactate threshold and VO_2 peak. Int J Sports Med 1990;11:267–272.
98 Saltin B: Physiological effects of physical conditioning. Med Sci Sports Exerc 1969;1:50–56.
99 Poole DC, Musch TI: Pulmonary and peripheral gas exchange during exercise; in Roca J, Rodriguez-Roisin R, Wagner PD (eds): Pulmonary and Peripheral Gas Exchange in Health and Disease, ed 1. New York, Dekker, 2000, pp 469–517.
100 Minotti JR, Johnson EC, Hudson TL, Zuroske G, Murata G, Fukushima E, Cagle TG, Chick TW, Massie BM, Icenogle MV: Skeletal muscle response to exercise training in congestive heart failure. J Clin Invest 1990; 86:751–758.
101 Hoppeler H, Howald H, Conley K, Lindstedt SL, Claassen H, Vock P, Weibel ER: Endurance training in humans: Aerobic capacity and structure of skeletal muscle. J Appl Physiol 1985;59:320–327.
102 Jubrias SA, Esselman PC, Price LB, Cress ME, Conley KE: Large energetic adaptations of elderly muscle to resistance and endurance training. J Appl Physiol 2001;90:1663–1670.

103 Orlander J, Aniansson A: Effect of physical training on skeletal muscle metabolism and ultrastructure in 70- to 75-year-old men. Acta Physiol Scand 1980;109:149–154.
104 Starritt EC, Angus D, Hargreaves M: Effect of short-term training on mitochondrial ATP production rate in human skeletal muscle. J Appl Physiol 1999;86:450–454.
105 Linke A, Schoene N, Gielen S, Hofer J, Erbs S, Schuler G, Hambrecht R: Endothelial dysfunction in patients with chronic heart failure: Systemic effects of lower-limb exercise training. J Am Coll Cardiol 2001;37:392–397.
106 Bruunsgaard H, Pedersen BK: Special feature for the Olympics: Effects of exercise on the immune system. Effects of exercise on the immune system in the elderly population. Immunol Cell Biol 2000;78:523–531.
107 McDonagh MJN, Davies CTM: Adaptive responses of mammalian skeletal muscle to exercise with high loads. Eur J Appl Physiol 1984;52:139–155.
108 Nelson ME, Fiatarone MA, Morganti CM, Trice I, Greenberg RA, Evans WJ: Effects of high-intensity strength training on multiple risk factors for osteoporotic fractures. A randomized controlled trial. JAMA 1994;272: 1909–1914.
109 Robertson MC, Devlin N, Gardner MM, Campbell AJ: Effectiveness and economic evaluation of a nurse delivered home exercise programme to prevent falls. 1. Randomised controlled trial. BMJ 2001;322:697–699.
110 Deschenes MR, Judelson DA, Kraemer WJ, Meskaitis VJ, Volek JS, Nindl BC, Harman FS, Deaver DR: Effects of resistance training on neuromuscular junction morphology. Muscle Nerve 2000;23:1576–1581.
111 Patten C, Kamen G, Rowland DM: Adaptations in maximal motor unit discharge rate to strength training in young and older adults. Muscle Nerve 2001;24:542–550.
112 Parise G, Yarasheski KE: The utility of resistance exercise training and amino acid supplementation for reversing age-associated decrements in muscle protein mass and function. Curr Opin Clin Nutr Metab Care 2000; 3:489–495.
113 Hasten DL, Pak-Loduca J, Obert KA, Yarasheski KE: Resistance exercise acutely increases MHC and mixed muscle protein synthesis rates in 78–84 and 23–32 year olds. Am J Physiol Endocrinol Metab 2000;278:E620–E626.
114 Chesley A, McDougall JD, Tarnopolski MA: Changes in human muscle protein synthesis after resistance exercise. J Appl Physiol 1992; 73:1383–1388.
115 Welle S, Bhatt K, Thompson C: Stimulation of myofibrillar synthesis by exercise is mediated by more efficient translation of mRNA. Am J Physiol Endocrinol Metab 1999;274:E673–E683.
116 Luthi JM, Howald H, Claassen H, Rosler K, Vock P, Hoppeler H: Structural changes in skeletal muscle tissue with heavy-resistance exercise. Int J Sports Med 1986;7:123–127.
117 Chilibeck P, Syrotuik DG, Bell GJ: The effect of strength training on estimates of mitochondrial density and distribution throughout muscle fibers. Eur J Appl Physiol 1999;80: 604–609.
118 LeMura LM, von Duvillard SP, Andreacci J, Klebez JM, Chelland SA, Russo J: Lipid and lipoprotein profiles, cardiovascular fitness, body composition, and diet during and after resistance, aerobic and combination training in young women. Eur J Appl Physiol 2000;82: 451–458.
119 Greiwe JS, Cheng B, Rubin DC, Yarasheski KE, Semenkovich CF: Resistance exercise decreases skeletal muscle tumor necrosis factor α in frail elderly humans. FASEB J 2001;15: 475–482.
120 Gordon A, Tyni-Lenne R, Jansson E, Jensen-Urstad M, Kaijser L: Beneficial effects of exercise training in heart failure patients with low cardiac output response to exercise – a comparison of two training models. J Intern Med 1999;246:175–182.
121 Simpson K, Killian K, McCartney N, Stubbing DG, Jones NL: Randomised controlled trial of weightlifting exercise in patients with chronic airflow limitation. Thorax 1992;47: 70–75.
122 Bernard S, Whittom F, LeBlanc P, Jobin J, Belleau R, Berube C, Carrier G, Maltais F: Aerobic and strength training in patients with chronic obstructive pulmonary disease. Am J Respir Crit Care Med 1999;159:896–901.
123 Rantanen T, Era P, Heikkinen E: Physical activity and the changes in maximal isometric strength in men and women from the age of 75 to 80 years. J Am Geriatr Soc 1997;45: 1439–1445.
124 Hughes VA, Frontera WR, Wood M, Evans WJ, Dallal GE, Roubenoff R, Fiatarone Singh MA: Longitudinal muscle strength changes in older adults: Influence of muscle mass, physical activity and health. J Gerontol A Biol Sci Med Sci 2001;56:B209–B217.
125 Akima H, Kubo K, Kanehisa H, Suzuki Y, Gunji A, Kukunaga T: Leg press resistance training during 20 days of 6° head down tilt bed rest prevents muscle deconditioning. Eur J Appl Physiol 2000;82:30–38.
126 Bamman MM, Clarke MSF, Feeback DL, Talmadge RJ, Stevens BR, Lieberman SA, Greenisen MC: Impact of resistance exercise during bed rest on skeletal muscle sarcopenia and myosin isoform distribution. J Appl Physiol 1998;84:157–163.
127 Hickson RC, Foster C, Pollock ML, Galassi TM, Rich S: Reduced training intensities and loss of aerobic power, endurance and cardiac growth. J Appl Physiol 1985;58:492–499.
128 Hickson RC, Rosenkoetter AM: Reduced training frequencies and maintenance of increased aerobic power. Med Sci Sports Exerc 1981;13:13–16.
129 Fortney S, Scneider VS, Greenleaf JF: The physiology of bed rest; in Fregley MJ, Blatteis CM (eds): Environmental Physiology. New York, Oxford University Press, 1996, pp 889–939.
130 Pawelczyk JA, Zuckerman JH, Blomqvist CG, Levine BD: Regulation of muscle sympathetic nerve activity after bed rest deconditioning. Am J Physiol Heart Circ Physiol 2001;280:H2230–H2239.
131 Linnarsson D: Pulmonary function and cardiopulmonary interactions at microgravity. Med Sci Sports Exerc 1996;28:S14–S17.
132 Teasell R, Dittmer DK: Complications of immobilization and bed rest. 2. Other complications. Can Fam Physician 1993;39:1440–1446.
133 Ferrando AA: Effects of inactivity and hormonal mediators on skeletal muscle during recovery from trauma. Curr Opin Clin Nutr Metab Care 2000;3:171–175.
134 Bikle DD, Halloran BP: The response of bone to unloading. J Bone Miner Metab 1999;17: 233–244.
135 DeRoshia CW, Greenleaf JE: Performance and mood-state parameters during 30-day 6° head-down bed rest with exercise training. Aviat Space Environ Med 1993;64:522–527.
136 Vallet G, Ahmaidi S, Serres I, Fabre C, Bourgouin D, Desplan J, Varray A, Prefaut C: Comparison of two training programmes in chronic airway limitation patients: Standardized versus individualized protocols. Eur Respir J 1997;10:114–122.
137 Horowitz MB, Littenberg B, Mahler DA: Dyspnea ratings for prescribing exercise intensity in patients with COPD. Chest 1996; 109:1169–1175.
138 Ferretti G, Girardis M, Moia C, Antonutto G: Effects of prolonged bed rest on cardiovascular oxygen transport during submaximal exercise in humans. Eur J Appl Physiol Occup Physiol 1998;78:398–402.

Marc Decramer, MD, PhD
Respiratory Division and
Respiratory Rehabilitation
University Hospital Gasthuisberg
Herestraat 49, B–3000 Leuven (Belgium)
Tel. +32 16 34 68 07, Fax +32 16 34 68 03
E-Mail marc.decramer@uz.kuleuven.ac.be

Weisman IM, Zeballos RJ (eds): Clinical Exercise Testing.
Prog Respir Res. Basel, Karger, 2002, vol 32, pp 72–80

Mechanisms and Measurement of Exertional Dyspnea

Donald A. Mahler[a] Gustavo Fierro-Carrion[a] John C. Baird[a–c]

[a]Dartmouth Medical School, Lebanon, N.H.;
[b]Psychological and Brain Sciences, Dartmouth College, Hanover, N.H., and
[c]Psychological Applications, Newport, N.H., USA

Summary

Dyspnea during physical activities is a common complaint of individuals with various respiratory diseases. One approach to examine and quantify this unpleasant sensation is to have the patient perform cardiopulmonary exercise testing (CPX) and provide ratings of breathlessness during exercise in the laboratory. Currently, the patient is instructed to give ratings of breathlessness each minute or increment of the CPX. However, computer technology has evolved to a point where a patient can provide continuous ratings throughout the exercise test. Investigations have demonstrated numerous clinical applications resulting from the measurement of dyspnea during CPX. As examples, bronchodilator therapy, pulmonary rehabilitation, oxygen, and bullectomy/volume reduction surgery have been shown to measurably reduce the severity of exertional dyspnea. Based on this extensive information, we recommend that the perception of breathlessness should be routinely measured as part of CPX in all symptomatic individuals.

Mechanisms of Exertional Dyspnea

What Is Exertional Dyspnea?

Dyspnea is a subjective experience of breathing discomfort comprised of qualitatively distinct sensations that can vary in intensity [1, 2]. The various phrases used to describe this sensation include 'breathlessness', 'shortness of breath', 'labored or difficult breathing' and 'an uncomfortable awareness of breathing' [3]. Clinicians as well as investigators generally believe that dyspnea is a sensory experience that is likely perceived similar to the perception of pain. In this article we review the possible mechanisms contributing to breathlessness based on a neurophysiological model. Then, we consider the principles of sensory psychophysics (stimulus → response relationship) that can be applied to the measurement of dyspnea during exercise testing. Information is provided on values obtained at peak exercise and as a continuum throughout the course of exercise. Finally, the clinical applications of measuring breathlessness as part of cardiopulmonary exercise testing (CPX) are considered in evaluating treatments such as bronchodilator therapy and pulmonary rehabilitation in patients with respiratory disease.

Neurophysiological Model

The mechanisms of dyspnea can be considered from a neurophysiological perspective [4]:

Receptor
↓
Afferent impulse
↓
Integration/processing in the CNS
↓
Efferent impulse
↓
Dyspnea

Receptors

The major receptor sites considered in the sensation of dyspnea include chemoreceptors, mechanoreceptors and lung receptors [3, 4].

Chemoreceptors

Hypoxemia stimulates respiration through its effects on the peripheral chemoreceptors, and may thereby cause breathlessness in patients with lung disease [2–4]. For example, the oxygen desaturation that may occur in many patients with chronic obstructive pulmonary disease (COPD), interstitial lung disease (ILD), and pulmonary vascular disease can stimulate the peripheral chemoreceptors and contribute to dyspnea. On the other hand, many patients with respiratory disease may experience dyspnea during exercise, but not develop hypoxemia.

Breathing carbon dioxide (CO_2) stimulates the central chemoreceptors and increases ventilation [4, 5]. An increase in dead space ventilation can develop during exertion in patients with severe respiratory impairment; alveolar ventilation may be therefore inadequate, resulting in hypercapnia. This enhances central respiratory drive and may cause breathlessness. Interestingly, patients with respiratory disease, especially COPD, may have hypercapnia at rest, but describe little if any dyspnea despite the increase in $PaCO_2$.

Taken as a whole, the foregoing suggests that chemoreceptors probably have limited contribution to the experience of exertional dyspnea.

Mechanoreceptors

There are a number of receptors distributed throughout the respiratory system that respond to mechanical stimuli.

Upper Airway Receptors. Clinical observations are supported by clinical research studies showing that upper airway and facial receptors modify the sensation of dyspnea [6]. Patients sometimes report a decrease in the intensity of their breathlessness when sitting by a fan or open window.

Chest Wall Receptors. The brain receives projections from a variety of receptors in the joints, tendons and muscles of the chest that influence ventilation. Mechanical stimuli, such as vibration, are known to activate these receptors, and may affect the sensation of breathlessness. For example, investigators have shown that in-phase chest wall vibration may reduce dyspnea in patients with COPD [7, 8].

Pulmonary Vascular Receptors. Receptors exist in the pulmonary arterial system that respond to increases in pressure and/or flow that result in increased ventilation. This process likely contributes to the sensation of dyspnea experienced by patients with pulmonary hypertension and acute pulmonary embolism.

Lung Receptors

The lung contains various types of receptors that transmit information to the central nervous system (CNS). Pulmonary stretch receptors in the airways respond to lung inflation; irritant receptors in the airway epithelium respond to a variety of mechanical and chemical stimuli and mediate bronchoconstriction, and C-fibers (unmyelinated nerve endings) located in the alveolar wall and blood vessels respond to interstitial congestion. Numerous studies suggest that afferent impulses from these vagal-mediated receptors may contribute to dyspnea [9–11]. For example, stimulation of vagal irritant receptors appears to intensify the sensation of breathlessness and may impart a sense of chest tightness or constriction.

Afferent Impulse

Various nerve pathways can transmit the information after stimulation of the receptor site(s) to the CNS. As mentioned earlier, the vagal nerve transmits afferent information from the lung receptors.

Integration/Processing in the CNS

Although afferent signals associated with breathlessness are received, integrated and processed in the CNS, little is actually known about these processes. However, it is believed that the motor cortex or brainstem respiratory neurons transmits a signal to the sensory cortex (i.e., corollary discharge) which may contribute to a 'sense of effort' to breathe [12]. This sensation increases whenever the central motor command is increased (e.g., the load placed on the respiratory muscles is increased), or whenever the respiratory muscles become weak or fatigued (e.g., prolonged increase in ventilation or dynamic hyperinflation which may occur with exercise).

Efferent Impulse

In response to afferent information, the CNS sends an efferent impulse via the phrenic nerve to the diaphragm and other respiratory muscles to increase respiration. How this impulse affects the level of ventilation, pattern of breathing, lung volume, flow rates, etc., is not completely understood. Clearly, the mechanisms of exertional dyspnea in patients with cardiorespiratory diseases are multifactorial and complex. Stimulation of one or more of the aforementioned receptors could potentially contribute to dyspnea at rest as well as during exercise. In 1963, Campbell and Howell [13] proposed the concept of length-tension inappropriateness as the cause of breathlessness. According to their theory, dyspnea arises from a disturbance in the relationship between the force or tension generated by the respiratory muscles and the resulting change in muscle length and lung volume. A current hypothesis proposes that a 'mismatch' occurs between afferent information to the CNS and the outgoing motor command to the respiratory muscles. In brief, this theory of 'neuroventilatory dissociation' suggests that the brain anticipates or expects a certain ventilatory response based on the associated afferent information [14]. Any dissociation or deviation from this system may cause and/or intensify the perception of dyspnea.

Measurement of Exertional Dyspnea

Psychophysical measurement pertains to the quantitative relationship between sensory experience and external stimulus events (outer psychophysics) as well as the relationship between sensory experience and physiological variables (inner psychophysics) [15, 16]. For example, the relationship between a person's breathlessness (sensory experience) and work performed in watts during cycle ergometry falls within the realm of outer psychophysics, whereas the relationship between breathlessness and oxygen consumption is considered a topic of inner psychophysics.

Another dichotomy in the field is the distinction between 'global' and 'local' processes. A global psychophysical method is employed when a person estimates the magnitude of breathlessness associated with each of a number of different magnitudes of a stimulus event (e.g., levels of work or oxygen consumption). A local method refers to a situation where the 'change' in breathlessness is the dependent variable associated with a change in stimulus magnitude. With global methods the investigator is interested in the quantitative relationship between breathlessness and the precipitating stimulus magnitude. Local methods focus on the amount of change in stimulus magnitude required to trigger a change in breathlessness for each of a number of different stimulus magnitudes [16]. Typically, these two aspects of breathlessness are measured using different procedures, though in the most recent applications breathlessness is continuously monitored over time and the patient provides ratings that can be analyzed from either perspectives.

The purposes of measuring exertional dyspnea include differentiating between people who have less dyspnea and those who have more dyspnea, and determining how dyspnea changes as a function of stimulus parameters and medical intervention.

What Is the Stimulus for Dyspnea during Exercise?

As described above, the exact mechanisms and precise stimuli for exertional breathlessness have not been completely identified. Nevertheless, for measurement purposes it is reasonable to consider that an exercise test performed on the cycle ergometer or treadmill (used to simulate a physical task) is a direct stimulus for both physiological and perceptual responses [17, 18]. During CPX the individual produces power, or generates work, which is a direct stimulus for both physiological and perceptual responses. At the present time it is reasonable to use such variables (e.g., power production, work, or oxygen consumption) as the putative 'stimulus' for provoking dyspnea during exertion [18–20].

Instruments Used to Measure Dyspnea during Exercise

Subjects generally provide ratings of dyspnea during exercise using a visual analog scale (VAS) or a category scale. In addition to rating the intensity of breathlessness, subjects can also be instructed to rate leg discomfort or chest pain if it is a predominant complaint.

VAS

The VAS is a continuous scale represented by either a vertical or horizontal line, usually 100 mm in length, with descriptors positioned as anchors [21]. For example, descriptors may be 'none' or 'no breathlessness' and 'very severe' or 'greatest breathlessness'. The subject places a mark on the VAS with a pen or can adjust a linear potentiometer (or the cursor on a computer screen) to indicate his/her level of dyspnea on the VAS displayed on a monitor.

0 to 10 category-ratio scale (CR-10)

The most widely used scale for enabling individuals to rate dyspnea during CPX is the category-ratio scale (CR-10) developed by Borg [22]. This scale consists of a vertical line labeled 0–10 with nonlinear spacing of verbal descriptors of severity corresponding to specific numbers that can be chosen by the subject to reflect presumed ratio properties of sensation or symptom intensity.

Table 1. Peak ratings of dyspnea on the CR-10 scale during cycle ergometry

Author (first author)	Ref.	Patients	Age (mean ± SD)	Diagnosis	Peak dyspnea rating
LeBlanc	45	18	NA	CRD	7.7 ± 2.0
Mahler	27	15	46 ± 16	Asthma	7.4 ± 1.9
Killian	26	97	64 ± 10	COPD	6 (median)
Dean	41	12	NA	COPD	8.5 ± 0.3
Mador	28	6	63 ± 6	COPD	6.8
O'Donnell	20	30	66 ± 1	COPD	5.3 ± 0.3
		30	69 ± 1	COPD	5.1 ± 0.3
Marciniuk	46	6	44 ± 15	ILD	4.0 ± 0.6
O'Donnell	33	12	64 ± 3	ILD	5.2 ± 1.4

NA = Not available; CRD = cardiorespiratory disease; COPD = chronic obstructive pulmonary disease.

Investigators have shown that the VAS and the CR-10 scale provide similar scores during incremental CPX in healthy subjects [23] and in patients with COPD [24]. However, the CR-10 scale has at least two advantages for measuring dyspnea during CPX. First, the presence of descriptors on the CR-10 scale permits comparisons among individuals under the assumption that the verbal descriptors on the scale correspond to the same subjective experience in different subjects. For example, two subjects may have different peak levels of cardiorespiratory fitness as measured by oxygen consumption, but nonetheless both may select the number '10' on the CR-10 scale as the proper indication of his or her subjective maximum breathlessness. Second, a numerical value or descriptor on the CR-10 scale may be easier to use as a dyspnea 'target' (as opposed to a measured length in mm on the VAS) for prescribing and monitoring exercise training [25].

Measurement of Dyspnea During Exercise

Peak Values

Initial investigations measured peak values of dyspnea on the VAS or the CR-10 scale during CPX. Although a wide range of values have been reported, both healthy individuals and patients with cardiorespiratory disease usually stop exercise on the cycle ergometer at submaximal (<100 mm on the VAS and <10 on the CR-10 scale) intensities of dyspnea and/or leg discomfort.

Most older subjects (both healthy individuals and patients with cardiorespiratory disease) reach 'symptom limitation' at ratings between 5 and 8 on the CR-10 scale (table 1). For example, Killian et al. [26] reported that 320 healthy subjects (63 ± 4 years) had a median dyspnea rating of 6 at peak exertion, with 25–75th percentile values of 5 and 9. Peak values for dyspnea were similar for patients with different severity of COPD. However, as expected, the peak power output on the cycle ergometer was almost twice as high in the healthy subjects compared with the patients with COPD. Mahler et al. [27] found that 15 patients with asthma (46 ± 4 years) gave a mean rating of 7.4 for dyspnea at peak exercise. Mador et al. [28] noted that 6 patients with COPD had mean ratings of 6.8 for 'breathing discomfort' on the CR-10 scale at maximal effort on the ergometer. However, O'Donnell et al. [20] observed somewhat lower values (5.1 ± 0.3) in 30 patients with COPD who stopped exercise because of breathlessness.

It is not clear why subjects terminate their exercise substantially below the maximum point on the scale inasmuch as they are instructed to exercise until they can no longer continue due to symptom limitation (i.e., reach their maximum breathlessness). Also, the existence of large individual variation in stopping points found in some studies brings into question the assumption that subjects all interpret the 'maximum' descriptor in the same manner.

An additional consideration during CPX is the determination of which symptom is more 'limiting' in the performance of an exercise task. It is generally believed that healthy individuals are more often limited by leg discomfort and/or general fatigue than by breathlessness. Of 40 patients with obstructive airway disease studied by Mahler and Harver [29], 18 patients noted higher ratings for 'leg fatigue' than for dyspnea, 14 reported dyspnea as the major symptom, and the remaining 8 patients indicated that leg fatigue and dyspnea were equal in intensity. Of 578 patients studied by Hamilton et al. [30], 265 (46%)

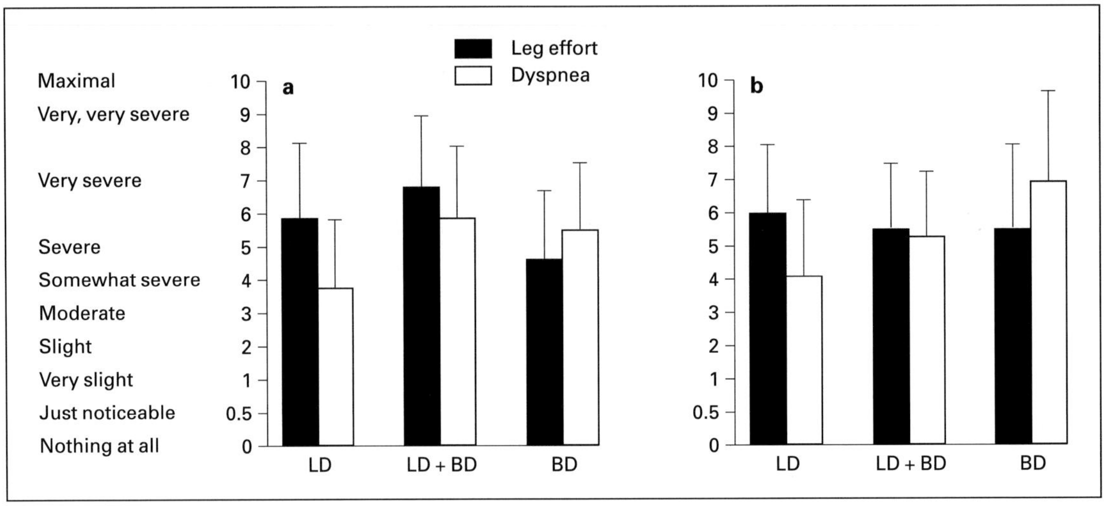

Fig. 1. Intensities of leg effort and dyspnea at peak exercise in patients with cardiac disease (**a**) and with pulmonary disease (**b**). LD = Leg discomfort; BD = breathing discomfort [from 32, with permission].

rated leg effort greater than dyspnea, 222 (38%) rated the intensity of leg effort and dyspnea as equal, and 91 (16%) rated the intensity of dyspnea greater than leg effort. Figure 1 shows the subjective ratings of leg effort and dyspnea at peak exercise in patients with a pulmonary diagnosis (n = 85) and with a cardiac diagnosis (n = 111) [30].

Together, these data suggest that healthy individuals and patients with lung disease experience similar intensities for dyspnea and for leg discomfort at peak exercise. Furthermore, either symptom may actually be a perceptual limit to an individual's exercise capacity. However, in those patients with more severe airflow obstruction, dyspnea was more frequently reported as being limiting compared with leg discomfort [26].

Although subjects are typically reliable in providing dyspnea ratings at peak exercise when tested at different time periods [17], Belman et al. [31] found that 9 patients with COPD gave lower ratings of breathlessness on the CR-10 scale with successive tests over 10 days while performing treadmill walking.

Continuum of Dyspnea Ratings

Although data on peak values of symptoms are clinically useful, there are clearly limits to such information, particularly when evaluating the effect of an intervention. Consequently, the next step in the development of methods for obtaining breathlessness ratings was to instruct patients to give ratings throughout the CPX. The most frequently applied exercise protocols incorporate an increase in power output on the cycle ergometer each 1–2 min (incremental test) or by a continuous increase (ramp test). In this procedure, the subject is instructed to provide ratings typically each minute 'on cue' during the CPX. Thus, a series of discrete dyspnea ratings is obtained throughout exertion.

The most common approach to examine the breathlessness continuum has been to determine the slope and intercept of the stimulus → response relationship over a range of stimulus values [18, 19]. In general, the slope of the regression between dyspnea ratings and power is higher in patients with respiratory disease compared with healthy individuals (fig. 2, 3) [17, 32, 33].

Continuous Measurement Using a Computerized System

In 1993, Harty et al. [34] described the methodology and results of the continuous measurement of breathlessness during exercise. Six healthy subjects used a potentiometer to give their ratings on a VAS displayed on a monitor.

In 2001, Mahler et al. [35] reported on a continuous method in which subjects throughout exercise moved a computer mouse that controlled the length of a bar whose lower edge coincided with a value along the CR-10 scale to represent the current level of perceived dyspnea (fig. 4). This approach allows the subject to provide ratings *spontaneously* and *continuously* while performing the CPX without waiting for a cue or request from the examiner.

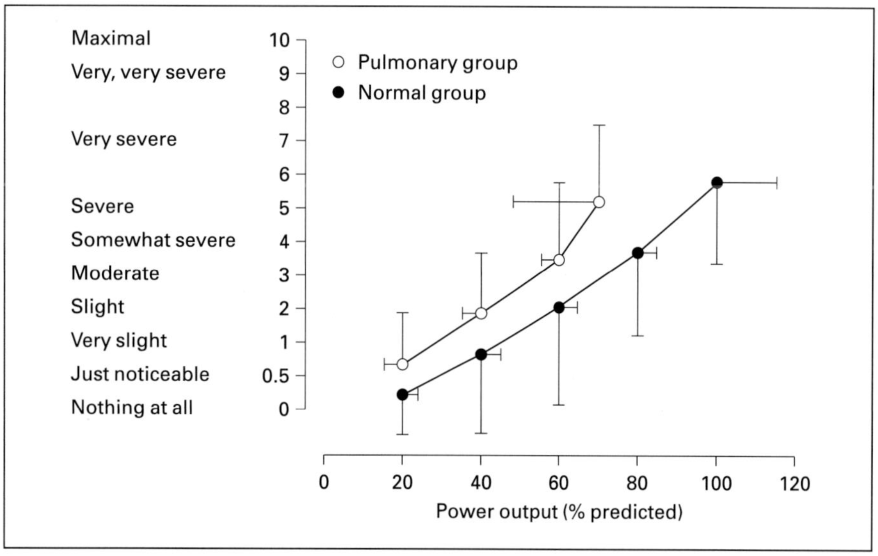

Fig. 2. Relationship between power output (% predicted) and dyspnea on the CR-10 scale in 85 patients with a pulmonary disease and 109 healthy normal individuals [from 32, with permission].

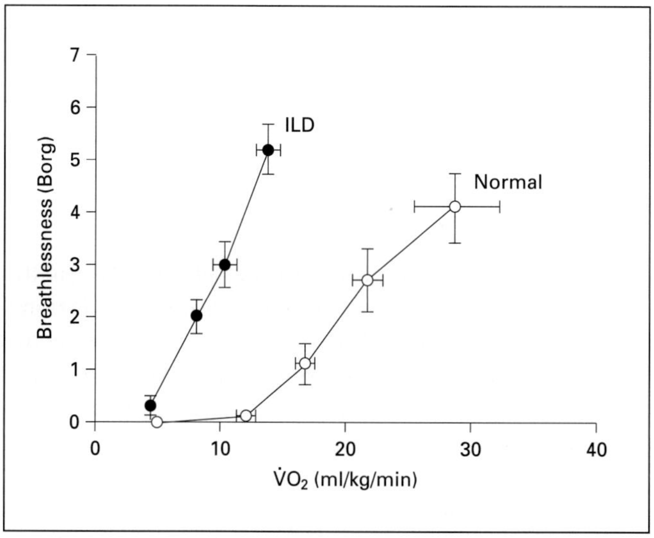

Fig. 3. Relationship between oxygen consumption (VO_2) and breathlessness on the CR-10 scale in 12 patients with interstitial lung disease (ILD) and 12 age-matched normal individuals [from 33, with permission].

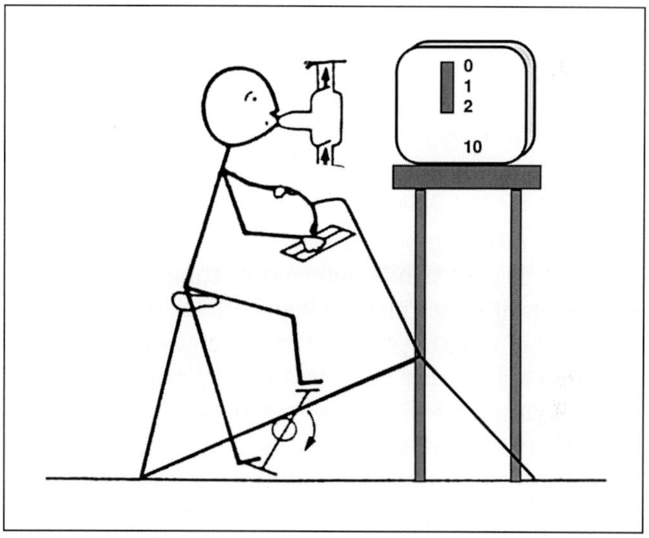

Fig. 4. Schematic diagram of subject pedaling on cycle ergometer with computerized system to enable the subject to provide continuous measurement of dyspnea during CPX. A mouse is positioned on a platform by the handlebars; the person can move the mouse in order to position the vertical bar to correspond to an intensity of dyspnea as measured on the CR-10 scale. The system is described in greater detail in Mahler et al. [35].

This method creates a more thorough mapping of the stimulus-response relationship because data can be recorded continuously throughout the course of exercise rather than only at discrete points in time selected by the investigator.

We compared the continuous method with the discrete method (rating each minute on 'cue') using the CR-10 scale presented on a computer screen. In healthy individuals and in patients with COPD, ratings of breathlessness using the continuous method were both reliable and comparable to those obtained by the discrete method during incremental CPX. The continuous method also was more responsive in showing the expected increase in dyspnea

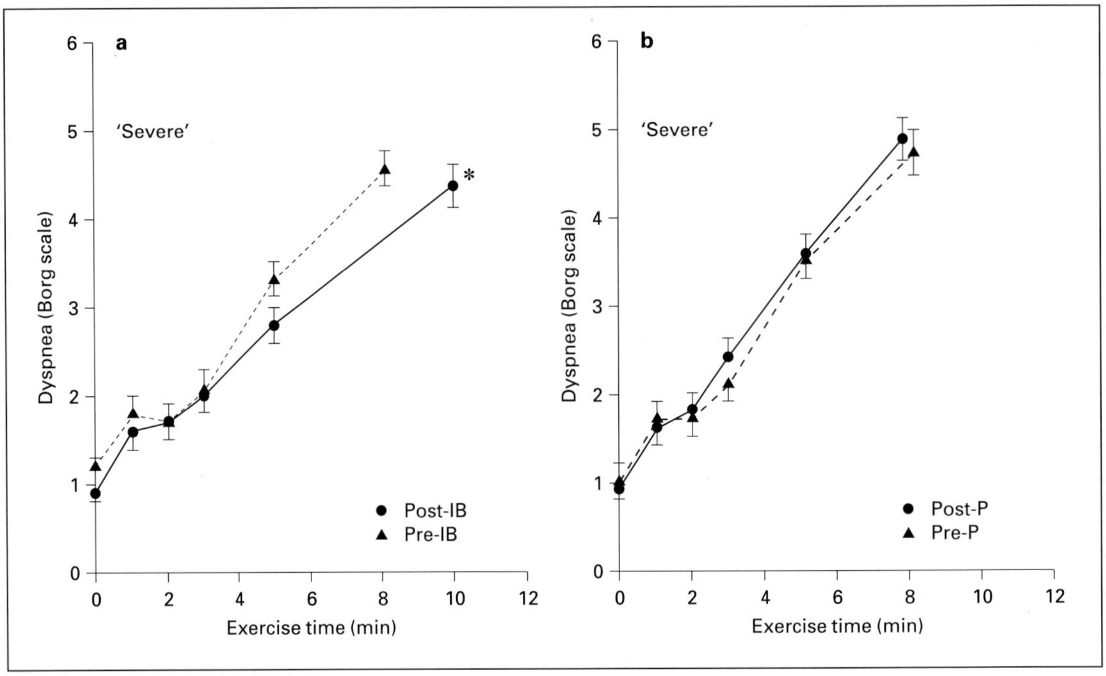

Fig. 5. Dyspnea ratings provided each minute during submaximal exercise at 50–60% of peak exercise capacity pre- and post-ipratropium bromide (IB) (**a**) and pre- and post-placebo (P) solution (**b**) in 29 patients with COPD. * $p < 0.05$ [from 36, with permission].

when an inspiratory load was added. Finally, patients with COPD gave significantly more ratings (mean = 157) with the continuous method than with the discrete method (mean = 5) during 5 min of an incremental CPX.

There are at least three important advantages of the continuous method for measuring dyspnea. First, the perception of breathlessness almost certainly changes throughout the entire course of exercise rather than only at arbitrary 1-min time intervals. Thus, the standard approach obtaining discrete ratings each minute may not accurately reflect the perceptual changes in dyspnea. Second, the continuous method enables subjects to provide substantially more dyspnea ratings compared with the discrete method. This is important because many patients with cardiopulmonary diseases may only be able to exercise for 4 or 5 min; consequently, only 4 or 5 dyspnea ratings can be obtained with the discrete method. Furthermore, statistical considerations become a concern when fitting a quantitative function to such a small number of data points. A third advantage of the continuous method is the ability to calculate 'just noticeable differences' (JNDs) and the Weber fraction which may offer new statistical indices for use in clinical measurement of dyspnea during CPX [35].

Clinical Applications

The following examples illustrate selected clinical applications in which patients provide ratings of exertional breathlessness during CPX. The exercise test simulates activities of daily living and provides the same standard stimulus for evaluating the efficacy of different treatments on the experience of dyspnea.

Bronchodilator Therapy

Mahler et al. [27] studied 15 patients with asthma during incremental CPX and examined responsiveness of the work → dyspnea relationship at a baseline visit and then after patients received a bronchodilator (metaproterenol) and a bronchoconstrictor (methacholine) prior to exercise testing. No differences were observed for the slope of work → dyspnea at the three testing periods; however, the intercept of work → dyspnea was significantly higher after bronchoconstriction. O'Donnell et al. [36] showed that dyspnea ratings were reduced with 500 μg of ipratropium bromide delivered via nebulizer as compared with placebo therapy during endurance exercise at 50–60% of peak work rate in 29 patients with COPD (fig. 5).

Pulmonary Rehabilitation

Studies have demonstrated the benefits of exercise training as part of a pulmonary rehabilitation program on reducing dyspnea during exercise [20, 37–39]. For example, Ries et al. [37] showed that breathlessness ratings on the CR-10 scale were significantly lower during endurance treadmill exercise in those with COPD who did exercise training compared with those who received only education. O'Donnell et al. [20] reported that the slope of oxygen consumption → breathlessness fell significantly in patients who performed 2.5 h of exercise training three times per week for 6 weeks compared with a control group. Similarly, Ramirez-Venegas et al. [38] demonstrated a reduction in the slope of power (W) → dyspnea relationship (pre: 0.09; post: 0.12) during incremental CPX after exercise training in 44 patients with COPD.

Oxygen

Oxygen therapy has been shown to reduce dyspnea ratings on the VAS and on the CR-10 scale during exercise [40, 41]. For example, O'Donnell et al. [40] observed that ratings of breathlessness on the CR-10 scale were significantly decreased in 11 patients with severe COPD when breathing 60% oxygen compared to when the same patients were breathing room air during incremental CPEX.

Bullectomy and Lung Volume Reduction Surgery

At least three different studies have reported lower ratings of breathlessness during exercise following bullectomy [42, 43] and after lung volume reduction surgery (LVRS) [44]. For example, Teramoto et al. [42] showed that the slope of VO_2-dyspnea was significantly decreased and the absolute threshold load of dyspnea (defined as the x-intercept of the regression line of VO_2-dyspnea relationship) was significantly increased after bullectomy in 8 patients with unilateral giant bulla. O'Donnell et al. [43] reported that ratings of breathlessness fell by 45% (from 6.1 ± 0.8 to 3.2 ± 0.7 on the CR-10 scale) at a standardized work rate (39% of predicted maximal work rate) during incremental exercise after unilateral bullectomy (n = 4) and after bullectomy plus ipsilateral lung reduction (n = 4). Finally, Martinez et al. [44] described reductions in dyspnea during exercise (from 7.1 ± 0.6 pre-LVRS to 3.5 ± 0.6 post-LVRS) in 12 patients with COPD selected for volume reduction surgery. The changes in dyspnea were significantly correlated with changes in end-expiratory lung volume (% predicted of total lung capacity).

References

1 O'Connell JM, Campbell AH: Respiratory mechanics in airways obstruction associated with inspiratory dyspnea. Thorax 1976;31:669–677.

2 Lane R, Cockcroft A, Adams L, Guz A: Arterial oxygen saturation and breathlessness in patients with chronic obstructive airways disease. Clin Sci 1987;72:693–698.

3 Swinburn CR, Wakefield JM, Jones PW: Relationship between ventilation and breathlessness during exercise in chronic obstructive airways disease is not altered by prevention of hypoxaemia. Clin Sci 1984;67:515–519.

4 Swinburn CR, Mould H, Stone TN, Corris PA, Gibson GJ: Symptomatic benefit of supplemental oxygen in hypoxemic patients with chronic lung disease. Am Rev Respir Dis 1991; 143:913–915.

5 Chonan T, Mulholland MB, Cherniack NS, Altose MD: Effects of voluntary constraining of thoracic displacement during hypercapnia. J Appl Physiol 1987;63:1822–1828.

6 Schwartzstein RM, Lahive K, Pope A, Weinberger SE, Weiss JW: Cold facial stimulation reduces breathlessness induced in normal subjects. Am Rev Respir Dis 1987;136:58–61.

7 Manning HL, Basner R, Ringler J, Rand C, Fencl V, Weinberger SE, Weiss JW, Schwartzstein RM: Effect of chest wall vibration on breathlessness in normal subjects. J Appl Physiol 1991;71:175–181.

8 Sibuya M, Yamada M, Kanamaru A, Tanaka K, Suzuki H, Noguchi E, Altose MD, Homma I: Effect of chest wall vibration on dyspnea in patients with chronic respiratory disease. Am J Respir Crit Care Med 1994;149:1235–1240.

9 Manning HL, Shea SA, Schwartzstein RM, Lansing RW, Brown R, Banzett RB: Reduced tidal volume increases 'air hunger' at fixed PCO_2 in ventilated quadriplegics. Respir Physiol 1992;90:19–30.

10 Davies SF, McQuaid KR, Iber C, McArthur CD, Path MJ, Beebe DS, Helseth HK: Extreme dyspnea from unilateral pulmonary venous obstruction. Demonstration of a vagal mechanism and relief by right vagotomy. Am Rev Respir Dis 1987;136:184–188.

11 Taguchi O, Kikuchi Y, Hida W, Iwase N, Satoh M, Chonan T, Takishima T: Effects of bronchoconstriction and external resistive loading on the sensation of dyspnea. J Appl Physiol 1991;71:2183–2190.

12 Killian KJ, Gandevia SC, Summer E, Campbell EJM: Effect of increased lung volume on perception of breathlessness. J Appl Physiol 1984;57:686–691.

13 Campbell EJM, Howell JBL: The sensation of breathlessness. Br Med Bull 1963;19:36–40.

14 O'Donnell DE: Exertional breathlessness in chronic respiratory disease; in Mahler DA (ed): Dyspnea. New York, Dekker, 1998, pp 97–147.

15 Baird JC, Noma E: Fundamentals of Scaling and Psychophysics. New York, Wiley Interscience, 1978.

16 Baird, JC: Sensory psychophysics; in Kotses H, Harver A (eds): Self-Management of Asthma. New York, Dekker, 1998, pp 231–267.

17 Mahler DA, Jones PW, Guyatt GH: Clinical measurement of dyspnea; in Mahler DA (ed): Dyspnea. New York, Dekker, 1998, pp 149–198.

18 Killian KJ: Th objective measure of breathlessness. Chest 1985;88(suppl):84S–90S.

19 Mahler DA: The measurement of dyspnea during exercise in patients with lung disease. Chest 1992;101(suppl):242S–247S.

20 O'Donnell DE, McGuire MA, Samis L, Webb KA: The impact of exercise reconditioning on breathlessness in severe chronic airflow limitation. Am J Respir Crit Care Med 1995;152: 2005–2013.

21 Gift AG: Visual analogue scales: Measurement of subjective phenomena. Nurs Res 1989;38: 286–288.
22 Borg GAV: Psychological bases of perceived exertion. Med Sci Sport Exerc 1982;14:377–381.
23 Wilson RC, Jones PW: A comparison of the visual analogue scale and modified Borg scale for the measurement of dyspnea during exercise. Clin Sci 1989;76:277–282.
24 Muza SR, Silverman MT, Gilmore GC, Hellerstein HK, Kelsen SG: Comparison of scales used to quantitate the sense of effort to breathe in patients with chronic obstructive pulmonary disease. Am Rev Respir Dis 1990;141:909–913.
25 Mejia R, Ward J, Lentine T, Mahler DA: Target dyspnea ratings predict expected oxygen consumption as well as target heart rate values. Am J Respir Crit Care Med 1999;159:1485–1489.
26 Killian KJ, LeBlanc P, Martin DH, Summers E, Jones NL, Campbell EJM: Exercise capacity and ventilatory, circulatory, and symptom limitation in patients with chronic airflow limitation. Am Rev Respir Dis 1992;146:935–940.
27 Mahler DA, Faryniarz K, Lentine T, Ward J, Olmstead E, O'Connor GT: Measurement of breathlessness during exercise in asthmatics: Predictor variables, reliability and resonsiveness. Am Rev Respir Dis 1991;144:39–44.
28 Mador MJ, Rodis A, Magalong VJ: Reproducibility of Borg scale measurements of dyspnea during exercise in patients with COPD. Chest 1995;107:1590–1597.
29 Mahler DA, Harver A: Prediction of peak oxygen consumption in obstructive airway disease. Med Sci Sports Exerc 1988;20:574–578.
30 Hamilton AL, Killian KJ, Summers E, Jones NL: Symptom intensity and subjective limitation to exercise in patients with cardiorespiratory disorders. Chest 1996;110:1255–1263.
31 Belman MJ, Brooks LR, Ross DJ, Mohsenifar Z: Variability of breathlessness measurement in patients with chronic obstructive pulmonary disease. Chest 1991;99:566–571.
32 Hamilton AL, Killian KJ, Summers E, Jones NL: Symptom intensity and subjective limitation to exercise in patients with cardiorespiratory disorders. Chest 1996;110:1255–1263.
33 O'Donnell DE, Chau LKL, Webb KA: Qualitative aspects of exertional dyspnea in patients with interstitial lung disease. J Appl Physiol 1998;84:2000–2009.
34 Harty HR, Heywood P, Adams L: Comparison between continuous and discrete measurements of breathlessness during exercise in normal subjects using a visual analogue scale. Clin Sci 1993;85:229–236.
35 Mahler DA, Mejia-Alfaro R, Ward J, Baird JC: Continuous measurement of breathlessness during exercise: Validity, reliability and responsiveness. J Appl Physiol 2001;90:2188–2196.
36 O'Donnell DE, Lam M, Webb KA: Spirometric correlates of improvement in exercise performance after anticholinergic therapy in chronic obstructive pulmonary disease. Am J Respir Crit Care Med 1999;160:542–549.
37 Ries AL, Kaplan RM, Limberg TM, Prewitt LM: Effects of pulmonary rehabilitation on physiologic and psychosocial outcomes in patients with chronic obstructive pulmonary disease. Ann Intern Med 1995;122:823–832.
38 Ramirez-Venegas A, Ward JL, Olmstead EM, Tosteson AN, Mahler DA: Effect of exercise training on dyspnea measures in patients with chronic obstructive pulmonary disease. J Cardiopulm Rehabil 1997;17:103–109.
39 Readon J, Awad E, Normandin E, Vale F, Clark B, ZuWallack RL: The effect of comprehensive outpatient pulmonary rehabilitation on dyspnea. Chest 1994;105:1046–1052.
40 O'Donnell DE, Douglas JB, Webb KA: Factors contributing to the relief of exertional breathlessness during hyperoxia in chronic airflow limitation. Am J Respir Crit Care Med 1997 155:530–535.
41 Dean NC, Brown JK, Himelman RB, Doherty JJ, Gold WM, Stulbarg MS: Oxygen may improve dyspnea and endurance in patients with chronic obstructive pulmonary disease and only mild hypoxemia. Am Rev Respir Dis 1992;146:941–945.
42 Teramoto S, Fukuchi Y, Nagase T, Matuse T, Shindo G, Orimo H: Quantitative assessment of dyspnea during exercise before and after bullectomy for giant bulla. Chest 1992;102:1362–1366.
43 O'Donnell DE, Webb KA, Bertley JC, Chau LKL, Conlan AA: Mechanisms of relief of exertional breathlessness following unilateral bullectomy and lung volume reduction surgery in emphysema. Chest 1996;110:18–27.
44 Martinez FJ, Montes de Oca M, Whyte RI, Stetz J, Gay SE, Celli BR: Lung-volume reduction improves dyspnea, dynamic hyperinflation and respiratory muscle function. Am J Respir Crit Care Med 1997;155:1984–1990.
45 LeBlanc P, Bowie DM, Summers E, Jones NL, Killian KJ: Breathlessness and exercise in patients with cardiorespiratory disease. Am Rev Respir Dis 1986;133:21–25.
46 Marciniuk DD, Watts RE, Gallagher CG: Reproducibility of incremental maximal cycle ergometer testing in patients with restrictive lung disease. Thorax 1993;48:894–898.

Donald A. Mahler, MD
Section of Pulmonary and Critical Care Medicine
Dartmouth-Hitchcock Medical Center
One Medical Center Drive
Lebanon, NH 03756-0001 (USA)
Tel. +1 603 650 5533, Fax +1 603 650 0580
E-Mail Donald.a.mahler@hitchcock.org

Weisman IM, Zeballos RJ (eds): Clinical Exercise Testing.
Prog Respir Res. Basel, Karger, 2002, vol 32, pp 81–88

Cardiopulmonary Exercise Testing in Unexplained Dyspnea

Steven E. Gay[a] Idelle M. Weisman[b] Kevin R. Flaherty[a] Fernando J. Martinez[a]

[a]University of Michigan Health System, Department of Internal Medicine, Division of Pulmonary and Critical Care Medicine, Ann Arbor, Mich., [b]Human Performance Laboratory, Department of Clinical Investigation, Pulmonary-Critical Care Service, William Beaumont Army Medical Center, El Paso, Tex., and Department of Medicine, Pulmonary-Critical Care Division, University of Texas Health Science Center at San Antonio, San Antonio, Tex., USA

Summary

The evaluation of unexplained dyspnea may be clarified and enhanced by evaluation with cardiopulmonary exercise testing. An organized, systematic and stepwise approach to the evaluation of dyspnea, beginning with the medical history and physical examination, and including specific laboratory, radiographic and physiologic testing, can help to clarify what can be a complex and potentially multifactorial problem. The utility of cardiopulmonary exercise testing lies in its sensitivity in differentiating between multiple etiologies of disease and its ability to study in greater detail the potential causes of disease and exercise limitation.

Dyspnea describes the sensation of breathlessness, feelings of air hunger, uncomfortable sensations of breathing, or awareness of respiratory distress [1–3]. A recent consensus statement from the American Thoracic Society defined dyspnea as '... a term used to characterize a subjective experience of breathing discomfort that consists of qualitatively distinct sensations that vary in intensity. The experience drives from interactions among multiple physiological, psychological, social, and environmental factors and may induce secondary physiological and behavioral responses' [4].

Breathlessness is an extremely common symptom; one large study identified dyspnea as the third most frequent complaint (following fatigue and back pain) from outpatients evaluated in medical clinics [5]. The causes of acute dyspnea can often be distinguished by history, clinical examination, chest radiography or physiologic testing [6–9]. However, the evaluation of dyspnea present for at least 1 month (chronic dyspnea) can be very challenging.

The etiologies of chronic dyspnea identified in three studies are listed in table 1. Airway disease (asthma or chronic obstructive pulmonary disease (COPD)) represents the majority of cases, followed by cardiovascular disease, interstitial lung disease (ILD), deconditioning, psychogenic disorders, gastroesophageal reflux, neuromuscular disease and pulmonary vascular disease. It should be appreciated that a referral bias is likely present in these studies which originated from pulmonary referral clinics. As such, physicians specializing in cardiovascular disease will likely identify a higher proportion of cardiovascular disease in their population of patients [10]. Similar data are lacking from a primary care setting.

The opinions or assertions contained herein are the private views of the authors and are not to be construed as official or as reflecting the views of the Department of the Army or the Department of Defense.

Table 1. Primary etiology of chronic dyspnea in three published studies and the number of patients evaluated with comprehensive cardiopulmonary exercise testing

Study	Patients n	Patients %	Number evaluated with CPET
Pratter et al. [15]			
Asthma	25	29	15
COPD	12	14	
Interstitial lung disease	12	14	
Cardiomyopathy	9	11	
Upper airway	7	8	
Psychogenic	4	5	
Deconditioning	4	5	
Gastroesophageal reflux	3	4	
Extrapulmonary	3	4	
Miscellaneous	5	6	
DePaso et al. [31]			
Hyperventilation syndrome	14	19	15
Unexplained	14	19	
Asthma	12	17	
Cardiac disease	10	14	
Pulmonary vascular disease	4	6	
Interstitial lung disease	2	3	
Chronic obstructive disease	3	4	
Neuromuscular disease	3	4	
Gastroesophageal	3	4	
Thyroid disease	2	3	
Deconditioning	2	3	
Upper airway	2	3	
Miscellaneous	1	1	
Martinez et al. [33]			
Deconditioning	14	28	50
Asthma	12	24	
Psychogenic	9	18	
Cardiac disease	7	14	
Unexplained	7	14	
Interstitial lung disease	4	8	
Gastroesophageal reflux	1	2	
Miscellaneous	1	2	

Evaluation of Chronic Dyspnea

Several groups have suggested a stepwise approach to the evaluation of patients with unexplained exertional dyspnea [6, 11]. These approaches take the most common causes of dyspnea into consideration during the evaluation process. Table 2 enumerates such an approach; figure 1 illustrates an adaptation of these published recommendations [9].

Table 2. Potential sequence of diagnostic testing in the evaluation of chronic dyspnea

Step	Suggested diagnostic studies
Initial evaluation	History and physical examination Chest radiograph Electrocardiogram Laboratory studies Spirometry/diffusing capacity Arterial blood gas
Initial diagnostic testing	*Pulmonary function tests:* Lung volumes MVV Mouth respiratory pressures Bronchial provocation testing *Cardiopulmonary exercise testing* *Echocardiography*
Subsequent diagnostic testing	*Functional cardiac testing:* Exercise thallium Exercise radionuclide ventriculography Exercise echocardiography Cardiac catheterization *Pulmonary vascular evaluation:* Ventilation/perfusion lung scanning Pulmonary angiography *Pulmonary parenchymal evaluation:* High resolution computed tomography of chest Lung biopsy *Gastroesophageal reflux evaluation*

Initial Evaluation

Medical History and Physical Examination

Different descriptors of dyspnea exist in patients with various types of cardiopulmonary disease [12, 13]. Therefore an evaluation should always begin with a detailed history and physical examination. Interestingly, a preliminary report of 11 patients suggested that a 15-item questionnaire, which assessed dyspnea descriptors, may provide additional complementary information to the medical history [14]. The value of this form of evaluation in patients presenting with breathlessness requires further prospective validation.

The timing of symptoms should be sought from every patient. An acute onset of symptoms may suggest bronchoconstriction, pulmonary embolism, cardiac ischemia, or airway obstruction due to a foreign body or secretion. In contrast, chronic symptoms are more likely to reflect slowly progressive disorders such as COPD, congestive heart failure (CHF), or ILD. Precipitating factors such as body position may provide additional diagnostic clues.

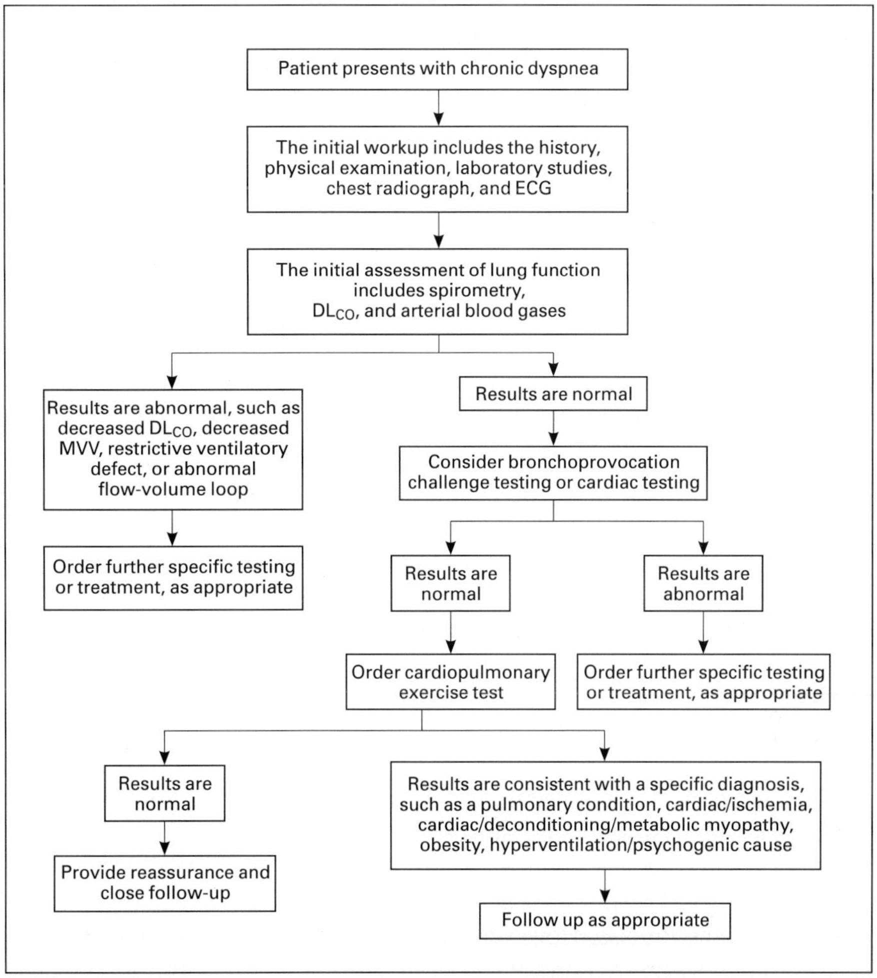

Fig. 1. Algorithm for the evaluation of chronic dyspnea [from 9, with permission].

Orthopnea is common in patients with CHF, severe COPD, ascites, obesity, anterior mediastinal masses and respiratory muscle weakness. Similarly, trepopnea (dyspnea in one lateral position but not in the other) can be seen with patients with unilateral lung disease, unilateral pleural effusion, and unilateral obstruction of the airway. Platypnea (dyspnea in the upright position, which may be relieved by recumbency) can be seen in patients with an intracardiac shunt, parenchymal lung shunts or hepatopulmonary syndrome [9].

Associated symptoms, such as cough, wheezing, or sputum production, can provide additional information in the evaluation process. Cough supports a diagnosis of airway disease, ILD, or gastroesophageal reflux disease. Similarly, wheezing suggests asthma, COPD, or CHF. In a prospective study of 100 patients evaluated for chronic breathlessness in a subspecialty clinic, Pratter et al. [15] reported the positive and negative predictive values for a history of wheezing and the diagnosis of asthma as 42 and 83% respectively. Past medical history, concurrent conditions, previous surgeries, social information (including cigarette smoking, previous and current occupation, family/living status), and medication history should also be reviewed. In the study of Pratter et al. [15] a smoking history had an excellent negative predictive value (100%) for excluding the diagnosis of COPD, however, only 20% of patients with a smoking history had COPD.

A detailed physical examination with special attention to the heart and lungs, is essential. Other organ systems pertinent to the history should also be investigated. After completing the history and physical examination, physicians may be able to generate a list of probable causes for chronic dyspnea, which can be used to direct diagnostic testing. For example, a strong history of cardiac risk factors or appropriate symptoms may lead to further, specific cardiac testing. In contrast, a strong suspicion of respiratory disease may lead to further pulmonary specific testing. This approach may allow for a rapid and cost-effective narrowing of the evaluation of chronic dyspnea.

Initial Diagnostic Testing

Laboratory/Radiographic Testing

Routine laboratory testing such as a complete blood count, thyroid function and renal testing, may be helpful in screening for basic systemic disorders (anemia, hypo-/hyperthyroidism, and metabolic acidosis) which can cause dyspnea [9]. Furthermore, the presence of a pneumothorax, hyperinflation, interstitial fibrosis, pulmonary edema, pulmonary artery enlargement, cardiomegaly, or diaphragm elevation can provide additional clues to the cause of chronic dyspnea. Although chest radiographs are helpful in determining the presence of certain abnormalities, the absence of changes should not rule out potential disorders. Mild ILD, for example, may not be seen on chest x-ray but may be suggested by pulmonary function testing [16].

Pulmonary Function Testing

The high prevalence of respiratory disease in patients presenting with dyspnea makes spirometry and flow-volume loop analysis essential during the initial work-up of chronic dyspnea [9]. Spirometry can be used to diagnose obstructive lung disease. However, the suggestion of restrictive lung disease requires further evaluation of lung volumes and respiratory muscle strength to differentiate ILD from respiratory muscle weakness. Evaluation of lung volumes by body plethysmography or by gas dilution techniques [17, 18] can give an accurate assessment of the presence/severity of restrictive lung disease. Similarly, the measurement of maximal inspiratory and maximal expiratory pressures is a useful tool to screen for respiratory muscle dysfunction. In fact, in patients with neuromuscular disease, the earliest physiologic abnormality is a decrease in respiratory pressure measured at the mouth [19, 20]. As such, syndromes of respiratory muscle weakness may be uncovered with this simple test. Unfortunately, in the setting of patients presenting with dyspnea, the sensitivity and specificity of this test is unknown. The measurement of maximum ventilatory ventilation can serve as an additional surrogate measurement of impaired respiratory muscle function [21]. Data from our institution have confirmed that an isolated decrement in MVV (compared to that expected for the measured $FEV_1 \times 40$) is seen in patients with mitochondrial myopathy presenting with unexplained exertional intolerance and involving the respiratory musculature [22]. The evaluation of a decreased MVV should also include assessment for upper airway abnormalities [23]. Important information can be obtained by examining the flow-volume curve to look for evidence of poor effort, vocal cord dysfunction, and extrathoracic airway obstruction [23]. Although a decreased MVV can be a useful clue to the etiology of chronic dyspnea, the effort dependence limits the diagnostic accuracy of this study.

Measurement of the DL_{CO} assesses the ability of the alveolar-arterial interface to transfer gas [24]. There is potential utility to the identification of an isolated reduction in DL_{CO} as this finding may be suggestive of several possible etiologies of dyspnea (see below) [24]. Interestingly, in an *asymptomatic* patient, an isolated reduction in DL_{CO} has not been shown to be clinically significant and does not demand further evaluation [25]. In addition, a decreased DL_{CO} may identify a group of patients more likely to demonstrate abnormal gas exchange during CPET (see below) [26].

Subsequent Diagnostic Testing

The results from the history, physical exam, and initial testing can be used to direct further testing if the etiology of the dyspnea remains elusive. For example, if the initial evaluation suggests a cardiac etiology, then further evaluation for CHF or cardiac ischemia is warranted. If, on the other hand, initial pulmonary function testing demonstrates an isolated decrease in DL_{CO}, further evaluation for pulmonary hypertension (echocardiography, right heart catheterization) [27], ILD with emphysema (high-resolution computed tomography) [28, 29] or imaging for recurrent pulmonary emboli can be pursued [30].

If the initial evaluation does not suggest a likely disorder, the age of the patient can be used to guide further testing. For a young patient, particularly if dyspnea is intermittent, there is a greater likelihood of asthma [31]. Methacholine challenge testing (MCT) allows for a sensitive, but not specific tool to evaluate for the presence of asthma [32]. MCT can also be used in older patients with a recent series identifying airway hyperreactivity in patients with a median age of 54 years [33].

In older individuals or those with potential cardiovascular risk factors, specific cardiac testing should be considered. In a recent evaluation of ambulatory and inpatient university-based family practice patients, the frequency of CHF increased with age [34]; 74% of the patients were older than 65 years. Importantly, 40% of the patients had preserved systolic function, a condition that was more commonly seen in women. This condition, diastolic heart failure, is more likely to be seen in older patients particularly in the presence of hypertension, diabetes mellitus, obesity or valvular heart disease [35]. A recent report has documented the presence of exertional pulmonary hypertension in a small series of patients evaluated for dyspnea [36]. A separate report described 103 consecutive patients evaluated in an emergency room setting with new onset dyspnea; 14 patients had pericardial effusions with 4 demonstrating clinically significant effusions (mean age 54 years) [37]. As such, some patients may be best evaluated with specific cardiac studies early in the evaluation process.

Cardiopulmonary Exercise Testing

Cardiopulmonary exercise testing (CPET) is a diagnostic modality that is ideally suited for the evaluation of unexplained dyspnea. Appropriate analysis of the patterns of response, as described elsewhere in this volume (see chapter 25), can suggest various disorders that can contribute to the sensation of breathlessness. Interestingly, in many series of unexplained dyspnea the utilization of CPET is infrequent. In 100 consecutive patients evaluated at a tertiary referral center for chronic dyspnea CPET was used in the evaluation of only 15 patients [15]. CPET was felt to be particularly useful in diagnosing psychogenic dyspnea (n = 4) and deconditioning (n = 4). In a subsequent study of 77 patients referred to a tertiary referral pulmonary clinic with unexplained dyspnea, CPET was utilized in 15 patients [31]. An abnormal study was noted in 4 patients but was only felt to be diagnostic or direct further evaluation in 2 of these subjects. [31] In a prospective study of 50 patients with unexplained dyspnea, Martinez et al. [33] examined the diagnostic value of CPET. Seven patients had a cardiac cause for their symptoms, 5 of whom demonstrated electrocardiographic changes of ischemia during CPET. In 17 patients, a pulmonary process was felt to be the cause of dyspnea; 9 of these patients demonstrated diagnostic CPETs (4 with exertional bronchospasm and 5 with gas exchange defects). The largest group of subjects (n = 24) demonstrated a pattern consistent with poor conditioning or occult cardiovascular disease. In 14 of these patients obesity and/or deconditioning were felt to be causal while 3 had cardiovascular disease and 7 had hyperactive airways disease confirmed with additional testing. Importantly, these investigators noted that CPET was useful in identifying a cardiac or pulmonary process, although it was insensitive in distinguishing deconditioning from a cardiac limitation. This latter group formed the largest group of patients. Sridhar et al. [38] described results of 100 randomly chosen CPETs; unexplained dyspnea was the indication for testing in 32 patients. The most frequent exercise pattern was 'inappropriate hyperventilation' (n = 14); 9 additional patients demonstrated a normal exercise response while 3 demonstrated ventilatory limitation, 2 demonstrated a cardiac limitation and 4 were felt to have deconditioning. The authors concluded that CPET provided information in many patients that negated the need for further testing.

Given the distribution of etiologies of dyspnea (table 1), CPET should be optimally suited to serve an important diagnostic role in the evaluation of this symptom. In fact, figure 2 demonstrates possible diagnostic categories derived from CPET in patients evaluated for dyspnea [11, 39]. Numerous chapters in this monograph provide specific data regarding the pattern of response in cardiac, respiratory, and myopathic disorders.

A review of the available literature suggests that a completely normal study does not exclude early disease but should serve to reassure the patient that a major disorder is not likely present [33, 38]. Most patients with psychogenic dyspnea will have a normal response to exercise although an abnormal pattern of ventilation may be instructive [11]. Figure 3 demonstrates an erratic pattern of respiratory flow generation during the course of a maximal CPET in a patient with psychogenic dyspnea. Similarly, a hyperventilation syndrome may be suggested during CPET [40], although this diagnosis is generally one of exclusion. Abnormal electrocardiographic tracings can suggest the presence of ischemic heart disease although other findings on CPET are nonspecific. One prospective study has demonstrated the similar response of patients with deconditioning and those with non-ischemic heart disease [33], therefore additional testing is likely indicated.

The diagnostic difficulty between diagnosing cardiovascular disease, deconditioning, and metabolic myopathies using CPET has been highlighted by recent data that confirm a similar hyperdynamic and hyperventilatory response in patients with abnormal peripheral muscle oxygen utilization [41, 42]. Patients with histologically or enzymatically confirmed mitochondrial disease can present with unexplained dyspnea and decreased maximal VO_2, a low anaerobic threshold and an abnormally steep heart rate response [22, 41–43]. Data from our institution confirm that metabolic myopathies represented 8.5% (28/331) of cases of unexplained exertional limitation evaluated in a tertiary specialty clinic over a 4-year period. Interestingly, these patients can demonstrate significant improvement in exercise capacity after pulmonary rehabilitation [44]. This finding has led some to sug-

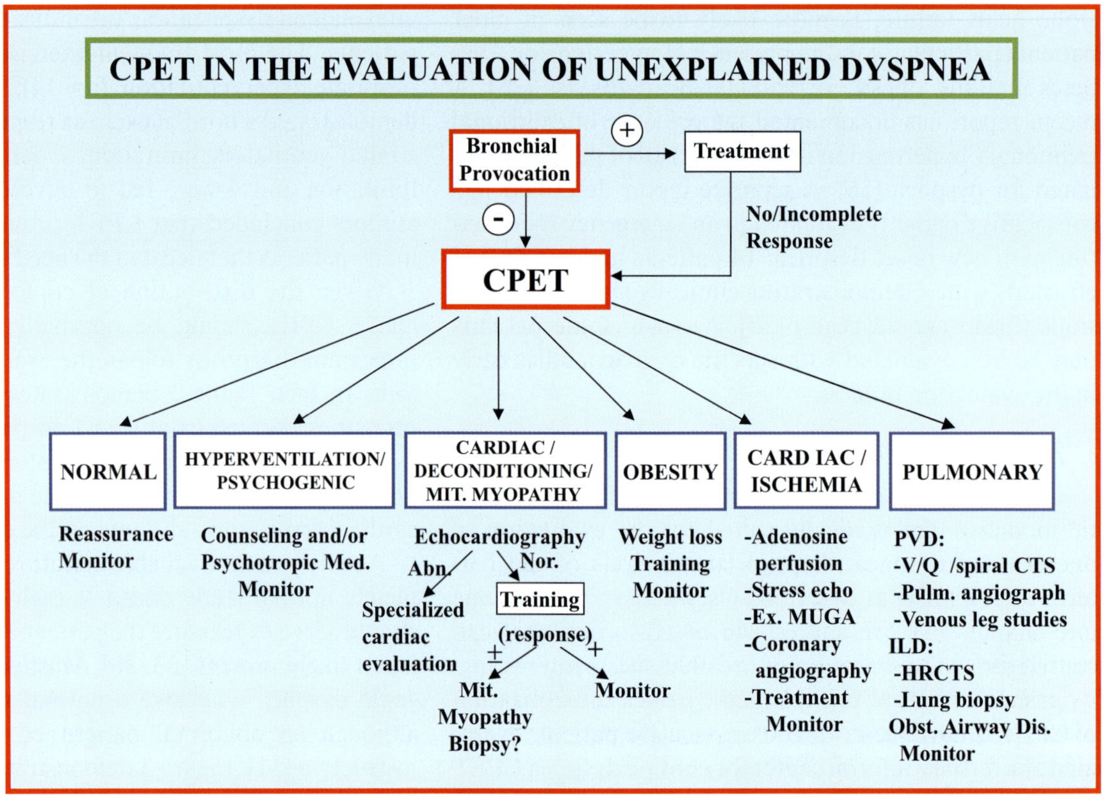

Fig. 2. Results from CPET which may help guide subsequent evaluation of unexplained dyspnea. CPET = Cardiopulmonary exercise test; ILD = interstitial lung disease; HRCTS = high-resolution computed tomography scan; PVD = pulmonary vascular disease; V/Q = ventilation/perfusion, +/– or incomplete resolution on the arm under treatment [from 39, with permission].

gest that an aggressive pulmonary rehabilitation program be considered in patients with suspected mitochondrial disease before muscle biopsy is performed [39]. Further data are required to address these evolving concepts.

CPET can be used to identify potential pulmonary disorders in patients presenting with dyspnea. Evaluation of potential pulmonary etiologies for unexplained dyspnea should include consideration of exercise-induced reactive airway disease, which may become apparent from measurement of flow volume loops during or after exercise, evaluation of gas exchange abnormalities from parenchymal lung disease and consideration of pulmonary hypertension manifest only during exercise. Measurement of arterial blood gases can provide useful information in identifying parenchymal lung disease [45, 46] or pulmonary vascular disease (pulmonary dead space (V_D/V_T) abnormality) [47]. Importantly, a decreased DL_{CO} appears to identify a group of patients more likely to demonstrate abnormal gas exchange during CPET [26]; those patients with a decreased DL_{CO} may be best assessed with collection of arterial blood samples during CPET.

Additional data collected during CPET can have important diagnostic significance. Measurement of pleural and diaphragmatic pressures can identify unexpected respiratory muscle dysfunction [48]. Serial spirometry after exercise may identify patients with exercise-induced bronchospasm, although the sensitivity of CPET in this setting appears to be less than other forms of bronchoprovocation testing [49, 50]. The addition of tidal flow volume loop analysis may improve diagnostic accuracy, although specific data are lacking [51]. Interestingly, examination of vocal cord function during exercise or flow-volume loops during and after exercise may identify patients with vocal cord dysfunction [52, 53]. A recent report identified vocal cord dysfunction in 5/33 young military personnel evaluated for exertional dyspnea [52].

As highlighted by the above studies, the utility of CPET in the evaluation of chronic dyspnea is decreased

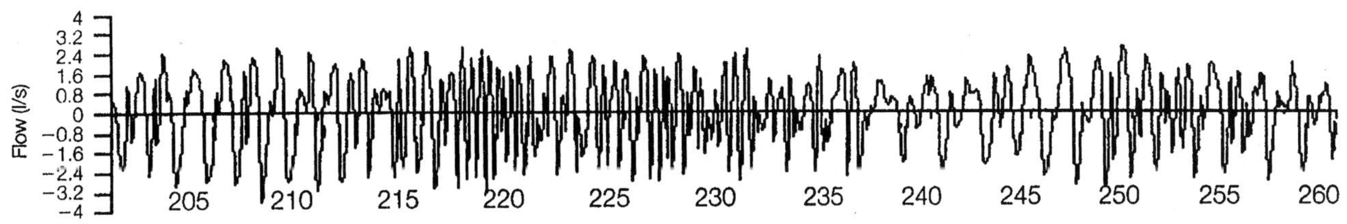

Fig. 3. Tidal inspiratory and expiratory flows during the final minute of a maximal cardiopulmonary exercise test demonstrate an erratic pattern of respiratory efforts. Further testing revealed no specific cardiopulmonary pathology and the patient's symptoms abated with psychotherapy. The most likely diagnosis was psychogenic dyspnea [from 9, with permission].

by its lack of specificity. Nonetheless, it can serve as a decision node in the overall evaluation of chronic dyspnea as outlined in figures 1 and 2. It is notable that figures 1 and 2 support a scheme in which bronchoprovocation testing precedes CPET in the evaluation of unexplained dyspnea, as it appears that bronchoprovocation testing is more sensitive than CPET in the diagnosis of hyperactive airways disease [50]. Importantly, as 10% of patients in some series [33] may have more than one diagnosis, both bronchoprovocation testing and CPET may be necessary in such scenarios (see case 1 in the chapter An Integrative Approach to the Interpretation of Cardiopulmonary Exercise Testing, pp 300–322). It is evident that further prospective study is required to better define the role of physiologic testing in the evaluation of unexplained dyspnea.

References

1 Wasserman K, Casaburi R: Dyspnea: Physiological and pathophysiological mechanisms. Annu Rev Med 1988;39:503–515.
2 Mahler DA, Harver A, Lentine T, Scott JA, Beck K, Schwartzstein RM: Descriptors of breathlessness in cardiorespiratory diseases. Am J Respir Crit Care Med 1996;154:1357–1363.
3 Simon PM, Schwartzstein RM, Weiss JW, Lahive K, Fencl V, Teghtsoonian M, Weinberger SE: Distinguishable sensations of breathlessness induced in normal volunteers. Am Rev Respir Dis 1989;140:1021–1027.
4 Society American Thoracic. Standardization of Spirometry, 1994 Update. American Thoracic Society. Am J Respir Crit Care Med 1995;152: 1107–1136.
5 Kroenke K, Arrington ME, Mangelsdorff AD: The prevalence of symptoms in medical outpatients and the adequacy of therapy. Arch Intern Med 1990;150:1685–1689.
6 Mahler DA: Diagnosis of dyspnea; in Mahler DA (ed): Dyspnea. New York, Dekker, 1998, pp 221–259.
7 Ailani RK, Ravakhah K, DiGiovine B, Jacobsen G, Tun T, Epstein D, West BC: Dyspnea differentiation index: A new method for the rapid separation of cardiac vs. pulmonary dyspnea. Chest 1999;116:1100–1104.
8 McNamara RM, Cionni DJ: Utility of the peak expiratory flow rate in the differentiation of acute dyspnea. Cardiac vs. pulmonary origin. Chest 1992;101:129–132.
9 Alhamad EH, Gay SE, Flaherty KR, Martinez FJ: Evaluating chronic dyspnea: A stepwise approach. J Respir Dis 2001;22:79–88.
10 Cook DG, Shaper AG: Breathlessness, angina pectoris and coronary artery disease. Am J Cardiol 1989;63:921–924.
11 Weisman IM, Zeballos RJ: Clinical evaluation of unexplained dyspnea. Cardiologia 1996;41: 621–634.
12 Elliott MW, Adams L, Cockcroft A, Macrae KD, Murphy K, Guz A: The language of breathlessness. Use of verbal descriptions by patients with cardiopulmonary disease. Am Rev Respir Dis 1991;144:826–832.
13 Simon PM, Schwartzstein RM, Weiss JW, Fencl V, Teghtsoonian M, Weinberger SE: Distinguishable types of dyspnea in patients with shortness of breath. Am Rev Respir Dis 1990; 142:1009–1014.
14 Scott JA, Mahler DA: Prospective evaluation of a descriptor model to diagnose the etiology of dyspnea. Chest 1995;188S.
15 Pratter MR, Curley FJ, Dubois J, Irwin RS: Cause and evaluation of chronic dyspnea in a pulmonary disease clinic. Arch Intern Med 1989;149:2277–2282.
16 Orens JB, Kazerooni EA, Martinez FJ, Curtis JL, Gross BH, Flint A III Lynch JP: The sensitivity of high-resolution CT in detecting idiopathic pulmonary fibrosis proved by open lung biopsy: A prospective study. Chest 1995;108: 190–115.
17 Aaron SD, Dales RE, Cardinal P: How accurate is spirometry at predicting restrictive pulmonary impairment? Chest 1999;115:869–873.
18 Irvin CG: Lung volumes. Semin Respir Med 1998;19:325–334.
19 Demedts M, Beckers J, Rochette F, Bulcke J: Pulmonary function in moderate neuromuscular disease without respiratory complaints. Eur J Respir Dis 1982;63:62–67.
20 Martinez FJ: Neuromuscular diseases of the chest; in Goldstein R, O'Connell J, Karlinsky J (eds): A Practical Approach to Pulmonary Medicine. Philadelphia, Lippincott-Raven, 1997, pp 323–344.
21 Celli BR: Clinical and physiologic evaluation of respiratory muscle function. Clin Chest Med 1989;10:199–214.
22 Flaherty KR, Wald J, Weisman KM, Zeballos RJ, Schork A, Blaivas M, Rubenfire M, Martinez FJ: Unexplained exertional limitation: Characterization of patients with a mitochondrial myopathy. Am J Respir Crit Care Med 2001;164:425–432.

23 Martinez FJ: Pulmonary function testing in the evaluation of upper airway obstruction; in Norton M (ed): Atlas of the Difficult Airway. St Louis, Mosby, 1996, pp 125–133.
24 Crapo RO: Carbon monoxide diffusing capacity (transfer factor). Semin Respir Crit Care Med 1998;19:335–347.
25 Ansari A, Collier J, Mohsenifar Z: Isolated reduction in single-breath diffusing capacity in young, healthy, asymptomatic women. Am J Med Sci 1995;310:226–228.
26 Mohsenifar Z, Collier J, Belman MJ, Koerner SK: Isolated reduction in single-breath diffusing capacity in the evaluation of exertional dyspnea. Chest 1992;101:965–969.
27 Rubin LJ: Primary pulmonary hypertension. N Engl J Med 1997;336:111–117.
28 Hansell DM: High-resolution computed tomography in the evaluation of fibrosing alveolitis. Clin Chest Med 1999;20:739–760.
29 Klein JS, Gamsu G, Webb WR, Golden JA, Müller NL: High-resolution CT diagnosis of emphysema in symptomatic patients with normal chest radiographs and isolated low diffusing capacity. Radiology 1992;182:817–821.
30 Fedullo PF, Auger WR, Channick RN, Kerr KM, Rubin LJ: Chronic thromboembolic pulmonary hypertension. Clin Chest Med 2001; 22:561–581.
31 DePaso WJ, Winterbauer RH, Lusk JA, Dreis DF, Springmeyer SC: Chronic dyspnea unexplained by history, physical examination, chest roentgenogram, and spirometry. Analysis of a seven-year experience. Chest 1991;100:1293–1299.
32 Sterk PJ: Bronchoprovocation testing. Semin Respir Med 1998;19:317–324.
33 Martinez FJ, Stanopoulos I, Acero R, Becker FS, Pickering R, Beamis JF: Graded comprehensive cardiopulmonary exercise testing in the evaluation of dyspnea unexplained by routine evaluation. Chest 1994;105:168–174.
34 Diller PM, Smucker DR, David B, Graham RJ: Congestive heart failure due to diastolic or systolic dysfunction: Frequency and patient characteristics in an ambulatory setting. Arch Fam Med 1999;8:414–420.
35 Vasan RS, Benjamin EJ, Levy RD: Prevalence, clinical features and prognosis of diastolic heart failure: An epidemiologic perspective. J Am Coll Cardiol 1995;26:1565–1576.
36 James KB, Maurer J, Wolski K, Lutton SR, Haas G, Schilz R, Rubin D, Young JB: Exercise hemodynamic findings in patients with exertional dyspnea. Tex Heart Inst J 2000;27:100–105.
37 Blaivas M: Incidence of pericardial effusion in patients presenting to the emergency department with unexplained dyspnea. Acad Emerg Med 2001;8:1143–1146.
38 Sridhar MK, Carter R, Banham SW, Moran F: An evaluation of integrated cardiopulmonary exercise testing in a pulmonary function laboratory. Scott Med J 1995;40:113–116.
39 Weisman IM, Zeballos RJ: A step approach to the evaluation of unexplained dyspnea: The role of cardiopulmonary exercise testing. Pulm Perspect 1998;15:8–11.
40 Gardner WN: The pathophysiology of hyperventilation disorders. Chest 1996;109:516–534.
41 Hooper RG, Thomas AR, Kearl RA: Mitochondrial enzyme deficiency causing exercise limitation in normal-appearing adults. Chest 1995;107:317–322.
42 Dandurand RJ, Matthews PM, Arnold DL, Eidelman DH: Mitochondrial disease. Pulmonary function, exercise performance, and blood lactate levels. Chest 1995;108:182–189.
43 Elliott DL, Buist NRM, Goldberg L, Kennaway NG, Powell BR, Kuehl KS: Metabolic myopathies: Evaluation by graded exercise testing. Medicine 1989;68:163–172.
44 Taivassalo T, DeStefano N, Argov Z, et al: Effects of aerobic training in patients with mitochondrial myopathies. Neurology 1998;50: 1055–1060.
45 Risk C, Epler GR, Gaensler EA: Exercise alveolar-arterial oxygen pressure difference in interstitial lung disease. Chest 1984;85:69–74.
46 Keogh BA, Lakatos E, Price D, Crystal RG: Importance of the lower respiratory tract in oxygen transfer. Exercise testing in patients with interstitial and destructive lung diseases. Am Rev Respir Dis 1984;129(suppl):S76–S80.
47 Wasserman K, Hansen JE, Sue DY, Casaburi R, Whipp BJ: Principles of Exercise Testing and Interpretation. Including Pathophysiology and Clinical Applications. Philadelphia, Lippincott Williams & Wilkins, 1999.
48 Knobil K, Becker FS, Harper P, Graf LB, Wolf GT, Martinez FJ: Dyspnea in a patient years after severe poliomyelitis. The role of cardiopulmonary exercise testing. Chest 1994;105: 777–781.
49 Eliasson AH, Phillips YY, Rajagopal KR: Sensitivity and specificity of bronchial provocation testing. An evaluation of four techniques in exercise-induced bronchospasm. Chest 1992;102:347–355.
50 Zeballos RJ, Weisman IM, Connery SM, Bradley JP: Standard treadmill (STE) vs. incremental cycle ergometry in the evaluation of airway hyperreactivity in unexplained dyspnea. Am Rev Respir Crit Care Med 1999;159:A419.
51 Johnson B, Weisman IM, Zeballos RJ, Beck KC: Emerging concepts in the evaluation of ventilatory limitation during exercise: The exercise tidal flow-volume loop. Chest 1999;116: 488–503.
52 Morris MJ, Deal LE, Bean DR, Grbach VX, Morgan JA: Vocal cord dysfunction in patients with exertional dyspnea. Chest 1999;116: 1676–1682.
53 Bacharier LB, Strunk RC: Vocal cord dysfunction: A practical approach to diagnosis. J Respir Dis 2001;22:93–103.

Fernando J. Martinez, MD
1500 E. Medical Center Drive
3916 Taubman Center
Ann Arbor, MI 48109 (USA)
Tel. +1 734 763 2540, Fax +1 734 936 5048
E-Mail fmartine@umich.edu

Weisman IM, Zeballos RJ (eds): Clinical Exercise Testing.
Prog Respir Res. Basel, Karger, 2002, vol 32, pp 89–98

Respiratory System Responses to Exercise in Aging

Bruce D. Johnson

Division of Cardiovascular Diseases, Department of Internal Medicine, Mayo Clinic and Foundation, Rochester, Minn., USA

Summary

Aging results in a progressive fall in vital capacity and maximal expiratory flows, at a rate which may accelerate in the more advanced years of life. In addition, there is an apparent reduction in pulmonary capillary blood volume, a gradual rise in pulmonary vascular pressures, and an altered ventilation distribution as aging progresses. These changes result in a reduction in ventilatory reserve and in theory would make the older adult more susceptible to gas exchange abnormalities during exercise. Nevertheless, the healthy older adult is generally able to maintain an appropriate alveolar ventilation to maintain arterial oxygenation and reduce arterial carbon dioxide levels, even during heavy exercise. The primary limitation resulting from the age-related changes in the pulmonary system may be related to the large work and cost of breathing which could limit exercise performance by competing for blood flow with the locomotory muscles.

The large capacities of the respiratory system allow for significant erosion in function between maturity and senescence with minimal impact on normal breathing. Only during moderate to heavy exercise does it appear that the aged-induced changes significantly impact normal breathing, and then primarily through an effect on breathing strategy, work and cost of breathing rather than on alveolar to arterial gas exchange [1–4]. The focus of this review will be the impact of age-related changes in the respiratory system on the response to exercise. For a formal review of baseline changes in the pulmonary system with aging, the reader is referred to several previous papers [5–9].

Table 1 summarizes the changes in lung and chest wall function, gas exchange and ventilatory control with aging and the impact of these age-related changes on the response to exercise in the healthy, active, older adult.

Pulmonary Mechanics

With the decline in pulmonary function (due primarily to a loss of lung elastic recoil), older subjects have a reduced ability to increase tidal volume (V_T) and to increase flow rates during exercise. In the average 70-year-old subject, the reduction amounts to a 30% loss in vital capacity (VC) and forced expiratory volume in 1 s (FEV_1) relative to the 20-year-old adult [4, 9, 10]. The relative reduction in flow rates is particularly great over the lower lung volumes (functional residual capacity, FRC, and below) and thus limits the ability to increase flow in the older adult over this lung volume range [1]. Interestingly, ventilatory (V_E) demand tends to fall with aging commensurate with the fall in metabolic demand so that it may be theorized that the relative demand/capacity balance may be similar to the average fit young adult. It is this relationship of demand to capacity that in part determines the adequacy of the ventilatory compensation to exercise in the older adult. Interestingly, recent studies have suggested that the decline in pulmonary function with aging may accelerate beyond age 50–60 years and that this decline in

Table 1. Influence of age-related changes in the respiratory system on the response to heavy exercise

Baseline change (or proposed change)	Result	Response to exercise in the older adult
Pulmonary Mechanics		
↓ Elastic recoil ↑ Chest wall stiffness ↓ Respiratory muscle strength ↓ Intervertebral space	↓ Lung volumes (TLC, VC) ↓ Flow rates ↓ Pressure generation capacity	↑ Expiratory flow limitation Altered regulation of end-expiratory lung volume ↓ Expiratory and inspiratory pressure reserve ↑ V_T/VC ↑ Work and oxygen cost of breathing ↑ Competition for blood flow between locomotor and respiratory muscles
Gas Exchange/Hemodynamics		
↓ Elastic recoil (nonuniform) ↑ Alveolar duct diameter ↓ Alveolar septa ↑ Stiffness of pulmonary arteries and capillaries Diastolic dysfunction	↓ Pulmonary capillary blood volume ↓ Surface area ↑ VA/Qc inhomogeneity ↑ Pulmonary pressures	↑ Dead space ventilation ↑ V_E to maintain alveolar PO_2 Arterial PO_2 maintained within 5 mm Hg resting values Alveolar to arterial PO_2 difference ↑ threefold
Ventilatory Control		
↓ Integration of sensory inputs in CNS ↓ Perceptual sensitivity to inspiratory and expiratory loads ↓ Inspiratory neuromuscular output	↓ Response to chemical and mechanical stimuli	V_E response generally adequate to maintain PaO_2 near resting values and to ↓ $PaCO_2$ below resting values

function is not modified by habitual physical activity nor high aerobic capacity [4, 7]. Thus in advanced age, the loss in *capacity* may begin to play a role in limiting human performance, especially in the elderly that maintain relatively high levels of activity [2–4].

Ventilatory Demand

Ventilatory demand is dependent foremost on metabolic demand (quantified by measurements of oxygen consumption, VO_2, or carbon dioxide production, VCO_2), but also on the dead space ventilation (VD) and regulation of arterial CO_2 levels ($PaCO_2$). This relationship is summarized in the following equation: $V_E = (K \cdot VCO_2)/[PaCO_2 \cdot (1 - VD/VT)]$ (K = the constant 0.863 and represents the factor needed to transform fractional gas concentration to partial pressure and to express gas volumes at body temperature and pressure saturated with water vapor). Many studies have evaluated changes in maximal oxygen consumption with aging and most demonstrate a decline of approximately 0.4–0.6%/year beyond the age of 30–35 and attribute the decline primarily to a reduced cardiac output as a result of a decline in heart rate, although a loss of muscle mass and altered mitochondrial function may play a role [11–14]. Thus the average 25- to 30-year-old may have a peak exercise VO_2 of 45 ml/kg/min and the average 70-year-old, 25 ml/kg/min. This results in a comparable decline in VCO_2 and thus it can be predicted (from the above equation) that the peak ventilation necessary for maintaining normal alveolar oxygen levels during peak exercise (assumes a similar dead space to tidal volume ratio, VD/VT) will fall by approximately 30–40% or a decrease from 120 l/min for the normally active 30-year-old to 70 l/min for the average fit 70-year-old adult. However, given the increase in dead space ventilation with aging (↑ 0.1–0.6%/year beyond age 25–30), it is expected the decline in ventilatory demand for the average 70-year-old will only be 25–30% [9, 15]. With increased fitness it can subsequently be predicted that for every 500 ml increase in metabolic demand (~50 W on a cycle ergometer), the ventilatory requirements will increase by ~15 l/min. The ventilatory demands would further increase as pH falls with heavy exercise and arterial CO_2 is reduced in an attempt to compensate for the acidosis.

Breathing Pattern

The typical response to exercise is to increase both the frequency of breathing and the tidal volume. Most studies

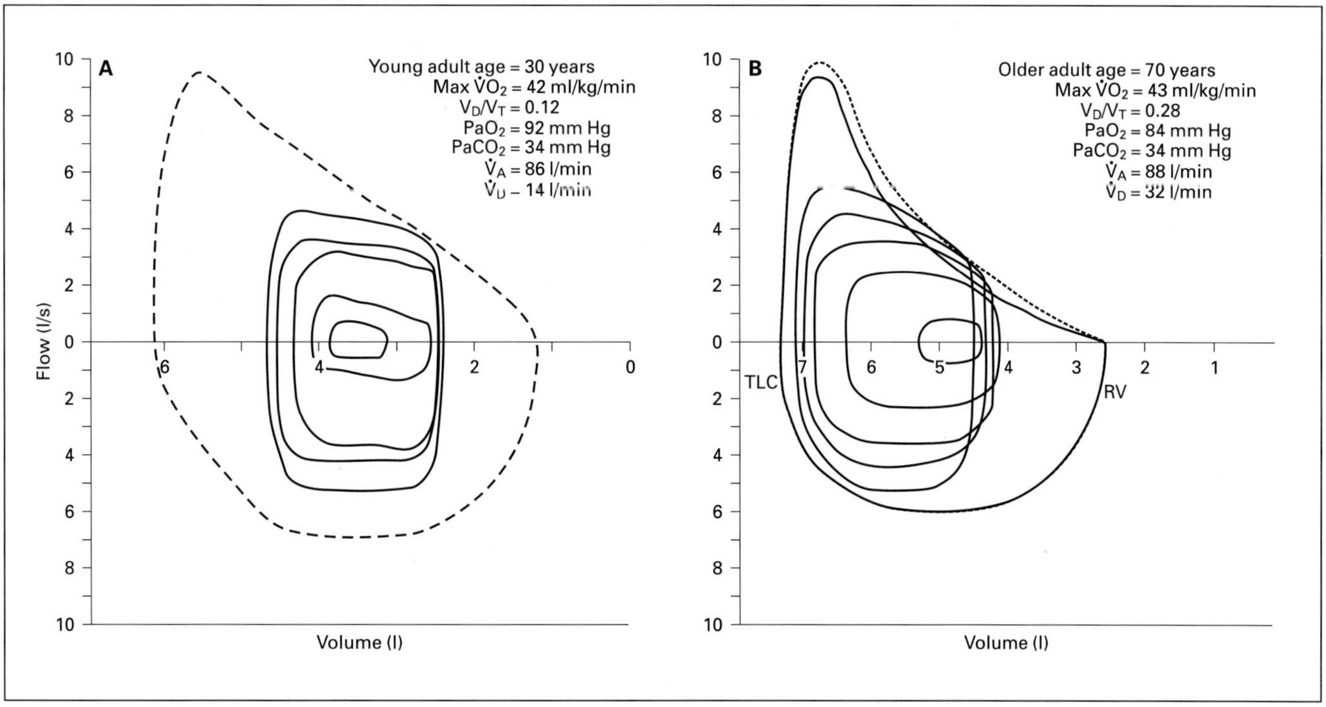

Fig. 1. Ventilatory response to exercise in young untrained adults (**A**) and older active adults (**B**) matched for exercise capacity. Tidal breathing exercise flow-volume loops at increasing work intensities are plotted according to a measured end-expiratory lung volume within the maximal volitional flow-volume envelope (MFVL). Additional mean gas exchange parameters are given for both groups. Dotted or dashed segments of the MFVL represent the expiratory flow obtained immediately post-exercise. From Johnson BD, Badr MS, Dempsey JA: Impact of the aging pulmonary system on the response to exercise; in Weisman IM, Zeballos RJ (eds): Clinics in Chest Medicine. Philadelphia, Saunders, 1994, vol 15, pp 229–246, with permission.

have demonstrated a primary increase in tidal volume early in exercise in healthy adults followed by a primary frequency response, especially in heavy and maximal exercise [16]. The aged tend to achieve a tidal volume that reaches a greater percent of their VC than their younger counterparts [1, 9].

Several factors likely determine the peak V_T chosen during exercise. Previous work by McParland et al. [17]. added dead space during exercise and found that most subjects will attempt to preserve gas exchange (eliminate CO_2 and maintain alveolar O_2) by increasing the tidal breath, suggesting a given tidal breath may be optimal for preserving gas exchange. On the other hand, lung inflation (stretch receptors in the lung) and the inspiratory elastic load (chest wall receptors) may act to limit the tidal breath so that the work and oxygen cost of breathing are not excessive. Of course this is dependent a great deal on where the subject breathes on the pressure-volume relationship of the lung and chest wall, i.e., regulation of end-expiratory lung volume (EELV). Thus in the aged adult, the increased lung compliance facilitates achieving a higher lung volume during exercise (end inspiratory lung volume, EILV) while the reduced compliance of the chest wall inhibits large tidal breaths (especially at a high percentage of total lung capacity (TLC), ↑ EELV).

Regulation of End Expiratory Lung Volume

Figure 1 demonstrates an example of the flow and volume response to progressive exercise in young adults relative to older 'fit' subjects (similar exercise capacity as the young average fit adults (VO_2max = 43 ml/kg/min) [1, 18–20]. Shown is the resting tidal breathing flow volume loop in the young and older adult and tidal breathing loops associated with progressive exercise relative to the volitional maximal flow-volume envelope (MFVL). In the young adult, tidal volume increases during exercise by encroachment on the inspiratory and expiratory reserve volumes. The encroachment on the expiratory reserve volume is accomplished by a reduction in EELV below the resting relaxation volume (i.e., FRC). The reduction

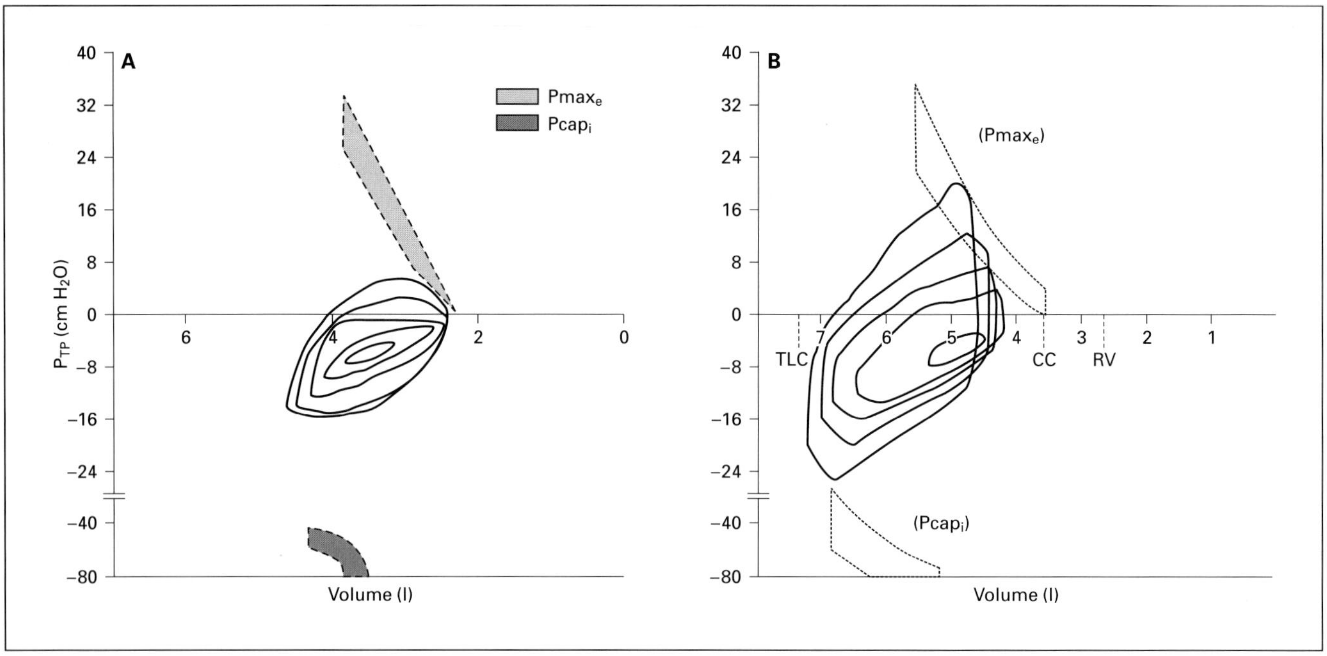

Fig. 2. Corresponding (to the flow-volume data shown in figure 1) tidal pressure-volume responses to progressive exercise in young untrained adults (**A**) and older fit adults (**B**). $Pmax_e$ = Maximal effective pressure generation; $Pcap_i$ = capacity for inspiratory pressure generation (determined at the flow and volume where peak inspiratory pressure occurred). From Johnson BD: Age-associated changes in pulmonary reserve; in Evans JG, Williams TF, Beattie LB, et al. (eds): Oxford Textbook of Geriatric Medicine, ed 2. Oxford, Oxford University Press, 2000, pp 483–497, with permission.

in EELV is thought to increase inspiratory muscle length thereby optimizing the length-tension relationship of the inspiratory muscles so that for a given neural input, greater force production occurs [21]. The drop in EELV also allows the tidal breath during exercise to stay on the linear portion of the pressure-volume relationship of the lung and chest wall, thus minimizing the elastic work and oxygen cost of breathing. The fall in EELV tends to progress with exercise intensity and averages 0.5–1.0 l in an average fit, young adult at peak exercise [19, 22].

In the older subjects (age 70 years), EELV typically decreases in a similar fashion with the onset of exercise as in the young adult. However, due to expiratory flow limitation (i.e., tidal flow volume breath that meets the expiratory boundary of the MFVL) particularly near the end of each tidal breath, the majority of older subjects subsequently fail to decrease EELV further or actually increase EELV to avoid further expiratory flow limitation [1, 2, 4]. On average, significant expiratory flow limitation begins to occur at a ventilation of ~40 l/min, 40–50% of VO_2max. Thus in the older adult, EILV encroaches to a greater extent on TLC than in the younger adult and the potential benefits from an increased inspiratory muscle length through a decrease in EELV are compromised [1–4].

Expiratory Flow and Pressure Development

As noted, expiratory flow reaches the maximal available flows over a significant portion of the tidal breath in the aged subjects beginning at a ventilation of ~40 l/min. This is in contrast with young adults who do not achieve this level of expiratory flow constraint until a ventilation of 100–120 l/min or near-peak exercise.

Figure 2 gives the corresponding tidal pleural-pressure-volume response in the young and older adults (relative to the flow-volume loops shown in figure 1). As shown, the expiratory pleural pressures become positive early in exercise in the older adults suggesting significant expiratory muscle recruitment and reach the maximal effective pressures (expiratory pressures that produce maximal flow, $Pmax_e$) over a significant portion of the tidal breath near peak exercise. This is in contrast to the young adult where expiratory pleural pressures do not become positive until near-maximal exercise and then only near EELV. The increase in expiratory pleural pressure development in the aged is out of proportion to the rise in expiratory flow so that resistance during expiration increases relative to the young adult at a similar level of ventilation [2]. Interestingly, despite the large positive pleural pressure produced on expiration and the degree of expiratory flow limitation, the older subject typically does not produce wasted effort (i.e., pressures in excess of effective pressures) suggesting a precise degree of expiratory muscle regulation during heavy exercise [2].

Inspiratory Flow and Pressure Development

Both inspiratory flow (muscle shortening velocity) and lung volume (muscle length, expressed as a percent of TLC) increase during exercise causing the capacity for pleural pressure generation ($Pcap_i$) to decline [2]. Despite an increase in peak inspiratory flow to 4 l/s (fig. 1) and peak inspiratory pressures that reach 75% of TLC (fig. 2), at peak exercise the average fit young adult only approaches 50% of the capacity of the inspiratory muscles to produce pressure [23]. Thus substantial reserve remains to increase ventilation through greater inspiratory pressure generation. In contrast the older adult, at a similar level of ventilation, approaches 80–90% of their dynamic capacity for pleural pressure generation ($Pcap_i$) [2]. The cause of the reduced pressure generating capacity in the older adult is primarily due to the rise in EELV causing peak inspiratory pressure and EILV to reach much higher lung volumes (95% TLC). Thus, the strategy used to limit expiratory flow limitation, by increasing EELV, results in encroachment on TLC and the inspiratory capacity for pressure generation. Indirectly this is the result of the loss of elastic recoil.

Work and Cost of Breathing during Exercise

With low levels of exercise (ventilation <40 l/min) little difference is noted in breathing pattern and strategy between the young and older adult and therefore, the work and cost associated with breathing are small. As expiratory flow limitation occurs and breathing strategy is modified by increasing EELV and producing large expiratory pressures, the work and cost of breathing accelerates. Figure 3 demonstrates the work and O_2 cost of breathing in our average fit, young adults and young athletes relative to older fit subjects [2, 19]. As shown, the work and cost associated with breathing accelerate in the older adults and by peak exercise these values are 50–60% higher than the young adult (at a similar ventilation). The increased metabolic demands of the younger athlete however result in a work and cost that exceeds the fit older adults, but at a ventilation that is 50 l/min greater than our older subjects. The cost of breathing was estimated at 13% of the total body VO_2 in the older subjects (range 7–23%), 6% in the young average fit subjects (range 5–8%) at a similar ventilation and 13% (range 10–16%) in the young athletes at peak exercise [2, 19, 24]. This represents a significant demand for blood flow to the respiratory muscles during exercise, which could theoretically compromise blood flow to the working locomotor muscles. Previous work by Saltin [25] has suggested that leg blood flow measurements at a given work intensity are reduced in the older subject, while extraction across the vascular bed is increased. Recent work by Proctor et al. [13] has confirmed that leg blood flow is reduced with aging for a given work intensity in older subjects (age = 63, n = 6) matched with young adults (age = 27, n = 6) for muscle mass, fitness and hemoglobin levels. Although speculative, it is likely that at least part of the reduction in leg blood flow with aging may be related to the increased work and cost of breathing in the older subjects. Work by Harms and colleagues [26–28] has suggested that the respiratory muscles may preferentially recruit blood flow at the expense of the locomotor muscles. Figure 4 shows leg blood flow relative to whole body VO_2 in older relative to younger subjects (fig. 4a) along with an estimate of the overall blood flow distribution if the majority of the decline in leg blood flow with aging is due to the enhanced work and cost of breathing (fig. 4b) [13].

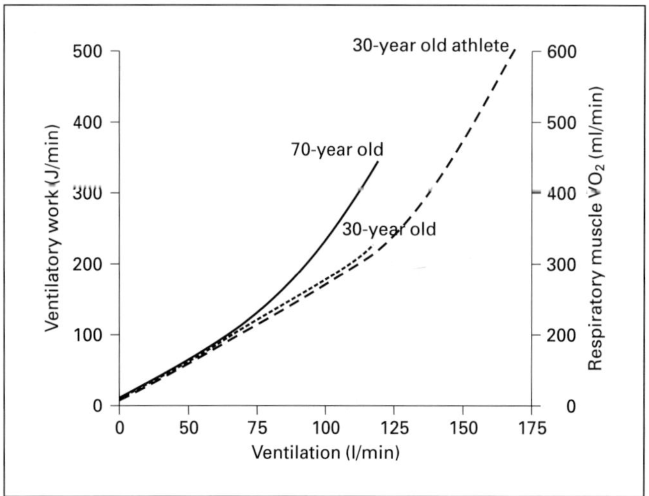

Fig. 3. Ventilatory work and the oxygen cost of breathing during progressive exercise in 30-year-old untrained adults (dotted line), 26-year-old endurance athletes (dashed line), and 70-year-old moderately fit older adults (solid line).

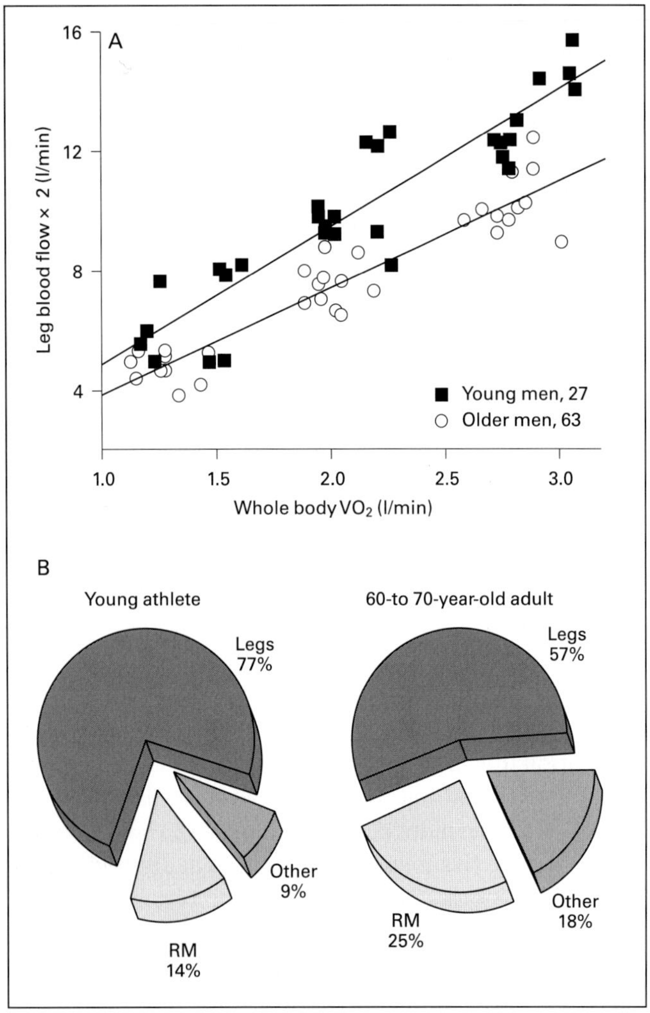

Fig. 4. A Leg blood flow during cycle ergometry in young and older adults matched for muscle mass, fitness and hemoglobin. For a given oxygen consumption, leg blood flow is reduced in the older adults. It is hypothesized that some of the blood flow may be going to support the demands of the respiratory muscles in the older adults due to the high work and cost of breathing [13]. **B** Do the respiratory muscles preferentially 'steal' blood flow from the locomotor muscles? Estimated demands of the respiratory muscles (RM) relative to total cardiac output with age [estimated from 13, 26–28].

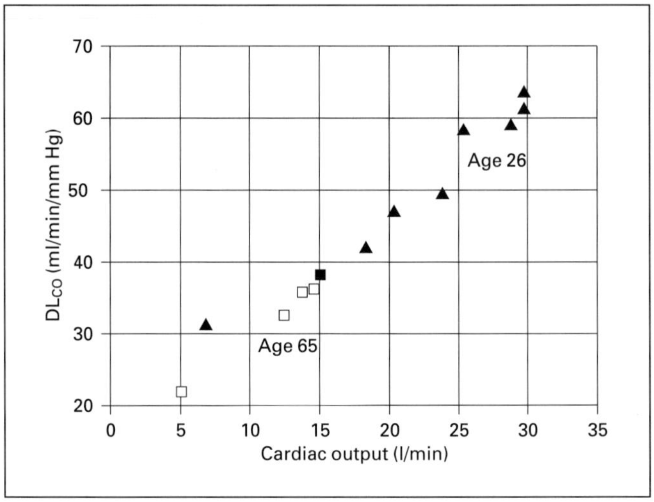

Fig. 5. Diffusing capacity of the lungs for carbon monoxide (DL_{CO}) obtained by rebreathing at rest and during exercise relative to cardiac output in young, highly trained (triangles, n = 8) adults relative to older, average fit (squares, n = 7) healthy adults. DL_{CO} is reduced at rest in the older adults, but increases in a linear fashion with progressive exercise similar to the young adults. From Johnson BD: Age-associated changes in pulmonary reserve; in Evans JG, Williams TF, Beattie LB, et al. (eds): Oxford Textbook of Geriatric Medicine, ed 2. Oxford, Oxford University Press, 2000, pp 483–497, with permission.

Pulmonary Gas Exchange

The changes in ventilation-perfusion relationships, reduced surface area for diffusion, a stiffening of the pulmonary vasculature and increased dead space ventilation would theoretically limit the adaptations available to maintain gas exchange homeostasis in the elderly [9]. However, as will be demonstrated, despite these age-related changes, the reserve available to the respiratory system to meet the demands of heavy exercise generally remain sufficient.

Dead Space and Alveolar Ventilation

In the limited studies that have measured this directly (with arterial blood gases), VD/VT drops with exercise similar to the decrease observed in the young adult [9, 29]. However, because baseline values are elevated, the values at peak exercise remain significantly elevated. The effect of the increased VD/VT on total ventilation becomes significant, especially as breathing frequency begins to increase during heavy and maximal exercise. In the young adult, at an average breathing frequency of 35 breaths per minute (bpm), VD approaches 7% of the total V_E, and 13% in young athletes at a breathing frequency of 60 bpm. In the aged adults, it approaches 30% of the V_E by peak exercise [9].

Lung Diffusion (Effective Alveolar-Capillary Surface Area)

We have measured the diffusing capacity of the lungs for carbon monoxide (DL_{CO}) using the rebreathe technique in young endurance athletes and in a limited number of healthy older subjects (age = 62, n = 9) of average

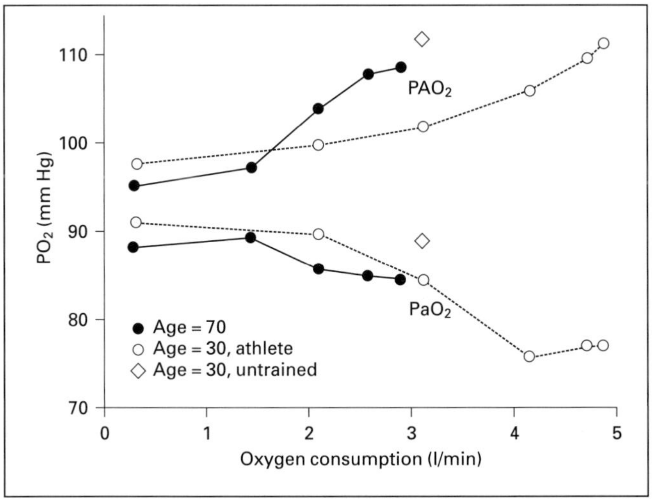

Fig. 6. Alveolar (PAO_2) and arterial oxygen (PaO_2) tensions during progressive exercise in young untrained adults (diamonds, maximum shown only), young endurance trained adults (open circles), and moderately fit older adults (solid circles) [9, 29]. From Johnson BD, Badr MS, Dempsey JA: Impact of the aging pulmonary system on the response to exercise; in Weisman IM, Zeballos RJ (eds): Clinics in Chest Medicine. Philadelphia, Saunders, 1994, vol 15, pp 229–246, with permission.

fitness (VO_2max = 24 ml/kg/min). The relationship of DL_{CO} to cardiac output is shown in figure 5 for the old (squares) and younger (triangles) subjects. Similar to what has been described using the single breath technique, DL_{CO} is reduced at rest in the older subjects using the rebreathe technique. With increasing work intensities during exercise, DL_{CO} increases in a linear fashion with the rise in cardiac output in both the young and older adults; although the older adults are at a significantly reduced metabolic demand. This would imply that despite the potential for mild changes in ventilation distribution, a reduced pulmonary capillary blood volume and a stiffening of the pulmonary vasculature in the older adults, that these changes are relatively mild and not sufficient to affect the recruitment of effective alveolar-capillary surface area for gas exchange during exercise.

Alveolar to Arterial Gas Exchange

Figure 6 shows the average changes in PaO_2 in the 70-year-old subjects relative to the average fit young adult and the young trained athlete. Arterial blood gas homeostasis is remarkably maintained during exercise despite the resting changes in the aging lung. The mild ventilation distribution abnormalities with aging are likely corrected with the increased inspiratory flow rates such as occur with the increased ventilatory demands of exercise. The older adult begins to widen the alveolar to arterial oxygen difference (Aa DO_2) at 40–50% of VO_2max and widens to a similar extent during maximal exercise (approximately threefold) as the young average fit adult at a similar oxygen consumption. On average, in a subgroup of 19 subjects studied in our laboratory, arterial oxygen partial pressures (PaO_2) remained within 5 mm Hg of resting values during maximal exercise [9, 29]. Other studies however have suggested that a large percentage of older, athletic subjects become hypoxemic during progressive exercise [30, 31]. We believe however that this relatively high incidence of hypoxemia in this population may in part reflect non-steady-state exercise with inadequate time for complete respiratory compensation.

Our 19 older fit adults did demonstrate a great deal of variability in the arterial PO_2 during exercise with approximately 30% of subjects demonstrating a 10 mm Hg drop or greater from rest during exercise (PaO_2 <75 mm Hg) at exercise intensities requiring a VO_2 of 40 ml/kg/min. Hypoxemia of this magnitude is rarely observed in healthy young adults at a similar metabolic demand, however, a significant number of young endurance athletes will become hypoxemic at VO_2max values near 65 ml/kg/min or greater [2, 32]. The reason for the hypoxemia in young athletes has been studied in great detail [19, 32, 33] and to date it is accepted that 50% is attributed to a worsening of interregional ventilation-perfusion matching (VA/Qc), and 50% to a diffusion limitation for oxygen and due to a small shunt from the bronchial and thebesian circulation. It can be theorized that the small reduction in pulmonary capillary blood volume in the older adult would increase the transit time of blood through the pulmonary capillaries at a lower cardiac output than in the younger adult. This combined with a greater potential for interregional VA/Qc inequalities may contribute to the hypoxemia at the lower metabolic demands with aging. It should be noted however that for the average level of fitness for a 70-year-old adult, little hypoxemia is noted attesting to the moderate reserve still available for gas exchange, even in the later years of life.

Pulmonary Vasculature

Several studies have examined the hemodynamic changes in the pulmonary vasculature in the healthy aged subjects [34–36]. The majority of data available describes changes in pulmonary arterial pressure (Ppa), pulmonary wedge pressure (Ppw) and the pulmonary vascular resis-

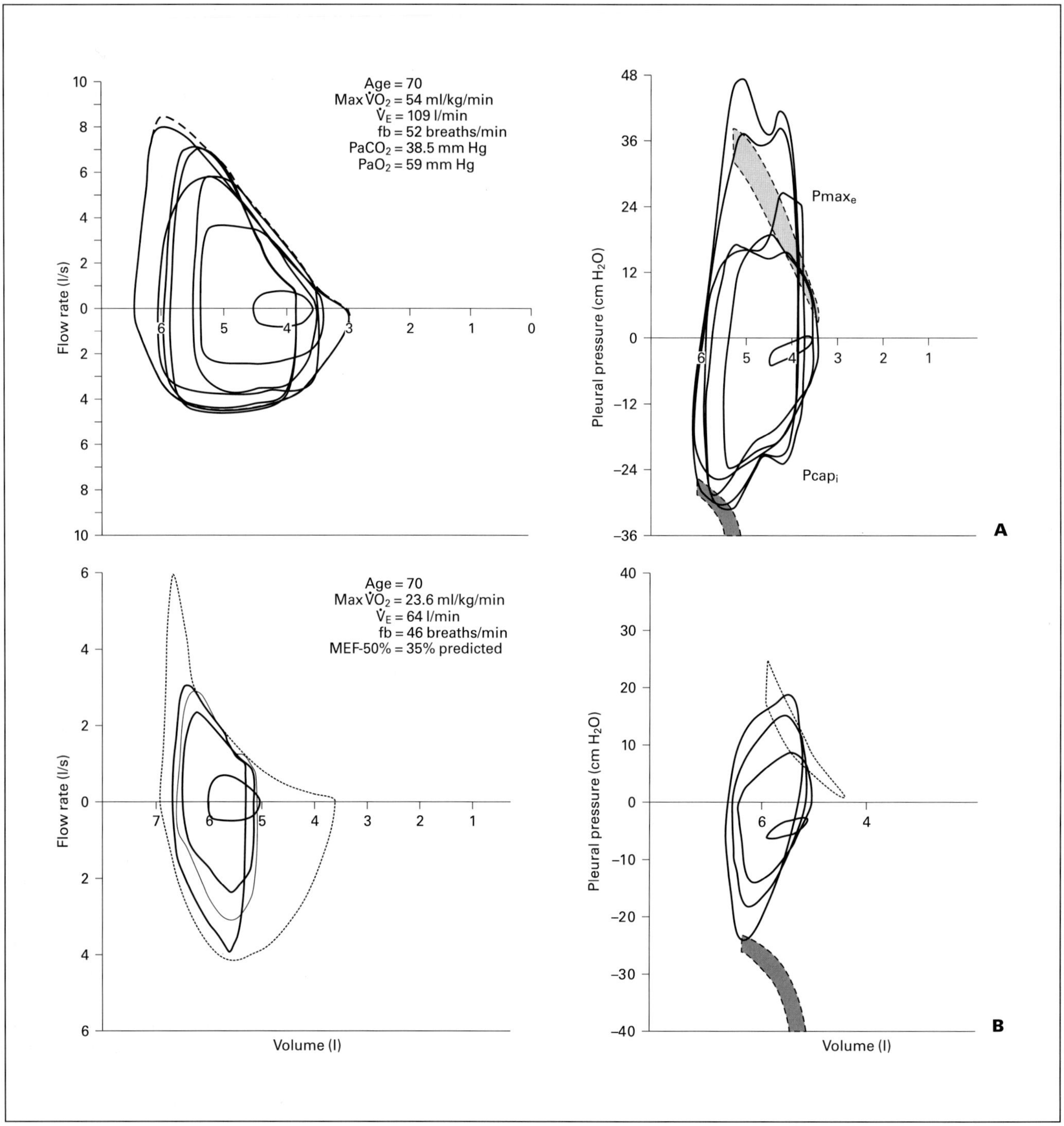

Fig. 7. Demand exceeds capacity. Subject RA (**A**) demonstrated the usual age-related declines in lung function (i.e., FEF-50% = 100% predicted, DL_{CO} = 109% of predicted). With progressive exercise, the mechanical limits to V_E are reached at a submaximal exercise load. During both heavy (but submaximal) and maximal exercise, the maximal effective expiratory pressures were significantly exceeded, the capacity for inspiratory pressure development was reached at peak pressure, the cost of breathing approached an estimated 23% of the total body VO_2, PaO_2 fell to 59 mm Hg, and $PaCO_2$ rose throughout the final workload. **B** A subject of similar age with normal ventilatory demands but with reduced capacities (FEF 50% = 50% predicted for age). A similar degree of ventilatory constraint is observed relative to the subject in **A**, however at a significantly reduced ventilatory and metabolic demand. From Johnson BD: Age-associated changes in pulmonary reserve; in Evans JG, Williams TF, Beattie LB, et al. (eds): Oxford Textbook of Geriatric Medicine, ed 2. Oxford, Oxford University Press, 2000, pp 483–497, with permission.

tance (PVR = Ppa – Ppw/blood flow) with exercise [36]. At rest, in the supine position, Ppa's are only slightly elevated in the older adults as are Ppw's and the estimated PVR. To increase blood flow through the lung, one must increase vascular driving pressure from the pulmonary artery to the left atrium. During heavy exercise in the older subjects, the Ppa increases (i.e., 100% from rest) out of proportion to those determined at a similar VO_2 and cardiac output in younger adults (50%). Similarly, Ppw increases 120% in the older subjects versus only 25% in the younger adults. The pressure difference, Ppa-Ppw, was similar in both groups and therefore, PVR was similar between ages. Although the older adults were more hypertensive than the younger ones at a given VO_2 and cardiac output, the younger adults were able to achieve much higher metabolic work rates and therefore reach Ppa's and Ppw's similar to those achieved in the older adults at lower workloads [36]. Measurements obtained in the sitting position at rest and during exercise reveal similar trends between the old and young, although differences are not as striking as while supine.

Advanced Age

Few studies have examined pulmonary mechanics, gas exchange and ventilatory control in subjects that make it to the more advanced years of life (age >80). Cross-sectional studies clearly represent some bias as there is a selection process to find healthy subjects in this age group. In general however, there appears to be a progressive loss of pulmonary function that may accelerate with aging [3, 4]. DeLorey and Babb [3] recently reported on 11 elderly subjects (peak VO_2, 133% of age predicted) with an average age of 88 years. These subjects demonstrated greater expiratory flow limitation than 70-year-old subjects, despite a reduced exercise capacity (peak work rate only 53 W) and no decrease in EELV typically observed in 70-year-old subjects with light exercise. These elderly subjects also demonstrated a blunted ventilatory response to exercise at the higher work intensities. Despite this apparent enhanced degree of mechanical constraint to breathing, it appeared (based on noninvasive data) that the ventilatory compensation for the metabolic demand was generally appropriate. Whether or not the enhanced mechanical constraint with advanced age contributed to reduced exercise tolerance in these subjects remains unclear, however it is likely that the increased work and cost of breathing in the presence of age-related changes in cardiac reserve would further compromise locomotor blood flow.

Scaling of Demand to Capacity

It is interesting that maximal oxygen consumption, cardiac output, FEV_1 and lung diffusion surface area appear to decline at similar annual rates with aging. All of these physiological measurements likely represent the general influence of aging. As a result, maximal metabolic demands generally do not exceed capacities. Only when the aging process is accelerated (reduced capacities, i.e., disease) or when demand is retained at exceedingly high levels (increased fitness), does the aging pulmonary system appear to significantly alter normal response to exercise. Within the older subjects tested in our laboratory, several did truly reach the limits of the lung and respiratory muscles for producing flow, volume and pressure, and as previously noted, there were several subjects who also demonstrated significantly reduced PaO_2 with progressive exercise, at metabolic loads where this is rarely observed in the young adult. Figure 7A shows an example of an extremely fit older subject (VO_2 = 215% of age predicted) with normal pulmonary function for age. In this particular subject, ventilation did not increase over the final two exercise loads or with an increased inspired CO_2. Aa DO_2 widened, primarily due to a drop in PaO_2. $PaCO_2$ actually began to increase over the final workload as would be expected if the ventilatory response was not adequate. The other extreme is also shown in figure 7B where fitness was average for age, but lung function had declined faster than the normal rate so that FEV_1 was 50% of age predicted. This subject also reaches the mechanical limits of the lung and chest wall, but due to low capacity rather than accentuated demand.

In summary, demand and capacity appear to fall together with aging so that the response to exercise is generally adequate. It does appear that the loss in lung mechanics may have a more profound effect on exercise performance relative to gas exchange, as even ventilations of 40–70 l/min will result in significant expiratory flow limitation, large increases in the work of breathing and the potential for significant blood flow competition between the locomotor muscles and the respiratory muscles. Although the arterial hypoxemia occurs in the older adults, the incidence does not appear to be enhanced in healthy, fit, older adults, but does occur at lower workloads than typically observed in the young athlete.

Acknowledgments

The author would like to thank Audrey Schroeder for preparation of the manuscript. Supported by the Mayo Foundation and HHS Grant No. M01-RR00585.

References

1 Johnson BD, Reddan WG, Pegelow DF, Seow KC, Dempsey JA: Flow limitation and regulation of functional residual capacity during exercise in a physically active aging population. Am Rev Respir Dis 1991;143:960–967.

2 Johnson BD, Reddan WG, Seow KC, Dempsey JA: Mechanical constraints on exercise hyperpnea in a fit aging population. Am Rev Respir Dis 1991;143:968–977.

3 DeLorey DS, Babb TG: Progressive mechanical ventilatory constraints with aging. Am J Respir Crit Care Med 1999;160:169–177.

4 McClaran SR, Babcock MA, Pegelow DF, Reddan WG, Dempsey JA: Longitudinal effects of aging on lung function at rest and exercise in healthy active fit elderly adults. J Appl Physiol 1995;78:1957–1968.

5 Knudson RJ, Lebowitz MD, Holberg CJ, Burrows B: Changes in the normal maximal expiratory flow-volume curve with growth and aging. Am Rev Respir Dis 1983;127:725–734.

6 Vollmer WM, Johnson LR, McCamant LE, Buist AS: Longitudinal versus cross-sectional estimation of lung function decline – further insights. Stat Med 1988;7:685–696.

7 Ware JH, Dockery DW, Louis TA, Xu XP, Ferris BG Jr, Speizer FE: Longitudinal and cross-sectional estimates of pulmonary function decline in never-smoking adults. Am J Epidemiol 1990;132:685–700.

8 Knudson R: Physiology of the aging lung; in Crystal R, West J (eds): The Lung. New York, Raven Press, 1991, pp 1749–1759.

9 Johnson BD, Dempsey J: Demand versus capacity during exercise in the aging pulmonary system; in Hollozy J (ed): Exercise and Sports Science Reviews. Baltimore, Williams & Wilkins, 1991, vol 19, pp 171–210.

10 Knudson RJ, Slatin RC, Lebowitz MD, Burrows B: The maximal expiratory flow-volume curve. Normal standards, variability, and effects of age. Am Rev Respir Dis 1976;113:587–600.

11 Bruce RA, Kusumi F, Hosmer D: Maximal oxygen intake and nomographic assessment of functional aerobic impairment in cardiovascular disease. Am Heart J 1973;85:546–562.

12 Jones NL, Makrides L, Hitchcock C, Chypchar T, McCartney N: Normal standards for an incremental progressive cycle ergometer test. Am Rev Respir Dis 1985;131:700–708.

13 Proctor DN, Beck KC, Shen PH, Eickhoff TJ, Halliwill JR, Joyner MJ: Influence of age and gender on cardiac output-VO_2 relationships during submaximal cycle ergometry. J Appl Physiol 1998;84:599–605.

14 Short K, Nair K: Does aging adversely affect muscle mitochondrial function? Exerc Sport Sci Rev 2001;29:118–123.

15 Raine J, Bishop J: Aa difference in O_2 tension and physiologial dead space in normal man. J Appl Physiol 1963;18:284–288.

16 Younes M, Kivinen G: Respiratory mechanics and breathing pattern during and following maximal exercise. J Appl Physiol 1984;57:1773–1782.

17 McParland C, Mink J, Gallagher CG: Respiratory adaptations to dead space loading during maximal incremental exercise. J Appl Physiol 1991;70:55–62.

18 Johnson BD, Scanlon PD, Beck KC: Regulation of ventilatory capacity during exercise in asthmatics. J Appl Physiol 1995;79:892–901.

19 Johnson BD, Saupe KW, Dempsey JA: Mechanical constraints on exercise hyperpnea in endurance athletes. J Appl Physiol 1992;73:874–886.

20 Johnson BD, Beck KC, Olson LJ, O'Malley KA, Allison TG, Squires RW, Gau GT: Ventilatory constraints during exercise in patients with chronic heart failure. Chest 2000;117:321–332.

21 Road J, Newman S, Derenne JP, Grassino A: In vivo length-force relationship of canine diaphragm. J Appl Physiol 1986;60:63–70.

22 Johnson BD, Seow KC, Pegelow DF, Dempsey JA: Adaptation of the inert gas FRC technique for use in heavy exercise. J Appl Physiol 1990;68:802–809.

23 Leblanc P, Summers E, Inman MD, Jones NL, Campbell EJ, Killian KJ: Inspiratory muscles during exercise: A problem of supply and demand. J Appl Physiol 1988;64:2482–2489.

24 Aaron EA, Seow KC, Johnson BD, Dempsey JA: Oxygen cost of exercise hyperpnea: Implications for performance. J Appl Physiol 1992;72:1818–1825.

25 Saltin B: The aging endurance athlete; in Sutton J, Brock R (eds): Sports Medicine for the Mature Athlete. Indianapolis, Benchmark Press, 1986, pp 59–80.

26 Harms CA, Wetter TJ, McClaran SR, Pegelow DF, Nickele GA, Nelson WB, Hanson P, Dempsey JA: Effects of respiratory muscle work on cardiac output and its distribution during maximal exercise. J Appl Physiol 1998;85:609–618.

27 Harms CA, Dempsey JA: Cardiovascular consequences of exercise hyperpnea. Exerc Sport Sci Rev 1999;27:37–62.

28 Harms CA, Wetter TJ, St Croix CM, Pegelow DF, Dempsey JA: Effects of respiratory muscle work on exercise performance. J Appl Physiol 2000;89:131–138.

29 Dempsey J, Johnson B, Pegelow D, Reddan W, Bahr S: Aging effects on exercise-induced arterial hypoxemia and expiratory flow limitation. Med Sci Sports Exerc 1993;18:S184.

30 Prefaut C, Anselme F, Caillaud C, Masse-Biron J: Exercise-induced hypoxemia in older athletes. J Appl Physiol 1994;76:120–126.

31 Prefaut C, Durand F, Mucci P, Caillaud C: Exercise-induced arterial hypoxaemia in athletes: A review. Sports Med 2000;30:47–61.

32 Dempsey JA: J.B. Wolffe memorial lecture. Is the lung built for exercise? Med Sci Sports Exerc 1986;18:143–155.

33 Wagner PD, Laravuso RB, Uhl RR, West JB: Continuous distributions of ventilation-perfusion ratios in normal subjects breathing air and 100% O_2. J Clin Invest 1974;54:54–68.

34 Ekelund LG: Circulatory and respiratory adaptation during prolonged exercise of moderate intensity in the sitting position. Acta Physiol Scand 1967;69:327–340.

35 Ekelund LG: Circulatory and respiratory adaptation during prolonged exercise. Acta Physiol Scand Suppl 1967;292:1–38.

36 Reeves J, Dempsey J, Grover R: Pulmonary circulation during exercise; in Weir E, Reeves J (eds): Pulmonary Vascular Physiology and Pathophysiology. New York, Dekker, 1989, pp 107–133.

Bruce D. Johnson, PhD
Division of Cardiovascular Diseases
Mayo Clinic and Foundation
200 1st Street, SW
Rochester, MN 55905 (USA)
Tel. +1 507 284 4375, Fax +1 507 255 4861
E-Mail johnson.bruce@mayo.edu

Weisman IM, Zeballos RJ (eds): Clinical Exercise Testing.
Prog Respir Res. Basel, Karger, 2002, vol 32, pp 99–108

Evolving Role of Cardiopulmonary Exercise Testing in Heart Failure and Cardiac Transplantation

Piergiuseppe Agostoni Marco Guazzi

Centro Cardiologico Monzino, IRCCS, Istituto di Cardiologia, Università di Milano, CNR, Milan, Italy

Summary

Heart failure (HF) is a multiorgan syndrome and the cardiopulmonary exercise test (CPET) provides an overall assessment of functional capacity and prognosis. From a prognostic point of view, useful information is obtained from peak VO_2 and VE/VCO_2 slope. These are independent predictors of survival in patients with HF and can be combined with other prognostic elements. Furthermore, CPET allows to identify the organ which is most responsible for HF severity and to target therapy on. Indeed, the following are classical aspects of CPET in HF: (a) reduction in workload achieved, (b) reduction in peak exercise VO_2, (c) reduction in VO_2 at anaerobic threshold, (d) reduction in VO_2/work rate relationship, (e) reduction in oxygen pulse, (f) reduction in rest to peak heart rate differences, (g) reduction in tidal volume at peak exercise and anaerobic threshold, (h) increase in VE/VCO_2 slope, (i) reduction in expiratory flow reserve and (l) increase in peak exercise functional respiratory capacity.

Heart failure (HF) is a multiorgan syndrome. The cardiopulmonary exercise test (CPET) provides an overall assessment of functional capacity, permitting evaluation of disease severity, progression, prognosis and therapeutic interventions. Furthermore, the CPET test is also able to target an individual organ system and prioritize which dysfunctional component impacts exercise capacity in HF to the greatest extent. This is important not only from a pathophysiological point of view, but also because it will allow guiding therapy. Indeed, at the present time, many anti-failure treatments are available and often just added on top of the others with patients receiving several pills of different sources (or various nonpharmacological interventions) without a clear idea of what and in whom something has to be preferred. However, anti-failure treatments have different targets and therefore may be chosen in consideration of the more altered body function. This is a new concept, which is at its beginning in clinical practice and, we believe, will greatly improve anti-failure treatment efficacy. This will generate the concept of a personalized anti-failure treatment and, consequently, will significantly increase the clinical use of CPET in HF patients. Last but not least, CPET provides information about the prognosis of patients and provides criteria for enrolling and removal of patients from heart transplant lists.

Exercise Modalities Used in the Evaluation of HF

Methods

Both cycloergometer and treadmill are extensively used and provide reliable and reproducible data. However, several differences have to be taken into account when comparing cycloergometer with treadmill data. First of all, with exercise on the treadmill the muscle mass

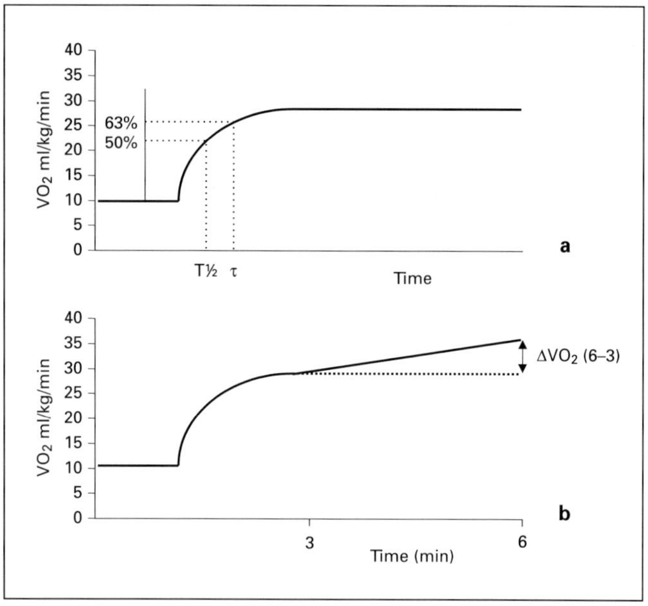

Fig. 1. Measurements obtainable from a constant workload exercise test performed below (**a**) or above (**b**) the anaerobic threshold.

involved is greater so that VO_2 at peak exercise is ~10% greater than with the cycloergometer albeit maximal heart rate is the same [1]; second the work performed can be only roughly estimated so that it is not possible to precisely calculate the external work or other parameters that are derived, such as the VO_2/work relationship; third because the subject is jumping while on the treadmill it is almost impossible to obtain invasive hemodynamic data which might be relevant on some occasions; fourth the treadmill is thought to be more dangerous than the cycloergometer, and finally a cycloergometer occupies a smaller amount of space.

Protocols and Measurements

Among the various types of exercise protocol utilized for evaluating HF, two are the most frequently used, namely constant and incremental workload. The former can be performed below or above the anaerobic threshold. In the first case, information can only be detected at the beginning of exercise and is related to the time needed for the body to adequately adapt VO_2 to the increased workload. Indeed, patients with HF have an impaired ability to utilize oxygen which, at the onset of exercise, depends on the rate of increase in cardiac output. Thus the VO_2 dynamics at the beginning of a step increase in workload is slower the more severe the exercise impairment [2]. However, it is impossible to precisely detect the moment when the VO_2 increase is 100% because the relationship is asymptotic. Accordingly, several mathematical suggestions have been proposed such as the time when 50% of VO_2 increase ($T_{1/2}$) is reached or the time constant (τ) which, in a first-degree system, is at 63% of the response (fig. 1). Other but conceptually similar variables are the time lag between the onset of exercise and R (VCO_2/VO_2) = 1 and the value of R at the 4th minute of exercise. Recently, Belardinelli et al. [3] showed a good correlation between these parameters and peak VO_2. If the constant workload exercise is performed above AT it is possible to analyze also the VO_2 increment between the 3rd and the 6th minute of constant workload (fig. 1). All the above-reported parameters are correlated with the exercise performance and can be used with no need of a maximal exercise test [4]. Incremental workload protocols can be with continuous or almost continuous workload increment (ramp or with intervals of 1 min or less) or 'truly incremental' with each level of exercise long enough to attain a steady state. This incremental protocol allows to perform special measurements during the steady state including hemodynamics and flow/volume curve, while the ramp protocol is more appropriate to build the VO_2/work relationship and to identify peak VO_2. Several parameters have been used to assess exercise capacity in HF including the work performed at peak exercise or exercise tolerance in an incremental protocol or distance procured in a certain amount of time typically 6 or 12 min. However, respiratory gas analysis offers the gold standard of measurements of exercise capacity, the peak VO_2, and several ancillary parameters as VO_2 at anaerobic threshold and the VO_2/work relationship. Peak VO_2 is the highest VO_2 measured during an incremental protocol. Because of intra-breath variability it is usually reported as a mean over 30 s. Peak VO_2 is used instead of VO_2max which is almost impossible to obtain in HF patients. VO_2max is defined as a plateauing in the increase of VO_2 despite increasing of workload. It is of note that because the arteriovenous oxygen difference both at peak exercise and at anaerobic threshold is almost fix, VO_2 reflects mainly cardiac output. Indeed during exercise the oxygen content has a specific behavior in HF patients. In the systemic artery, oxygen content increases above the anaerobic threshold because of an increase in hemoglobin (the oxygen/hemoglobin saturation curve is on the flat part so that PO_2 changes do not significantly effect oxygen content) [5]. Exercise-induced hemoconcentration is likely due to an oncotic effect of increased intracellular lactates and lactate metabolites, but a role of spleen contraction cannot be excluded [6]. In the pulmonary artery the oxygen content reduces progressively throughout the exercise due to a reduction of PO_2 and, above anaerobic threshold, due to a shift on the oxy/hemoglobin dissociation curve [7]. In the femoral vein during exercise the reduction of oxygen content is due to PO_2 changes below anaerobic threshold and due to the Bohr effect above it. Indeed PO_2 reduces up to the anaerobic threshold while oxy/hemoglobin saturation reduces through the entire test [5, 7]. Because PO_2 reduction during a progressive exercise test reaches a well-defined value (~ 18 mm Hg), by knowing hemoglobin the oxygen content at anaerobic threshold can be easily estimated. This is not the case with central mixed venous blood because in the pulmonary artery, blood comes from the entire circulation including blood from organs not actively involved with exercise. However, the percentage of blood coming from the exercising muscles versus all body blood flow is progressively greater the more severe the disease so that the arteriovenous oxygen difference is, at a given workload, progressively greater [5]. Therefore, by knowing VO_2 and hemoglobin, it is possible to estimate the arteriovenous oxygen difference [8].

For VO_2 determination a preliminary test for familiarization of the patient with the laboratory and the technique is mandatory [9]. Weber and Janicki [10] reported a frequently utilized classification of HF severity based on peak VO_2 which does not consider age, sex and fitness (table 1). Furthermore, the Weber and Janicki classification reports VO_2 normalized for body weight but does not take into account obese subjects. Indeed in obesity the correction for body weight does not consider that fat has a very low oxygen consumption and VO_2/kg underestimates the true VO_2 [11]. Other classifications have been proposed based on a percentage of VO_2max [12] but are not very popular.

VO_2 at anaerobic threshold is a good indicator of exercise capacity [13]. The value of VO_2 at anaerobic threshold is unrelated to patient motivation and does not need a maximal effort albeit the patients have to perform an effort above the anaerobic threshold. Indeed to calculate anaerobic threshold, data above it are needed. The best way to calculate anaerobic threshold is the so-called V-slope plot in which VCO_2 and VO_2 are plotted against each other [14]. To obtain a correct measure, data at the beginning of exercise, which are or might be influenced by psychologically-induced hyperventilation, and at the end of exercise, when ventilation can be further increased because of thermodynamic reasons, have to be withdrawn. Afterwards, two linear relations can be identified with the slope of the first between 0.95 and 0.99 and the slope of the second well above 1. However, in HF a gradual modification of peripheral muscle metabolism can occur so that anaerobic threshold can be difficult to calculate. Therefore it is strongly recommended to confirm the anaerobic threshold value calculated with the V-slope. Two methods are used. The first is the increase in the so-called ventilatory equivalent for oxygen (VE/VO_2) with a constant ventilatory equivalent for CO_2 (VE/VCO_2) and second an increase in end-expiratory oxygen pressure with a constant end-expiratory pressure for CO_2. However, VO_2 at anaerobic threshold is rarely utilized by itself to quantify exercise capacity but, more often, is used as an accessory tool to confirm the value of peak VO_2 [15]. As an alternative to anaerobic threshold the calculation of the VO_2 when the respiratory ratio (VCO_2/VO_2) became = 1 has been proposed [15] but this is not the anaerobic threshold.

Table 1. Functional classification based on peak exercise O_2 uptake and anaerobic threshold [10]

Functional class	Peak VO_2 ml/min/kg	VO_2 at anaerobic threshold, ml/min/kg
A	>20	>14
B	16–20	11–14
C	10–15	8–11
D	<10	<8

The VO_2/work relationship is an index of cardiovascular performance used to assess HF. In HF this relationship flattens [16]. Sometimes the VO_2/work relationship shows two slopes with the first in the normal range (~ 10 ml/min/W) and the second reduced. This suggests inadequate oxygen availability to the exercising muscle possibly due to effort induced cardiac ischemia.

CPET in Evaluation of HF Prognosis and Selection/Follow-Up of Patients on Heart Transplant Lists

Serial assessment by cardiopulmonary exercise test provides very relevant information concerning prognosis and risk stratification of HF. As initially demonstrated by the V-HeFT I and II trials, peak VO_2 has emerged as a strong prognostic indicator [17]. Mancini et al. [18] have proposed peak VO_2 as a critical decision-making parameter to detect the optimal timepoint for heart transplantation. Szlachcic et al. [19] reported a 77% annual mortality rate in those patients with a peak VO_2 <10 ml/min/kg compared to 21% in those with a peak VO_2 between 10 and 18 ml/min/kg. More recent studies report a mortality rate of respectively 36 or 15% in case the peak VO_2 was below or above 13 ml/min/kg [20]. However, improvement in HF treatment has progressively increased survival of HF patients so that it is important to frequently re-evaluate prognosis of such patients [21]. Since VO_2 is dependent on several determinants such as the muscular mass, age, sex and training effect, it has emerged that considering the percent predicted peak VO_2 (% peak VO_2) rather than the absolute value bears a better prognostic power [12, 22, 23]. It has been suggested, however, that to correctly evaluate a low VO_2 an objective exercise limitation has to be evident [24]. In other words, it is mandatory to know that peak VO_2 is a real peak VO_2. Furthermore, exercise capacity might improve in the follow-up despite a low peak VO_2 on initial testing. Stevenson et al. [25] showed that it was possible to safely withdraw from a heart transplant waiting list 29% of ambulatory patients who had in the follow-up an improvement in peak VO_2 that indicates improvement in prognosis and functional capacity. Accordingly, serial assessment of HF status is needed [26].

Moreover, the survival analysis has been performed considering additional parameters such as the heart rate, blood pressure and respiratory quotient other than peak VO_2, % peak VO_2 and VO_2 at the anaerobic threshold [27]. Patients with a peak VO_2 <14 ml/min/kg, systolic arterial blood pressure <120 mm Hg or a % peak VO_2 <50 showed the worse prognosis. Specifically, in patients with a systolic blood pressure <120 mm Hg the 3-year survival rate was 55% compared to 83% in those showing a systolic blood pressure >120 mm Hg.

A controversial issue regards the relative importance and the potential additive contribution of combining CPET evaluation with simultaneous hemodynamic evaluation. Chomsky et al. [28] reported an improved predictive power when peak VO_2 was combined with invasive cardiac output evaluation. Opposite results were reported in another study [29]. At present, although there is general consensus in identifying patients with a peak VO_2 <10 ml/min/kg as a subgroup at very high risk and highest priority for transplantation [30], and patients with a peak VO_2 >18 ml/min/kg as those with a very good 2-year prognosis, uncertainty still exists when considering patients whose peak VO_2 is between these cut-off values. Interestingly, a peak VO_2 of 14 ml/min/kg, although initially proposed as an important cut-off value, no longer appears as valuable in this respect [31–33]. In any case, VO_2 has to be measured and not only estimated from workload [33].

A recent re-analysis aimed at evaluating the prognostic significance of peak VO_2 revealed that in the presence of severe HF it is important to figure out any clinical contraindication to perform a test, and a lack of the prognostic power of peak VO_2 is observed in those with severe HF while it is maintained in less severe patients [34]. However, in the female population the cardiopulmonary exercise test lacks predictive [23, 34] and decisional power [35]. In this regard, significant gender-related differences in the exercise response have been reported despite comparable hemodynamic impairment [36]. It is also interesting to note that in most of the studies in which peak VO_2 was evaluated, the average population age range was between 49 and 59.5 years [37].

Recently, it has been shown that abnormalities occur in the ventilatory response to exercise, and particularly an increased slope of the ventilation to carbon dioxide production (VE/VCO_2) is a powerful independent prognostic indicator [38–41]. In a population of 470 patients undergoing CPET, Robbins et al. [42] demonstrated that an increased VE/VCO_2 slope (>44) is a relevant prognostic indicator whose power increased when combined to a reduced chronotropic index. Recently, Ponikowski et al. [40] analyzed 123 patients with a peak VO_2 >18 ml/min/kg. In this subset of patients the authors found that those with a steeper VE/VCO_2 (>34), the 3-year survival rate was 57% compared to 93% in those with a normal VE/VCO_2.

Limiting Factor to Exercise in HF

Several organs can be the limiting factor of exercise in HF. As a consequence, there is not a single parameter measured at rest which can predict exercise capacity. For instance the lack of correlation between left ventricle ejection fraction at rest and peak VO_2 has been known for many years [17, 43]. Albeit the interplay between each organ is relevant, we will analyze independently each function to identify specific targets for treatment.

The Heart

The heart is the organ from which HF starts. However, when HF is overt, it may not be the leading cause of exercise limitation. In the presence of exercise limitation a prevalence of cardiac dysfunction is suggested by a reduced VO_2 at anaerobic threshold, a decreased heart rate difference between rest and peak exercise, oxygen pulse and slope of VO_2/work relationship. Indeed, because oxygen delivery to the muscle is reduced, energy is produced by anaerobic pathways even at low workload loads which determines an early appearance of anaerobic threshold. The difference between rest and peak exercise heart rates is reduced because resting heart rate is higher than in normal subjects, with the exception of patients treated with β-blockers, and because peak exercise heart rate is low due to chronotropic incompetence or treatments such as digitalis, β-blockers, amiodarone, or a combination of such drugs. The oxygen pulse is clinically utilized as an index of stroke volume. In reality the oxygen pulse is stroke volume × the arteriovenous oxygen difference and therefore it is related to stroke volume if the arteriovenous oxygen difference is normal. Therefore, before utilizing the oxygen pulse as an index of stroke volume, anemia and hypoxia have to be excluded. A low VO_2/work relationship slope through the exercise or in the second part of exercise is also an index of reduced cardiac output.

The Circulation

Alteration in peripheral circulation can participate to limiting exercise capacity in HF. However, those patients with the greatest HF severity have the greatest capability to redistribute blood flow toward the exercising muscle. As a consequence, HF patients, for instance, compensate for the reduced kidney blood flow by increasing oxygen extraction, thereby keeping kidney VO_2 constant. It has been suggested that this is due to a local vascular tone regulation possibly mediated by hemoglobin-desaturation-induced NO release. In HF, fluid accumulates both inside the vascular wall and in the tissue increasing the distance between capillary and mitochondria. This should also make more difficult oxygen flow toward the mitochondria. At the present time, no specific parameters derived from CPET can be used to suggest a peripheral circulatory alteration in HF.

The Muscular Fibers

The muscular fibers undergo relevant changes in HF. Indeed a switch in fiber type has been claimed but both types are grossly atrophic with variation and inhomogeneity of fiber size, reversion to neonatal isoform of myosin, altered morphology of mitochondria and enzymes function [44]. It is likely that these muscular alterations are due to cytokine activation including tumor necrosis factor or development of insulin resistance. This has allowed the formulation of a 'muscular hypothesis' to explain symptoms and progression of HF. This hypothesis states that due to inactivity, malnutrition and increase of inflammatory status, HF patients develop a skeletal and respiratory myopathy which not only induces fatigue and dyspnea by itself, but also through an increased ergoreflex activity (sympathetic activity) increases ventilation and peripheral vasoconstriction. In this regard it is of note that in some HF patients the PO_2 in the femoral increase in the second part of exercise suggests recruitment of muscular fibers with a low VO_2/blood flow relationship. Accordingly, elements which suggest that the peripheral muscles are the major cause of exercise limitation are symptoms such as leg pain and fatigue and a reduced VO_2/work slope; increased ventilation can also be considered as incompatible with the suggestion of muscular origin of exercise ventilation. However, a great deal of information is lacking as regards the inflammatory status of HF [45, 46].

The Sympathetic Neuroendocrine System

Inappropriate activation of the sympathetic neuroendocrine system in HF has been known for many years. Indeed, Cohn et al. [47] showed that the norepinephrine plasma level was increased in HF and that the norepinephrine plasma level can be used to assess prognosis. Furthermore, improvement of norepinephrine kinetics during exercise was paralleled by improvement in exercise parameters [48] and β-blocking agents, used to reduce sympathetic hyperactivity, are now utilized in ~30% of HF patients in western countries.

The Lungs

Respiratory function is severely impaired in HF because of mechanical and diffusion alterations. The former is classically characterized by an increase in ventilation due to reduction in tidal volume and increase in respiratory rate [49]. This increase in ventilation is observed relative to work rate, VO_2 and VCO_2. Recently, however, Johnson et al. [50] showed, using pulmonary flow/volume curves, that the expiratory flow reserve was dramatically reduced through exercise and that the only way that HF patients have to keep increasing ventilation is through an increment in functional respiratory capacity (FRC) during exercise. Parameters suggestive of lung mechanical alteration during exercise are: (a) increase in ventilation for a given work rate, (b) reduced tidal volume, (c) increased dead space to tidal volume ratio and (d) increase in respiratory rate. Also, lung diffusion is altered in HF. Indeed, albeit the capillary blood volume increase during exercise, this is not enough to compensate the specific membrane diffusive capability reduction. This is likely due to increase in fibrosis and cellular content at the alveolar-capillary membrane. Furthermore, lung diffusion increase during exercise is blunted in HF. Another role of the lung in HF is to regulate the

Table 2. Effects of different drug classes on CPET variables in CHF

	Vasodilators	Ca^{2+} blockers	ACE inhibitors	AT_1 blockers	β-Blockers
Exercise time	↑↑	↔	↑	↑	↔
Peak VO_2	↑↑	↔	↑	↑	↔
Peak VE	↔	↔	↑	↔	↔
Peak VT	↔	↔	↑	↔	↔
VE/VCO_2	↔	↔	↓	↔	↓
O_2 pulse	↑	↔	↔	↑	↔
VO_2/WR	↑	↔	↔	↑	↔

norepinephrine plasma level. Indeed, in normal subjects at rest, blood flow through the lung is associated with a reduction of norepinephrine plasma level. This is also true during exercise up to a norepineprhirene plasma value of ~1,300 pg ml^{-1}, when the lung capability to clear norepinephrine is lost and actually blood flow through the lung is associated with an increase of plasma norepinephrine [51].

Typical CPET Response in HF

As a consequence of the limiting factors to exercise in HF, it is possible to summarize the following as classical CPET responses in HF: (a) reduction in workload achieved, (b) reduction in peak exercise VO_2, (c) reduction in VO_2 at anaerobic threshold, (d) reduction in VO_2/work rate relationship, (e) reduction in oxygen pulse, (f) reduction in rest to peak heart rate differences, (g) reduction in tidal volume at peak exercise and anaerobic threshold, (h) increase in VE/VCO_2 slope, (i) reduction in expiratory flow reserve and (l) increase in peak exercise FRC.

Use of CPET in the Assessment of Therapeutic Intervention in HF

A systematic analysis of cardiovascular, ventilatory and peripheral variables and the relative contribution of each of them in the overall exercise performance represents a step forward in exploring the mechanisms whereby various treatment strategies can be beneficial. Table 2 summarizes the effect on CPET parameters of the various anti-failure drugs.

Pharmacological Interventions

Vasodilator Drugs. The Veterans Administration Studies (V-HeFT I and V-HeFT II) showed that a vasodilator regimen such as the combination of hydralazine + isosorbide dinitrate is capable of reducing mortality and improving peak VO_2 [43, 52]. An overall improvement in cardiac output response and peripheral blood flow distribution are mechanisms likely involved in the observed peak VO_2 amelioration. The V-HeFT I changes in peak VO_2 with the hydralazine + isosorbide dinitrate combination were not duplicated by the α_1-blocker prazosin [53]. The somewhat surprising contrast between a better angiotensin-converting enzyme (ACE) inhibitor-mediated effect on mortality, and a superior efficacy of the hydralazine + isosorbide dinitrate combination on peak VO_2, may be justified by the different mortality rate and dropouts from exercise testing in the two treatment arms [43].

Whether Ca^{2+} channel blockers may have favorable effects on the exercise capacity of HF patients remains controversial. Nifedipine has a positive action in acute pulmonary edema, particularly in the presence of systemic hypertension, but its long-term use has adverse clinical events which fail to benefit from VO_2 and exercise performance [54, 55]. Nevertheless, nonvascular-selective dihydropiridine Ca^{2+} antagonists which promote less sympathetic activation and are hypothesized to better modulate vascular compliance, might produce a more efficient ventricular unloading [56]. However, large trials have failed to show any positive effect of amlodipine [57, 58].

ACE Inhibitors. ACE inhibition is one of the most effective pharmacological remedies for improving exercise capacity in HF [59, 60]. In a wide meta-analysis of 35 double-blind trials, involving 3,411 patients receiving chronic ACE inhibition, Naragh et al. [59] reported a significant improvement in patients' symptoms in 76% of the studies with a prolongation of exercise duration in 66%. The therapeutic properties of ACE inhibitors are class-dependent and there seems to be no significant relationship with their pharmacokinetics and tissue ACE specificity [59]. ACE inhibition improves cardiac performance and reverses, at least in part, peripheral abnormalities. Hence, amelioration of functional capacity with ACE inhibitors in HF patients has been interpreted as related to structural or functional improvements involving heart [61], peripheral circulation [60] or skeletal muscles [62]. The relevance of an influence on lungs and ventilatory abnormalities observed during exercise has recently been investigated [44, 63]. The pathophysiology is based on the concepts that lung microvessels are the major site of conversion of angiotensin I to angiotensin II and ACE is highly concentrated on the luminal surface of the pulmonary vasculature [64] and its blockade reduces the exposure to angiotensin II and enhances local vasodilator prostaglandins, mainly prostacyclin (PGI_2) and NO production. In both short- [45] and long-term [63] prospective studies of HF patients, enalapril (20 mg/day) enhanced the alveolar-capillary gas diffusion and this was paralleled by an improvement in exercise ventilation-perfusion matching, VE/VCO_2 relationship and VO_2 at peak and at any paired-matched exercise load [63, 65]. Moreover, the observation that the improvement in exercise capacity and DL_{CO} with enalapril may be attenuated by administration of acetylsalicylic acid supports the interpretation that overexpression of the bradykinin pathway, and specifically stimulation of PGI_2 production by ACE inhibition, may mediate of this effect.

AT_1 Receptor Blockers. Despite encouraging premises the recent introduction of AT1 receptor blockers failed to show consistent advantages over ACE inhibitors [66]. In spite of this, AT_1 receptor blockers possess some pharmacological properties that make these compounds attractive, especially when combined with ACE inhibitors. AT_1 receptor blockers possess a greater ability than ACE inhibitors in blocking the angiotensin II stimulation of AT_1 receptors and in enhancing the AT_2 receptor activation. On the other hand, it is now clear that part of the effects of ACE inhibitors are due to an increased bradykinin-mediated availability of endothelium-dependent factors, such as NO and PGI_2. AT_1 receptor blockade with losartan in HF patients results in hemodynamic changes similar to those with ACE inhibition [67–69]. Combination of these two drugs is safe, well tolerated and produced a significantly greater overall effect on peak VO_2 [68–69]. Analyzing CPET variables of cardiac, ventilatory and peripheral performance [69], differences between the two classes of drugs have been noted regarding lung function (i.e. reduction of VE vs. VCO_2 slope and VD/VT while on enalapril) and O_2 utilization (i.e. increased rate of VO_2/watt relationship while on losartan) that were synergistic in improving peak VO_2 when the two classes of drugs were combined.

β-Adrenergic Receptor Blockers. Although chronic β-receptor blockade has been shown to improve functional and biological properties of the failing heart and increases life expectancy [70], changes in peak VO_2 and maximal exercise performance do not seem to benefit from β-blockers [71–75].

Hormones. Several hormones like growth hormone and thyroxine have been proposed as additive therapeutic tools in HF. Albeit thyroxine has been shown to improve exercise capacity [76, 77] and increase peak VO_2 and VO_2 at anaerobic threshold, the mechanisms are still unclear.

Other Drugs. Several other drugs are very effectively used for HF treatment, such as digitalis [78] and diuretics, however their specific action on cardiopulmonary parameters is almost unknown.

Nonpharmacological Interventions

Cardiac Surgery. Several surgical procedures have been applied to treat HF. At the present time only mitral valve repair, dynamic cardiomyoplasty and left ventricular size reduction, the so-called Batista operation, are still under evaluation. Mitral valve repair is not a standardized surgical procedure, which has produced inconsistent results with some very successful cases and some failures. From an exercise evaluation point of view, a successful operation should produce an increase in peak and anaerobic threshold VO_2, peak oxygen pulse and slope of the VO_2/work relationship. However, no such data have been published. The dynamic cardiomyoplasty consists of wrapping the left ventricle with a thoracic flat muscle, the latissimus dorsi. This should allow to increase the force of the failing left ventricle. No positive consistent results have been reported. Finally, left ventricular size reduction should not only allow to reduce left ventricle size and improve function, but also reduce the lung restrictive syndrome because it increases the thoracic volume available for the lung [79]. More promising are chronic left ventricle assist devices, but their evaluation as not-bridge-to-heart-transplant tools is at the very beginning [80]. Preliminary data, however, suggest the possibility that chronic left ventricular assist devices can reverse ventricular remodeling and induce some degree of recovery of myocardial properties in heart previously considered to have irreversible end-stage HF [81]. Whether this improvement will last after the device has been removed is still unknown.

Ultrafiltration. Ultrafiltration is a dialytic technique utilized in HF to reduce excessive body fluid. Ultrafiltration is a safe procedure. In brief, a venovenous bypass is needed through which blood is propelled by a peristaltic pump to a filter which allows separation of blood from plasma fluid (which contains molecules with a weight of <50,000 daltons) so that the oncotic power of blood is increased after the filtered blood flows back into the venous circulation. The beauty of the technique is that it allows, in contrast to diuretics, a normotonic reduction of body fluid which does not interfere with the balance of intra- and extracellular fluids [48]. Cardiopulmonary exercise testing has been extensively used to test the efficacy of the technique and has allowed to understand some of the physiological insights of exercise in HF patients. Indeed, ultrafiltration improves exercise capacity, in terms of exercise tolerance, VO_2 at peak exercise and anaerobic threshold, through an increase in ventilation due to an increase in tidal volume. Ultrafiltration induces an increase in dynamic lung compliance and, as a consequence, reduces the external constraint on the heart [82]. Interestingly, while ultrafiltration has allowed to show an increase in lung mechanical properties, it has not shown any effect on lung diffusion, suggesting that, in chronic HF, the often demonstrated lung diffusion abnormalities are not related to an increased fluid content along the alveolar-capillary membrane but probably to an increase in connective tissue [83].

Pacing. The use of pacemakers has been proposed to improve cardiac function in HF. Two types of pacing techniques have been studied, namely (a) atrioventricular synchronous pacing and (b) biventricular pacing. Albeit several studies have shown that at rest atrioventricular synchrony improves cardiac output [84], evaluation with different atrioventricular intervals was not able to show consistent results. Biventricular pacing is a new pacing technique that allows simultaneous stimulation of both ventricles. Initial results are promising but large and long-term studies are lacking and it is unknown which patients are the best candidates for biventricular pacing. Furthermore, it is unclear whether the relevant event is biventricular stimulation or left ventricle stimulation by itself.

References

1 Myers J, Buchanan N, Walsh D, Kraemer M, McAuley P, Hamilton-Wessler M, Froelicher V: Comparison of the ramp versus standard exercise protocols. J Am Coll Cardiol 1991;17:1334–1342.
2 Koike A, Yajima T, Adachi H, Shimizu N, Kano H, Sugimoto K, Niwa A, Marumo F, Hiroe M: Evaluation of exercise capacity using submaximal exercise at a constant work rate in patients with cardiovascular disease. Circulation 1995;81:1719–1724.
3 Belardinelli R, Zhang YY, Wasserman K, Purcaro A., Agostoni PG: A four-minute submaximal constant work rate exercise test to assess cardiovascular functional class in chronic heart failure. Am J Cardiol 1998;81:1210–1214.
4 Sietsema KE, Daly JA, Wasserman K: Early dynamics of O_2 uptake and heart rate as affected by exercise work rate. J Appl Physiol 1989;67:2535–2541.
5 Perego GB, Marenzi M, Guazzi M, Sganzerla P, Assanelli E, Palermo P, Conconi B, Lauri G, Agostoni PG: Contribution of PO_2, P_{50}, and Hb to changes in arteriovenous O_2 content during exercise in heart failure. J Appl Physiol 1996;80623–631.
6 Agostoni PG, Wasserman K, Guazzi M, Cattadori G, Palermo P, Marenzi G, Guazzi MD: Exercise-induced hemoconcentration in heart failure due to dilated cardiomyopathy. Am J Cardiol 1999;83:278–280.
7 Agostoni PG, Wasserman K, Perego GB, Marenzi G, Guazzi M, Assanelli E, Lauri G, Guazzi MD: Oxygen transport to muscle during exercise in chronic congestive heart failure secondary to idiopathic dilated cardiomyopathy. Am J Cardiol 1997;79:29–33.
8 Agostoni PG, Wasserman K, Perego GB, Guazzi M., Cattadori G, Palermo P, Lauri G, Marenzi G: Non-invasive measurement of stroke volume during exercise in heart failure patients. Clin Sci 2000;98:545–551.
9 Elborn JS, Stanford CF, Nicholls DP: Reproducibility of cardiopulmonary parameters during exercise in patients with chronic cardiac failure. The need for a preliminary test. Eur Heart J 1990;11:75–81.
10 Weber KT, Janicki JS: Cardiopulmonary exercise testing for evaluation of chronic cardiac failure. Am J Cardiol 1985;55:22A–31A.
11 Agostoni PG, Bussotti M, Palermo P, Melzi G, Lomanto M: La valutazione dell'insufficienza cardiaca. Cardiologia 1998;43:305–308.
12 Stelken AM, Younis LT, Jennison SH, Miller DD, Miller LW, Shaw LJ, Kargl D, Chaitman BR: Prognostic value of cardiopulmonary exercise testing using percent achieved of predicted peak oxygen uptake for patients with ischemic and dilated cardiomyopathy. J Am Coll Cardiol 1996;27:345–352.
13 Sullivan MJ, Cobb FR: The anaerobic threshold in chronic heart failure. Relation to blood lactate, ventilatory basis, reproducibility, and response to exercise training. Circulation 1990; 81(suppl 2):47–58.
14 Beaver WL, Wasserman K, Whipp BJ: Improved detection of lactate threshold during exercise using a log-log transformation. J Appl Physiol 1985;59:1936–1940.
15 Cohen-Solal A, Aupetit JF, Gueret P, Kolsky H, Zannad F: Can anaerobic threshold be used as an end-point for therapeutic trials in heart failure? Lesson from a multicentre randomized placebo-controlled trial. Eur Heart J 1994;15:236–241.
16 Cohen-Solal A Chabernaud JM, Gourgon R: Comparison of oxygen uptake during bicycle exercise in patients with chronic heart failure and in normal subjects. J Am Coll Cardiol 1990;16:80–85.
17 Cohn JN, Johnson GR, Shabetai R, Loeb H, Tristani F, Rector T, Smith R, Fletcher R: Ejection fraction, peak exercise oxygen consumption, cardiothoracic ratio, ventricular arrhythmias, and plasma norepinephrine as determinants of prognosis in heart failure. The V-HeFT VA Cooperative Studies Group. Circulation 1993;87:VI5–V16.
18 Mancini DM, Eisen H, Kussmaul W, Mull R, Edmunds LH, Wilson JR: Value of peak exercise oxygen consumption for optimal timing of cardiac transplantation in ambulatory patients with heart failure. Circulation 1991;83:778–786.
19 Szlachcic J, Massie BM, Kramer BL, Topic N, Tubau J: Correlates and prognostic implication of exercise capacity in chronic congestive heart failure. Am J Cardiol 1985;55:1037–1042.
20 Miller LW: Listing criteria for cardiac transplantation: Results of an American Society of Transplant Physicians-National Institutes of Health conference. Transplantation 1998;66:947–951.
21 Stevenson WG, Stevenson LW, Middlekauff HR, Fonarow GC, Hamilton MA, Woo MA, Saxon LA, Natterson PD, Steimle A, Walden JA, Tillisch JH: Improving surviving for patients with advanced heart failure: A study of 737 consecutive patients. J Am Coll Cardiol 1995;26:1417–1423.
22 Likoff MJ, Chandler SL, Kay HR: Clinical determinants of mortality in chronic congestive heart failure secondary to idiopathic dilated or to ischemic cardiomyopathy. Am J Cardiol 1987;59:634–638.
23 Aaronson KD, Mancini DM: Is percentage of predicted maximal exercise oxygen consumption a better predictor of survival than peak exercise oxygen consumption for patients with severe heart failure? J Heart Lung Transplant 1995;14:981–989.

24 Ramos-Barbòn D, Fitchett D, Gibbons WJ, Latter DA, Levy RD: Maximal exercise testing for the selection of heart transplantation candidates. Limitation of peak oxygen consumption. Chest 1999;115:410–417.
25 Stevenson LW, Steimle AE, Fonarow G, Kermani M, Kermani D, Hamilton MA, Moriguchi JD, Walden J, Tillisch JH, Drinkwater DC, Laks H: Improvement in exercise capacity of candidates awaiting heart transplantation. J Am Coll Cardiol 1995;25:163–170.
26 Stevenson LW: Selection and management of candidates for heart transplantation. Curr Opin Cardiol 1996;11:166–173.
27 Osada N, Chaitman BR, Miller LW, Yip D, Cishek MB, Wolford TL, Donohue TJ: Cardiopulmonary exercise testing identifies low risk patients with heart failure and severely impaired exercise capacity considered for heart transplantation. J Am Coll Cardiol 1998;31: 577–582.
28 Chomsky DB, Lang CC, Rayos GH, Shyr Y, Yeoh TK, Pierson RN, Davis SF, Wilson JR: Hemodynamic exercise testing. A valuable tool in the selection of cardiac transplantation candidates. Circulation 1996;94:3176–3183.
29 Mancini D, Katz S, Donchez L, Aaronson K: Coupling of hemodynamic measurements with oxygen consumption during exercise does not improve risk stratification in patients with heart failure. Circulation 1996;94:2492–2496.
30 Mancini D, LeJemtel T, Aaronson K: Peak VO_2: A simple yet enduring standard. Circulation 2000;101:1080–1082.
31 Kao W, Winkel E, Costanzo MR: Candidate evaluation and selection for heart transplantation. Curr Opin Cardiol 1995;10:159–168.
32 Pina IL: Optimal candidates for heart transplantation: Is 14 the magic number? J Am Coll Cardiol 1995;26:436–437.
33 Myers J, Gullestad L, Vagelos R, Do D, Bellin D, Ross H, Fowler MB: Clinical, hemodynamic, and cardiopulmonary exercise test determinants of survival in patients referred for evaluation of heart failure. Ann Intern Med 1998;129:286–293.
34 Opasich C, Pinna GD, Bobbio M, Sisti M, Demichelis B, Febo O, Forni G, Riccardi R, Riccardi PG, Capomolla S, Cobelli F, Tavazzi L: Peak exercise oxygen consumption in chronic heart failure: Toward efficient use in the individual patient. J Am Coll Cardiol 1998; 31:766–775.
35 Richards DR, Mehra MR, Ventura HO, Lavie CJ, Smart FW, Stapleton DD, Milani RV: Usefulness of peak oxygen consumption in predicting outcome of heart failure in women versus men. Am J Cardiol 1997;80:1236–1238.
36 Guazzi M, Pontone G, Brambilla R, Agostoni PG, Guazzi MD: Gender differences in cardiopulmonary exercise testing response in patients with chronic heart failure. Eur J Heart Failure 2001;ABS (in press).
37 Myers J, Gullestad L: The role of exercise testing and gas-exchange measurement in the prognostic assessment of patients with heart failure. Curr Opin Cardiol 1998;13:145–155.
38 Chua TP, Ponikowski P, Harrington D, Anker SD, Webb-Peploe K, Clark AL, Poole-Wilson PA, Coats AJ: Clinical correlates and prognostic significance of the ventilatory response to exercise in chronic heart failure. J Am Coll Cardiol 1997;29:1585–1590.
39 Kleber FX, Vietzke G, Wernecke KD, Bauer U, Opitz C, Wensel R, Sperfeld A, Glaser S: Impairment of ventilatory efficiency in heart failure: Prognostic impact. Circulation 2000; 101:2803–2809.
40 Ponikowski P, Francis DP, Piepoli MF, Davies LC, Chua TP, Davos CH, Florea V, Banasiak W, Poole-Wilson PA, Coats AJ, Anker SD: Enhanced ventilatory response to exercise in patients with chronic heart failure and preserved exercise tolerance: Marker of abnormal cardiorespiratory reflex control and predictor of poor prognosis. Circulation 2001;103:967–972.
41 Johnson RL: Gas exchange efficiency in congestive heart failure. Circulation 2000;101: 2774–2776.
42 Robbins M, Francis G, Pashkow FJ, Snader CE, Hoercher K, Young JB, Lauer MS: Ventilatory and heart rate responses to exercise: Better predictors of heart failure mortality than peak oxygen consumption. Circulation 1999; 100:2411–2477.
43 Ziesche S, Cobb FR, Cohn JN, Johnson G, Tristani F for the VeFT VA Cooperatives Studies Group: Hydralazine and isosorbide dinitrate combination improves exercise tolerance in heart failure. Results from V-HeFT I and V-HeFT II. Circulation 1993,87:VI-56–VI-64.
44 Poole-Wilson PA: The relation between muscle function and increased ventilation in heart failure; in Wasserman K (ed): Exercise Gas Exchange in Heart Disease. Armonk/NY, Futura, 1996, pp 83–93.
45 Guazzi M, Marenzi GC, Alimento M, Contini M, Agostoni PG: Improvement of alveolar-capillary membrane diffusing capacity with enalapril in chronic heart failure and counteracting effect of aspirin. Circulation 1997;95:1930–1936.
46 Cugno M, Agostoni PG, Brunner HR, Gardinali M, Agostoni A, Nussberger J: Plasma bradykinin levels in human chronic congestive heart failure. Clin Sci 2000;99:461–466.
47 Cohn JN, Levine TB, Olivari MT, Garberg V, Lura D, Francis GS, Simon AB, Rector T: Plasma norepinephrine as a guide to prognosis in patients with chronic congestive heart failure. N Engl J Med 1984;311:819–823.
48 Agostoni PG, Marenzi GC, Pepi M, Doria E, Salvioni A, Perego G, Lauri G, Giraldi F, Grazi S, Guazzi MD: Isolated ultrafiltration in moderate congestive heart failure. J Am Coll Cardiol 1993;21:424–431.
49 Wasserman K, Zhang YY, Gitt A, Belardinelli R, Koike A, Lubarsky L, Agostoni PG: Lung function and exercise gas exchange in chronic heart failure. Circulation 1997;96:2221–2227.
50 Johnson BD, Weisman IM, Zeballos RJ, Beck KC: Emerging concepts in the evaluation of ventilatory limitation during exercise. The exercise tidal flow-volume loop. Chest 1999;116: 488–503.
51 Marenzi G, Agostoni PG, Guazzi M, Lauri G, Assanelli E, Guazzi MD: The noradrenaline plasma concentration and its gradient across the lung. Eur J Clin Invest 2000;30:660–667.
52 Cohn JN, Johnson GR, Shabetai R, Loeb H, Tristani F, Rector T, Smith R, Fletcher R: Ejection fraction, peak exercise oxygen consumption, cardiothoracic ratio, ventricular arrhythmias and plasma norepinephrine as determinants of prognosis in heart failure. The V-HeFT VA Cooperative Studies Group. Circulation 1993;87:VI5–V16.
53 Fink LI, Wilson JR, Ferraro N: Exercise ventilation and pulmonary artery wedge pressure in chronic stable congestive heart failure. Am J Cardiol 1986;57:249–253.
54 Elkayam U, Amin J, Mehra A, Vasquez J, Weber L, Rahimtoola SH: A prospective, randomized, double-blind, crossover study to compare the efficacy and safety of chronic nifedipine therapy with that of isosorbide dinitrate and their combination in the treatment of chronic congestive heart failure. Circulation 1990;82:1954–1961.
55 Agostoni PG, De Cesare N, Doria E, Polese A, Tamborini G, Guazzi MD: Afterload reduction: A comparison of captopril and nifedipine in dilated cardiomyopathy. Br Heart J 1986;55: 391–399.
56 Packer M, Nicod P, Khanderia R: Randomized, multicenter, double-blind, placebo-controlled evaluation of amlodipine in patients with mild-to-moderate heart failure (abstract). J Am Coll Cardiol 1996:274A.
57 Cohn JN, Zieshe SM, Smith R, Anand I, Dunkman WB, Loeb H, Cintron G, Boden W, Baruch L, Rochin P, Loss L: Effect of calcium antagonist felodipine as supplementary vasodilator therapy in patients with chronic heart failure treated with enalapril: V-HeFT III. Circulation 1997;96:856–863.
58 Udelson JE, DeAbate CA, Berk M, Neuberg G, Packer M, Vijay NK, Gorwitt J, Smith WB, Kukin ML, LeJemtel T, Levine TB, Konstam MA: Effects of amlodipine on exercise tolerance, quality of life, and left ventricular function in patients with heart failure from left ventricular systolic dysfunction. Am Heart J 2000; 139:503–510.
59 Naragh N, Swedberg K, Cleland JFG: What is the ideal study design for evaluation of treatment for heart failure? Insight from trials assessing the effects of ACE inhibitors on exercise capacity. Eur Heart J 1996;17:120–134.
60 Mancini DM, Davis L, Wexler JP, Chadwick B, Lejemtel TH: Dependence of enhanced maximal exercise performance on increased peak skeletal muscle perfusion during long-term captopril therapy in heart failure. J Am Coll Cardiol 1987;10:845–850.
61 Cohn JN: Structural basis for heart failure: Ventricular remodeling and its pathophysiological inhibition. Circulation 1995;91:2504–2507.

62 Wilson IR, Ferraro N: Effect of the renin-angiotensin system on limb circulation and metabolism during exercise in patients with chronic heart failure. J Am Coll Cardiol 1985; 6:556–563.
63 Guazzi M, Melzi G, Marenzi GC, Agostoni PG: ACE inhibition facilitates alveolar-capillary gas transfer, and improves ventilation/perfusion coupling in patients with left ventricular dysfunction. Clin Pharmacol Ther 1999;65: 319–327.
64 Pieruzzi F, Abassi ZA, Keiser HR: Expression of renin-angiotensin system components in the heart, kidneys and lungs of rats with experimental heart failure. Circulation 1995;92: 3105–3112.
65 Kitaoka H, Takata J, Hitomi N, Furuno T, Seo H, Chikamori T, Doi YL: Effect of angiotensin-converting enzyme inhibitor (enalapril or imidapril) on ventilation during exercise in patients with chronic heart failure secondary to idiopathic dilated cardiomyopathy. Am J Cardiol 2000;85:758–760.
66 Pitt B, Poole-Wilson PA, Segal R, Martinez FA, Dickstein K, Camm AJ, Konstam MA, Riegger G, Klinger GH, Neaton J, Sharma D, Thiyagarajan B: Effect of losartan compared with captopril on mortality in patients with symptomatic heart failure: Randomised trial – the Losartan Heart Failure Survival Study ELITE II. Lancet 2000;355:1582–1587.
67 Lang RM, Elkayam U, Yellen LG, Krauss D, McKelvie RS, Vaughan DE, Ney DE, Makris L, Chang PI: Comparative effects of losartan and enalapril on exercise capacity and clinical status in patients with heart failure. J Am Coll Cardiol 1997;30:983–991.
68 Hamroff G, Katz SD, Mancini D, Blaufarb I, Bijou R, Patel R, Joundeau G, Olivari MT, Thomas S, LeJemtel TH: Addition of angiotensin II receptor blockade to maximal angiotensin-converting enzyme inhibition improves exercise capacity in patients with severe congestive heart failure. Circulation 1999;99:990–992.
69 Guazzi M, Palermo P, Pontone G, Susini F, Agostoni PG: Synergistic efficacy of enalapril and losartan on exercise performance and oxygen consumption at peak exercise in congestive heart failure. Am J Cardiol 1999;84:1038–1043.
70 Eichhorn EJ, Bristow MR: Medical therapy can improve the biological properties of the chronically failing heart. A new era in the treatment of heart failure. Circulation 1996;94:2285–2296.
71 Waagstein F, Bristow MR, Swedberg K, Camerini F, Fowler MB, Silver MA, Gilbert EM, Johnson MR, Goss FG, Hjalmarson A: Beneficial effects of metoprolol in idiopathic dilated cardiomyopathy. Metoprolol in Dilated Cardiomyopathy (MDC) Trial Study Group. Lancet 1993;342:1441–1446.
72 Australia/New Zealand Heart Failure Research Collaborative Group: Effects of Carvedilol, a vasodilator β-blocker, in patients with congestive heart failure due to ischemic heart disease. Circulation 1995;92:212–218.
73 Packer M, Colucci WS, Sackner-Bernstein JD, Liang CS, Goldscher DA, Freeman I, Kukin ML, Kinhal V, Udelson JE, Klapholz M, Gottlieb SS, Pearle D, Cody RJ, Gregory JJ, Kantrowitz NE, LeJemtel TH, Young ST, Lukas MA, Shusterman NH: Double-blind, placebo-controlled study of the effects of Carvedilol in patients with moderate to severe heart failure. The PRECISE Trial. Prospective Randomized Evaluation of Carvedilol on Symptoms and Exercise. Circulation 1996;94:2793–2799.
74 Colucci WS, Packer M, Bristow MR, Gilbert EM, Cohn JN, Fowler MB, Krueger SK, Hershberger R, Uretsky BF, Bowers JA, Sackner-Bernstein JD, Young ST, Holcslaw TL, Lukas MA: Carvedilol inhibits clinical progression in patients with mild symptoms of heart failure. US Carvedilol Heart Failure Study Group. Circulation 1996;94:2800–2806.
75 Engelmeier RS, O'Connell JB, Walsh R, Rad N, Scanlon PJ, Gunnar RM: Improvement in symptoms and exercise tolerance by metoprolol in patients with dilated cardiomyopathy: A double-blind, randomized, placebo-controlled trial. Circulation 1985;75:536–546.
76 Moruzzi P, Doria E, Agostoni PG, Capacchione V, Sganzerla P: Usefulness of *L*-thyroxine to improve cardiac and exercise performance in idiopathic dilated cardiomyopathy. Am J Cardiol 1994;73:374–378.
77 Moruzzi P, Doria E, Agostoni PG: Medium-term effectiveness of *L*-thyroxine treatment in idiopathic dilated cardiomyopathy. Am J Med 1996;101:461–467.
78 Sullivan M, Atwood JE, Myers J, Feuer J, Hall P, Kellerman B, Forbes S, Froelicher V: Increased exercise capacity after digoxin administration in patients with heart failure. J Am Coll Cardiol 1989;13:1138–1143.
79 Agostoni PG, Cattadori G, Guazzi M, Palermo P, Bussotti M, Marenzi G: Cardiomegaly as a possible cause of lung dysfunction in patients with heart failure. Am Heart J 2000;140:24.
80 Jaski BE, Lingle RJ, Reardon LC, Dembitsky WP: Left ventricular assist device as a bridge to patient and myocardial recovery. Prog Cardiovasc Dis 2000;43:5–18.
81 Burkhoff D, Holmes JW, Madigan J, Barbone A, Oz MC: Left ventricular assist device-induced reverse ventricular remodeling. Prog Cardiovasc Dis 2000;43:19–26.
82 Agostoni PG, Marenzi GC, Sganzerla P, Assanelli E, Guazzi M, Perego GB, Lauri G, Doria E, Pepi M, Guazzi MD: Lung-heart interaction as a substrate for the improvement in exercise capacity following body fluid volume depletion in moderate congestive heart failure. Am J Cardiol 1995;76:793–798.
83 Agostoni PG, Guazzi M, Bussotti M, Grazi M, Palermo P, Marenzi G: Lack of improvement of lung diffusing capacity following fluid withdrawal by ultrafiltration in chronic heart failure. J Am Coll Cardiol 2000;36:1600–1604.
84 Linde C, Gadler F, Edner M, Nordlander R, Rosenqvist M, Rydén L: Results of atrioventricular synchronous pacing with optimized delay in patients with severe congestive heart failure. Am J Cardiol 1995;75:919–923.

Piergiuseppe Agostoni, MD, PhD
Chief Heart Failure Unit
Centro Cardiologico Monzino, IRCCS
Istituto di Cardiologia
Università di Milano, CNR
via Parea 4, I–20138 Milan (Italy)
Tel. +39 02 58002299, Fax +39 02 50011039
E-Mail Piergiuseppe.Agostoni@
cardiologicomonzino.it

Weisman IM, Zeballos RJ (eds): Clinical Exercise Testing.
Prog Respir Res. Basel, Karger, 2002, vol 32, pp 109–119

Noninvasive Exercise Testing Modalities for Ischemia

Katherine Strelich David S. Bach

Department of Medicine, Division of Cardiology, University of Michigan, Ann Arbor, Mich., USA

Summary

Cardiovascular disease is the leading cause of mortality in the United States and accounts for nearly 1 million deaths each year. Because revascularization and medical treatment of coronary artery disease (CAD) can improve outcome, early recognition and diagnosis are essential. In patients with an intermediate probability of CAD based on risk factor assessment and symptoms, noninvasive diagnostic testing is appropriate. Exercise treadmill testing is the most widely available testing modality and provides important information regarding functional status and prognosis. However, the sensitivity and specificity for the diagnosis of CAD are relatively low, especially in certain patient populations. The use of cardiac imaging, including nuclear perfusion imaging and echocardiography, improves the diagnostic accuracy of exercise testing and allows further characterization of ischemia. Among patients unable to exercise adequately, pharmacologic stress with dobutamine or a vasodilating agent provides a useful alternative to exercise, and is equally powerful in establishing a diagnosis of CAD.

Cardiovascular disease is the leading cause of mortality in the United States and accounts for nearly 1 million deaths each year [1]. Because revascularization and medical treatment of coronary artery disease (CAD) can improve outcome, early recognition and diagnosis is essential. Clinical factors such as age, sex, the presence of typical angina, and cardiovascular risk factors are helpful in predicting the likelihood of CAD in many patients. However, diagnostic testing is helpful in establishing the presence of CAD for patients at intermediate risk, and in guiding management in patients with known CAD.

The concept of stratifying patients into low-, intermediate- and high-risk groups based on clinical parameters was first introduced by Diamond and Forrester [2] in 1979. They described a method based on Bayes theorem of conditional probability in which the pre-test probability of disease was incorporated with the results of diagnostic testing to determine the post-test probability of disease. It was recognized that although the accuracy of a diagnostic test is defined by its sensitivity and specificity, its usefulness is highly dependant on the prevalence of disease in the tested population, which can be estimated based on clinical characteristics. For example, in a 65-year-old man with typical angina, the probability of CAD is so high [2, 3] that further testing will do little to change the probability of disease. In such patients, a negative test result is more likely to be falsely negative than to accurately exclude CAD. Conversely, the probability of CAD in a 50-year-old woman with atypical chest pain is intermediate and will be influenced by further testing.

This concept underscores the importance of patient selection when ordering tests for the diagnosis of CAD. Equally important is knowing the strengths and limitations of the testing modalities available. This article describes the most common methods of noninvasive test-

Table 1. Contraindications to exercise testing

Absolute	
Acute myocardial infarction (with 2 days)	
Unstable angina	
Uncontrolled cardiac arrhythmias	
Symptomatic, severe aortic stenosis	
Uncontrolled symptomatic heart failure	
Acute pulmonary embolus	
Acute aortic dissection	
Acute myocarditis or pericarditis	
Thrombosis of lower extremity	
Physical disability that would preclude safe and adequate test performance	
Relative	
Left main coronary stenosis	
Moderate aortic stenosis	
Electrolyte abnormalities	
Systemic hypertension (SBP > 200 mm Hg, DBP > 110 mm Hg)	
Severe pulmonary hypertension	
Tachyarrhythmias or bradyarrhythmias	
Hypertrophic cardiomyopathy with outflow tract obstruction	
High degree AV block	

Modified from Fletcher et al. [6] and Gibbons et al. [3].

ing and reviews their diagnostic performance in different patient populations. Although stress testing is done in a wide variety of clinical settings, the present review focuses on the utility of stress testing in the detection of ischemia and the diagnosis of obstructive CAD.

Exercise Treadmill Test

Exercise testing with ECG monitoring (ETT) is a well-established, widely available, and low cost method of testing for CAD. Data from the National Ambulatory Medical Care Surveys indicated that 6.2 million exercise stress tests were ordered in the outpatient setting in 1991 and 1992 [4]. Only 27% of these patients had known CAD, suggesting that most outpatient stress tests are ordered for diagnostic purposes.

Class I indications for an exercise stress test, as outlined in ACC/AHA guidelines [3], are to diagnose obstructive CAD in adult patients with an intermediate pretest probability of disease (including those with complete right bundle branch block (RBBB) or <1 mm resting ST-segment depression); and for risk assessment/prognosis in patients with known or suspected CAD undergoing initial evaluation, or who present with a change in clinical status. In patients with a baseline ECG documenting pre-excitation syndrome (Wolf-Parkinson-White), electronically paced rhythm, >1 mm ST-segment depression, or left bundle branch block (LBBB), ETT without imaging should not be done for the diagnosis of CAD, but may be helpful in the assessment of risk and prognosis.

Although exercise testing is generally safe, myocardial infarction (MI) and sudden cardiac death occur at a reported rate of approximately 1 per 2,500 tests [5]. The risk is higher in patients with recent MI and in those being evaluated for malignant ventricular arrhythmias [6]. In patients with CAD, the relative risk of a cardiac event occurring during exercise stress test is 60–100 times higher than during normal daily activity. The relative and absolute contraindications to exercise testing are outlined in table 1.

Overview of the Procedure

A standard exercise test consists of a physical stress (treadmill, upright or supine bicycle) during continuous ECG monitoring. Treadmill testing is the most common method of stress, at least in part because most patients can achieve maximal exertion with walking, whereas leg fatigue may precede maximal exertion with bicycle ergometry. Several treadmill protocols are used, including Bruce, Naughton, Cornell, and Ramp. The specifics of each test are beyond the scope of the present discussion. However, the goal of the practitioner is to select a protocol that is individualized to the patient. The optimum protocol should last 6–12 min [7] during which time the patient reaches peak exertion in a controlled manner.

A resting ECG is obtained in supine and standing positions prior to starting the test. Since modified limb lead placement is used, the baseline ECG may differ slightly from prior ECGs. Blood pressure is checked throughout the procedure at predetermined intervals. Heart rate and rhythm are continuously monitored by either a 3- or 12-lead ECG, and a 12-lead ECG is printed at least at the end of each stage. Throughout the test, the patient is typically questioned regarding perceived level of exertion based on the Borg scale [8], and symptoms of dyspnea or angina.

Exercise testing is often stopped when the patient reaches 85% of age-predicted maximum heart rate, but the ideal endpoint is that of maximal effort as perceived by the patient. Symptom-limited testing is especially useful when assessing functional capacity. However, there are several clinical and hemodynamic parameters that should prompt early termination of the study (table 2). Hemodynamic and ECG monitoring are continued into the post-exercise period for 6–8 min or until any ECG changes have returned to baseline.

Interpretation

Interpretation of the exercise stress test involves assessment of symptoms, exercise capacity, hemodynamic response and ECG response. Overall functional capacity is best communicated in metabolic equivalents (METS) achieved, rather than duration of exercise.

The product of peak heart rate and blood pressure (pressure-rate product) is a measure of the level of hemodynamic stress obtained. For a diagnostic test, the peak heart rate should exceed 85% of the age-predicted maximum. Blood pressure response during exercise can provide valuable diagnostic and prognostic information independent of ECG results. Exercise-induced hypotension, defined as a drop in blood pressure during exercise below pre-test standing blood pressure, or a decrease in SBP >20 mm Hg during the test, has been associated with an increased risk of cardiac events and the presence of severe CAD [9–11]. The mechanism of hypotension is likely exercise-induced ischemia and LV dysfunction. However, there is a subset of patients without CAD who develop hypotension during testing. This may be related to peripheral vasodilation or an as yet undefined mechanism [11].

The ECG response to exercise, specifically ST-segment shifts, has received the most attention when assessing the diagnostic utility of ETT. In patients with a normal baseline ECG, a positive test is most commonly defined as ≥ 1 mm horizontal or down-sloping ST-segment depression measured 60–80 ms from the j-point. Patients with up-sloping ST-segment depression have been shown to have an increased probability of CAD [12], although the initial study in which this was shown used 2 mm ST-segment depression as the threshold for a positive test. In addition, data from a recent meta-analysis showed that when upsloping ST-segment depression was considered a positive test, sensitivity did not improve and specificity was significantly reduced [13]. ACC/AHA guidelines recommend using the more conservative definition of horizontal and down-sloping ST-segment depression as a positive test.

Several studies evaluating the diagnostic utility of single lead systems and a study by Miranda et al. [14] suggest that exercise-induced ST-segment depression in the precordial leads is more accurate than is ST-segment depression in the inferior leads. In this relatively small study of 173 men, the specificity of ST-segment depression in lead II was only 44%. ST-segment depression limited to the inferior leads is uncommon, but is more suggestive of a false-positive test.

Table 2. Indications for terminating exercise test[1]

Absolute
Drop in SPB > 10 mm Hg from baseline when accompanied by other evidence of ischemia
Moderate to severe angina
Central nervous system symptoms (ataxia, dizziness, near syncope)
Signs of poor perfusion
Sustained ventricular tachycardia
Technical difficulties
Subjects desire to stop
ST-segment elevation (≥ 1 mm) in leads AVR, V1 and leads without diagnostic Q waves
Relative
Drop in SPB ≥ 10 mm Hg from baseline in the absence of other evidence of ischemia
ST-segment depression > 2 mm Hg or marked axis shift
Arrhythmias other than sustained ventricular tachycardia (heart block, supraventricular tachycardia, ventricular triplets, multifocal PVCs)
Increasing chest pain
Hypertensive response (SBP > 250 and/or DBP > 115 mm Hg)
Fatigue, SOB, claudication, wheezing

1 Modified from Fletcher et al. [6] and Gibbons et al. [3].

Exercise-induced ST-segment elevation is abnormal. In leads AVR and V1, ST-segment elevation likely represents ischemia, and in regions of prior MI may represent aneurysm or dyskinetic wall motion [6]. ST-segment elevation in the absence of prior MI is rare, and represents transmural ischemia caused by spasm or a critical stenosis [3]. Unlike ST-segment depression, ST-segment elevation accurately correlates with the region of ischemia [15]. An analysis of the Coronary Artery Surgery Study (CASS) [16] confirmed the suspicion that ST-segment elevation during exercise is predictive of CAD and a marker of poor prognosis.

The significance of premature ventricular complexes (PVCs) and other ventricular arrhythmias during exercise has been evaluated in several populations undergoing stress testing [17–22]. Early studies suggested a higher prevalence of CAD and an increased risk of cardiovascular events in patients who developed ventricular arrhythmias during exercise. However, the prognostic implication of frequent PVCs was not fully appreciated until Jouven et al. [22] published results from exercise testing in over 6,000 asymptomatic French men. Subjects underwent ETT between 1967 and 1972 and were prospectively classified as having or not having frequent PVCs (a run of 2 or more consecutive PVCs or PVCs constituting more

Table 3. Diagnostic performance of exercise treadmill testing

Group	Year	Total patients	Sensitivity %	Specificity %	Accuracy %
Meta-analysis of standard ETT [13]	1989	24,047	68	77	73
Meta-analysis without work-up bias [13]	1989	>1,000	50	90	69
Meta-analysis for mutivessel disease [23]	1989	12,030	81	66	N/A
ETT without work-up bias (VA group) [24]	1998	814	45	85	N/A
Meta-analysis of ETT in women [35]	1999	4,113	61	70	N/A

than 10% of all ventricular beats in any of the 30-second ECG recordings). At 23 years, subjects with frequent PVCs had an increased risk of death from cardiovascular causes compared with men without frequent PVCs (relative risk 2.67; 95% confidence interval 1.76–4.07). Frequent PVCs remained a strong predictor of risk even after multivariate analysis controlled for standard risk factors. Further, exercise-induced ST-segment depression and frequent PVCs were equally and independently predictive of cardiovascular death.

Sensitivity and Specificity

The sensitivity and specificity of exercise stress testing are summarized in table 3. The prevalence of disease in the population studied, the patients excluded from analysis, and the level at which a test is defined as positive all influence sensitivity and specificity of the test. This is true of exercise stress testing, and can partially explain disparate results in the literature. Meta-analysis performed by Gianrossi et al. [13] on 147 consecutively published reports involving 24,047 patients who had undergone exercise stress testing and coronary angiography demonstrated a mean sensitivity of 68% (range 23–100%) and a mean specificity of 77% (range 17–100%). Sensitivity was slightly higher when studies that enrolled patients with LVH or digoxin use were excluded from analysis (mean sensitivity 72%).

In a companion paper [23], the accuracy of ETT in detecting multivessel or left main disease was evaluated. Again, wide variability was found, although the overall sensitivity was improved. The mean sensitivity of ETT in patients with multivessel disease was 81% (range 40–100%); sensitivity was 86% (range 20–100%) in those with triple vessel or left main disease. Mean specificity was 66% (range 17–100%) in those with multivessel disease and 53% (range 17–100%) in those with triple vessel or left main disease. The decline in specificity can be anticipated in that the absence of disease is defined as absence of multivessel CAD, including those with single-vessel disease.

Assessment of the diagnostic accuracy of a test is influenced by work-up bias. Work-up bias (or post-test referral bias) occurs when the diagnostic gold standard of angiography is more likely performed among patients with a positive noninvasive test. This typically results in a sensitivity that is higher and specificity that is lower than would be seen in an unbiased population. Only three studies in the meta-analysis performed by Gianrossi et al. [13] eliminated work-up bias. However, the results were striking in that sensitivity decreased to 50% and specificity increased to 90%. These results are similar to those from a recent study specifically designed to eliminate work-up bias [24]. In this VA cooperative study, 814 consecutive subjects presenting with chest pain, but without known CAD, agreed to undergo both ETT and coronary angiography. In this population, mean sensitivity was 45% and specificity 85%. These markers of test performance most accurately reflect the sensitivity and specificity of ETT in the outpatient setting.

Prognosis

Even though exercise testing is not a highly accurate method of diagnosing obstructive CAD, information obtained is predictive of outcomes. The most commonly applied method of establishing prognosis is the Duke prognostic score [25]. The score is calculated as

Exercise time (Bruce protocol) – (5 × ST deviation) – (4 × anginal index),

where exercise time is measured in minutes, ST-segment deviation in millimeters, and anginal score defined as 0 = no angina, 1 = nonlimiting angina, 2 = limiting angina. This score was developed and validated in 2,842 patients who underwent both cardiac catheterization and ETT at

Duke University between 1969 and 1981. The Duke prognostic score was later applied prospectively to 613 patients and found to be predictive of outcome [26]. Low-risk patients (score > +5) had an average yearly mortality rate of 0.25%, whereas high-risk patients (score < –10) had an average yearly mortality of 5%. A commonly used nomogram based on the Duke prognostic score predicts annual and 5-year mortality based on ST-segment deviation, angina and exercise duration (minutes and METS).

Special Considerations

The diagnostic accuracy of ETT has been independently evaluated in several special populations. These include women and those with baseline ECG abnormalities including LBBB, RBBB, left ventricular hypertrophy (LVH), digoxin use, and resting ST-segment depression. Among patients with LBBB, the ST-segment response to exercise is not different between those with and without CAD [27]. As such, an alternative method of testing should be performed for the diagnosis of CAD, in patients with LBBB.

In patients with RBBB, exercise-induced ST-segment depression in leads V1–V3 is common and does not predict the presence of CAD [28, 29]. It has been recommended that consideration for ischemia should be limited to ST-segment depression in the inferior leads and V5–V6, although data supporting this approach are conflicting. Most published reports in patients with RBBB are small and have a reported sensitivity of 0–53%. The largest study to date included 133 patients [30], with a sensitivity of 27% and a specificity of 87%. The low sensitivity in this study was supported by the results of a meta-analysis on exercise testing [23] in which the sensitivity of predicting multivessel and left main disease increased when patients with RBBB were excluded. The impact on test sensitivity should be considered when patients with RBBB undergo stress testing for the diagnosis of CAD.

In patients with baseline ST-segment abnormalities secondary to digoxin use or LVH, the sensitivity of ST-segment depression is reduced and an alternative method of testing should be performed [3, 31]. However, in those with isolated resting ST-segment depression of <1 mm, exercise stress testing is a reasonable option. Among such patients, the sensitivity [32] and prognostic value [33] of ETT are preserved, with an acceptable test specificity.

A lower diagnostic accuracy of exercise stress testing in women was first noted in 1975 by Sketch et al. [34], and has been observed in several studies since that time. A recent meta-analysis of stress testing in women by Kwok et al. [35] supports this finding. Nineteen studies comprising 4,113 women were included. The weighted mean sensitivity of ETT for the detection of CAD was 61% (95% confidence interval 54–68%), and mean specificity was 70% (95% confidence interval 64–75%). Several explanations for reduced accuracy of stress testing in women have been proposed, including a lower prevalence of disease, increased presence of resting ST-segment abnormalities, mitral valve prolapse and post-test referral bias. However, even when the prevalence of disease is the same [36] and work-up bias is considered [37], ETT remains less accurate in women than in men.

Limitations

There are several limitations of ETT. Sensitivity is relatively low, especially among patients with single-vessel disease and in women. Elderly patients and those with significant comorbidities are often unable to achieve an adequate level of stress. In addition, ischemia when present is not localized, and information on overall LV function is not available.

The diagnostic accuracy of exercise testing is improved with the addition of an imaging modality, including either nuclear scintigraphy or echocardiography. ACC/AHA guidelines recommend stress imaging as the initial test in patients with baseline ECG abnormalities (LBBB, pre-excitation, >1 mm ST-segment depression) and in patients with a history of revascularization [38]. In patients unable to exercise to an adequate level, pharmacological stress is recommended. Alternatives to standard exercise testing are discussed below.

Stress Myocardial Perfusion Imaging

The most important clinical application of myocardial perfusion imaging is its use in combination with stress to assess the presence and extent of ischemic heart disease. The first scintigraphic images of myocardial blood flow were obtained in 1964 by Carr et al. [39] using cesium-131. But it was in 1974, when thallium-201 became widely available, that myocardial perfusion imaging started to gain widespread acceptance.

The two most commonly used radiopharmaceuticals for myocardial perfusion imaging are thallium-201 and technetium-99m (^{99m}Tc) sestamibi. Thallium-201 is a potassium analog with a biologic half-life of 58 h. The initial myocardial accumulation and distribution of thallium-201 is dependent on flow, but over time, there is redistribution to all viable myocardial cells. ^{99m}Tc sestamibi is a lipophilic monovalent cation that enters myocardial cells by passive diffusion. The half-life of 6 h is much shorter than thallium-201, and there is no cellular redistribution over time. The decision of which radionuclide to use depends on the purpose of the test. Sestamibi can be given in a larger bolus, which makes first-pass angiography possible, and results in higher emission counts and less scatter. In obese patients and women with a large amount of breast tissue, higher emission counts with sestamibi may result in improved image quality. However, thallium-201 is ideal when assessing myocardial viability.

Imaging is done with either planar or tomographic (SPECT) techniques. SPECT is generally more accurate than planar imaging for the diagnosis of CAD, for detection of single-vessel disease, and for localization of the vascular territory involved [40].

Overview of the Procedure

Exercise. Exercise is performed under a standard protocol with ECG and hemodynamic monitoring. When the patient nears peak exercise, either thallium-201 or ^{99m}Tc sestamibi is injected and the patient is asked to exercise for another 30–60 s to allow distribution of the radionuclide at peak exercise. Stress images are obtained within a few minutes with thallium and in 60–90 min with sestamibi. When thallium is used, redistribution takes place spontaneously and rest/redistribution images are obtained 4–6 h after the initial injection. A second small injection (reinjection technique) of thallium can be given 30 min before rest images, which improves the accuracy of the test [41]. ^{99m}Tc sestamibi is typically administered in a 2-day protocol, with stress images taken the second day and after a second injection of sestamibi. However, newer protocols allow for complete sestamibi imaging within a single day [42].

Vasodilation. Coronary vasodilation serves as an alternative method of stress among patients who are unable to exercise. Either dipyridamole, which blocks the cellular reabsorption of adenosine, or adenosine is infused intravenously. Pharmacologic vasodilation results in a 4- to 5-fold increase in coronary blood flow in normal coronary arteries. However, the response is attenuated in diseased vessels. The resultant heterogeneity of blood flow is detected on myocardial perfusion imaging. Unlike exercise or dobutamine stress, ischemia is only rarely induced with vasodilation, occurring secondary to a coronary 'steal' phenomenon in the setting of a very high-grade stenosis.

The safety and side effect profiles of dipyridamole and adenosine have been evaluated in thousands of patients. Side effects with both dipyridamole and adenosine are common, occurring in approximately 50 and 80% of patients, respectively [43–46]. Death and nonfatal MI are extremely rare [47], although bronchospasm and respiratory arrest have been observed in patients with reactive airway disease or severe COPD. Transient atrial-ventricular conduction disturbances can occur. In a series of 9,256 patients receiving adenosine, the incidence of first-, second- and third-degree heart block was 2.8, 4.1 and 0.8%, respectively [46]. More frequent minor side effects include chest pain, headache, dizziness, shortness of breath, flushing, hypotension and nausea. Side effects can be readily reversed with discontinuation of the drug and administration of aminophylline if necessary.

Absolute contraindications to dipyridamole and adenosine are unstable angina, severe asthma, allergy to either drug or aminophylline and advanced heart block. Relative contraindications include baseline hypotension, aortic or mitral stenosis and carotid artery stenosis.

Dobutamine. When contraindications to vasodilators are present, dobutamine can be used as the pharmacologic stress in conjunction with myocardial perfusion imaging. Dobutamine is a β_1-agonist that increases myocardial oxygen demand by increasing myocardial contractility, and to a lesser degree heart rate and blood pressure. Normally there is a resultant 2- to 3-fold increase in coronary blood flow, and inhomogeneous myocardial perfusion can be detected in patients with significant CAD [48]. Dobutamine is infused at increasing doses of 5, 10, 20, 30 μg/kg/min in 3-min stages. Thallium-201 or ^{99m}Tc sestamibi is injected during the final stage of infusion.

Interpretation

Stress and rest images are reviewed for fixed and reversible perfusion defects. The images are viewed in short-axis, vertical and horizontal long-axis planes. Fixed perfusion defects represent prior MI, whereas reversible defects represent areas of viable myocardium subtended by a stenotic coronary artery. Images can be analyzed qualitatively or quantitatively, the latter yielding improved sensitivity with both planar [49] and SPECT [49] techniques. Attenuation artifacts caused by overlying diaphragmatic and breast soft tissues must be considered in interpreting the images.

The number, size and location of perfusion defects reflect the extent and location of coronary stenoses. Multivessel disease is suggested when two distinct vascular territories are involved. Severe diffuse obstructive coronary disease is also suggested by increased lung uptake of thallium-201 following stress [50] or LV cavity dilation with stress [51].

Sensitivity and Specificity

Data reflecting the accuracy of myocardial perfusion imaging for the detection of CAD is summarized in table 4. Most early experience in the diagnostic accuracy of myocardial perfusion imaging was with thallium-201, but the accuracy of ^{99m}Tc sestamibi is felt to be comparable. For thallium-201 planar scintigraphy, the average reported sensitivity and specificity using visual analysis is 83 and 88% respectively, and 90 and 80% with quantitative analysis. SPECT imaging results in an average sensitivity of 89% and specificity of 76% with visual analysis, and a sensitivity averaging 90% and specificity of 70% with quantitative techniques [52]. The sensitivity and specificity of dipyridamole and adenosine stress are similar to exercise. Data on dobutamine perfusion imaging are limited. However, in a report from Hays et al. [53] comprising 144 patients, the overall sensitivity with dobutamine thallium-201 was 86% with a specificity of 90%.

Prognosis

The size and number of perfusion defects [54], LV cavity dilation with stress, and increased lung uptake of thallium predict increased risk of future cardiac events [52]. Normal perfusion following stress, among patients with or without known CAD, is associated with a low risk of MI or death (0.9% per year) [55].

Special Considerations

The presence of LBBB is associated with a high rate of false-positive tests when using exercise or dobutamine myocardial perfusion imaging. Both fixed and reversible septal defects occur in up to 84% of patients with LBBB and normal coronary arteries [56]. Perfusion imaging with dipyridamole and adenosine is more accurate, and is preferred in patients with LBBB [38]. A recent report by Kucuk et al. [57] suggests that patients with RBBB may have an increased proportion of false-positive tests, with perfusion abnormalities in the inferoseptal wall.

The diagnostic accuracy of thallium-201 SPECT is lower in women than in men [35]. Possible explanations include smaller heart size, lower prevalence of disease and the presence of breast attenuation artifact. To evaluate the potential benefit of sestamibi in reducing breast artifact, a prospective study of 115 women was performed comparing thallium-201 with ^{99m}Tc sestamibi SPECT. The sensitivity was comparable (84 and 80%), but specificity was improved with sestamibi (67 vs. 84%) [58]. These data suggest ^{99m}Tc sestamibi may be preferable for the detection of CAD in women when using myocardial perfusion imaging.

Table 4. Diagnostic performance of myocardial perfusion imaging

Test	Sensitivity %	Specificity %
Exercise thallium[1]		
Planar	83	88
Quantitative	90	80
SPECT		
Quantitative	89	76
Normalcy rate[2]	89	89
Exercise thallium in women [35]	78	64
Dipyridamole thallium (planar and SPECT)[1]	90	70
Dobutamine thallium [53]	86	90

1 Adapted from ACC/AHA guidelines for clinical use of cardiac radionuclide imaging [52].

2 Normalcy is a surrogate for specificity adjusted for post-test referral bias.

Stress Echocardiography

Stress echocardiography was first proposed as a diagnostic modality in 1979 [59], but limitations in early generation two-dimensional echocardiography and difficulties in videotape analysis prevented widespread use. In the mid-1980s, advances in image quality and the ability to digitize images led to the advancement of stress echocardiography. The two most common methods of stress are exercise and dobutamine, although vasodilator stress is advocated by some.

Overview of the Procedure

Exercise Echocardiography. Exercise echocardiography is most commonly performed in combination with treadmill [60–62] or bicycle ergometry [63]. Most reports suggest that both methods of stress provide accurate diagnostic information. However, bicycle stress may result in a slightly higher test sensitivity, likely because images can be obtained throughout exercise [64]. Following treadmill stress, the subject is quickly positioned in the left lateral decubitus position and echocardiographic images obtained. Because heart rate may decrease rapidly after cessation of exercise, it is important to obtain post-stress images within 30–90 s.

Test endpoints, contraindications and risks of exercise echocardiography are the same as for standard exercise testing.

Dobutamine Echocardiography. Echocardiographic images are obtained at baseline and during dobutamine

Table 5. Diagnostic performance of stress echocardiography

Group	Sensitivity %	Specificity %
Exercise echocardiography[1]	85	86
Exercise echocardiography in women [35]	86	79
Dobutamine echocardiography[1]	82	85

[1] Adapted from the ACC/AHA guidelines for the clinical application of echocardiography [73].

infusion. Specific infusion protocols may vary, although a typical protocol uses 3-min stages at doses of 10, 20, 30 and 40 μg/kg/min. If the target heart rate is not achieved, protocols may allow for an infusion of 50 μg/kg/min [65] and/or the addition of atropine boluses. Heart rate, blood pressure and heart rhythm are monitored throughout the study. Dobutamine infusion is typically stopped when 85% age-predicted maximum heart rate is achieved, or when the end of the infusion protocol is reached. However, the test is stopped earlier if the patient develops significant arrhythmia, moderate or severe angina, new wall motion abnormalities, hypotension, left ventricular outflow tract obstruction, or severe noncardiac side effects such as headache or nausea.

The risks and side effects of dobutamine-atropine echocardiography have been reported from three large centers comprising over 8,000 patients [65–67]. In this population, no deaths were reported, and MI occurred in only 2 patients. In the series by Secknus and Marwick [66], 3,011 consecutive patients were evaluated. They reported test-limiting side effects in 7.6% of patients, including ventricular tachycardia (0.9%), supraventricular tachycardia (0.7%), severe hypertension (0.7%) and hypotension or LVOT obstruction (3.8%). Noncardiac side effects limited the test in 1.6% of patients and angina in 3.5%. They found that the percentage of diagnostic studies increased with the use of atropine, but that risk did not increase with a more aggressive protocol. Contraindications to dobutamine include systemic hypertension (SBP > 200 mm Hg or DBP > 110 mm Hg), unstable angina, uncontrolled arrhythmia, or recent MI (within 2 days).

Interpretation

Study interpretation involves the analysis of regional LV wall motion and systolic thickening at various stages of stress. Image digitization greatly enhances the ability to discern subtle changes between stages by allowing side-by-side comparisons using a quad-screen format. For purposes of analysis, the LV is conventionally divided into 16 segments, and wall motion graded as normal, hypokinetic, akinetic, or dyskinetic. A hyperdynamic response to exercise or dobutamine is normal, and worsening of wall motion in one or more segments is considered an abnormal test and indicative of ischemia. In order to avoid false-positive tests, some advocate a threshold of two abnormal segments for the diagnosis of ischemia when a wall motion abnormality is confined to a single basal segment in the inferior or posterior wall [68]. A definite target heart rate is laboratory-dependent, but some argue that a test should be interpreted as nondiagnostic if the heart rate does not exceed 85% age-predicted maximum [69] or if all walls are not adequately seen.

The development of ST-segment depression during dobutamine infusion in patients with a normal baseline ECG is only moderately predictive of CAD and adds very little to the diagnostic accuracy of the test [70, 71]. Hypotension during dobutamine stress echocardiography has not been shown to predict the presence of CAD, but was found to be independently predictive of perioperative events in a group of patients undergoing DSE for preoperative risk assessment [72].

Sensitivity and Specificity

The sensitivity and specificity of stress echocardiography is summarized in table 5. There have been numerous published series on the diagnostic and prognostic accuracy of stress echocardiography. Similar to data reflecting the efficacy of ETT, referral bias and heterogeneity of the populations studied confound published reports. Based on 40 studies, ACC/AHA guidelines for echocardiography [73] report an overall sensitivity and specificity of exercise echocardiography of 85 and 86% respectively. The overall accuracy of dobutamine stress echocardiography is similar, with a sensitivity and specificity of 82 and 85%, respectively. The sensitivity for stress echocardiography is higher in patients with multivessel than with single-vessel disease.

A few studies have compared exercise and dobutamine echocardiography in the same patients [74–76]. In these reports, test accuracy was not significantly different, but several observations were made: the pressure-rate product was higher in patients following exercise, ST-segment depression on ECG was more common with exercise, and a larger ischemic burden was induced with exercise.

Prognosis

Several findings on stress echocardiography have been associated with a poor prognosis. Specifically, LV cavity dilation with stress, a combination of fixed and inducible wall motion abnormalities indicative of mixed ischemia and scar, and impaired overall LV function are predictive of future cardiac events [77]. Conversely, a negative test predicts a low risk for future cardiac events [78]. Preoperative assessment of perioperative risk prior to noncardiac surgery has been evaluated in several patient populations. In general, a negative stress echocardiogram carries a negative predictive value of 93–100% [79] for freedom from adverse perioperative cardiac events.

Special Considerations

The diagnostic utility of stress echocardiography has been demonstrated in patients with prior MI and resting wall motion abnormalities [62], among patients with renal failure [80], paced rhythms [81], dilated cardiomyopathy [82], LVH [83] and LBBB [84].

Choosing the Appropriate Test

It is important to select the appropriate test for each patient when referring for stress testing. The first consideration is regarding the information sought with the stress test. For the diagnosis of CAD, ETT is recommended as the first test in patients with an intermediate pre-test likelihood of disease, assuming an ability to exercise adequately and a normal resting ECG. Despite previously cited data reflecting the lower accuracy for detection of CAD in women, there are no compelling data to support an alternative strategy for testing. If a patient cannot exercise, then either vasodilator radionuclide imaging or dobutamine stress echocardiography is an acceptable alternative. In patients who are able to exercise but have ECG abnormalities that make ETT unreliable, exercise testing with either nuclear scintigraphy or echocardiography result in a sensitivity of 85–90% for the detection of CAD. However, the specificity of testing may be slightly higher with dobutamine echocardiography [85]. Among patients with LBBB, both exercise echocardiography and exercise thallium are associated with a high number of false-positive tests. As such, pharmacologic stress with either dobutamine echocardiography or vasodilator perfusion imaging may be preferred in these patients.

Among patients with known CAD, stress testing may be employed to further characterize the location, extent and significance of disease. If a stress test is performed for these indications, then an imaging modality is essential. Stress echocardiography and nuclear scintigraphy perform equally well for the localization and characterization of CAD in all but the left circumflex territory, in which SPECT perfusion imaging is better [86].

It is important to recognize the prognostic power associated with functional capacity. Specifically, although the ability to diagnose, localize, and further characterize the extent of CAD has improved over time, the ability to exercise to a high workload remains one of the best predictors of survival and freedom from morbid cardiac events.

References

1 Singh G, Matthews T, Clarke S, Yannicos T, Smith B: Annual summary of births, marriages, divorces and deaths: United States, 1994. Monthly Vital Statist Rep 1995;43.

2 Diamond GA, Forrester JS: Analysis of probability as an aid in the clinical diagnosis of coronary artery disease. N Engl J Med 1979;300: 1350–1358.

3 Gibbons RJ, Balady GJ, Beasley JW, et al: ACC/AHA Guidelines for Exercise Testing. A report of the American College of Cardiology/American Heart Association Task Force on Practice Guidelines (Committee on Exercise Testing). J Am Coll Card 1997;30:260–311.

4 Cohen MC, Stafford RS, Misra B: Stress testing: National patterns and predictors of test ordering. Am Heart J 1999;138:1019–1024.

5 Stuart RJ Jr, Ellestad MH: National survey of exercise stress testing facilities. Chest 1980;77: 94–97.

6 Fletcher GF, Balady G, Froelicher VF, Hartley LH, Haskell WL, Pollock ML: Exercise standards. A statement for healthcare professionals from the American Heart Association. Writing Group. Circulation 1995;91:580–615.

7 Myers J, Froelicher VF: Optimizing the exercise test for pharmacological investigations. Circulation 1990;82:1839–1846.

8 Borg GA: Psychophysical bases of perceived exertion. Med Sci Sports Exerc 1982;14:377–381.

9 Sanmarco ME, Pontius S, Selvester RH: Abnormal blood pressure response and marked ischemic ST-segment depression as predictors of severe coronary artery disease. Circulation 1980;61:572–578.

10 Weiner DA, McCabe CH, Cutler SS, Ryan TJ: Decrease in systolic blood pressure during exercise testing: Reproducibility, response to coronary bypass surgery and prognostic significance. Am J Cardiol 1982;49:1627–1631.

11 Dubach P, Froelicher VF, Klein J, Oakes D, Grover-McKay M, Friis R: Exercise-induced hypotension in a male population. Criteria, causes and prognosis. Circulation 1988;78: 1380–1387.

12 Stuart RJ, Ellestad MH: Upsloping ST segments in exercise stress testing. Six-year follow-up study of 438 patients and correlation with 248 angiograms. Am J Cardiol 1976;37:19–22.

13 Gianrossi R, Detrano R, Mulvihill D, et al: Exercise-induced ST depression in the diagnosis of coronary artery disease. A meta-analysis. Circulation 1989;80:87–98.

14 Miranda CP, Liu J, Kadar A, et al: Usefulness of exercise-induced ST-segment depression in the inferior leads during exercise testing as a marker for coronary artery disease. Am J Cardiol 1992;69:303–307.

15 Mark DB, Hlatky MA, Lee KL, Harrell FE Jr, Califf RM, Pryor DB: Localizing coronary artery obstructions with the exercise treadmill test. Ann Intern Med 1987;106:53–55.

16 Bruce RA, Fisher LD, Pettinger M, Weiner DA, Chaitman BR: ST segment elevation with exercise: A marker for poor ventricular function and poor prognosis. Coronary Artery Surgery Study (CASS) confirmation of Seattle Heart Watch results. Circulation 1988;77:897–905.

17 Nair CK, Aronow WS, Sketch MH, et al: Diagnostic and prognostic significance of exercise-induced premature ventricular complexes in men and women: A four-year follow-up. J Am Coll Cardiol 1983;1:1201–1206.

18 Califf RM, McKinnis RA, McNeer JF, et al: Prognostic value of ventricular arrhythmias associated with treadmill exercise testing in patients studied with cardiac catheterization for suspected ischemic heart disease. J Am Coll Cardiol 1983;2:1060–1067.

19 Marieb MA, Beller GA, Gibson RS, Lerman BB, Kaul S: Clinical relevance of exercise-induced ventricular arrhythmias in suspected coronary artery disease. Am J Cardiol 1990;66: 172–178.

20 Schweikert RA, Pashkow FJ, Snader CE, Marwick TH, Lauer MS: Association of exercise-induced ventricular ectopic activity with thallium myocardial perfusion and angiographic coronary artery disease in stable, low-risk populations. Am J Cardiol 1999;83:530–534.

21 Elhendy A, Sozzi FB, van Domburg RT, Bax JJ, Valkema R, Roelandt JR: Relation between exercise-induced ventricular arrhythmias and myocardial perfusion abnormalities in patients with intermediate pretest probability of coronary artery disease. Eur J Nucl Med 2000;27: 327–332.

22 Jouven X, Zureik M, Desnos M, Courbon D, Ducimetiere P: Long-term outcome in asymptomatic men with exercise-induced premature ventricular depolarizations. N Engl J Med 2000;343:826–833.

23 Detrano R, Gianrossi R, Mulvihill D, et al: Exercise-induced ST segment depression in the diagnosis of multivessel coronary disease: A meta analysis. J Am Coll Cardiol 1989;14: 1501–1508.

24 Froelicher VF, Lehmann KG, Thomas R, et al: The electrocardiographic exercise test in a population with reduced work-up bias: Diagnostic performance, computerized interpretation, and multivariable prediction. Veterans Affairs Cooperative Study in Health Services #016 (QUEXTA) Study Group. Quantitative Exercise Testing and Angiography. Ann Intern Med 1998;128:965–974.

25 Mark DB, Hlatky MA, Harrell FE Jr, Lee KL, Califf RM, Pryor DB: Exercise treadmill score for predicting prognosis in coronary artery disease. Ann Intern Med 1987;106:793–800.

26 Mark DB, Shaw L, Harrell FE Jr, et al: Prognostic value of a treadmill exercise score in outpatients with suspected coronary artery disease. N Engl J Med 1991;325:849–853.

27 Whinnery JE, Froelicher VF Jr, Stewart AJ, Longo MR Jr, Triebwasser JH, Lancaster MC: The electrocardiographic response to maximal treadmill exercise of asymptomatic men with left bundle branch block. Am Heart J 1977;94: 316–324.

28 Whinnery JE, Froelicher VF: Exercise testing in right bundle-branch block. Chest 1977;72: 684–685.

29 Tanaka T, Friedman MJ, Okada RD, Buckels LJ, Marcus FI: Diagnostic value of exercise-induced ST segment depression in patients with right bundle branch block. Am J Cardiol 1978;41:670–673.

30 Yen RS, Miranda C, Froelicher VF: Diagnostic and prognostic accuracy of the exercise electrocardiogram in patients with preexisting right bundle branch block. Am Heart J 1994;127: 1521–1525.

31 Sundqvist K, Atterhog JH, Jogestrand T: Effect of digoxin on the electrocardiogram at rest and during exercise in healthy subjects. Am J Cardiol 1986;57:661–665.

32 Fearon WF, Lee DP, Froelicher VF: The effect of resting ST segment depression on the diagnostic characteristics of the exercise treadmill test. J Am Coll Cardiol 2000;35:1206–1211.

33 Kwok JM, Miller TD, Christian TF, Hodge DO, Gibbons RJ: Prognostic value of a treadmill exercise score in symptomatic patients with nonspecific ST-T abnormalities on resting ECG. JAMA 1999;282:1047–1053.

34 Sketch MH, Mohiuddin SM, Lynch JD, Zencka AE, Runco V: Significant sex differences in the correlation of electrocardiographic exercise testing and coronary arteriograms. Am J Cardiol 1975;36:169–173.

35 Kwok Y, Kim C, Grady D, Segal M, Redberg R: Meta-analysis of exercise testing to detect coronary artery disease in women. Am J Cardiol 1999;83:660–666.

36 Weiner DA, Ryan TJ, McCabe CH, et al: Exercise stress testing. Correlations among history of angina, ST-segment response and prevalence of coronary-artery disease in the Coronary Artery Surgery Study (CASS). N Engl J Med 1979; 301:230–235.

37 Morise AP, Diamond GA: Comparison of the sensitivity and specificity of exercise electrocardiography in biased and unbiased populations of men and women. Am Heart J 1995; 130:741–747.

38 Gibbons RJ, Chatterjee K, Daley J, et al: ACC/AHA/ACP-ASIM guidelines for the management of patients with chronic stable angina: A report of the American College of Cardiology/American Heart Association Task Force on Practice Guidelines (Committee on Management of Patients with Chronic Stable Angina). J Am Coll Cardiol 1999;33:2092–2197.

39 Carr EA, Gleason G, Shaw J: The direct diagnosis of myocardial infarction by photoscanning after administration of cesium-131. Am Heart J 1964;68:62.

40 Fintel DJ, Links JM, Brinker JA, Frank TL, Parker M, Becker LC: Improved diagnostic performance of exercise thallium-201 single photon emission computed tomography over planar imaging in the diagnosis of coronary artery disease: A receiver operating characteristic analysis. J Am Coll Cardiol 1989;13:600–612.

41 Maublant JC, Lipiecki J, Citron B, et al: Reinjection as an alternative to rest imaging for detection of exercise-induced ischemia with thallium-201 emission tomography. Am Heart J 1993;125:330–335.

42 Heo J, Powers J, Iskandrian AE: Exercise-rest same-day SPECT sestamibi imaging to detect coronary artery disease. J Nucl Med 1997;38: 200–203.

43 Laarman GJ, Niemeyer MG, van der Wall EE, et al: Dipyridamole thallium testing: Noncardiac side effects, cardiac effects, electrocardiographic changes and hemodynamic changes after dipyridamole infusion with and without exercise. Int J Cardiol 1988;20:231–238.

44 Abreu A, Mahmarian JJ, Nishimura S, Boyce TM, Verani MS: Tolerance and safety of pharmacologic coronary vasodilation with adenosine in association with thallium-201 scintigraphy in patients with suspected coronary artery disease. J Am Coll Cardiol 1991;18:730–735.

45 Verani MS: Adenosine thallium-201 myocardial perfusion scintigraphy. Am Heart J 1991; 122:269–278.

46 Cerqueira MD, Verani MS, Schwaiger M, Heo J, Iskandrian AS: Safety profile of adenosine stress perfusion imaging: Results from the Adenoscan Multicenter Trial Registry. J Am Coll Cardiol 1994;23:384–389.

47 Ranhosky A, Kempthorne-Rawson J: The safety of intravenous dipyridamole thallium myocardial perfusion imaging. Intravenous Dipyridamole Thallium Imaging Study Group. Circulation 1990;81:1205–1209.

48 Meyer SL, Curry GC, Donsky MS, Twieg DB, Parkey RW, Willerson JT: Influence of dobutamine on hemodynamics and coronary blood flow in patients with and without coronary artery disease. Am J Cardiol 1976;38:103–108.

49 Mahmarian JJ, Verani MS: Exercise thallium-201 perfusion scintigraphy in the assessment of coronary artery disease. Am J Cardiol 1991;67: 2D–11D.

50 Nishimura S, Mahmarian JJ, Verani MS: Significance of increased lung thallium uptake during adenosine thallium-201 scintigraphy. J Nucl Med 1992;33:1600–1607.

51 Weiss AT, Berman DS, Lew AS, et al: Transient ischemic dilation of the left ventricle on stress thallium-201 scintigraphy: A marker of severe and extensive coronary artery disease. J Am Coll Cardiol 1987;9:752–759.

52 Ritchie JL, Bateman TM, Bonow RO, et al: Guidelines for clinical use of cardiac radionuclide imaging. Report of the American College of Cardiology/American Heart Association Task Force on Assessment of Diagnostic and Therapeutic Cardiovascular Procedures (Committee on Radionuclide Imaging), developed in collaboration with the American Society of Nuclear Cardiology. J Am Coll Cardiol 1995;25: 521–547.
53 Hays JT, Mahmarian JJ, Cochran AJ, Verani MS: Dobutamine thallium-201 tomography for evaluating patients with suspected coronary artery disease unable to undergo exercise or vasodilator pharmacologic stress testing. J Am Coll Cardiol 1993;21:1583–1590.
54 Iskandrian AS, Chae SC, Heo J, Stanberry CD, Wasserleben V, Cave V: Independent and incremental prognostic value of exercise single-photon emission computed tomographic thallium imaging in coronary artery disease. J Am Coll Cardiol 1993;22:665–670.
55 Brown KA: Prognostic value of thallium-201 myocardial perfusion imaging. A diagnostic tool comes of age. Circulation 1991;83:363–381.
56 Caner B, Rezaghi C, Uysal U, et al: Dobutamine thallium-201 myocardial SPECT in patients with left bundle branch block and normal coronary arteries. J Nucl Med 1997;38:424–427.
57 Kucuk NO, Arican P, Ibis E, et al: False-positive results obtained with stress myocardial SPECT in patients with right bundle branch block. Clin Nucl Med 2000;25:585–587.
58 Taillefer R, DePuey EG, Udelson JE, Beller GA, Latour Y, Reeves F: Comparative diagnostic accuracy of Tl-201 and Tc-99m sestamibi SPECT imaging (perfusion and ECG-gated SPECT) in detecting coronary artery disease in women. J Am Coll Cardiol 1997;29:69–77.
59 Wann LS, Faris JV, Childress RH, Dillon JC, Weyman AE, Feigenbaum H: Exercise cross-sectional echocardiography in ischemic heart disease. Circulation 1979;60:1300–1308.
60 Robertson WS, Feigenbaum H, Armstrong WF, Dillon JC, O'Donnell J, McHenry PW: Exercise echocardiography: A clinically practical addition in the evaluation of coronary artery disease. J Am Coll Cardiol 1983;2:1085–1091.
61 Armstrong WF, O'Donnell J, Dillon JC, McHenry PL, Morris SN, Feigenbaum H: Complementary value of two-dimensional exercise echocardiography to routine treadmill exercise testing. Ann Intern Med 1986;105: 829–835.
62 Armstrong WF, O'Donnell J, Ryan T, Feigenbaum H: Effect of prior myocardial infarction and extent and location of coronary disease on accuracy of exercise echocardiography. J Am Coll Cardiol 1987;10:531–538.
63 Presti CF, Armstrong WF, Feigenbaum H: Comparison of echocardiography at peak exercise and after bicycle exercise in evaluation of patients with known or suspected coronary artery disease. J Am Soc Echocardiogr 1988;1: 119–126.
64 Sawada SG, Ryan T, Fineberg NS, et al: Exercise echocardiographic detection of coronary artery disease in women. J Am Coll Cardiol 1989;14:1440–1447.
65 Mertes H, Sawada SG, Ryan T, et al: Symptoms, adverse effects and complications associated with dobutamine stress echocardiography. Experience in 1,118 patients. Circulation 1993; 88:15–19.
66 Secknus MA, Marwick TH: Evolution of dobutamine echocardiography protocols and indications: Safety and side effects in 3,011 studies over 5 years. J Am Coll Cardiol 1997;29:1234–1240.
67 Mathias W Jr, Arruda A, Santos FC, et al: Safety of dobutamine-atropine stress echocardiography: A prospective experience of 4,033 consecutive studies. J Am Soci Echocardiogr 1999; 12:785–791.
68 Bach DS, Muller DW, Gros BJ, Armstrong WF: False-positive dobutamine stress echocardiograms: Characterization of clinical, echocardiographic and angiographic findings. J Am Coll Cardiol 1994;24:928–933.
69 Ballal RS, Secknus MA, Mehta R, Kapadia S, Lauer MS, Marwick TH: Cardiac outcomes in coronary patients with submaximum dobutamine stress echocardiography. Am J Cardiol 1997;80:725–729.
70 Daoud EG, Pitt A, Armstrong WF: Electrocardiographic response during dobutamine stress echocardiography. Am Heart J 1995;129:672–677.
71 Shaheen J, Luria D, Klutstein MW, Rosenmann D, Tzivoni D: Diagnostic value of 12-lead electrocardiogram during dobutamine echocardiographic studies. Am Heart J 1998; 136:1061–1064.
72 Day SM, Younger JG, Karavite D, Bach DS, Armstrong WF, Eagle KA: Usefulness of hypotension during dobutamine echocardiography in predicting perioperative cardiac events. Am J Cardiol 2000;85:478–483.
73 Cheitlin MD, Alpert JS, Armstrong WF, et al: ACC/AHA Guidelines for the Clinical Application of Echocardiography. A report of the American College of Cardiology/American Heart Association Task Force on Practice Guidelines (Committee on Clinical Application of Echocardiography). Developed in collaboration with the American Society of Echocardiography. Circulation 1997;95:1686–744.
74 Cohen JL, Ottenweller JE, George AK, Duvvuri S: Comparison of dobutamine and exercise echocardiography for detecting coronary artery disease. Am J Cardiol 1993;72:1226–1231.
75 Rallidis L, Cokkinos P, Tousoulis D, Nihoyannopoulos P: Comparison of dobutamine and treadmill exercise echocardiography in inducing ischemia in patients with coronary artery disease. J Am Coll Cardiol 1997;30:1660–1668.
76 Attenhofer CH, Pellikka PA, Oh JK, Roger VL, Sohn DW, Seward JB: Comparison of ischemic response during exercise and dobutamine echocardiography in patients with left main coronary artery disease. J Am Coll Cardiol 1996;27: 1171–1177.
77 Marcovitz PA, Shayna V, Horn RA, Hepner A, Armstrong WF: Value of dobutamine stress echocardiography in determining the prognosis of patients with known or suspected coronary artery disease. Am J Cardiol 1996;78:404–408.
78 Geleijnse ML, Elhendy A, van Domburg RT, Cornel JH, Roelandt JR, Fioretti PM: Prognostic implications of a normal dobutamine-atropine stress echocardiogram in patients with chest pain. J Am Soc Echocardiogr 1998;11: 606–611.
79 Eagle KA, Brundage BH, Chaitman BR, et al: Guidelines for perioperative cardiovascular evaluation for noncardiac surgery. Report of the American College of Cardiology/American Heart Association Task Force on Practice Guidelines (Committee on Perioperative Cardiovascular Evaluation for Noncardiac Surgery). J Am Coll Cardiol 1996;27:910–948.
80 Herzog CA, Marwick TH, Pheley AM, White CW, Rao VK, Dick CD: Dobutamine stress echocardiography for the detection of significant coronary artery disease in renal transplant candidates. Am J Kidney Dis 1999;33:1080–1090.
81 Oral H, Armstrong WF, Bach DS: Preserved diagnostic utility of dobutamine stress echocardiography in pacemaker-dependent patients with absolute chronotropic incompetence. Am Heart J 1999;138:364–368.
82 Sharp SM, Sawada SG, Segar DS, et al: Dobutamine stress echocardiography: Detection of coronary artery disease in patients with dilated cardiomyopathy. J Am Coll Cardiol 1994;24: 934–939.
83 Fragasso G, Lu C, Dabrowski P, Pagnotta P, Sheiban I, Chierchia SL: Comparison of stress/rest myocardial perfusion tomography, dipyridamole and dobutamine stress echocardiography for the detection of coronary disease in hypertensive patients with chest pain and positive exercise test. J Am Coll Cardiol 1999;34: 441–447.
84 Mairesse GH, Marwick TH, Arnese M, et al: Improved identification of coronary artery disease in patients with left bundle branch block by use of dobutamine stress echocardiography and comparison with myocardial perfusion tomography. Am J Cardiol 1995;76:321–325.
85 Fleischmann KE, Hunink MG, Kuntz KM, Douglas PS: Exercise echocardiography or exercise SPECT imaging? A meta-analysis of diagnostic test performance. JAMA 1998;280: 913–920.
86 O'Keefe JH Jr, Bateman TM, Gibbons RJ: Exercise echocardiography vs. exercise SPECT testing. JAMA 1999;282:1621–1622.

Katherine Strelich, MD
UH B1F245-0022, 1500 E. Medical Center Dr.
University of Michigan
Ann Arbor, MI 48109 (USA)
Tel. +1 734 936 9678, Fax +1 734 763 7390
E-Mail kstrelic@umich.edu

Weisman IM, Zeballos RJ (eds): Clinical Exercise Testing.
Prog Respir Res. Basel, Karger, 2002, vol 32, pp 120–137

Role of Cardiac Rehabilitation in Heart Failure and Cardiac Transplantation

Randy W. Braith David G. Edwards

Center for Exercise Science, College of Health and Human Performance, College of Medicine, University of Florida, Gainesville, Fla., USA

Summary

Exercise training increases functional capacity and improves symptoms in selected patients with compensated stable heart failure and moderate to severe left ventricular (LV) systolic dysfunction. These favorable outcomes usually occur without deterioration in LV function. Peripheral adaptations, particularly in skeletal muscle and peripheral circulation, appear to mediate the improvement in exercise tolerance rather than adaptations in the cardiac musculature. Patients who have a combination of LV dysfunction and residual myocardial ischemia, however, may not benefit from exercise training. Exercise training appears to optimize the symptomatic and functional benefits of ACE inhibitor therapy. The most consistent benefits occur with exercise training at least 3 times per week for 12 or more weeks. The duration of aerobic exercise training sessions can vary from 20 to 40 min, at an intensity of 50–85% of peak HR on the graded exercise test or 40–70% of VO_2peak. Resistance exercise training appears to be a safe modality for heart transplant recipients (HTR) and is an effective countermeasure for steroid-induced osteoporosis and skeletal muscle myopathy when introduced early in the post-transplantation period. Exercise training also elicits a beneficial evolution of heart rate responsiveness during physical activity and significant increases in peak heart rate. These benefits are not seen in HTR who do not participate in structured exercise training. However, the mechanism(s) responsible for improved peak HR, VO_2peak cardiac index, and total exercise time are incompletely understood. There is evidence that enhanced leg strength confers a 'permissive' effect, allowing the cardiac allograft to approach optimal levels of function. Thus, increased exercise tolerance in HTR may be related to greater skeletal muscle hypertrophy and strength rather than central adaptations or intrinsic cardiac mechanisms.

Role of Cardiac Rehabilitation in Heart Failure and Cardiac Transplantation

Heart failure is a condition associated with a high morbidity and mortality and is the final pathway of many cardiovascular problems. The incidence of newly diagnosed heart failure patients is now pandemic. Thus, the socioeconomic impact of this syndrome is important. It is essential, therefore, to focus attention on interventions that may elicit significant decrements in morbidity and mortality in this expanding patient population. There is growing clinical consensus that stable, compensated chronic heart failure (CHF) patients respond favorably to exercise training. Exercise-trained CHF patients not only 'do better' through reduction in CHF symptoms, but there is recent evidence that exercise may alter the clinical course of CHF.

Heart transplantation improves the survival rate for patients with severe symptoms of CHF and an ejection fraction of 20% or less. However, with dramatic improvements in immunosuppressive drug management, short-term survival is no longer the pivotal issue for most heart transplant recipients (HTR). Rather, a return to function-

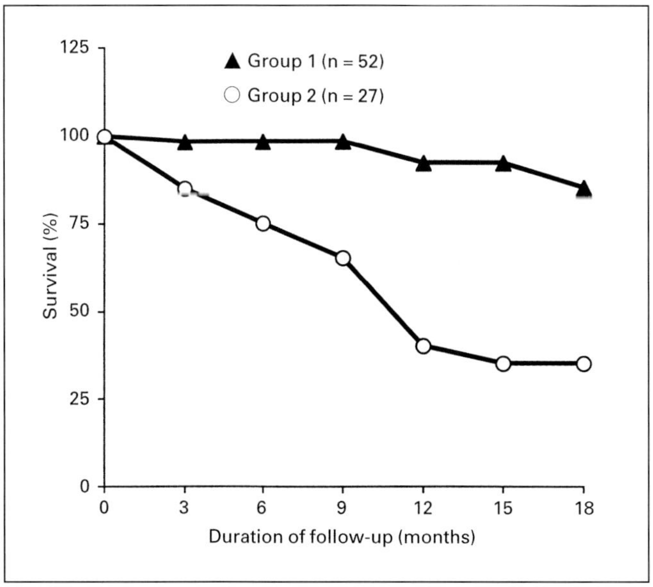

Fig. 1. Survival curves for heart failure patients with preserved exercise capacity (▲; group 1) and those with markedly impaired exercise capacity (○; group2). Group 1: n = 52; age = 47 years; New York Heart Association (NYHA) class = 3; VO_2peak = 19.0 ml/kg/min. Group 2: n = 27; age = 53 years; NYHA class = 3; VO_2peak = 10.5 ml/kg/min. Adapted with permission from Mancini et al. [1].

al lifestyle with good quality of life is now the desired procedural outcome. To achieve this outcome, aggressive exercise rehabilitation is essential. There is recent convincing evidence that exercise training is an effective adjunct therapy in postoperative management of end-stage CHF patients who undergo orthotopic heart transplantation.

This chapter will explore recent advances in Exercise Physiology for both heart failure and heart transplantation patients. Included are reviews of the factors contributing to exercise intolerance in both patient populations and a summary of results from exercise rehabilitation studies in these patients. Current recommendations for exercise testing and exercise prescription are also provided.

Chronic Heart Failure Patients

Fatigue and activity intolerance are uniform complaints of patients with CHF. Exercise tolerance, as assessed by peak oxygen consumption (VO_2peak), is a powerful predictor of survival in these patients [1] (fig. 1). Because of safety concerns, CHF patients were excluded from exercise rehabilitation programs prior to 1980. In acute or unstable CHF, rest can improve hemodynamics and reduce ventricular volumes, both of which are beneficial in acute or unstable CHF. However, *prolonged* rest is neither necessary nor beneficial. Over the past decade, exercise rehabilitation has been used increasingly to attain functional and symptomatic improvement in CHF. The risk of myocardial infarction (MI) or life-threatening arrhythmia in selected CHF patients is not significantly higher with exercise than is the risk conferred by their heart failure.

Mechanisms of Exercise Intolerance in CHF

Impaired Left Ventricular (LV) Function. Although the primary pathophysiologic features of CHF are central hemodynamic abnormalities, exercise tolerance is not directly related to the degree of cardiac dysfunction. Left ventricular ejection fraction (LVEF) is important in assessing myocardial systolic dysfunction but is of little value in predicting a patient's ability to exercise and is not a sensitive index for determining the beneficial effects of exercise rehabilitation in CHF. Additionally, pharmacological augmentation of cardiac output through administration of inotropes does not immediately increase blood flow to exercising muscle and does not immediately elicit increases in VO_2peak, clearly suggesting that forward cardiac output is not the singular factor contributing to exercise intolerance in CHF.

CHF patients with preserved LV systolic function also have significant exercise intolerance. In these patients, abnormalities in LV diastolic function prevent augmentation of stroke volume via the Frank Starling mechanism; the result is diminished cardiac output and severe exercise intolerance. In diastolic failure patients, increased LV filling pressure during exercise is not accompanied by increases in end-diastolic volume and patients are unable to increase VO_2peak [2]. The weak relationship between LVEF and exercise tolerance in CHF has led to interest in peripheral mechanisms to explain exercise intolerance.

Baroreflex Desensitization and Sympathetic Activation. In the acute phase of low-output CHF, arterial and cardiopulmonary baroreflexes are activated to help maintain systemic blood pressure. However, sensitivity of both arterial and cardiac baroreceptors become diminished, resulting in unrestrained sympathetic excitation. Sympathetic hyperactivation is observed at rest and during exercise [3, 4]. Resting plasma norepinephrine levels are 2- to 3-fold higher in CHF patients compared to healthy controls and muscle sympathetic nerve activity is dramatically increased in CHF patients. CHF patients become tachycardic with loss of heart rate (HR) variability and peripheral vascular vasodilation is prevented by excessive sympathetic vasoconstrictor tone. The loss of baroreflex sensitivity and elevated levels of circulating norepinephrine are closely correlated with disease severity and overall survival.

Neurohormonal Activation. Neurohormonal mechanisms play a central role in the progression of CHF [3, 4]. In acute heart failure, neurohormonal activation is a desirable compensatory mechanism that facilitates vasoconstriction and plasma volume expansion that act to maintain forward cardiac output and systemic blood pressure. However, sustained neurohormonal arousal further complicates heart failure and is associated with poor long-term prognosis in CHF. Activation of the sympathetic nervous system, the renin-angiotensin-aldosterone system (RAAS), and hypersecretion of pituitary arginine vasopressin (AVP) have adverse hemodynamic consequences in heart failure because they enhance vasoconstriction and promote fluid retention. Prolonged neurohormonal activation exerts a direct deleterious effect on the heart that is *independent* of the hemodynamic actions of these systems. High concentrations of angiotensin II (ANG II) induce necrosis of cardiac myocytes [5], adversely influence matrix structure of myocardium [6], increase sympathetic drive and impair baroreceptor restraint on sympathetic drive [7]. Large multicenter clinical trials have provided compelling evidence that pharmacological suppression of neurohormonal activation, rather than stimulation of the failing myocardium, improves symptoms and survival in CHF [8, 9]. These observations support the need for more therapeutic strategies directed at modulation of neurohormonal activation in CHF.

Impaired Vasodilatation. Sympathetic stimulation and neurohormonal activation are potent sources of vasoconstriction in CHF. However, peripheral α-adrenergic blockade and angiotensin-converting enzyme (ACE) inhibitor therapy do not immediately restore vasodilating capacity in CHF patients, indicating that intrinsic vascular abnormalities contribute to impaired vasodilatory capacity. Vascular stiffness, caused by increased sodium and water content within vascular tissue, may be responsible for up to one third of vasodilatory impairment in CHF. Acute diuretic therapy improves muscle blood flow but continued diuresis does not restore normal vasodilatory capacity, despite further reductions in fluid volume. There is now compelling evidence of endothelial dysfunction in both peripheral and coronary vessels in patients with CHF [10, 11]. The consequences of endothelial dysfunction in CHF are reduced peripheral perfusion and increased LV load. The mechanism of endothelial dysfunction is likely a combination of increased sympathetic tone and vasoconstrictor activity, reduced production of nitric oxide (NO) and inactivation of NO by superoxide.

Skeletal Muscle Abnormalities. Exercise intolerance in CHF patients has been attributed to underperfusion of exercising muscle. However, increasing blood supply to skeletal muscle does not result in an immediate improvement in VO_2peak in these patients, suggesting that skeletal muscle abnormalities exist that are unrelated to blood flow [12]. Indeed, recent studies have shown that reductions in skeletal muscle blood flow, skeletal muscle mass (13–15% reduction), aerobic enzyme activity and an increased percentage of fast type IIb fibers (more glycolytic; less fatigue-resistant) act in concert to induce early anaerobic metabolism during exercise and limit exercise tolerance in patients with CHF [13]. Studies using ^{31}P magnetic resonance spectroscopy (^{31}P-MRS) revealed abnormalities of skeletal muscle metabolism manifested by a greater magnitude (and increased rate) of phosphocreatine (P_{Cr}) depletion and a decreased pH in patients with CHF [13, 14].

Morphological data from biopsy studies corroborate that there is pronounced and selective atrophy in highly oxidative, fatigue-resistant, type I muscle fibers resulting in a shift in fiber type distribution toward the glycolytic, less fatigue-resistant, type II muscle fibers. One laboratory has reported a significant correlation between the percent distribution of the three myosin heavy chain (MHC) isoforms in the gastrocnemius (namely MHCI = slow aerobic; MHCIIa = fast oxidative; MHCIIb = fast glycolytic), the severity of CHF, and VO_2peak [15].

Pulmonary Abnormalities. Exertional dyspnea is a prominent symptom in CHF and a variety of abnormalities in pulmonary function are believed to be exacerbated by CHF. Exertional dyspnea had been attributed to increases in LV filling pressure and pulmonary capillary wedge pressure (PCWP); however, recent hemodynamic studies have failed to correlate dyspnea symptoms with measurements of PCWP [16]. Dyspnea in nonedematous CHF patients may be as much or more related to deconditioning and skeletal muscle metabolic abnormalities than to pulmonary congestion. In a group of CHF patients studied before and after exercise training, PCWP was unchanged by training, despite a 23% increase in VO_2max and a reduction in dyspnea symptoms [16]. Respiratory muscle fatigue also contributes to dyspnea in CHF patients. Exercise has been shown to induce deoxygenation of accessory respiratory muscles in patients with CHF, implying that decreased cardiac output during exercise results in deoxygenation of accessory respiratory muscles [17].

Exercise Training Adaptations in CHF Patients

Oxygen Consumption (VO_2peak). Training-induced improvements in VO_2peak are a consistent finding in CHF patients and range from 1.4 to 7 ml/kg/min. In their pioneering CHF training study, Sullivan et al. [18] reported a 23% increase in VO_2peak (16.8 vs. 20.6 ml/kg/min) in CHF patients (LVEF 24 ± 10%) after 4 months of exercise training consisting of 4 h of monitored exercise per week. There were no changes in rest or exercise pulmonary wedge pressure, stroke volume, cardiac output, or LVEF. Braith et al. [3] recently reported a 25% increase in VO_2peak in CHF patients (NYHA class II or III; LVEF 30%; age = 61 ± 7 years) who participated in a program of supervised treadmill walking 3 days/week for 16 weeks at 40–70% of VO_2peak.

CHF patients whose LVEF is less than 40% after a recent large MI, but remain free of anginal symptoms, can safely engage in an exercise program and increase their VO_2peak. However, CHF patients with anginal symptoms on a treadmill test may not achieve improvements in VO_2peak because of a limited exercise training intensity.

Myocardial Remodeling. The influence of exercise training on myocardial wall thinning and the 'remodeling' process in post-MI patients generates considerable debate. Early animal and human post-MI studies reported a deterioration in LV function [19, 20]. Recent studies, however, have not confirmed those findings [18, 21]. Sullivan et al. [18] reported no change in rest and exercise radionuclide measurements of LVEF, LV end-diastolic volume, and LV end-systolic volume in CHF patients after 4–6 months of exercise training. A multicenter randomized trial found that a 6-month training program consisting of aggressive stationary cycling and walking did not result in further ventricular enlargement or deterioration after training in patients recovering from an anterior MI [21]. Jette et al. [22] used restriction (to anterior MIs), stratification (by LVEF <30% and >30%), and a controlled randomized design to overcome biases that have plagued most earlier exercise studies. Radionuclide ventriculography and echocardiography revealed that training did not cause further deterioration in ventricular function. Dubach et al. [23] recently used magnetic resonance imaging (MRI) before and after 8 weeks of high-intensity cardiac rehabilitation. The MRI detected no deleterious effects of exercise training on supine resting LV volume, function, or wall thickness regardless of infarct area. In aggregate, the experience to date indicates that selected CHF patients without clinical complications can benefit from exercise training without negative effects on LV volume, function, or wall thickness.

Baroreflex and Sympathetic Activation. The mechanisms responsible for exercise-induced improvements in baroreflex sensitivity are not clearly understood, perhaps due to the complexity of the neural circuitry. Nonetheless, markers of autonomic nervous system function in CHF patients show a significant shift away from sympathetic activity toward greater dominance of vagal parasympathetic tone after exercise training. One study found a 30% improvement in baroreflex sensitivity in 70 CHF patients after exercise training [24]. Improved baroreceptor sensitivity was correlated with decreased sympathetic and neurohormonal activation, and an increase in parasympathetic activity and HR variability. The clinical implication is that improved baroreflex function and vagal tone could diminish susceptibility to life-threatening arrhythmias in CHF patients.

Two principal mechanisms are recognized in neurohormonal activation in CHF patients and both may be modulated by endurance exercise training. Neuroendocrine hyperactivity in CHF may be triggered by baroreflex dysfunction caused by prolonged exposure to low cardiac output. The resulting loss of inhibitory baroreflex signals to the brainstem likely contributes to sympathetic excitation and elevated circulating neurohormones. An alternative but physiologically related mechanism for baroreflex and sympathetic activation in CHF is associated with the direct effects of circulating ANG II. Elevated ANG II exerts excitatory effects at the level of the brain, ganglionic transmission, and at adrenergic nerve terminals [25].

Thus, a reduction in circulating ANG II levels achieved through exercise training may be one approach toward improving baroreflex control of sympathetic activity [3].

Neurohumoral Systems. A recent study at the University of Florida was the first randomized controlled trial of intermediate-term exercise training to measure fluid regulatory hormone levels in CHF patients [3]. Nineteen clinically stable coronary disease patients with chronic (>4 months) symptoms of heart failure (NYHA II or III) were randomly assigned to a training group (n = 10; age = 61 ± 6; EF = 30 ± 6) or a control group (n = 9; age = 62 ± 7; EF = 29 ± 7). Exercise training consisted of supervised walking 3 times per week for 16 weeks at 40–70% of VO_2peak. Neurohormones were measured at rest and at VO_2peak before and after training. At study entry, values for ANG II, aldosterone, AVP and ANP did not differ between groups. After 16 weeks of training, all resting neurohormone levels were significantly reduced by approximately 30% in the exercise group but unchanged in the control group (fig. 2).

Vasodilatory Capacity. Recent studies have confirmed that the vascular endothelium is a therapeutic target to reduce symptoms of CHF. Hornig et al. [10] were the first to suggest that an exercise program can enhance vasodilatory capacity. In this cross-over trial, patients with CHF participated in 4 weeks of daily handgrip exercise at 70% of maximal voluntary contraction. Ultrasound was used to measure radial artery diameter during reactive hyperemia and during sodium nitroprusside infusion. Exercise training restored flow-dependent vasodilatory capacity but enhanced vasodilation was specific to the region trained and was lost after 6 weeks of cessation of training. Hambrecht et al. [26] went a step further and demonstrated that exercise training improves both basal endothelial NO formation and agonist-mediated endothelium-dependent vasodilation of the skeletal muscle vasculature in patients with CHF. Six months of home-based bicycle ergometry performed twice daily (total of 40 min) 5 days/week at 70% of VO_2peak improved femoral artery blood flow 23% in response to 90 μg/min acetylcholine. The inhibitory effect of N^G-monomethyl-*L*-arginine (*L*-NMMA) increased by 174%, indicating that exercise increases basal NO formation in resistance vessels. Importantly, the endothelium-dependent change in femoral blood flow was significantly ($p < 0.005$) correlated with VO_2peak. In a recent study, Hambrecht et al. [27] advanced this line of research in CHF patients by demonstrating that lower body exercise on a cycle ergometer leads to a correction of endothelial dysfunction of the upper extremity, indicating a systemic effect of local exercise training on endothelial function.

The expression of endothelial NO synthase (eNOS) is reduced in a canine model of heart failure but eNOS was restored to normal after a 10-day exercise training program [28]. The expression of eNOS is increased by shear stress in isolated endothelial cells. Thus, impaired endothelium-dependent vasodilation in CHF may be restored by repetitive increases in blood flow during exercise training which cause intermittent enhanced shear stress and, consequently, increased expression and activity of eNOS. These observations suggest that local mechanical forces play a key role in the beneficial effects of training. In addition to the regulation of eNOS, other shear-dependent mechanisms are likely involved as well; i.e., shear stress upregulates the expression of superoxide dismutase, a

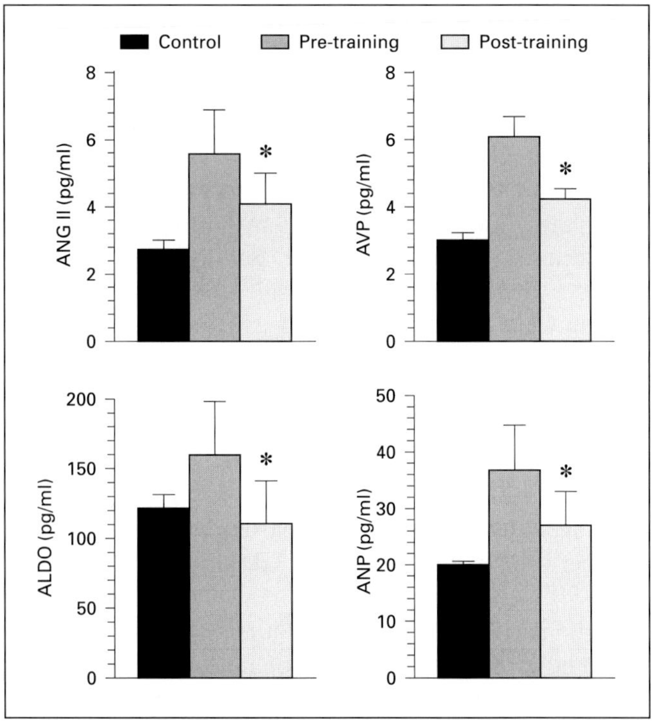

Fig. 2. Rest plasma levels of angiotensin II (ANG II), aldosterone (ALDO), arginine vasopressin (AVP) and atrial natriuretic peptide (ANP) in age-matched untrained healthy controls (n = 11) and heart failure patients (n = 10) before and after 16 weeks of exercise training. Values represent the mean ± SEM. Significance: * $p < 0.05$. Reprinted with permission from the American College of Cardiology [3].

radical-scavenging enzyme, but suppresses the expression and activity of ACE [29].

Skeletal Muscle Metabolism. Studies using ^{31}P-NMR spectroscopy and in-magnet exercise protocols have reported significant improvement in metabolic capacity following exercise training. Muscle endurance was increased up to 260% without any change in muscle mass, limb blood flow and cardiac output [30]. Rather, improved exercise tolerance was attributed to reduced depletion of P_{Cr}, higher muscle pH at submaximal workloads, and more rapid resynthesis of P_{Cr}, which is an indicator of mitochondrial oxidative phosphorylation [30].

Our laboratory assessed muscle metabolism by ^{31}P-NMR spectroscopy in the medial head of the gastrocnemius before and after a 4-month walking program [14]. The in-magnet exercise protocol consisted of repetitive plantar flexion at a low-intensity (25% of maximal voluntary contraction) and high-intensity (85%) workload. The results show a marked reduction (19%) in the inorganic

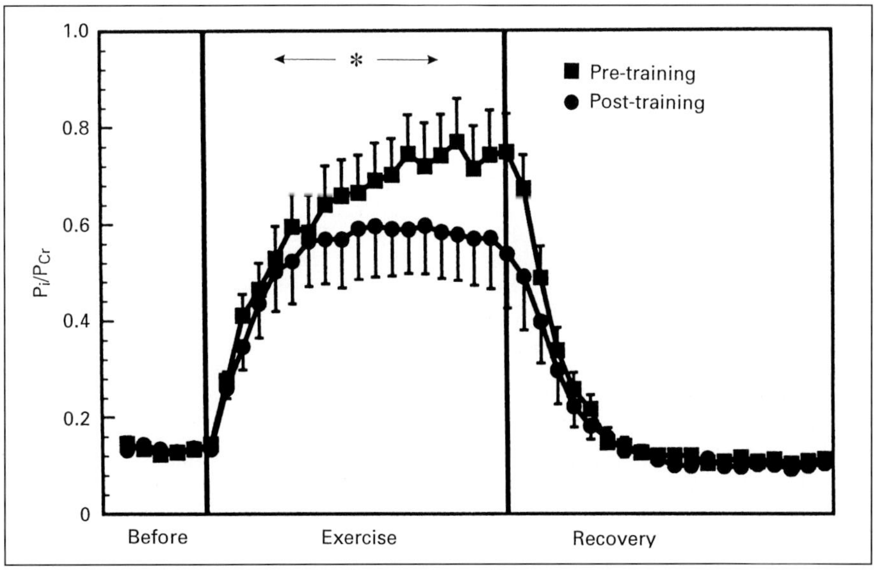

Fig. 3. The P_i:P_{Cr} ratio before, during and immediately following low-intensity plantar flexion (25% maximal voluntary contraction) in heart failure patients (n = 14) before (■) and after (●) 16 weeks of exercise training. The P_i:P_{Cr} ratio, as determined by ^{31}P-NMR spectroscopy, is an index of skeletal muscle oxidative capacity. Values represent the mean ± SEM. Significance: * $p < 0.05$. Modified from Kluess et al. [14].

phosphate/phosphocreatine ratio (P_i/P_{Cr}) during the low-intensity exercise, and a significant decrease (30%) in intramuscular diprotonated inorganic phosphate ($H_2PO_4^-$) during the high-intensity exercise (fig. 3). The 19% reduction in P_i/P_{Cr} during the low-intensity exercise protocol reflects an improved capacity of muscle to produce ATP from oxidative metabolic pathways. Additionally, significant improvements (28%) in P_{Cr} resynthesis following both the low- and high-intensity protocols, indicate improved recovery kinetics. In contrast, the skeletal muscle metabolic profile remained unchanged in the control group.

Clinical Outcomes. A decade has passed since the first prospective controlled trials of exercise training in CHF but valuable long-term follow-up data is lacking. Belardinelli et al. [31] recently provided the first longitudinal data which argues that exercise training results favorable clinical outcomes. The authors randomized 99 patients with moderate to severe CHF to supervised exercise rehabilitation or control for a period of 14 months. Subjects initially trained at 60% of VO_2peak 3 times per week for 8 weeks, then twice a week for 1 year. Changes were observed only in the training group. Both VO_2peak and thallium activity score improved ($p < 0.001$), 18 and 24%, respectively. Follow-up started after 14 months of exercise training and patients were monitored for an average of 1,214 ± 56 days (range 1,161–1,268 days). Follow-up ended at the time of study closure or with an adverse event. Exercise training was associated with both lower total all-cause mortality (9 vs. 20 deaths; risk reduction –63%; 95% CI, 17–84%; $p < 0.01$) and hospital readmission for heart failure (5 vs. 14 admissions; risk reduction –71%; 95% CI, 11–88%; $p < 0.02$). While the results of this important study do not prove that exercise reduces mortality in CHF patients (the study was not powered or designed to show these effects reliably), they do give encouragement that exercise training is a beneficial treatment in CHF.

Summary of Responses to Exercise. In selected patients with compensated stable CHF and moderate to severe LV systolic dysfunction, favorable outcomes usually occur without deterioration in LV function. Exercise training increases functional capacity and improves symptoms. Adaptations in skeletal muscle and the peripheral circulation appear to be responsible for the improvement in exercise tolerance rather than central adaptations. Patients who have a combination of LV dysfunction and residual myocardial ischemia, however, may not benefit from exercise training. The most consistent benefits occur with exercise training at least 3 times per week for 12 or more weeks. The duration of aerobic exercise training sessions can vary from 20 to 40 min, at an intensity of 50–85% of peak HR on the graded exercise test or 40–70% of VO_2peak.

Designing an Exercise Program for CHF Patients

Risk Stratification and Patient Screening. There is uniform encouragement for stratification of individuals into risk categories prior to engaging in an exercise program by the American Heart Association, American College of

Table 1. American Heart Association (AHA) risk stratification criteria

AHA classification	NYHA class	Exercise capacity	Angina/ischemia and clinical characteristics	ECG Monitoring
A Apparently Healthy			Less than 40 years of age Without symptoms, no major risk factors, and normal GXT	No supervision or monitoring required
B Known stable CAD, low risk for vigorous exercise	1 or 2	5–6 METS	Free of ischemia or angina at rest or on the GXT EF = 40–60%	Monitored and supervised only during prescribed sessions (6–12 sessions) Light resistance training may be included in comprehensive rehabilitation programs
C Stable CV disease with low risk for vigorous exercise but unable to self-regulate activity	1 or 2	5–6 METS	Same disease states and clinical characteristics as Class B but without the ability to self-monitor exercise	Medical supervision and ECG monitoring during prescribed sessions Nonmedical supervision of other exercise sessions
D Moderate to high risk for cardiac complications during exercise	≥3	<6 METS	Ischemia (≥4.0 mm ST depression) or angina during exercise Two or more previous MIs EF < 30%	Continuous ECG monitoring during rehabilitation until safety is established Medical supervision during all exercise sessions until safety is established
E Unstable disease with activity restriction	≥3	<6 METS	Unstable angina Uncompensated heart failure Uncontrollable arrhythmias	No activity is recommended for conditioning purposes Attention should be directed to restoring patient to Class D or higher

Sports Medicine, American Association for Cardiovascular and Pulmonary Rehabilitation, and the Centers for Disease Control. Using these risk strata, the AHA recommends that medically stable CHF patients may participate in exercise training programs (table 1). The majority of stable CHF patients will be classified as Class C patients but a significant number of patients with mild heart failure may be classified as Class B (i.e. an exercise capacity of 6 METS and LVEF of 40–60%) and be qualified to participate in comprehensive rehabilitation programs including light to moderate resistance training. Regardless of the classification, the exercise program should be individualized and medical supervision provided until safety is established.

Before starting an exercise program, CHF patients must be stable with fluid volume status controlled. CHF patients with an LVEF of less than 30% should be carefully screened for ischemia. Pre-training evaluation with a symptom-limited bicycle or treadmill graded exercise test is essential. Only patients free of unstable or exercise-induced ventricular arrhythmias should be considered for exercise training. Echocardiographic assessment of ventricular function and expired gas analysis for assessment of VO_2peak may also aid in preparing an exercise prescription. The patient selection process for exercise training is summarized in figure 4.

Initial Exercise Intensity. The initial exercise intensity should be customized for each patient. It may be necessary to use an interval training approach consisting of 2–6 min of low-level activities alternated with 1- to 2-min rest periods. Symptoms and general fatigue guide the determination of training frequency which may be 2–3 times a day during the early stages of the program. Warm-up and cool-down periods should be longer than normal for observation of possible arrhythmias. Because the chronotropic response to exercise is frequently abnormal, appropriate exercise intensity for CHF patients should be based on VO_2peak rather than HRpeak.

A starting exercise intensity of 40–60% of VO_2peak is recommended. Alternatively, the initial exercise intensity should be 10 beats below any significant symptoms including, angina, exertional hypotension, dysrhythmias and dyspnea. Continuous supervision may be necessary during the early stages of the program for all CHF patients and frequent monitoring of blood pressure and echocardiographic responses should be used in patients at higher risk (AHA Class C). Rating of perceived exertion should range from 11 to 14 ('light' to 'somewhat hard') on the Borg perceived exertion scale. Anginal symptoms should not exceed 2+ on the 0–4 angina scale ('moderate to bothersome') and exertional dyspnea should not exceed 2+ on the dyspnea scale ('mild, some difficulty') [32]. Initially, full resuscitation equipment should be available.

Exercise Program Progression. The duration of exercise should be gradually increased to 30 min, at an intensity approximating 70–85% of peak HR or 40–60% of

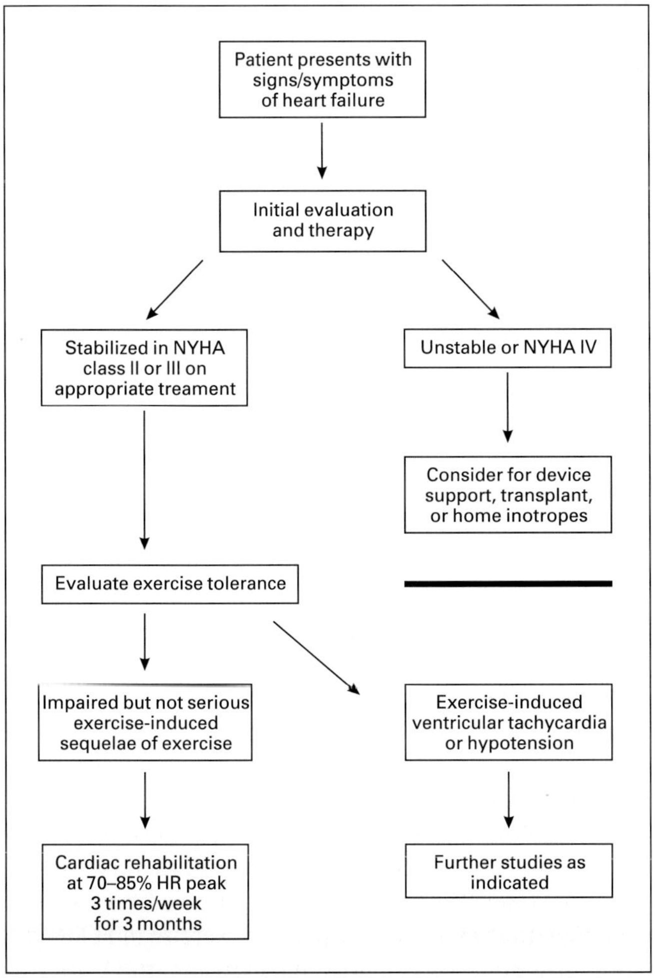

Fig. 4. Screening of patients with chronic heart failure for cardiac rehabilitation.

VO_2peak. The most consistent benefits occur with exercise training at least three times per week for 12 or more weeks. In selected patients, after a prolonged period (6–12 weeks) of supervised sessions without adverse events, exercise may continue away from the supervised environment (i.e. home program). The mode of exercise should be predominantly cardiovascular in nature, such as walking and cycling. Although the AHA does not have specific guidelines for a resistance training component for CHF patients, light to moderate resistance training is often integrated as part of a comprehensive rehabilitation program for low risk (AHA Class B) patients who have successfully completed at least 6–12 weeks of cardiovascular exercise training without adverse events.

Summary. New guidelines have been directed toward health professionals who are involved in regular exercise testing and exercise training [33]. Rehabilitation personnel must watch for symptoms of cardiac decompensation during exercise, including cough or dyspnea, hypotension, lightheadedness, cyanosis, angina and arrhythmias. Patient's body weight should be recorded prior to exercise and daily pulmonary auscultation for rales and shortness of breath is recommended. Patients should avoid exercise immediately after eating or taking a vasodilator. Fluid and electrolyte balance is vital. Patients who have potassium or magnesium deficiency should take supplements to replenish electrolytes before embarking on an exercise program.

Rehabilitation of Heart Transplant Recipients

The second half of the chapter will review the unique exercise rehabilitation challenges presented by HTR and summarize their adaptations to chronic exercise training. Most HTR have suffered preoperatively from chronic debilitating cardiac illness. Many of them have had prolonged pre-transplantation hospitalizations for inotropic support or a ventricular assist device. VO_2peak and related cardiovascular parameters regress approximately 26% within the first 1–3 weeks of sustained bed rest [33]. Consequently, extremely poor aerobic capacity, skeletal muscle myopathy and cardiac cachexia are not unusual occurrences in HTR who have required mechanical support or been confined to bed rest. In addition to exercise limitations attributable to antecedent heart failure, HTR must also contend with de novo exercise challenges conferred by chronic cardiac denervation and the multiple sequela resulting from immunosuppression therapy. Therefore, this section of the chapter will emphasize the following three factors that determine exercise performance in HTR: (1) altered anatomy and physiology of the transplanted heart; (2) the effects of previous cardiac illness and supportive care, and (3) the effects of immunosuppressive drug therapy, most notably chronic glucocorticoid use.

Central Factors Contributing to Exercise Intolerance in HTR

Heart Rate. The transplanted heart exhibits unique characteristics that heavily influence exercise performance [34]. Figure 5 illustrates typical resting and exercise responses of the transplanted heart. Resting HR is high with rates approaching 100 bpm early after transplantation and diminishing to 80–90 bpm late after transplantation. Elevated resting HR appears to reflect the

Fig. 5. A representation of the typical evolution in heart rate (HR) responses before, during and after exercise in heart transplant recipients when compared to normal age-matched control subjects: (a) resting HR is elevated, (b) chronotropic response at initiation of exercise is sluggish, (c) peak HR is attenuated, (d) peak HR often occurs early in recovery after conclusion of exercise, and (e) deceleration of HR is prolonged.

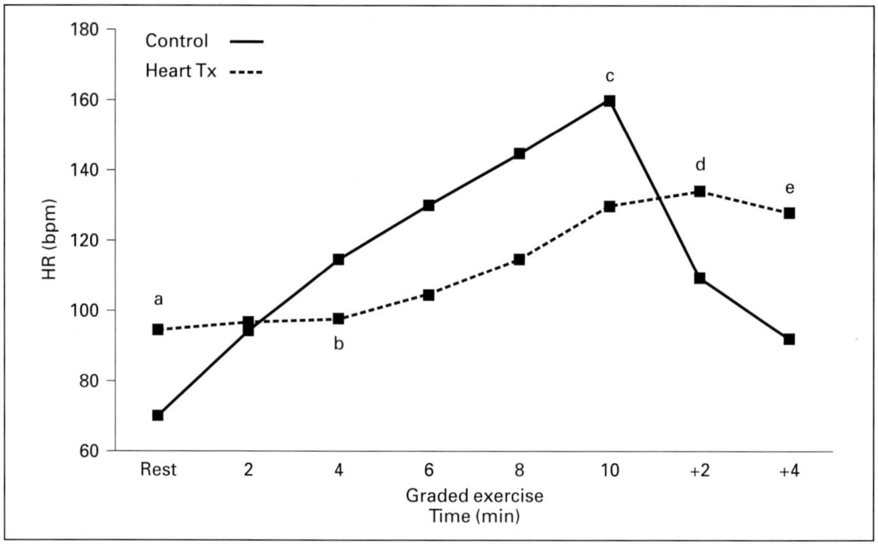

intrinsic depolarization rate of the SA node in the absence of parasympathetic innervation. Normal tachycardic responses at the onset of exercise are sluggish and rate acceleration during exercise is nearly entirely dependent upon the chronotropic effects of circulating catecholamines. Peak HR in untrained HTR is markedly reduced, being only 70–80% of age-matched norms. Peak HR is frequently observed during recovery from graded exercise testing because humoral catecholamine levels reach their zenith early after termination of exercise. Recovery HR decelerates very slowly due to high circulating catecholamine levels and the absence of parasympathetic inhibition. Peak HR does increase with time after transplantation but most of the improvement occurs during the first postoperative year [35–37]. Mandak et al. [37] and Givertz et al. [36] performed serial assessment of exercise capacity for up to 5 years in large cohorts of HTR (n = 60 and n = 57, respectively) and both studies concluded that no significant improvements in peak HR occurred after the first year.

The critical importance of HR reserve in exercise performance has been illustrated in recent studies [38, 39]. Richard et al. [38] reported that highly trained HTR achieved values for both peak HR (169 bpm) and VO_2peak (39 ml/kg/min) that were 95% of age-matched norms. Braith et al. [39] used a cross-over design to explore the efficacy of rate-responsive cardiac pacemakers as a therapy for chronotropic incompetence. Stable HTR who had a pacemaker implanted at the time of transplantation, completed two maximal Naughton treadmill tests. During one of the treadmill tests the pacemaker was programmed to be rate responsive but not in the other. Peak HR (+15%), VO_2peak (+20%) and total treadmill time (+17%) were significantly improved by rate responsive pacing.

Rehabilitation personnel must also recognize that β-adrenergic antagonists contribute to chronotropic incompetence and have an exaggerated effect on exercise capacity and systolic blood pressure in HTR. Leenen et al. [40] evaluated the HR responses to cycle exercise in HTR (n = 7) and patients with essential hypertension (n = 8) on placebo and β-blocker. Nonselective β-blockade (nadolol; 20 and 40 mg/day) decreased peak exercise HR by 60 and 70%, respectively, in HTR but only 10 and 20%, respectively, in the hypertensive group. Moreover, β-blockade diminished total exercise time by 2 min in HTR but had no effect in the hypertensive group.

Cardiac Output. Cardiac output at rest is normal [41, 42] or mildly reduced [34] in HTR. Both LV end-diastolic volume and stroke volume are reduced in HTR at rest (20–40%) but the elevated resting HR serves to maintain cardiac index within a normal range (albeit low-normal). LVEF is also normal at rest and normal or near normal during exercise [34].

Peak exercise cardiac output is diminished by 30–40% in HTR secondary to chronotropic incompetence and diastolic dysfunction [34]. The absence of sympathetic innervation appears to alter cardiac compliance, resulting in diastolic dysfunction and a leftward shift in the pressure-volume curve. Systolic function, in contrast, remains relatively normal after transplantation. Thus, despite normal contractile reserve and LVEF, the denervated heart be-

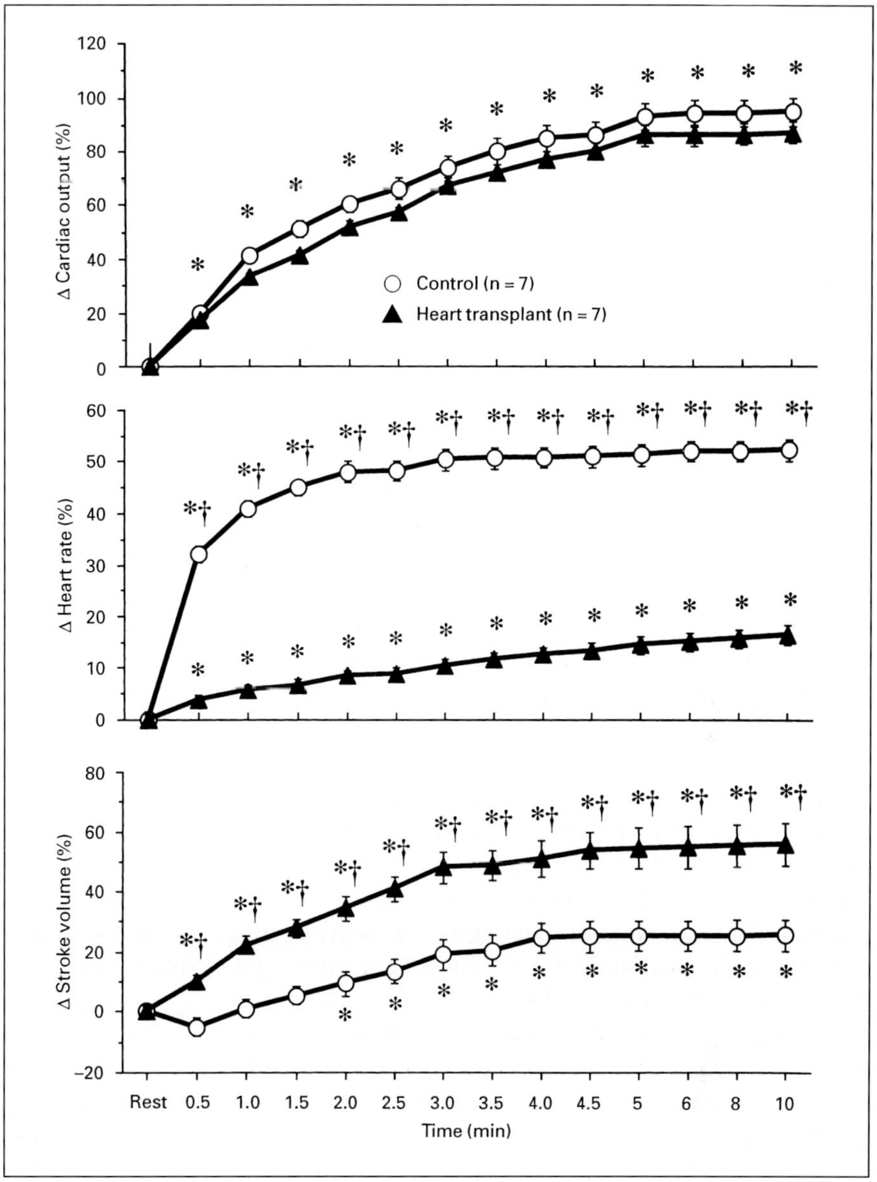

Fig. 6. Temporal pattern of relative changes (percent change from rest) in cardiac output, heart rate and stroke volume during 10 min of constant load cycle exercise at 40% peak power output in heart transplant recipients and age-matched control subjects. Values are expressed as mean value ± SEM. * $p < 0.05$ rest vs. exercise. † $p < 0.05$ transplant vs. control group. Reprinted with permission from the American College of Cardiology [42].

comes 'stiff' and diastolic volume and stroke volume at peak exercise are only ~80% of predicted [34]. The mechanism responsible for abnormal allograft compliance is unclear but diastolic dysfunction may be another consequence of autonomic denervation and it has been demonstrated that β-adrenergic tone is, in part, responsible for regulation of diastolic filling in normal subjects [36]. Exercise training does not elicit changes in rest or peak exercise cardiac output in most HTR [41, 43].

Despite chronotropic and inotropic limitations however, HTR are able to augment cardiac output during upright exercise but the mechanism differs from normally innervated persons. While immediate increases in HR augment cardiac output in the normal intact heart, augmentation of cardiac output in HTR is achieved by increases in stroke volume. Braith et al. [42] demonstrated that HTR augment stroke volume immediately (within 30 s) at the onset of exercise and achieved stroke volume values that were 61% greater than resting values (fig. 6). The adjustment in stroke volume was too rapid to be ascribed to catecholamines because humoral norepinephrine levels did not increase above baseline values until nearly 4 min after onset of exercise. Rather, it is likely that an increase in venous return, facilitated by the 'skeletal muscle pump,' may offset the altered inotropic state and diastolic dysfunction of the denervated heart. The 12–14% expansion of blood volume in HTR raises the possibility that volume expansion is a compensatory adaptation to cardiac denervation [42, 44]. Indeed, HTR may require an expanded blood volume to maintain cardiac output in the absence of cardiac autonomic nerves.

Hemodynamics. Intracardiac and pulmonary pressures are elevated in CHF patients. Transplantation improves the hemodynamic profile but right atrial, pulmonary artery (+40%), and PCWPs (+30–35%) [34] remain elevated, suggesting that hemodynamic changes associated with CHF may persist indefinitely. At peak exercise, PCWP (25–50% > normal) and right atrial pressure (80–100% > normal) are significantly elevated in HTR, even though absolute workload is substantially lower than age-matched control [34]. To date, only one small study has assessed the effect of exercise training on central hemodynamics in HTR (n = 7) and reported no changes in rest or exercise values for pulmonary artery, pulmonary capillary wedge, or right atrial pressures following 6 weeks of endurance exercise [43].

The impact of elevated cardiac and pulmonary pressures on exercise tolerance has been investigated in one study [45]. The investigators measured arterial blood gases and pH in HTR (n = 10) during 10 min of cycle exercise at 70% of peak power output. Arterial oxygen pressure declined to <80 mm Hg in 5 patients and <60 mm Hg in 3 patients. None of the preoperative right heart catheterization variables were significantly correlated with exercise-induced hypoxemia. However, postoperative mean pulmonary artery pressure was significantly related to exercise-induced hypoxemia ($r = 0.71$; $p = 0.03$) [45].

Pulmonary Spirometry. End-stage CHF patients have abnormal pulmonary diffusion capacity (DL_{CO}) and diminished spirometric parameters including, forced vital capacity (FVC), forced expiratory volume in 1 s (FEV_1), and total lung capacity (TLC) [45, 46]. In large part, the reduction in lung volumes is a consequence of cardiac hypertrophy, but other factors such as pleural effusions and interstitial edema likely contribute to the reduction in lung volumes. Most longitudinal studies report that abnormal spirometric parameters are completely reversed after heart transplantation. Thus, in the absence of established COPD, spirometric parameters should not restrict exercise tolerance in most HTR.

Pulmonary Diffusion. Numerous studies have shown that the abnormal DL_{CO} observed in CHF patients persists following heart transplantation [45–48]. However, few data are available concerning the impact of impaired DL_{CO} on exercise capacity. Braith et al. [45] collected serial arterial blood gases and found marked hypoxemia in 50% (5 of 10 subjects) of a small cohort of HTR during 10 min of cycle ergometry at 70% of peak power output (fig. 7). All subjects with exercise-induced hypoxemia (n = 5) had abnormal pulmonary diffusing capacity (<70% of predicted). In 3 of the 5 HTR who became hypoxemic, DL_{CO} was diminished to approximately 50% of predicted. Ville et al. [46] also measured arterial blood gases at maximal exercise in HTR with normal (n = 8; DL_{CO} 88% of norm) and abnormal (n = 9; DL_{CO} 52% of norm) diffusing capacity. Peak power, VO_2peak, peak oxygen pulse and peak minute ventilation were all significantly greater in the group with normal DL_{CO}. A strong correlation ($r = 0.81$) was found between DL_{CO} and VO_2peak. Stepwise regression analysis revealed that DL_{CO} explained 66% of the variance in VO_2peak in the HTR. Squires et al. [49] assessed arterial oxygen saturation (SaO_2) in a large (n = 50) group of HTR undergoing symptom-limited treadmill testing. Only 4 subjects (8%) experienced exercise-induced desaturation (>4%). DL_{CO} in subjects with exercise-induced desaturation (DL_{CO} = 62% of predicted) was lower than in subjects that did not desaturate (DL_{CO} = 69% of predicted). Thus, the available evidence indicates that, while abnormal DL_{CO} is prevalent in HTR, exercise-induced hypoxemia is not a consistent finding and occurs only in those patients exhibiting the greatest deficits (~50% of predicted) in DL_{CO}.

Peripheral Factors Contributing to Exercise Intolerance in HTR

Skeletal Muscle Metabolism. Abnormal skeletal muscle metabolism is not immediately resolved by heart transplantation. Rather, muscle atrophy, decreased mitochondrial content, decreased oxidative enzymes and the shift toward less fatigue-resistant type IIb fibers continue to contribute to exercise intolerance in HTR. Immunosuppression therapy, including both glucocorticoids and cyclosporine, further alters skeletal muscle metabolism after transplantation. Glucocorticoids promote muscle atrophy, particularly in type II fibers, by increasing the rate of protein catabolism and amino acid efflux while simultaneously decreasing the rate of protein synthesis [50]. Cyclosporine decreases oxidative enzymes in animals and may further complicate the loss of oxidative capacity in HTR [51].

Bussieres et al. [50] used a biopsy technique to longitudinally study skeletal muscle in HTR. Consistent with other studies, they reported a predominance of type II

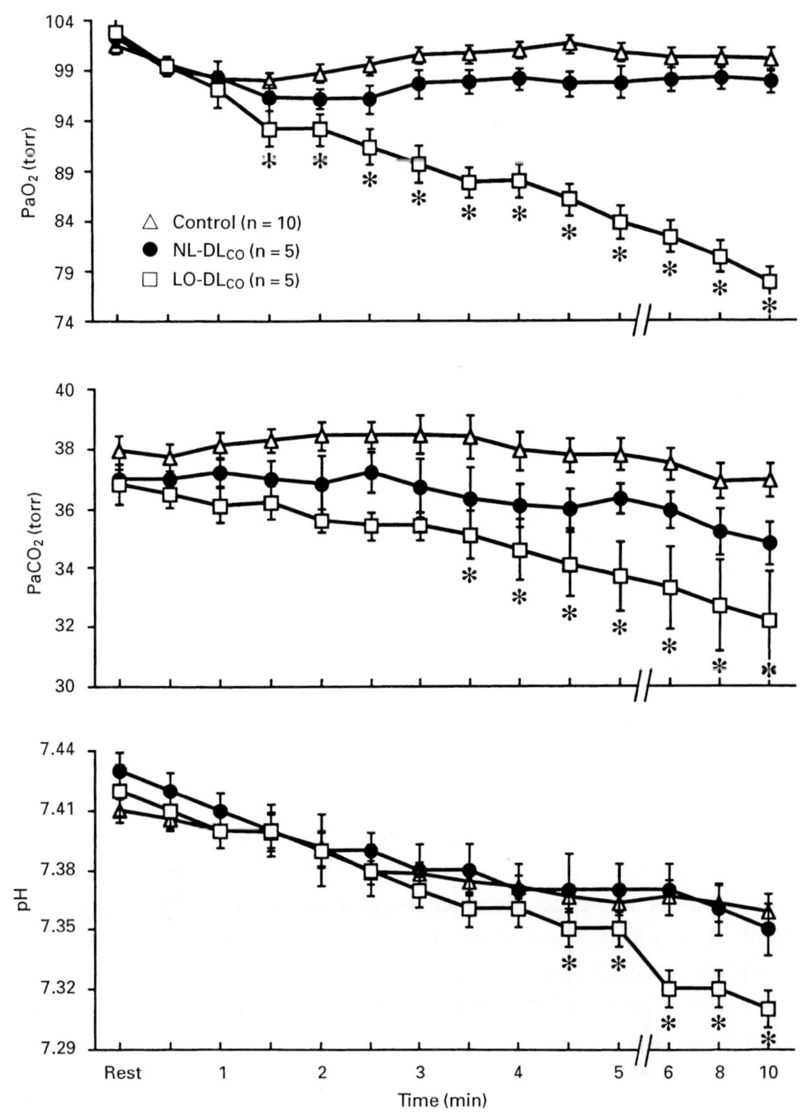

Fig. 7. Temporal pattern of arterial oxygen pressure (PaO_2), arterial carbon dioxide pressure ($PaCO_2$) and pH during 10 min of constant load cycle exercise at 70% of peak power output in patients with normal (NL-DL_{CO}) and very low (LO-DL_{CO}) pulmonary diffusion capacity and in normal age-matched control subjects. Values are expressed as mean value ± SEM. * $p < 0.05$ LO-DL_{CO} vs. control group and NL-DL_{CO} during exercise. Reprinted with permission from the American College of Cardiology [45].

fibers (66%) in CHF patients before transplantation. At 3 and 12 months after transplantation, both glycolytic and oxidative enzyme activity were increased. Surprisingly, however, no significant changes in fiber type were observed despite the significant changes in enzyme activity. Stratton et al. [30] used a cross-sectional design and ^{31}P-NMR spectroscopy to assess metabolism in the forearm flexor digitorum superficialis muscle of subjects before transplantation, and <6 or >6 months after transplantation. P_{Cr} depletion remained elevated and P_{Cr} resynthesis rate remained diminished in HTR studied late after transplantation (mean 15 months), indicating a sustained emphasis on anaerobic bioenergetic pathways. Additionally, capillary density and capillary/fiber ratio in skeletal muscle remain significantly reduced below age-matched norms (24 and 27%, respectively) in HTR late after transplantation [51, 52].

One important limitation of muscle metabolism studies to date is that they were conducted with untrained HTR and the patients were studied relatively early after transplantation. Thus, it is not known if a long-term program of endurance and/or resistance exercise training can normalize skeletal muscle metabolic responses to exercise and this remains a fertile area for future research.

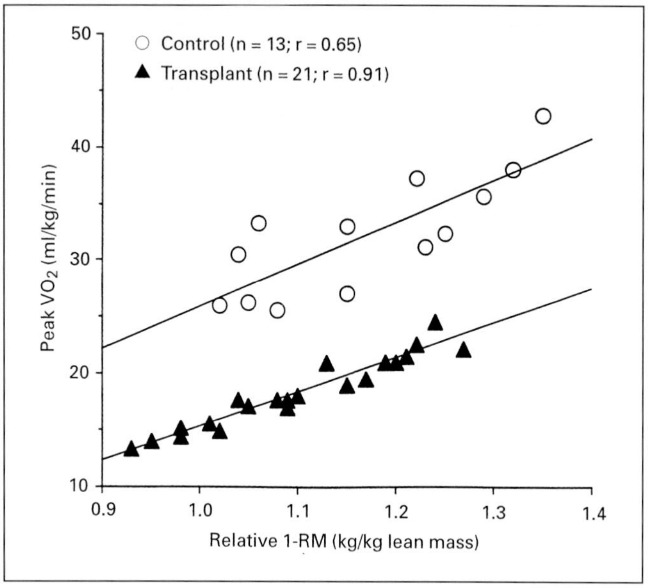

Fig. 8. The relationship between one repetition maximum (1-RM) strength of the knee extensors, corrected for lean body mass, and peak oxygen consumption (Peak VO_2) in heart transplant recipients and age-matched normal control subjects. Reprinted from Braith et al. [53], with permission from Elsevier Science.

Skeletal Muscle Strength. Muscle strength is an important determinant of exercise capacity in HTR. In fact, muscle weakness may preclude objective measurement of VO_2peak in HTR because treadmill and cycle testing devices place considerable demands on leg strength. HTR studied at the University of Florida consistently exhibit 1-RM knee extension strength values (normalized for lean body mass) that are only 60–70% of values achieved by age-matched sedentary control subjects [53]. The Florida group has shown that knee-extension strength is highly correlated with VO_2peak in HTR ($r = 0.90$) but not in age-matched control subjects ($r = 0.65$) (fig. 8). These data argue that steroid-induced weakness of leg muscles in HTR may be a primary factor limiting optimal performance of the transplanted heart. It is reasonable to speculate that training-induced improvements in peak HR, VO_2peak and treadmill time to exhaustion in HTR are a function of increased leg strength.

Resistance Exercise as Therapy for Skeletal Muscle Myopathy. Braith et al. [54] were the first to study the efficacy of progressive resistance training as a therapy to prevent the catabolic effects of glucocorticoids on skeletal muscle in HTR. The 6-month training regimen consisted of two components: (1) lumbar extensor training 1 day/week on a MedX (MedX Corp., Ocala, Fla., USA) lumbar extension machine, and (2) upper and lower body resistance training 2 days/week using MedX variable resistance machines. A single set consisting of 10–15 repetitions was completed for each exercise. The initial training weight represented 50% of one repetition maximum (1-RM). When 15 repetitions were successfully achieved, the weight was increased by 5–10% at the next training session. Fat-free mass decreased significantly and fat mass increased dramatically within only 2 months after transplantation, while total body mass remained unchanged (fig. 9). Fat-free mass in the resistance training group was

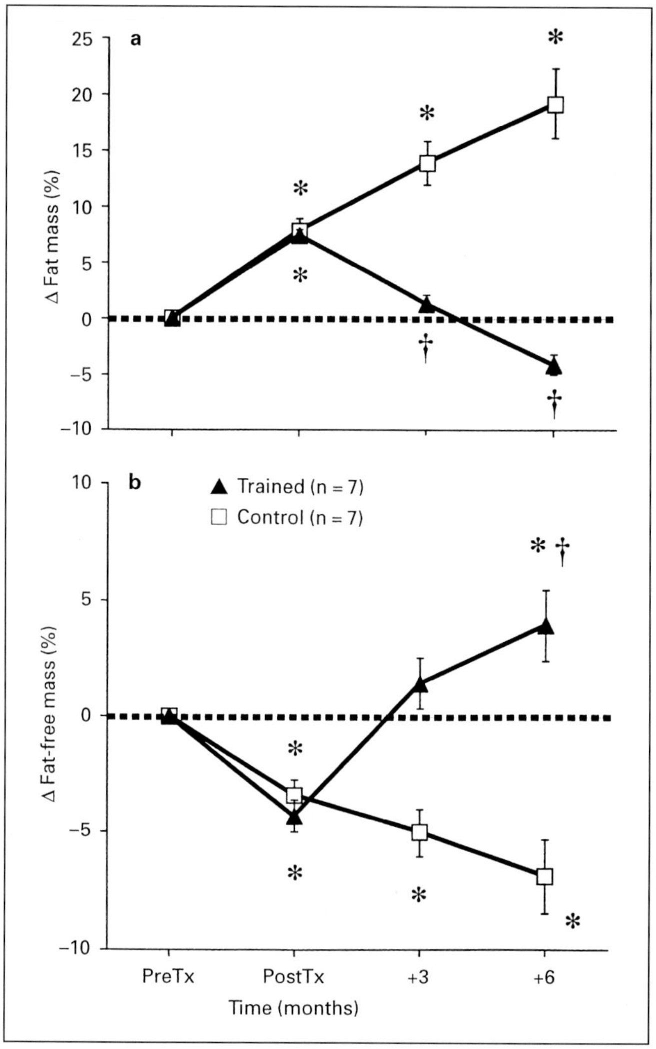

Fig. 9. Changes in fat mass (**a**) and fat-free mass (**b**) at 2 months after heart transplantation, and after 3 and 6 months of a resistance exercise program or control period. Data are mean value ± SEM. * $p < 0.05$ vs. pretransplantation (PreTx) value. † $p < 0.05$ trained group vs. control group. Adapted with permission from Braith et al. [54].

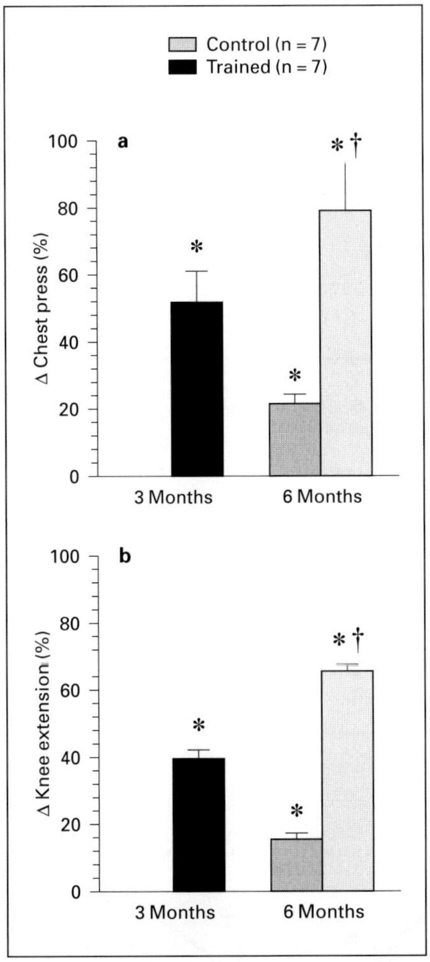

Fig. 10. Changes in chest press strength (**a**) and bilateral knee extension strength (**b**) after 3 and 6 months of a resistance exercise program or control period. Data are mean ± SEM. Controls did not train and were not tested at 3 months; * $p < 0.05$ vs. post-transplantation baseline value. † $p < 0.05$ trained group vs. control group. Adapted with permission from Braith et al. [54].

restored to pre-transplantation levels after 3 months of exercise and was increased to levels significantly greater than the pre-transplantation baseline after 6 months. When expressed in absolute terms, the control group lost 4 kg of fat-free mass (group mean) and gained 5.5 kg of fat mass. The resistance trained group increased fat-free mass (+2.2 kg; group mean) and reduced fat mass (–1.1 kg) during the study. Resistance exercise training also prevented steroid-induced deterioration of skeletal muscle strength. Improvements in muscle strength were observed in the control group but the magnitude of improvement in the training group was 4- to 6-fold greater than in the control group (fig. 10).

Peripheral Circulation. Cardiac transplantation does not immediately restore peripheral vasodilatory capacity. Endothelium-independent vasodilation (response to NO donors), but not endothelium-dependent vasodilation (response to acetylcholine or hyperemia), is well preserved in HTR, indicating that reduced vasodilatory capacity results from a defect in NO synthesis or availability rather than a defect in vascular smooth muscle [55]. Cyclosporine-induced endothelial damage is implicated as a causal mechanism for inadequate NO production and availability [56]. Cyclosporine also alters the balance of vasoactive substances by stimulating an increase in production of endothelin, a potent vasoconstrictor [56]. Exercise training improves endothelial function in CHF but it is not known if the same training benefits are possible in HTR immunosuppressed with cyclosporine.

Glucocorticoid-Induced Osteoporosis. Osteoporosis, defined by the World Health Organization as bone mineral density (BMD) that is 2.5 SD below predicted, is a frequent complication of chronic glucocorticoid therapy and exercise rehabilitation of HTR requires an understanding of the challenges conferred by abnormal bone metabolism. Trabecular or cancellous bone of the axial skeleton is lost more rapidly than cortical bone from the long bones of the appendicular skeleton. The lumbar vertebrae (trabecular bone) are particularly susceptible to osteoporosis, with bone losses of 10–20% observed as early as 2 months after transplantation. Bone loss from the femoral neck is also dramatic, ranging from 20 to 40% below age-matched norms. In contrast, total-body bone mineral loss is approximately 2–3% at 2 months post-transplant [57]. In HTR, there is radiologic evidence of long-bone fractures in up to 44% of patients early in the postoperative period [58]. More important clinically is the alarming prevalence (35%) of osteoporotic compression fractures in the lumbar vertebra in HTR [59].

Resistance Exercise as Therapy for Osteoporosis. Braith et al. [57] conducted the first controlled study to determine the efficacy of resistance exercise training as a therapy for defective bone metabolism in HTR. Eighteen HTR were randomly assigned to a training group or a nontraining control group. The 6-month training protocol was initiated at 2 months after transplantation and consisted of two components: (1) lumbar exercise 1 day/week on a MedX lumbar extension machine, and (2) upper and lower body training 2 days/week using MedX variable resistance machines. Subjects used the greatest resistance possible to complete a single set consisting of 10–15 repetitions for each exercise. The last repetition was considered volitional failure. The specific resistance exercises

Table 2. Order of exercises in the resistance training regimen used to prevent steroid-induced osteoporosis and skeletal muscle myopathy in heart transplant recipients

1	Lumbar extension
2	Chest press
3	Knee extension
4	Pullover
5	Tricep dip
6	Bicep curl
7	Shoulder press
8	Leg press

are outlined in table 2. BMD losses in the lumbar vertebra were 12.2 and 14.9% in the control and training groups, respectively, at only 2 months after transplantation (fig. 11). The main finding was that a 6-month program of specific variable resistance exercises was osteogenic and restored BMD toward pretransplantation levels.

Summary of Adaptations to Exercise Training. Resistance exercise training appears to be a safe modality for HTR and is an effective countermeasure for steroid-induced osteoporosis and skeletal muscle myopathy when introduced early in the post-transplantation period. Endurance exercise training also elicits a beneficial evolution of HR responsiveness during physical activity and significant increases in peak HR. These benefits are not seen in HTR who do not participate in exercise training. However, the mechanism(s) responsible for improved peak HR, VO_2peak and total exercise time are not completely understood. There is evidence that metabolic and strength adaptations in skeletal muscle confers a 'permissive' effect, allowing the transplanted human heart to approach optimal levels of function. Thus, increased exercise tolerance in HTR may be related to skeletal muscle strength and aerobic capacity rather than central adaptations or intrinsic cardiac mechanisms.

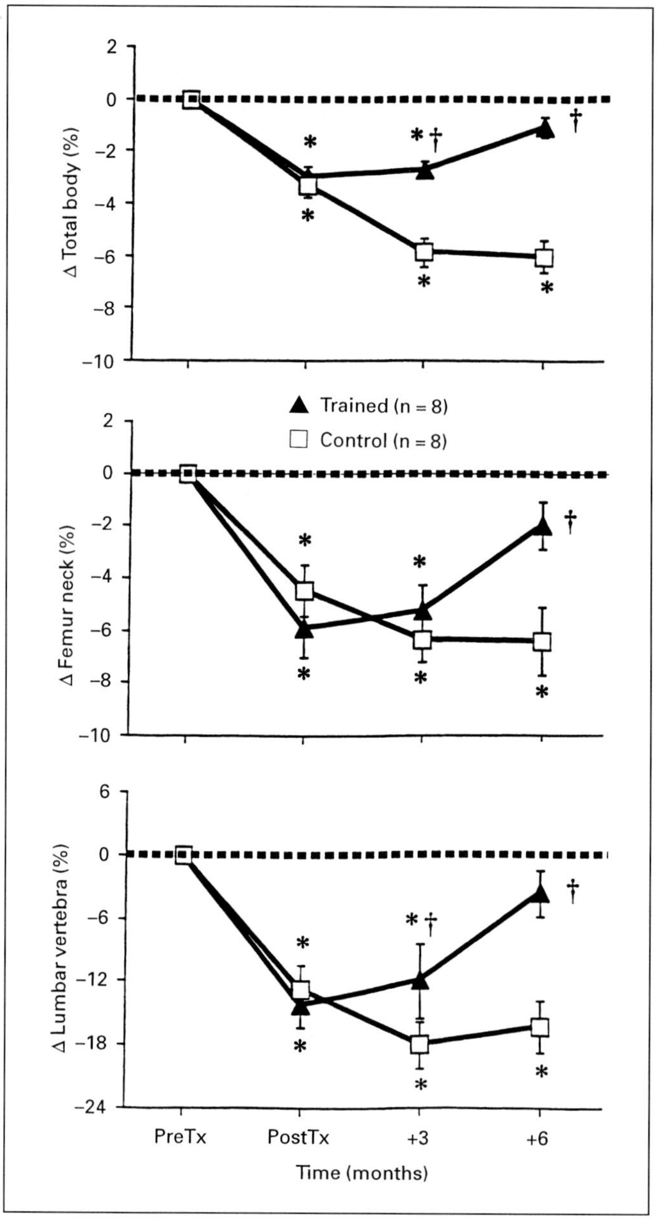

Fig. 11. Changes in bone mineral density of the total body, femur neck, and lumbar vertebra at 2 months after heart transplantation (PostTx) and after 3 and 6 months of a resistance exercise program or a control period. Data are mean value ± SEM. * $p < 0.05$ vs. pretransplantation (PreTx) value. † $p < 0.05$ trained group vs. control group. Reprinted with permission from the American College of Cardiology [57].

Designing an Exercise Program for Heart Transplant Recipients

Outpatient aerobic exercise training programs can often begin as early as the third postoperative week. Modalities for aerobic exercise can include walking, cycling, stair-stepping, arm ergometry and calisthenics. Resistance training programs should not be initiated until 6–8 weeks after transplantation, thereby permitting time for sternum healing and glucocorticoid taper. Furthermore, training should be discontinued during acute allograft rejection that requires enhanced glucocorticoid immunosuppression. The possibility of a coronary event is heightened during a rejection episode that requires bolus administration of glucocorticoids and the catabolic influence of the glucocorticoids on bone and skeletal muscle supersedes the beneficial effects of exercise.

Initial Exercise Intensity and Progression. Traditional exercise prescription, which is dependent upon HR responses to determine exercise intensity, are not applicable in some cardiac denervated HTR. Alternative methods to prescribe exercise intensity have proven to be adequate. Utilizing RPE of 12–14, corresponding to 60–80% of target HR, improves VO_2peak by 29% in 10 weeks [60]. Moreover, RPE of 12–14 accurately reflects the ventilatory threshold in HTR [61]. Thus, setting initial exercise intensity at slightly below an RPE of 12–14 establishes an entry level of work rate. RPE can subsequently be used to 'fine tune' further adjustments and progressions in the intensity of exercise.

Exercise Safety Precautions. Safety problems typically encountered with CAD patients in cardiac rehabilitation programs are associated with cardiac work and myocardial ischemia. In contrast, HTR are not limited by coronary underperfusion, provided they are free from acute rejection or allograft vascular disease. Rather, the rehabilitation staff must take special precautions to ensure adequate maintenance of systemic blood pressure. Approximately 25% of HTR experience transient hypotension during resistance exercise and this problem is exaggerated when the exercise requires lifting above the level of the heart (e.g. shoulder press). This hemodynamic problem is likely a consequence of autonomic sympathetic denervation. The denervated transplanted heart is almost entirely dependent upon preload and the 'Frank-Starling' mechanism for defending cardiac output and systemic blood pressure. The following maneuvers help sustain venous return and prevent blood pooling in patients who experienced hypotension: (1) Upper body exercises alternated with lower body exercises. (2) Symptomatic subjects walk 2 min between exercises or performed standing calf raises. (3) Conclude each resistance training session with a 5-min cool-down walk at low intensity on the treadmill.

Subjects with BMD deficits greater than 2 standard deviations from age-matched norms after transplantation are at great risk for fractures and resistance training may be contraindicated. HTR participating in resistance exercise programs must be carefully managed with conservative initial resistances and very gradual progressions in resistance loads.

Conclusion

The era of exercise training as a treatment for CHF has begun. In the decade following the pioneering work from Duke University there has been a profusion of small predominantly single-center studies and a litany of impressive physiological benefits that can be achieved. There is growing clinical consensus that stable, compensated CHF patients who engage in exercise training 'do better' through reduction in secondary peripheral manifestations of CHF syndrome. Moreover, there is recent exciting evidence that exercise training may actually alter the clinical course of CHF. Much remains to be done, however, and many unanswered questions remain. For example, it is not know whether training effects in CHF patients can be maintained over the long term and it is not clearly established whether training is feasible outside of specialized research and clinical environments.

During the past two decades, heart transplantation has evolved from a rarely performed experimental procedure to an accepted life extending therapy for end-stage heart failure patients. However, with dramatic improvements in organ preservation, surgery and immunosuppressive drug management, short-term survival is no longer the pivotal issue for most HTR. Rather, a return to functional lifestyle with good quality of life is now the desired procedural outcome. To achieve this outcome, aggressive exercise rehabilitation is essential.

References

1 Mancini DM, Eisen H, Kussmaul W, Mull R, Edmunds LH, Wilson JR: Value of peak exercise oxygen consumption for optimal timing of cardiac transplantation in ambulatory patients with heart failure. Circulation 1991;83:778–786.

2 Belardinelli R, Georgiou D, Cianci G, Berman N, Ginzton L, Purcaro A: Exercise training improves left ventricular diastolic filling in patients with dilated cardiomyopathy: Clinical and prognostic implications. Circulation 1995; 91:2775–2784.

3 Braith RW, Welsch MA, Feigenbaum MS, Kleuss HA, Pepine CJ: Neurohormone activation in heart failure is modified by endurance exercise. J Am Coll Cardiol 1999;34:1170–1175.

4 Cohn JN, Levine TB, Olivari MT, Garberg V, Lura D, Francis GS, Simon AB, Rector T: Plasma norepinephrine as a guide to prognosis in patients with chronic congestive heart failure. N Engl J Med 1984;311:819–823.

5 Tan LB, Jalil JE, Pick R, Janicki JS, Weber KT: Cardiac myocyte necrosis induced by angiotensin II. Circ Res 1991;69:1185–1195.

6 Weber KT: Extracellular matrix remodeling in heart failure: A role for de novo angiotensin II generation. Circulation 1997;96:4065–4082.

7 Grassi G, Cattaneo BM, Servavalle G, Lanfranchi A, Pozzi M, Morganti A, Carugo S, Mancia G: Effects of chronic ACE inhibition on sympathetic nerve traffic and baroreflex control of the circulation. Circulation 1997;96: 1173–1179.

8 The CONSENSUS Trail Study Group: Effects of enalapril on mortality in severe congestive heart failure: Results of the Cooperative North Scandinavian Enalapril Survival Study (CONSENSUS). N Engl J Med 1987;316:1429–1435.
9 The SOLVD Investigators: Effect of enalapril on survival in patients with reduced left ventricular ejection fraction and congestive heart failure. N Engl J Med 1991;325:293–302.
10 Hornig B, Maier V, Drexler H: Physical training improves endothelial function in patients with chronic heart failure. Circulation 1996;93: 210–214.
11 Drexler H: Endothelial dysfunction: Clinical implications. Prog Cardiovasc Dis 1997;39: 287–324.
12 Drexler H, Reide U, Munzel T, Konig H, Funke E, Just H: Alterations of skeletal muscle in chronic heart failure. Circulation 1992;85: 1751–1759.
13 Clark AL, Poole-Wilson PA, Coats AJ: Exercise limitation in chronic heart failure: Central role of the periphery. J Am Coll Cardiol 1996;28: 1092–1102.
14 Kluess HA, Welsch MA, Properzio AM, et al: Accelerated skeletal muscle metabolic recovery following exercise training in heart failure. Circulation 1996;94:I–192.
15 Vescovo G, Serafini F, Dalla Libera L, Leprotti C, Facchin L, Tenderini P, Ambrosio GB: Skeletal muscle myosin heavy chain composition in CHF: Correlation between the magnitude of the isoenzymatic shift, exercise capacity, and gas exchange measurements. Am Heart J 1998; 135:130–137.
16 Sullivan MJ, Higginbotham MB, Cobb FR: Exercise training in patients with chronic heart failure delays ventilatory anaerobic threshold and improves submaximal exercise performance. Circulation 1989;79:324–329.
17 Mancini DM, Henson D, LaManca J, Levine S: Respiratory muscle function and dyspnea in patients with chronic congestive heart failure. Circulation 1992;86:909–918.
18 Sullivan MJ, Higginbotham MB, Cobb FR: Exercise training in patients with severe left ventricular dysfunction: Hemodynamic and metabolic effects. Circulation 1988;78:506–515.
19 Gaudron P, Hu K, Schamberger R, Budin M, Walter B, Ertl G: Effect of endurance training early or late after coronary artery occlusion on left ventricular remodeling, hemodynamics and survival in rats with chronic transmural myocardial infarction. Circulation 1994;89: 402–412.
20 Jugdutt BI, Michorowski BL, Kappagoda CT: Exercise training after anterior Q wave myocardial infarction: Importance of regional left ventricular function and topography. J Am Coll Cardiol 1988;12:362–372.
21 Giannuzzi P, Tavazzi L, Temporelli PL, Corra U, Imparato A, Gattone M, Giordano A, Sala L, Schweiger C, Malinverni C: Long-term physical training and left ventricular remodeling after anterior myocardial infarction: Results of the Exercise in Anterior Myocardial Infarction (EAMI) trial. J Am Coll Cardiol 1993;22:1821–1829.
22 Jette M, Heller R, Landry F, Blumchen G: Randomized 4-week program in patients with impaired left ventricular function. Circulation 1991;84:1561–1567.
23 Dubach P, Myers J, Dziekan G, Goebbels U, Reinhart W, Vogt P, Ratti R, Muller P, Miettunen R, Buser P: Effect of exercise training on myocardial remodeling in patients with reduced left ventricular function after myocardial infarction. Circulation 1997;95:2060–2067.
24 La Rovere MT, Mortara A, Specchia G, Specchia G, Schwartz PJ: Myocardial infarction and baroreflex sensitivity: Clinical studies. J Ital Cardiol 1992;22:639–645.
25 Kaye DM, Lambert GW, Lefkovits J, Morris M, Jennings G, Esler MD: Neurochemical evidence of cardiac sympathetic activation and increased central nervous system norepinephrine turnover in severe congestive heart failure. J Am Coll Cardiol 1994;23:570–578.
26 Hambrecht R, Fiehn E, Weigle C, Gielen S, Hamann C, Kaiser R, Yu J, Adams V, Niebauer J, Schuler G: Regular physical exercise corrects endothelial dysfunction and improves exercise capacity in patients with chronic heart failure. Circulation 1998;98:2709–2715.
27 Linke A, Schoene N, Gielen S, Hofer J, Erbs S, Schuler G, Hambrecht R: Endothelial dysfunction in patients with chronic heart failure: Systemic effects of lower-limb exercise training. J Am Coll Cardiol 2001;37:392–397.
28 Smith C, Sun D, Hoegler C, Zhang X, Zhao G, Xu XB, Kobari Y, Pritchard K Jr, Sessa WC, Hintze TH: Reduced gene expression of vascular endothelial NO synthase and cyclooxygenase-1 in heart failure. Circ Res 1996;78:58–64.
29 Rieder M, Carmona R, Krieger J, Pritchard KA Jr, Greene AS: Suppression of angiotensin-converting-enzyme expression and activity by shear stress. Circ Res 1997;80:312–319.
30 Stratton J, Dunn J, Adamopoulos S, Kemp G, Coats A, Rajagopalan B: Training partially reverses skeletal muscle metabolic abnormalities during exercise in heart failure. J Appl Physiol 1994;76:1575–1582.
31 Belardinelli R, Georgiou D, Cianci G, Purcaro A: Randomized, controlled trial of long-term moderate exercise training in chronic heart failure: Effects on functional capacity, quality of life and clinical outcome. Circulation 1999;99: 1173–1182.
32 ACSM Guidelines for Exercise Testing and Prescription, ed 5. Baltimore, Williams & Wilkins, 1995.
33 Braith RW, Mills RM: Exercise training in patients with congestive heart failure: How to achieve benefits safely. Postgrad Med 1996;96: 119–130.
34 Kao AC, Vantrigt P, Shaeffer-Mccall GS, Shaw JP, Kuzil BB, Page RD, Higginbotham MB: Allograft diastolic dysfunction and chronotropic incompetence limit cardiac output response to exercise two to six years after heart transplantation. J Heart Lung Transplant 1995;14: 11–22.
35 Mercier J, Ville N, Wintrebert P, Caillaud C, Varray A, Albat B, Thevenet A, Prefaut C: Influence of post-surgery time after cardiac transplantation on exercise responses. Med Sci Sports Exerc 1996;28:171–175.
36 Givertz MM, Hartley LH, Colucci WS: Long-term sequential changes in exercise capacity and chronotropic responsiveness after cardiac transplantation. Circulation 1997;96:232–237.
37 Mandak J, Aaronson K, Mancini D: Serial assessment of exercise capacity after heart transplantation. J Heart Lung Transplant 1995;14:468–478.
38 Richard R, Verdier JC, Duvallet A, Rosier SP, Leger P, Nignan A, Rieu M: Chronotropic competence in endurance trained heart transplant recipients: Heart rate is not a limiting factor for exercise capacity. J Am Coll Cardiol 1999;33:192–197.
39 Braith RW, Clapp L, Brown T, Brown C, Schofield R, Mills RM, Hill JA: Rate-responsive pacing improves exercise tolerance in heart transplant recipients. J Cardiopulm Rehabil 2000;20:377–382.
40 Leenen FH, Davies RA, Fourney A: Role of cardiac β_2-receptors in cardiac responses to exercise in cardiac transplant patients. Circulation 1995;91:685–690.
41 Kavanagh T, Yacoub M, Mertens D, Kennedy J, Campbell RB, Sawyer P: Cardiorespiratory responses to exercise training after orthotopic cardiac transplantation. Circulation 1988;77: 162–171.
42 Braith RW, Plunkett MB, Mills RM: Cardiac output responses during exercise in volume-expanded heart transplant recipients. Am J Cardiol 1998;81:1–5.
43 Geny B, Saini J, Mettauer B, Piquard F, Follenius M, Epailly E, Schnedecker B, Eisenmann B, Haberey P, Lonsdorfer J: Effect of short-term endurance training on exercise capacity, hemodynamics and atrial natriuretic peptide secretion in heart transplant recipients. Eur J Appl Physiol 1996;73:259–266.
44 Braith RW, Mills RM, Wilcox CS, Convertino VA, Davis GL, Limacher MC, Wood CE: Fluid homeostasis after heart transplantation: The role of cardiac denervation. J Heart Lung Transplant 1996;15:872–880.
45 Braith RW, Limacher MC, Mills RM, Leggett SH, Pollock ML, Staples ED: Exercise-induced hypoxemia in heart transplant recipients. J Am Coll Cardiol 1993;22:768–776.
46 Ville N, Mercier J, Varray A, Albat B, Messner-Pellenc P, Prefaut C: Exercise tolerance in heart transplant patients with altered pulmonary diffusion capacity. Med Sci Sports Exerc 1998;30:339–344.
47 Egan JJ, Kalra S, Yonan N, Hasleton P, Brooks N, Woodcock A: Pulmonary diffusion abnormalities in heart transplant recipients. Chest 1993;104:1085–1089.
48 Ohar J, Osterloh J, Ahmed N, Miller L: Diffusing capacity decreases after heart transplantation. Chest 1993;103:857–861.
49 Squires RW, Hoffman CJ, James GA, et al: Arterial oxygen saturation during graded exercise testing after cardiac transplantation. J Cardiopulm Rehabil 1998;18:348.

50 Bussieres LM, Pflugfelder PW, Taylor AW, Noble EG, Kostuk WJ: Changes in skeletal muscle morphology and biochemistry after cardiac transplantation. Am J Cardiol 1997;79: 630–634.

51 Biring M, Fournier M, Ross D, Lewis MI: Cellular adaptations of skeletal muscle to cyclosporine. J Appl Physiol 1998;84:1967–1975.

52 Lampert E, Oyono-Enguelld S, Mettauer B, Freund H, Lonsdorfer J: Short endurance training improves lactate removal in patients with heart transplants. Med Sci Sports Exerc 1996;28:801–807.

53 Braith RW, Limacher MC, Leggett SH, Pollock ML: Skeletal muscle strength in heart transplant recipients. J Heart Lung Transplant 1993;12:1018–1023.

54 Braith RW, Welsch MA, Mills RM, Keller JW, Pollock ML: Resistance exercise prevents glucocorticoid-induced myopathy in heart transplant recipients. Med Sci Sports Exerc 1998;30: 483–489.

55 Andreassen AK, Gullestad L, Holm T, Simonsen S, Kvernebo K: Endothelium-dependent vasodilation of the skin microcirculation in heart transplant recipients. Clin Transplant 1998;12:324–332.

56 Gonzales-Santiago L, Lopez-Ongil S, Lamas S, Quereda C, Rodriguez-Puyol M, Rodriguez-Puyol D: Imbalance in endothelial vasoactive factors as a possible cause of cyclosporine toxicity: A role for endothelin-converting-enzyme. J Lab Clin Med 2000;136:395–401.

57 Braith RW, Mills RM, Welsch MA, Keller JW, Pollock ML: Resistance exercise training restores bone mineral density in heart transplant recipients. J Am Coll Cardiol 1996;28:1471–1477.

58 Rich GM, Mudge GH, Laffel GL, LeBoff MS: Cyclosporine A and prednisone associated osteoporosis in heart transplant recipients. J Heart and Lung Transplant 1992;11:950–958.

59 Shane E, Rivas MD, Silvergerg SJ, Kim TS, Staron RB, Bilezikian JP: Osteoporosis after cardiac transplantation. Am J Med 1993;94: 257–264.

60 Keteyian S, Shepard R, Ehrman J, Fedel F, Glick K, Rhoads K, Levine B: Cardiovascular responses of heart transplant patients to exercise training. J Appl Physiol 1991;70:2627–2631.

61 Brubaker P, Berry MJ, Brozena SC, Morley DL, Walter JD, Paolone AM, Bove AA: Relationship of lactate and ventilatory thresholds in cardiac transplant patients. Med Sci Sport Exerc 1993;25:191–196.

Randy W. Braith, PhD
Center for Exercise Science
College of Health and Human Performance
College of Medicine, University of Florida
PO Box 118206, Gainesville, FL 32611 (USA)
Tel. +1 352 392 9575/ext 1340
Fax +1 352 392 0316
E-Mail rbraith@hhp.ufl.edu

Weisman IM, Zeballos RJ (eds): Clinical Exercise Testing.
Prog Respir Res. Basel, Karger, 2002, vol 32, pp 138–158

Exercise Limitation and Clinical Exercise Testing in Chronic Obstructive Pulmonary Disease

Denis E. O'Donnell

Division of Respiratory and Critical Care Medicine, Department of Medicine, Queen's University, Kingston, Ont., Canada

Summary

Exercise intolerance in patients with chronic obstructive pulmonary disease (COPD) is the result of a complex interaction of factors that include ventilatory constraints, skeletal muscle dysfunction, and the distressing exertional symptoms of dyspnea and leg discomfort. Cardiopulmonary exercise testing can be used to uncover the various pathophysiological contributions to exercise intolerance, on an individual basis. Recent advances in the assessment of ventilatory constraints by quantitative flow-volume loop analysis during excercise and the measurement of exertional symptoms using validated scales, now permit a more rigorous evaluation of physiological impairment and disability. In severe COPD, ventilatory factors are often predominant. Thus, interventions that increase ventilatory capacity (i.e., bronchodilators) or that reduce ventilatory demand (i.e., exercise training and oxygen therapy) have been shown to improve exercise endurance. Additionally, pharmacological and surgical interventions that reduce dynamic lung overdistention during exercise effectively alleviate exertional dyspnea. Skeletal muscle weakness and deconditioning have been shown to respond favorably to targeted training. Comprehensive management strategies that incorporate pharmacological therapies and supervised exercise training can minimize exercise capabilities, and thus the health status of patients with advanced symptomatic disease.

Introduction

The inability to engage in the usual activities of daily living is one of the most distressing experiences of people afflicted with COPD. Exercise intolerance progresses relentlessly as the disease advances and can lead to virtual immobility and social isolation. Our understanding of the complex interface between physiological impairment and disability in COPD has increased considerably in recent years and is the main focus of this review. It has become clear that in COPD, exercise intolerance ultimately reflects integrated abnormalities of the ventilatory, cardiovascular, peripheral muscle, and neurosensory systems. Ventilatory limitation is the dominant contributor to exercise curtailment in more advanced disease and will be considered in detail. Important advances have been made in our ability to 'noninvasively' assess dynamic ventilatory mechanics in COPD during exercise and will be highlighted in this review. The derangements of ventilatory mechanics peculiar to this disease will be reviewed so as to better understand how these can be therapeutically manipulated to improve exercise performance. Recent important research into the role of peripheral muscle dysfunction in exercise limitation will be reviewed, as well as emerging concepts on the pathophysiology of cardiopulmonary-locomotor muscle interactions in COPD.

Exercise Limitation in COPD

Exercise limitation is multifactorial in COPD. Recognized contributing factors include: (1) ventilatory limitation due to impaired respiratory system mechanics and ventilatory muscle dysfunction; (2) metabolic and gas exchange abnormalities; (3) peripheral muscle dysfunction; (4) cardiac impairment; (5) intolerable exertional symptoms, and (6) any combination of these interdependent factors. The predominant contributing factors to exercise limitation vary among patients with COPD or, indeed, in a given patient over time. The more advanced the disease, the more of these factors come into play in a complex integrative manner.

Table 1. Typical abnormalities during exercise in COPD

Significant dyspnea and leg discomfort
Reduced peak VO_2 and work rate
Low maximal heart rate
Elevated submaximal ventilation
Low peak ventilation
High ratio of ventilation to maximal ventilatory capacity (V_E/MVC)
Blunted V_T response to exercise, with increased breathing frequency
High deadspace (V_D/V_T)
Variable arterial oxygen desaturation
$PaCO_2$ usually normal but may increase
Reduced dynamic IC with exercise (i.e., dynamic hyperinflation)
Reduced IRV at low work rates
High V_T/IC ratios at low work rates

Cardiopulmonary Exercise Testing (CPET) in COPD

CPET, using an incremental cycle ergometry protocol, has traditionally been used to evaluate exercise performance in COPD. Standard CPET measures the following physiological responses: metabolic load [oxygen uptake (VO_2) and carbon dioxide output (VCO_2)], power output, ventilation (V_E), breathing pattern, arterial oxygen saturation, heart rate, electrocardiogram, oxygen pulse, and blood pressure. Increasingly, exertional symptom assessment using validated scales (i.e. Borg and visual analogue scales) is being used during CPET and this constitutes an important advance [1, 2]. Common physiological responses to incremental cycle exercise in COPD are now well established (table 1). These patterns, however, are not specific for COPD: for example, similar patterns are observed in interstitial lung disease and pulmonary vascular disease. Thus, traditional CPET protocols do not allow diagnostic discrimination between various pulmonary conditions. However, conventional CPET has the potential to yield important clinical information on an individual basis: (1) it provides an accurate assessment of the patient's exercise capacity that cannot be predicted from resting physiological measurements; (2) it measures the perceptual responses to quantifiable physiological stimuli (i.e. VO_2, ventilation and power output); (3) it can provide insight into the pathophysiological mechanisms of exercise intolerance and dyspnea in a given patient (e.g. excessive ventilatory demand, arterial oxygen desaturation), and (4) it can identify other co-existent conditions that contribute to exercise limitation (i.e. cardiac disorders, intermittent claudication, musculoskeletal problems, etc.). The results of CPET can also assist in developing individualized exercise training protocols and sequential CPET can be used to evaluate the impact of therapeutic interventions in patients with COPD. One shortcoming of traditional CPET is that it gives little or no information about the prevailing dynamic ventilatory mechanics during exercise. This information is arguably important in the assessment of mechanisms of exercise intolerance in a given patient. In this regard, exercise flow-volume loops can provide a noninvasive assessment of dynamic mechanics, and allow greater refinement in the evaluation of the ventilatory constraints to exercise (see below) [3, 4] (fig. 1).

Serial IC measurements have been used to track end-expiratory lung volume (EELV) during exercise for more than 30 years [4–8] (fig. 1, 2). This approach is based on the reasonable assumption that TLC does not change appreciably during exercise in COPD, and that reductions in dynamic IC must, therefore, reflect increases in EELV or dynamic hyperinflation (DH) [6]. However, regardless of any possible changes in TLC with exercise, progressive reduction of an already diminished resting IC means that V_T becomes positioned closer to the actual TLC and the upper alinear extreme of the respiratory system's pressure-volume relationship, where there is increased elastic loading of the respiratory muscles (fig. 3). Reduction of IC as exercise progresses in COPD is likely a true reflection of shifts in EELV rather than simply the inability to generate maximal effort because of dyspnea or functional muscle weakness. In fact, several studies have established that dyspneic patients, even at the end of exhaustive exercise, are capable of generating maximal inspiratory efforts as assessed by peak inspiratory esophageal pressures [6, 8]. Moreover, we have recently shown that IC measurements during constant load cycle exercise are both highly reproducible and responsive in patients with severe COPD,

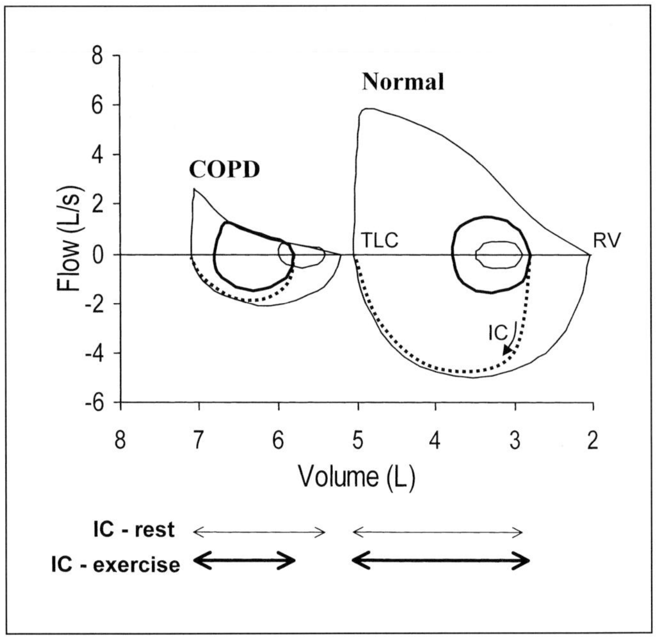

Fig. 1. In a normal healthy subject and in a typical patient with COPD, tidal flow-volume loops at rest and during exercise (peak exercise in COPD compared with exercise at a comparable metabolic load in the age-matched person) are shown in relation to their respective maximal flow-volume loops. In the COPD example, note expiratory flow limitation (tidal flows overlap the maximal curve) and an increase in end expiratory lung volume (EELV), as reflected by a decrease in IC during exercise. 'Minimal IRV' is the upper volume boundary that could be achieved during exercise.

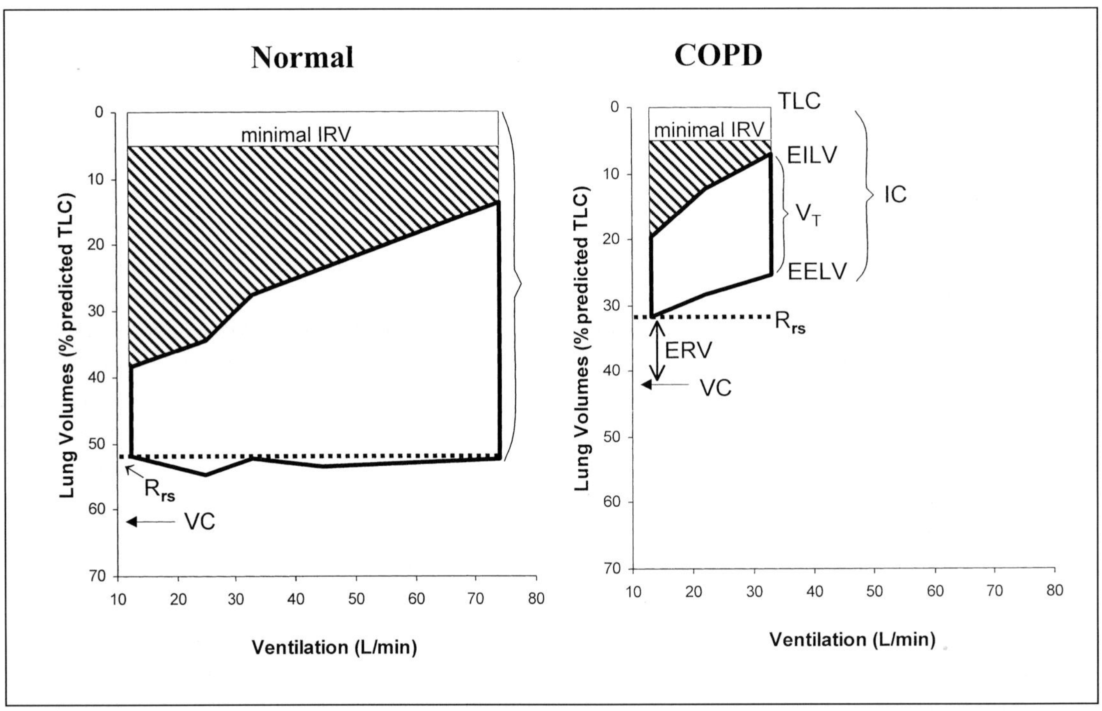

Fig. 2. Changes in operational lung volumes are shown as ventilation increases with exercise in COPD (n = 105) and in normal subjects (n = 25). 'Restrictive' constraints on tidal volume (V_T, solid area) expansion during exercise are significantly greater in the COPD group from both below (reduced IC) and above (minimal IRV, open area). R_{rs} = Relaxation volume of the respiratory system. From O'Donnell et al. [4] with permission.

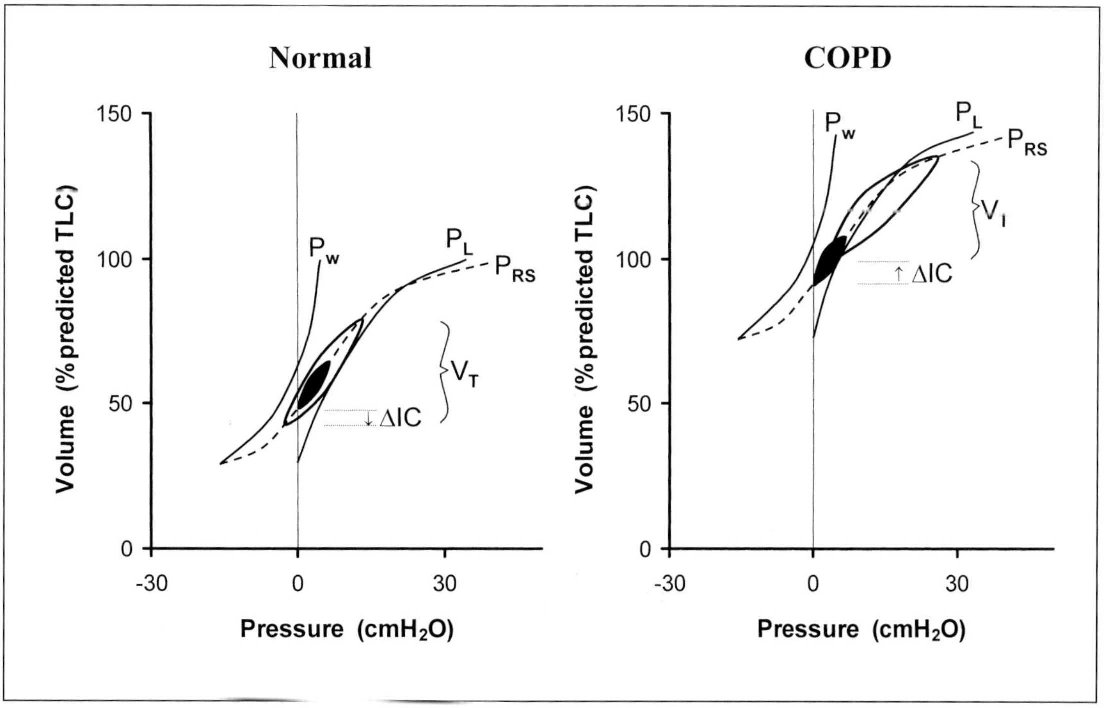

Fig. 3. Pressure-volume (P-V) relationships of the lung, chest wall, and total respiratory system in health and in COPD. Tidal pressure-volume curves during rest (filled area) and exercise (open area) are provided. Note that in COPD, because of resting and dynamic hyperinflation, V_T encroaches on the upper alinear extreme of the respiratory system's P-V curve where there is increased elastic loading.

provided due attention is taken with their measurement [12].

Changes in the dynamic volume components during exercise can be measured by a combination of serial IC and tidal volume measurements, and inspiratory lung volume (EILV) can be calculated by adding EELV to V_T (fig. 2). The operating lung volumes during exercise dictate the length-tension and the force-velocity characteristics of the ventilatory muscles, and influences breathing pattern and the quality and intensity of dyspnea (see below). Moreover, dynamic volume measurements give clear information about the extent of mechanical restriction during exercise in COPD (fig. 1, 2). Inspiratory reserve volume (IRV) during exercise, in particular, provides an indication of the existing constraints on V_T expansion. Similarly, the reserves of inspiratory flow can be evaluated by measuring the difference between tidal inspiratory flow rates and those generated at the same volume during a simultaneous maximal IC maneuver (fig. 1). In COPD, the pressure generating capacity of the inspiratory muscles and, thus, the ability to generate inspiratory flow, may be compromised when breathing at a high dynamic EELV compared with when a breath is initiated from RV at rest during the forced vital capacity (FVC) maneuver. Hence, maximal inspiratory flow rates during exercise IC maneuvers may be the more appropriate comparator to use when calculating inspiratory flow reserves than the FVC plot.

The crucial abnormality in COPD is expiratory flow limitation (EFL), and its presence during exercise can be evaluated by measuring the overlap of the tidal expiratory flow-volume curves with the maximal expiratory flow-volume curve [3, 13] (fig. 1). However, this assessment provides at best imprecise quantitative information about EFL. This 'overlap' method may become inaccurate because of errors in placement of the V_T curve on the absolute volume axis due to erroneous IC measurements. Additionally, in many incidences, tidal expiratory flow rates exceed those generated during the FVC maneuver. This occurs because of gas compression and airway compression effects, differences in volume history and in the uniformity of lung emptying during the maximal breath initiated from TLC compared with tidal breathing. Despite these reservations, it is clear that patients with more advanced COPD often have markedly reduced maximal expiratory flow rates at lower lung (operating) volumes and, therefore, show substantial overlap of the tidal and maximal curves. Expiratory flow limitation can reasonably be assumed to exist in this setting, particularly when there is attendant DH. In patients who demonstrate DH during exercise, tidal expiratory flow rates represent the maximal possible flows that can be generated at that volume.

The negative expiratory pressure test (NEP) has been developed by Milic-Emili and colleagues [14] in order to provide a more accurate determination of EFL. Under conditions of EFL, tidal expiratory flow rates are determined by the transpulmonary pressure and the resistance of the airways upstream from the flow-limiting segment, and are independent of downstream mouth pressure [13]. Therefore, negative pressure or suction (e.g. –5 to –12 cm H_2O) applied at the mouth does not increase expiratory flow rates apart from a brief transient increase at the onset of expiration, representing gas discharged from the upper airways (anatomical deadspace) [14–16]. By contrast in non-flow-limited patients, NEP results in consistent and substantial increases in tidal expiratory flow rates [14, 15]. The NEP test does not provide any quantitative information about the extent of EFL, merely whether or not it is present at rest. The absence of EFL at rest, as determined by the NEP test, certainly does not preclude the development of significant EFL and consequent DH at low exercise levels, particularly if ventilation is excessive.

Ventilatory Constraints on Exercise Performance in COPD

In patients with severe COPD, ventilatory limitation is often the predominant contributor to exercise intolerance. The patient is deemed to have ventilatory limitation if, at the breakpoint of exercise, he or she has reached estimated maximum ventilatory capacity (MVC), while at the same time cardiac and other physiological functions are operating below maximal capacity.

In practice, it is difficult to precisely determine if ventilatory limitation is the proximate boundary to exercise performance in a given individual. Attendant respiratory discomfort may limit exercise before actual physiological limitation occurs, and the relative importance of other nonventilatory factors is impossible to quantify with precision. Our assessment of the MVC, as estimated from resting spirometry (i.e. $FEV_{1.0} \times 35$ or 40) [17, 18] or from brief bursts of voluntary hyperventilation is inaccurate [3]. Prediction of the peak ventilation actually achieved during exercise from maximal voluntary ventilation at rest is problematic because the pattern of ventilatory muscle recruitment, the changes in intrathoracic pressures and in respired flows and volumes, and the extent of DH are often vastly different under the two conditions. While an increased ratio (i.e. >90%) of peak exercise ventilation (V_E) to the estimated MVC strongly suggests limiting ventilatory constraints, a preserved peak V_E/MVC ratio (i.e. <75% predicted) by no means excludes the possibility of significant ventilatory impairment during exercise [4]. Thus, simultaneous analysis of exercise flow-volume loops at the symptom-limited peak of exercise may show marked constraints on flow and volume generation in the presence of an apparently adequate ventilatory reserve as estimated from the peak V_E/MVC ratios [4]. In a recent study, 14% of a population sample of clinically stable patients with COPD (n = 105), with apparent ventilatory reserve at peak exercise (i.e. V_E/MVC <75% predicted) had coexisting limiting restrictive ventilatory constraints as indicated by an EILV >95% of the TLC (i.e. significantly reduced peak IRV) at the same time point [4].

An alternative approach to the evaluation of the role of ventilatory factors in exercise limitation is to determine the effects of interventions that selectively increase, or decrease, ventilatory demand or capacity on exercise performance. For example, the addition of hypercapnic stimulation, or external dead space, to the breathing circuit will increase ventilatory demand. In this regard, the inability to increase ventilation with earlier attainment of peak V_E and premature termination of exercise when an external dead space is added, indicates that ventilatory factors likely contribute importantly to poor exercise capacity in the unloaded condition. Similarly, we can conclude that ventilatory limitation contributes importantly to exercise intolerance in chronic pulmonary disease; by using an intervention that decreases ventilatory demand and delays peak ventilation (i.e. such as oxygen therapy), we can improve exercise tolerance [19]. If exercise performance is enhanced by unloading the ventilatory pump, either by mechanical ventilation or by breathing helium-oxygen mixtures, we can conclude that the load on the inspiratory muscles (or its perception by the patient) contributes to exercise limitation during nonassisted exercise [20, 21]. Studies of how exercise capacity can be increased in patients with COPD that have used therapeutic manipulation of the ventilatory demand-capacity relationship allow us to explore, in a novel manner, the nature of the existing ventilatory constraints to exercise (see below).

Ventilatory Mechanics in COPD

COPD is a heterogeneous disorder characterized by dysfunction of the small and large airways and by parenchymal and vascular destruction, in highly variable combinations. Although the most obvious physiological defect in COPD is expiratory flow limitation, due to combined reduced lung recoil (and airway tethering effects) as well as intrinsic airway narrowing, the most important mechanical consequence of this is a 'restrictive' ventilatory deficit due to DH [4, 22, 23] (fig. 2, 3). When expiratory flow limitation reaches a critical level, lung emptying becomes incomplete during resting tidal breathing, and lung volume fails to decline to its natural equilibrium point (i.e. the relaxation volume of the respiratory system). EELV, therefore, becomes dynamically and not statically determined, and represents a higher resting lung volume than in health [22] (fig. 2, 3). In flow-limited patients, EELV is therefore, a continuous variable which fluctuates widely with rest and activity. When V_E increases in flow-limited patients, as for example during exercise, increases in EELV (or DH) is inevitable (fig. 1–3). DH (and its negative mechanical consequences) can occur in the healthy elderly, but at much higher V_E and VO_2 levels than in COPD [3, 24, 25]. For practical purposes, the extent of DH during exercise depends on the extent of expiratory flow limitation, the level of baseline lung hyperinflation, the prevailing ventilatory demand, and the breathing pattern for a given ventilation [4].

The extent and pattern of DH development in COPD patients during exercise is highly variable. Clearly, some patients do not increase EELV during exercise, whereas others show dramatic increases (i.e. >1 l) [4, 8, 12]. We recently studied the pattern and magnitude of DH during incremental cycle exercise in 105 patients with COPD ($FEV_{1.0}$ = 37 ± 13% predicted; mean ± SD) [4] (fig. 1, 2). In contrast to age-matched healthy control subjects, the majority of this sample (80%) demonstrated significant increases in EELV above resting values: dynamic IC decreased significantly by 0.37 ± 0.39 l (or 14 ± 15% predicted) from rest [4]. Similar levels of DH have recently been reported in COPD patients after completing a 6-min walking test while breathing without an imposed mouthpiece [26]. For the same $FEV_{1.0}$, patients with lower diffusion capacity (D_LCO <50% predicted), and presumably more emphysema, had faster rates of DH at lower exercise levels, earlier attainment of critical volume constraints (peak V_T), greater exertional dyspnea, and lower peak V_E and VO_2 when compared with patients with a relatively preserved D_LCO [4]. In the latter group, the magnitude of rest to peak change in EELV was similar to that of the low D_LCO group, but air trapping occurred predominantly at a higher VO_2 and V_E at the end of exercise. Patients with predominant emphysema likely had faster rates of DH because of reduced elastic lung recoil (and airway tethering), and an increased propensity to expiratory flow limitation. In this group, DH is often further compounded by a greater ventilatory demand as a result of higher physiological dead space, reflecting greater ventilation-perfusion abnormalities [27]. The extent of DH during exercise is inversely correlated with the level of resting lung hyperinflation: patients who were severely hyperinflated at rest showed minimal further DH during exercise [4].

Tidal Volume Restriction and Exercise Intolerance

An important mechanical consequence of DH is severe mechanical constraints on tidal volume expansion during exercise: V_T is truncated from below by the increasing EELV and constrained from above by the TLC envelope and the relatively reduced IRV (fig. 2). Thus, compared with age-matched healthy individuals, COPD patients at comparable low work rates and V_E showed substantially greater increases in dynamic EILV, a greater ratio of V_T to IC, and marked reduction in the IRV (fig. 2). In 105 COPD patients, the EILV was found to be 94 ± 5% of TLC at a peak symptom-limited VO_2 of only 12.6 ± 5.0 ml/kg/min – this indicates that the diaphragm is maximally shortened at this volume and greatly compromised in its ability to generate greater inspiratory pressures [4].

The resting IC and, in particular, the dynamic IC during exercise (and not the resting VC) represent the true operating limits for V_T expansion in any given patient. Therefore, when V_T approximates the peak dynamic IC during exercise or the dynamic EILV encroaches on the TLC envelope, further volume expansion is impossible, even in the face of increased central drive and electrical activation of the diaphragm [28]. (fig. 2)

In our study, using multiple regression analysis with symptom-limited peak VO_2 as the dependent variable, and several relevant physiological measurements as independent variables (including $FEV_{1.0}$/FVC ratio and V_E/MVC), peak V_T (standardized as % predicted VC) emerged as the strongest contributory variable, explaining 47% of the variance [4] (fig. 4). Peak V_T, in turn, correlated strongly with both the resting and peak dynamic IC (fig. 4). It is noteworthy that this correlation was particularly strong (r = 0.9) in approximately 80% of the sample, who had a diminished resting and peak dynamic IC (i.e. <70% predicted) (fig. 4). Studies by Tantucci et al. [29] have provided evidence that such patients with a dimin-

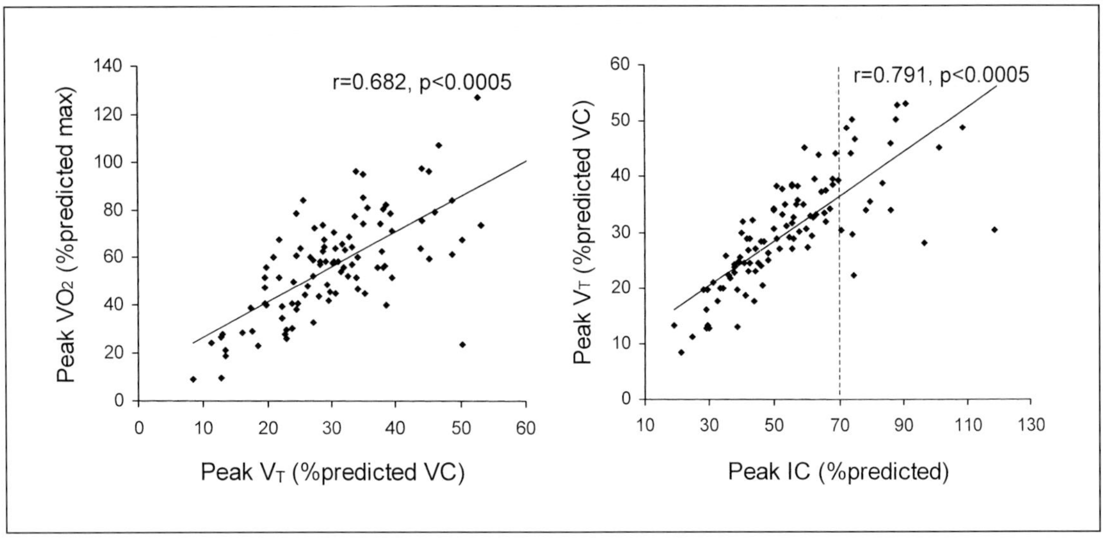

Fig. 4. In COPD (n = 105), the best correlate of peak oxygen consumption (VO_2) was the peak tidal volume attained (V_T standardized as % predicted vital capacity). In turn, the strongest correlate of peak V_T was the peak inspiratory capacity (IC). Adapted from O'Donnell et al. [4], with permission.

ished resting IC have demonstrable resting expiratory flow limitation by the negative expiratory pressure (NEP) technique. Recent studies have confirmed that in patients with COPD, a reduced resting IC with evidence of resting expiratory flow limitation, have poorer exercise performance when compared with those with a better preserved resting IC with no evidence of expiratory flow limitation at rest [4, 14, 30].

Table 2. Negative effects of dynamic hyperinflation during exercise

↑ Elastic/threshold loads Inspiratory muscle weakness	↑ P_{es}/PI_{max} 'effort'
Reduced V_T expansion → tachypnea	↓ C_L dyn ↑ V_D/V_T ↑ $PaCO_2$
Early ventilatory limitation to exercise ↑ Exertional dyspnea ↓ Cardiovascular function	

DH and Inspiratory Muscle Dysfunction

While DH serves to maximize tidal expiratory flow rates during exercise, it has serious consequences with respect to dynamic ventilatory mechanics, inspiratory muscle function, perceived respiratory discomfort, and probably, cardiac function (table 2). As already noted, DH resulted in 'high-end' pressure-volume mechanics in contrast to health, where the relationship between pressure and volume is relatively constant throughout exercise (fig. 3). This results in increased elastic loading of muscles already burdened with increased resistive work. The combined elastic and resistive loads on the ventilatory muscles substantially increase the mechanical work and the oxygen cost of breathing at a given ventilation compared with health. It has been estimated that at a peak exercise V_E of approximately 30 liters/min, ventilatory work may approach 200 J/min and respiratory muscle VO_2 may be as much as 300 ml/min in severe, mechanically compromised, COPD patients [31]. In patients with poor exercise performance (peak symptom-limited VO_2 <1 liter/min) this represents a much higher fraction (approximately 1/3) of the total body VO_2, at this low ventilation, compared with health [31].

Another more recently recognized mechanical consequence of DH is inspiratory muscle threshold loading (ITL) [32, 32]. Since, in flow-limited patients, inspiration begins before tidal lung emptying is complete, the inspiratory muscles must first counterbalance the combined inward (expiratory) recoil at the lung and chest wall before inspiratory flow is initiated. This phenomenon (i.e. reduced lung emptying) is associated with positive intrapulmonary pressures at the end of quiet expiration (i.e. auto-

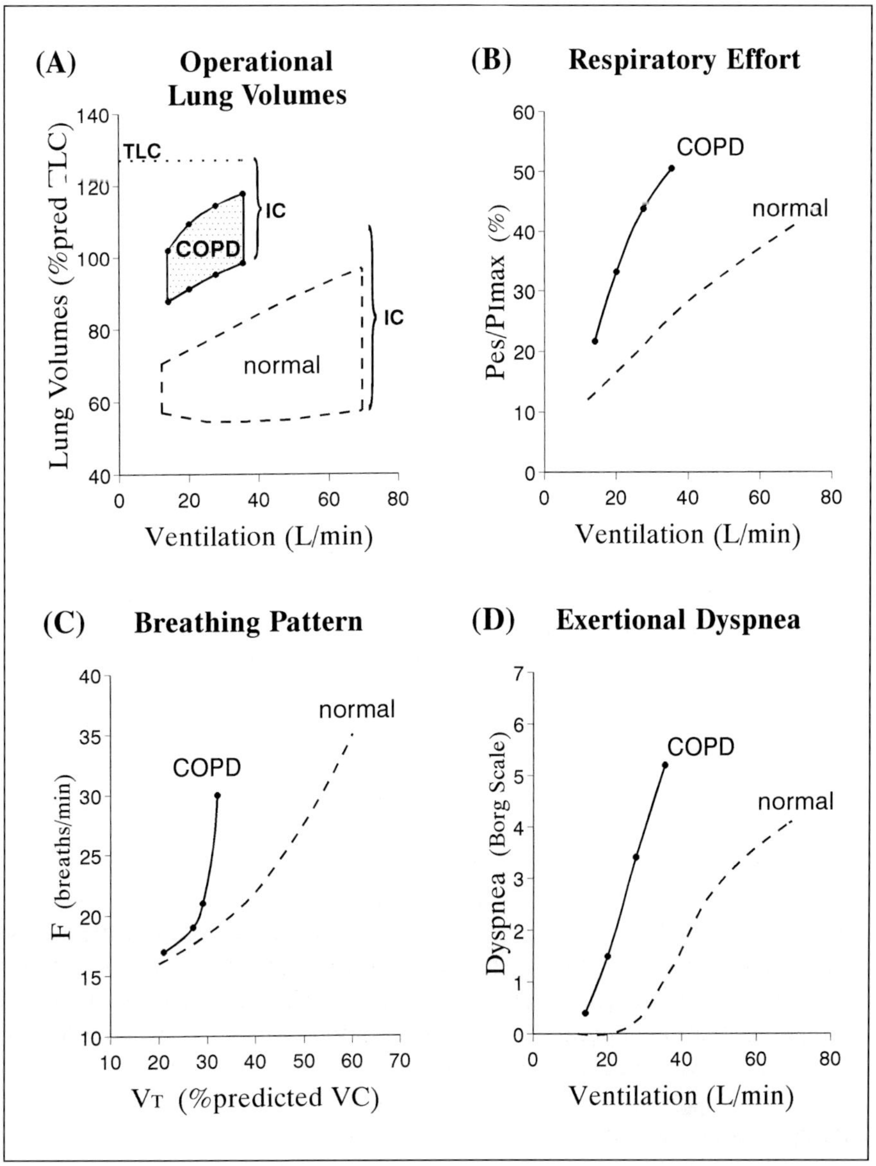

Fig. 5. Behavior of (**A**) operational lung volumes, (**B**) respiratory effort (Pes/PI_{max}), and (**D**) exertional dyspnea as ventilation increases throughout exercise in normals and COPD. In COPD, tidal volume (V_T) takes up a larger proportion of the reduced inspiratory capacity (IC), and the inspiratory reserve volume (IRV) is decreased at any given ventilation – these mechanical constraints on tidal volume expansion are further compounded because of dynamic hyperinflation during exercise. **C** Due to a truncated V_T response to exercise, patients with COPD must rely more on increasing breathing frequency (F) to generate increases in ventilation. Adapted from O'Donnell et al. [35], with permission.

PEEP or intrinsic PEEP) and may have important implications for dyspnea causation [32]. The ITL, which is present throughout inspiration and which may occur at rest in flow-limited patients, further increases in conjunction with DH during exercise and can be substantial [35].

The tachypnea associated with an increased elastic load causes increased velocity of muscle shortening during exercise and results in further functional inspiratory muscle weakness [22]. Exercise tachypnea also results in reduced dynamic lung compliance, which has an exaggerated frequency dependence in COPD [22]. DH alters the length-tension relationship of the inspiratory muscles, particularly the diaphragm, and compromises its ability to generate pressure. Because of weakened inspiratory muscles, and the intrinsic mechanical loads already described, tidal inspiratory pressures represent a high fraction of their maximal force generating capacity [34, 35–37] (fig. 5). Moreover, DH results in a disproportionate increase in the end-expiratory ribcage volume, which likely decreases the effectiveness of sternocleidomastoid and scalene muscle activity [5]. Therefore, DH may alter the pattern of ventilatory muscle recruitment to a more inefficient pattern, with negative implications for muscle energetics [5].

Table 3. Correlates of change (Δ) in standardized Borg dyspnea ratings during exercise in COPD

Author, year	Intervention	n	Independent variable	Significance
O'Donnell, 1999	ipratropium bromide	29	ΔIC% predicted at isotime exercise	$r = -0.33$, $p < 0.05$
Belman, 1996	albuterol	13	ΔEILV/TLC at isotime exercise	$r = 0.749$, $p < 0.01$
Martinez, 1997	LVRS	12	ΔEELV/predicted TLC at isotime exercise	$r = 0.75$, $p < 0.01$
O'Donnell, 1996	LVRS	8	ΔEELV/predicted TLC at isotime exercise	$r = 0.84$, $p < 0.05$

LVRS = Lung volume reduction surgery; IC = inspiratory capacity; EELV = end-expiratory lung volume; EILV = end-inspiratory lung volumes; TLC = total lung capacity.

The net effect of DH during exercise in COPD is, therefore, that the V_T response to increasing exercise is progressively constrained despite near maximal inspiratory efforts [8]. The ratio of tidal esophageal pressure (relative to maximum [P_{es}/PI_{max}]) to tidal volume (V_T/VC or V_T/predicted IC) is significantly higher at any given work rate or ventilation in COPD, compared with health.

Dynamic Hyperinflation and Dyspnea

Dyspnea intensity during exercise has been shown to correlate well with concomitant measures of dynamic lung hyperinflation [35, 38]. In a multiple regression analysis with Borg ratings of dyspnea intensity as the dependent variable, versus a number of independent physiological variables, the change in EILV (expressed as % of TLC) during exercise emerged as the strongest independent correlate ($r = 0.63$, $p = 0.001$) in 23 patients with advanced COPD (average $FEV_{1.0}$, 36% predicted) [38]. The change in EELV and change in V_T (components of EILV) emerged as significant contributors to exertional breathlessness and together with increased breathing frequency accounted for 61% of the variance in exercise Borg ratings [38]. A second study showed equally strong correlations between the intensity of perceived inspiratory difficulty during exercise and EILV/TLC ($r = 0.69$, $p < 0.01$) [35]. Dyspnea intensity also correlates well with the ratio of effort (P_{es}/PI_{max}) to tidal volume response [V_T/VC]) [35]. This increased effort-displacement ratio in COPD ultimately reflects neuromechanical dissociation (or uncoupling) of the ventilatory pump.

Current evidence suggests that breathlessness is not only a function of the amplitude of central motor output, but is also importantly modulated by peripheral feedback from a host of respiratory mechanoreceptors (for comprehensive reviews see [39–42]). Thus, the psychophysical basis of neuromechanical dissociation likely resides in the complex central processing and integration of signals that mediate (1) central motor command output [43–45], and (2) sensory feedback from various mechanoreceptors that provide precise instantaneous proprioceptive information about muscle displacement (muscle spindles and joint receptors), tension development (Golgi tendon organs), and change in respired volume or flow (lung and airway mechanoreceptors) [46–55]. Awareness of the disparity between effort and ventilatory output may elicit patterned psychological and neurohumoral responses that culminate in respiratory distress, which is an important affective dimension of perceived inspiratory difficulty.

Further indirect evidence of the importance of DH in contributing to exertional dyspnea in COPD has come from a number of studies that have shown that dyspnea was effectively ameliorated by interventions that reduced operational lung volumes (either pharmacologically or surgically), or that counterbalanced the negative effects of DH on the inspiratory muscles (continuous positive airway pressure) [20, 56–62] (table 3). Consistently strong correlations have been reported between reduced Borg ratings of dyspnea and reduced DH during exercise in a number of studies following various bronchodilators and lung volume reduction surgery [20, 56–62].

Ventilatory Limitation and Gas Exchange Abnormalities in COPD

Arterial hypoxemia during exercise commonly occurs in patients with severe COPD as a result of the effect of a fall in mixed venous oxygen tension ($P\bar{v}O_2$) on low venti-

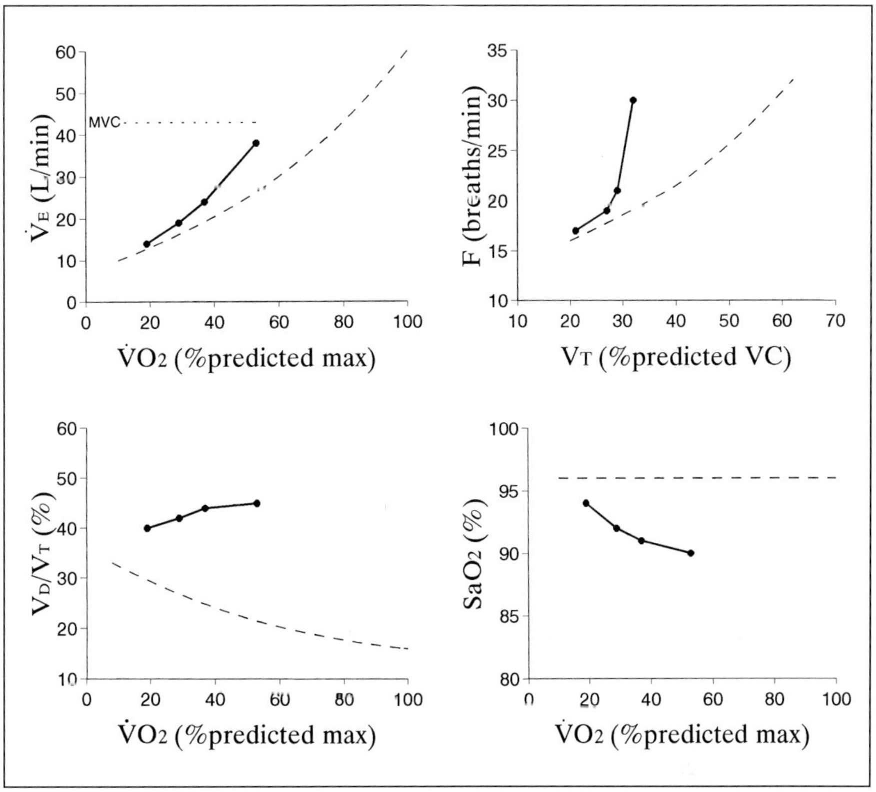

Fig. 6. Plots of ventilation (V_E), physiological deadspace (V_D/V_T) and arterial oxygen saturation (SaO_2) versus VO_2 and breathing pattern (F/V_T) in COPD (solid lines) and in age-matched healthy subjects (dotted lines). See text for abbreviations.

lation-perfusion lung units, and shunting [63]. In severe COPD, both the ability to increase lung perfusion and to distribute inspired ventilation throughout the lungs during exercise is compromised [63]. Resting physiological dead space is often increased, reflecting ventilation-perfusion inequalities, and fails to decline further during exercise as is the case in health [63, 64] (fig. 6). To maintain appropriate alveolar ventilation and blood gas homeostasis in the face of increased physiological dead space (V_D/V_T), minute ventilation must increase. In this regard, several studies have confirmed high submaximal ventilation levels during exercise in COPD compared with health [27, 65, 66] (fig. 6).

In more advanced COPD, arterial hypoxemia during exercise occurs as a result of alveolar hypoventilation [67, 68]. The reduced exercise ventilation relative to metabolic demand, may reflect reduced output of the central controller ('won't breathe' hypothesis), or a preserved or amplified central respiratory drive in the presence of an impaired mechanical/ventilatory muscle response ('can't breathe' hypothesis) [69–71]. It has further been postulated that CO_2 retention during exercise may result from the 'behavioral' adoption of a shallow breathing pattern, which would serve to minimize intrathoracic pressure perturbations, reduce respiratory discomfort, and possibly obviate the development of respiratory muscle fatigue ('wise fighter' hypothesis) [67].

The evidence that CO_2 retention during exercise is the result of reduced central or peripheral chemosensitivity is inconclusive. The resting ventilatory response to hypoxic or hypercapnic stimulation fails to predict exercise CO_2 retention in COPD [72, 73]. Moreover, studies that have measured mouth occlusion pressure in the first 0.1 s of inspiration ($P_{0.1}$) during chemical stimulation tests have shown that this index of central drive is not different in patients who are hypercapnic compared with those who are eucapnic during exercise [74, 75].

Theoretically, the imbalance between inspiratory muscle load and capacity may predispose patients with COPD to inspiratory muscle fatigue or frank task failure and consequent CO_2 retention [67]. However, Montes de Oca and Celli [76] have recently shown that maximal inspiratory pressure generation, the pattern of ventilatory muscle recruitment, and breathing pattern were not different in those who maintained eucapnia and those who developed hypercapnia during exercise thereby, casting doubt on fatigue, or its avoidance by the adoption of a rapid shallow breathing pattern, as the explanation for CO_2 retention.

In a recent study conducted in our laboratory, patients with COPD who retained CO_2 during exercise could not be distinguished from nonretainers on the basis of resting $FEV_{1.0}$, resting lung volumes, resting P_aCO_2, or V_D/V_T. Similarly, breathing pattern responses and measured V_D/V_T during exercise were not different between the two groups [77]. The rapid shallow breathing pattern, which is invariable in advanced COPD during exercise, is likely largely dictated by restrictive mechanics and the increased elastic load, rather than being behaviorally mediated (fig. 3). CO_2 retainers showed greater DH and earlier attainment of their peak alveolar ventilation than non-CO_2 retainers. In the group as a whole, there was a good correlation between the EELV/TLC and the P_aCO_2 measured simultaneously during exercise ($r = 0.68$, $p < 0.005$) and EELV contributed to 41% of the variance in P_aCO_2 after accounting for repeated measurements [77]. We concluded that CO_2 retention occurred, in part, because of greater dynamic mechanical constraints in the setting of a fixed high physiological dead space during exercise.

Increased Ventilatory Demand during Exercise in COPD

The effects of the above-outlined mechanical derangements in COPD are often amplified by concomitantly increased ventilatory demand. A high V_D/V_T that fails to decline with exercise, is the primary stimulus for increased submaximal ventilation in this population (fig. 6). Other factors contributing to increased submaximal ventilation include early lactic acidosis, hypoxemia, high metabolic demands of breathing, low arterial CO_2 set points and other nonmetabolic sources of ventilatory stimulation (i.e. anxiety). As we have seen, the extent of DH and its consequent negative sensory consequences in flow-limited patients will vary with ventilatory demand. There is abundant evidence that increased ventilatory demand contributes to dyspnea causation in COPD: dyspnea intensity during exercise has been shown to correlate strongly with the change in V_E or with V_E expressed as a fraction of maximal ventilatory capacity [38]. Flow-limited patients with the highest ventilation will develop limiting ventilatory constraints on flow and volume generation, and greater dyspnea early in exercise [4]. For a given $FEV_{1.0}$, patients who have greater ventilatory demands have been shown in one study to have more severe chronic activity-related dyspnea [27]. Moreover, exertional dyspnea relief and improved exercise endurance following interventions such as exercise training [78], oxygen therapy [19], and opiates [79] has been shown to result, in part, from the attendant reduction in submaximal ventilation (see below).

Inspiratory Muscle Weakness during Exercise in COPD

Reduced ventilatory capacity, due to reduced ventilatory muscle strength could, theoretically, contribute to ventilatory limitation in patients with advanced COPD [35–37]. We have seen that DH during exercise can contribute to functional inspiratory muscle weakness by altering length-tension and force-velocity characteristics of the inspiratory muscles. Additionally, factors such as chronic hypoxia and hypercapnia, steroid over-usage, electrolytic disturbances, and malnutrition could predispose to ventilatory muscle weakness in COPD. However, the evidence that a weakened ventilatory pump is a common contributor to exercise intolerance is inconclusive [80–83]. The prevalence of inspiratory muscle weakness in COPD patients has not been established and may not be as pervasive as previously thought. In fact, there is evidence that functional muscle strength is remarkably preserved in some patients with advanced chronic ventilatory insufficiency [84]. Biopsies of the diaphragm in patients with advanced COPD have shown several adaptations to chronic intrinsic mechanical loading. These include: (1) reduction of sarcomere length, which enhances the capacity of the muscles to generate pressure at high lung volumes [85]; (2) increase in the proportion of Type I fibres, which are slow-twitch and fatigue resistant [86], and (3) increase in mitochondrial concentration, which improves oxidative capacity [87].

To the extent that inspiratory muscle weakness contributes to exercise limitation in COPD, then targeted strengthening of these muscles should improve exercise performance. The results of studies on the effectiveness of specific inspiratory muscle training using a variety of techniques (i.e. voluntary isocapnic hyperventilation, inspiratory resistive loading, and inspiratory threshold loading) have been inconsistent. A meta-analysis of 17 clinical studies concluded that there is insufficient evidence to recommend specific inspiratory muscle training for routine clinical purposes [88].

Notwithstanding this negative meta-analysis, a few important controlled studies have shown that inspiratory muscle training using targeted resistive or inspiratory threshold loading, improved dyspnea and exercise endurance in patients with COPD, and that these improvements correlated with physiological improvements (i.e. increased static maximal inspiratory pressure [MIP]) [89–91]. It would appear, therefore, that a subset of patients with COPD do have critical inspiratory muscle weakness which can contribute to exercise intolerance and dyspnea.

Inspiratory Muscle Fatigue in COPD

The imbalance between energy supply and demand could predispose to inspiratory muscle fatigue during exercise in COPD [81]. However, to date, the evidence that contractile fatigue contributes to exercise intolerance in COPD is not convincing. Bye et al. [80], demonstrated a change in the diaphragmatic electromyogram (EMG) power spectrum (i.e. a fall in the high/low ratio) during exercise in some COPD patients during exercise. This 'fatiguing' pattern was partially reversed after giving supplemental oxygen, suggesting fatigue may have contributed to exercise intolerance when breathing room air. However, other explanations are equally plausible. Oxygen, for example, has been shown to reduce submaximal ventilation and consequently, DH, which together delay the onset of critical ventilatory limitation [19, 92–94]. These effects could collectively influence EMG signal recordings, independent of the existence of inspiratory muscle fatigue.

Kyroussos et al. [82, 95], demonstrated a slowing of maximal sniff inspiratory muscle relaxation rates following exhaustive exercise in patients with COPD, and suggested that this may be an indicator of incipient inspiratory muscle fatigue. These authors showed a reduction of this slowing effect and improved exercise endurance following pressure support (PS = 15 cm H_2O) in 6 patients with severe COPD ($FEV_{1.0}$ = 22% predicted) compared with unassisted control [95]. These results indicate that PS successfully reduced the load on the inspiratory muscles and, therefore, we can conclude that this load, or its perception by the patient, contributed to exercise intolerance during unassisted walking. However, the extent to which inspiratory muscle fatigue was delayed by PS remains conjectural.

Mador et al. [96], measured twitch trans-diaphragmatic pressures in patients with moderate to severe COPD during high intensity constant load cycle exercise to tolerance. The results of this study indicated that the majority of these patients showed no evidence of contractile fatigue of the diaphragm following symptom-limited exercise. In reality, many patients with COPD may stop exercise because of intolerable exertional symptoms well before fatigue or contractile failure actually develops. As already mentioned, there is also increasing evidence that the diaphragm may adapt to chronic intrinsic loading by becoming more resistant to fatigue [84–87].

Expiratory Muscle Activity during Exercise in COPD

In the presence of expiratory flow limitation, tidal expiratory flow rates are independent of expiratory transpulmonary pressures beyond a critical level [13]. In fact, increasing expiratory effort beyond this level not only fails to increase expiratory flow, but results in dynamic airway compression of airways downstream from the flow-limiting segment [13]. Expiratory muscle recruitment appears to be highly variable in COPD during exercise [4–8, 97, 98]. During constant-load exercise, some patients allow expiratory transpulmonary pressures to reach, but not exceed, the critical flow-limiting pressure, thus attenuating dynamic airway compression and its consequences [98]. However, other studies have shown marked expiratory muscle activity (i.e., expiratory pleural pressures >20 cm H_2O), particularly at high work rates in some COPD patients [35, 95]. Expiratory muscle recruitment during exercise is advantageous in health, through optimization of diaphragmatic length and of dynamic ventilatory mechanics (fig. 2). These important advantages are lost in COPD. Increased abdominal pressure generation (relative to expiratory intercostal activity) should increase diaphragmatic length at end-expiration and, therefore, assist the inspiratory muscles. However, the extent to which this expiratory/inspiratory synergy exists in COPD has not been fully established [23]. Moreover, any increase in EILV (or V_T) as a result of inspiratory muscle activity augmented in this manner would be expected to have a net negative effect: an increase in the EILV at a fixed expiratory timing (T_E) (not unusual in COPD) will result in further DH.

Aggravation of dynamic airway compression during forced expiratory efforts may have deleterious sensory consequences and/or may reflexly increase ventilation with attendant aggravation of DH [15, 16]. Increased expiratory muscle action, in the setting of expiratory flow limitation, will reduce the velocity of shortening (V_T/T_E) of these muscles [99]. The consequent amplified abdominal and intrathoracic pressure development throughout expiration will compromise cardiac output by reducing venous return and by increasing pulmonary vascular resistance through intrathoracic compression of alveolar vessels.

It would appear, therefore, that the deleterious effects of vigorous expiratory muscle contraction on cardiac performance outweigh potential beneficial effects on inspiratory muscle function in many patients with COPD.

Peripheral Muscle Dysfunction and Exercise Intolerance in COPD

Recently, there has been heightened interest in the role of abnormalities of peripheral muscle structure and function in exercise limitation in COPD [for excellent comprehensive reviews see 100, 101]. The importance of increased leg effort as an exercise-limiting symptom in COPD was first highlighted by Killian et al. [102]. These authors studied the intensity of exertional symptoms during incremental exercise in a sample of 97 patients with COPD ($FEV_{1.0}$ = 46.6% predicted). They found that 43% of the sample rated leg effort (by Borg scale) higher than dyspnea, 26% rated dyspnea intensity greater than leg effort, and the remainder (31%) noted the intensity of leg effort and dyspnea equally. The authors extended this study to show that the distribution of exercise-limiting symptoms in COPD was remarkably similar to that of healthy individuals and patients with congestive heart failure (CHF) at the end of incremental exercise [104].

We recently studied the distribution of exercise-limiting symptoms in 105 clinically stable patients ($FEV_{1.0}$ 37% predicted) with poor exercise performance, who were referred to respirology clinics at our institution [4] Severe breathing discomfort was the primary symptom limiting incremental cycle exercise in 61% of this sample; combined dyspnea and leg discomfort limited exercise in 19%, and only 18% stopped primarily because of leg discomfort [4]. This frequency distribution of exercise limiting symptoms was very similar to that found in a previous study in 125 patients entering a pulmonary rehabilitation program [104]. We demonstrated that patients who stopped exercise primarily because of dyspnea, had greater levels of DH, greater ventilatory constraints and poorer exercise performance than the minority who stopped mainly because of leg discomfort [4].

Peripheral muscle dysfunction is a potentially reversible cause of exercise curtailment in COPD and is currently the focus of intense study [105–114]. Abnormalities of peripheral muscle structure and function have now been extensively documented in COPD [100, 101, 104]. Many of these abnormalities ultimately represent the effects of reduced activity levels or immobility because of overwhelming dyspnea. These abnormalities include: loss of muscle mass and mitochrondrial (aerobic) potential and compromised oxidative phosphorylation which results in an exaggerated dependence on high-energy phosphate transfer and anaerobic glycolysis [105, 110]. Severe peripheral muscle weakness due in part to disuse atrophy has been reported in several studies [105, 107]. In a number of studies, lactate thresholds (i.e. the VO_2 at which lactate begins to increase) have been shown to be lower in COPD than in health. Casaburi [111] has reported a mean lactacte threshold in 33 COPD patients of being 0.7 liters/min, equivalent to a slow walking pace; as compared with 1.2 liters/min in age-matched healthy individuals. VO_2 kinetics at the peripheral muscle level have also been shown to be slower in COPD than in health [112]. Thus, in exercising COPD patients there is excessive accumulation of metabolic byproducts that impair contractility and increase the propensity to fatigue. The early metabolic acidosis (and increased CO_2 production through acid buffering effects) may stimulate increased ventilation and hasten the onset of critical ventilatory limitation. Moreover, an acidic milieu, with an altered ionic status (e.g. increased potassium) of the active peripheral muscle may also stimulate resident metabo-receptors, which may have important effects on ventilatory and sympathetic stimulation, as has been demonstrated in patients with CHF [100, 115].

Muscle biopsies in COPD have shown reduced capillarization with preserved or decreased capillary to fiber ratios [108–110]. These muscles show consistent reductions in type I slow-twitch, high oxidative, low tension, fatigue-resistant muscle fibers [108–110]. There is an increased preponderance of type II fiber, which would be expected to be associated with an increased velocity of contraction, a reduced mechanical efficiency, and increased fatigability [116]. General muscle wasting (cachexia) in COPD has been associated with low circulating levels of anabolic steroids, growth hormone, and altered circadian rhythms of leptin production in COPD [117–120]. It has recently been shown that exercise in COPD patients accelerated free radical formation [121]. If these are not scavenged by antioxidants, they can result in extensive damage to membranes and the cation cycling proteins [122]. Other well-recognized factors that contribute to peripheral muscle weakness in COPD, under certain circumstances, include: chronic oral steroid therapy, malnutrition, and the effects of hypoxia, hypercapnia and acidosis.

Exercise training has been shown to improve peripheral muscle function and perceived leg discomfort in both moderate and severe COPD [123–125] (fig. 14). Measurable improvements in peripheral muscle function, including strength and endurance, have been consistently reported [66, 78, 126, 127]. Quadriceps muscle biopsies have confirmed increased aerobic enzyme concentrations and increased capillary density after supervised training [124]. VO_2 kinetics are faster after training and blood lactate levels are lower at a standardized work [125]. Perceived leg discomfort is significantly less at any given work rate following exercise training and contributes to improved exercise endurance, particularly in patients where leg discomfort was the primary locus of sensory limitation prior to program entry [66, 78].

Ventilatory-Locomotor Muscle Competiton during Exercise in COPD

The above outlined structural abnormalities of the peripheral muscle are not unique to COPD – identical abnormalities have been reported in CHF [100]. In addition to the metabolic abnormalities of the muscle, other factors may also contribute to locomotor dysfunction in COPD. Simon et al. [128], demonstrated that at least in some patients (6 of 14) with COPD ($FEV_{1.0}$ = 35% predicted), leg VO_2, leg blood flow and O_2 extraction plateaued as exercise increased, despite progressive increases in total whole body VO_2. This suggests a ventilatory 'steal' effect, at least in some patients, such that blood was diverted away from the competing locomotor muscles to the ventilatory muscles when cardiac output had reached its maximal level. Harms et al. [129], demonstrated this 'steal' phenomenon in highly trained athletes at the extremes of endurance, when maximal VO_2 had plateaued. In these high-performance athletes, unloading of the ventilatory muscles using proportional assist ventilation (PAV) caused a significant increase in blood flow to the leg, with increased leg VO_2 [129].

The concept of ventilatory-locomotor competition for a limited availability of energy supplies during exercise in COPD was bolstered by a recent study by Richardson et al. [21]. These authors showed that in the absence of ventilatory competition, 'isolated' small muscle mass exercise resulted in a 2.2-fold greater muscle mass specific power output than during whole body exercise, indicating substantial metabolic reserve. Improved power output occurred, presumably because of greater blood perfusion and energy supplies to the small muscles, than during whole body exercise where there was competition with the ventilatory muscles. Given the high oxygen cost of breathing at a given ventilation in severe COPD during exercise (see above), and compromised cardiac function (in part as a result of the effects of DH and excessive expiratory muscle recruitment), reduced blood flow to the exercising locomotor muscles may very well contribute to exercise intolerance.

Cardiovascular Factors

The effect of COPD on cardiac performance during exercise is complex and multifactorial, and has received relatively little attention. Severe lung hyperinflation and excessive expiratory muscle recruitment can impair venous return and reduce right ventricular preload in COPD. Several studies have demonstrated increased pulmonary vascular resistance during exercise in COPD [130–132]. This results from emphysematous vascular destruction with reduced area, or compliance, of the pulmonary vascular bed and, in some cases, from critical hypoxemia as a result of alveolar hypoventilation [133, 134]. Pulmonary artery pressures and right-ventricular afterload are generally much higher than in health at a given cardiac output in COPD [133, 134]. Right-ventricular afterload during exercise is also increased because of the increased pulmonary vascular resistance associated with breathing at lung volumes close to TLC (i.e. DH) [132–135]. Earlier studies have shown that right-ventricular ejection fraction failed to increase despite a rise in right-ventricular end-diastolic pressure in COPD during exercise [131]. The left-ventricular ejection fraction is generally preserved in COPD in the absence of concomitant ischemic heart disease or hypertension [135, 136]. Left ventricular diastolic function may be impaired because of ventricular interdependence: increased tension or displacement of the right ventricle (because of increased pulmonary vascular resistance) may impede left diastolic filling [135, 136]. Left-ventricular afterload is increased during exercise because the left-ventricular transmural pressure gradient is increased as a result of progressively negative intrathoracic pressure generation. Cardiac output has been found to increase normally with VO_2 during submaximal exercise in COPD, despite the increased pulmonary vascular resistance, but peak cardiac output (and VO_2) reaches a lower maximal value than in health [130, 137]. Stroke volume is generally smaller and heart rate correspondingly higher, at a given VO_2 in COPD compared with health [130]. Reduced peak cardiac output was shown to correlate well with the extent of prevailing expiratory flow limitation [138, 139]. Morrison et al. [137], found that peak symptom-limited VO_2 correlated strongly with reduced cardiac output in COPD: reduced cardiac output alone accounted for 63% of variance in exercise performance. Montes de Oca [140] showed a statistical correlation between oxygen pulse (VO_2/heart rate), which is a crude measure of stroke volume, and the magnitude of pleural pressure swings during exercise.

Improving Exercise Performance in COPD

Quantitative flow-volume loop analysis during constant-load exercise testing (at approximately 60% of the achievable peak work rate [or VO_2]) allows a noninvasive assessment of ventilatory mechanics in COPD [12]. Changes in dynamic IC correlate strongly with the elastic load and this measurement is, therefore, a useful surrogate for direct esophageal pressure measurements [8, 56]. Furthermore, comparison of exercise flow-volume loops before and after therapeutic interventions at a standardized time, using a constant-load endurance protocol, provide valuable insights into the mechanisms of improved exercise performance and symptoms [12]. To improve exercise capacity in symptomatic COPD patients, therapeutic interventions must either increase ventilatory capacity (i.e. the maximal flow-volume envelope), delay the rate of DH (i.e. the shift of exercise tidal flow-volume loops towards TLC), or a combination of both. The effect of a few common therapeutic interventions on exercise performance in COPD is described below.

Bronchodilator Therapy

Bronchodilator therapy is the first step in the management of patients with symptomatic COPD. All classes of bronchodilator therapy (i.e. inhaled β_2-agonists, inhaled anticholinergics, and oral theophyllines) have been shown to improve exertional dyspnea and increase exercise capacity in COPD patients when tested in placebo-controlled studies [141–144]. Constant load endurance cycle exercise protocols have been shown to be more responsive to the effects of bronchodilators than incremental protocols or the six-minute walk distance test [145]. The mechanisms of improved exercise endurance following bronchodilators are complex and not fully elucidated. From the available literature on the topic it is clear that meaningful improvement in symptoms, activity levels and quality of life can occur in the presence of only modest changes in $FEV_{1.0}$ after bronchodilator therapy [141–144].

Bronchodilators improve dynamic small airway function and lung emptying, and reduce the resistive and elastic loads on the respiratory muscles. Belman et al. [56], in an elegant mechanical study, showed that relief of exertional dyspnea following albuterol (salbutamol) therapy in advanced COPD correlated well with reduction in operating lung volumes as well as a reduction in inspiratory effort required for a given tidal volume, the latter an indication of improved neuromechanical coupling of the respiratory system. In that study, important reductions in lung volume occurred in the presence of only minimal changes in $FEV_{1.0}$ [56]. This likely reflects the fact that $FEV_{1.0}$ provides at best a crude estimation of the extent of prevailing expiratory flow limitation, which is a primary determinant of DH. In severe hyperinflated COPD, improvement in lung volumes, which reflects increased conductance of the small airways are likely more relevant measurements for the assessment of bronchodilator efficacy than traditional $FEV_{1.0}$ measurements [146, 147].

We have shown [12] in a placebo-controlled study that relief of exertional dyspnea and improved exercise endurance following acute anticholinergic therapy (nebulized ipratropium bromide [IB], 500 μg) in advanced COPD correlated best with improvement in dynamic IC measurements which reflect reductions in the EELV. IC-derived measures such as EILV, the IRV, and the V_T/IC ratio, also correlated well with reduced exertional dyspnea measured by the Borg scale [12]. Because of the bronchodilator-induced increase in expiratory flow rates over the tidal volume range, more effective lung emptying was achieved at rest (fig. 7). Patients, therefore, could maintain the same, or greater, ventilation while breathing at lower lung volumes, with a more efficient breathing pattern, and reduced exertional dyspnea. During bronchodilator therapy the IRV was significantly increased at both submaximal levels and at peak exercise, despite a 32% increase in exercise endurance [12] (fig. 7). Because of this delay in ventilatory limitation, dyspnea was displaced by leg discomfort as the primary exercise-limiting symptom in many of the study patients.

Increased IC and IRV following bronchodilators meant that V_T at end-exercise was positioned on a lower, more linear portion, of the respiratory system's pressure-volume relationship, where there is reduced elastic and inspiratory threshold loading of the inspiratory muscle (fig. 3). Therefore, less pressure is required by the inspiratory muscles for a greater V_T response [56]. Evidence is accumulating that relatively small changes in resting IC (i.e. in the order of 0.3–0.4 l) or in plethysmographic lung volumes, can translate into clinically important improvements in exercise endurance in severe COPD [56, 58]. Similar close correlations between reduced operating lung volumes and dyspnea relief have been shown after surgical volume reduction [59, 60] (table 3).

Oxygen Therapy during Exercise

Since the extent of DH during exercise in flow-limited COPD patients depends on the ventilation and the breathing pattern for a given ventilation, it follows that therapeutic interventions that reduce submaximal ventilation during exercise, such as supplemental oxygen therapy, exercise training, and opiates, should delay the rate of DH and the onset of critical ventilatory constraints that limit exercise. These interventions do not typically affect the maximal flow-volume loop envelope (as is the case of bronchodilators), but merely alter the time course for the development of restrictive ventilatory mechanics. In a placebo-controlled, crossover study, where patients with advanced COPD received either 60% oxygen or room air, we have recently shown that hyperoxia more than doubled the time to reach ventilatory limitation [92] (fig. 8). In this study, the improvements in dyspnea and exercise endurance during hyperoxia were explained, in large measure, by the effects of reduced ventilatory demand (i.e. by reducing hypoxic drive and the metabolic load) on operational lung volumes [92]. At a standardized submaximal work rate, V_E was decreased by approximately 3 liters·min^{-1} and the inspiratory reserve volume increased by 0.3 liters during 60% oxygen compared with room air [92] (fig. 8).

The effects of oxygen therapy on exercise performance are complex: in addition to delaying ventilatory limitation, oxygen also improves the metabolic load, peripheral muscle function (and reduced leg discomfort), and cardiac function [148–153]. The relative importance of these various factors in contributing to improved exercise endurance in a given individual is difficult to evaluate, but in patients with unequivocal ventilatory limitation on room air, O_2-induced changes in operational lung volumes and dyspnea appear to be most important [92].

A Comprehensive Approach to Improving Exercise Intolerance in COPD

To optimize exercise performance in advanced COPD, a step-by-step, integrated approach to management achieves best results. Combination bronchodilator therapy should be carefully optimized to achieve sustained 24-hour lung volume reduction. Oxygen therapy, in selected individuals, provides further performance enhancement [149–154]. Exercise training remains the pivotal intervention to maximize activity levels and is reviewed elsewhere in this volume. These combined therapies cause a myriad of relatively small changes in a number of physiological parameters (i.e. resting and operating lung volumes, submaximal V_E, strength and endurance of the inspiratory muscles) which culminate in meaningful clinical improvement [66, 78, 154].

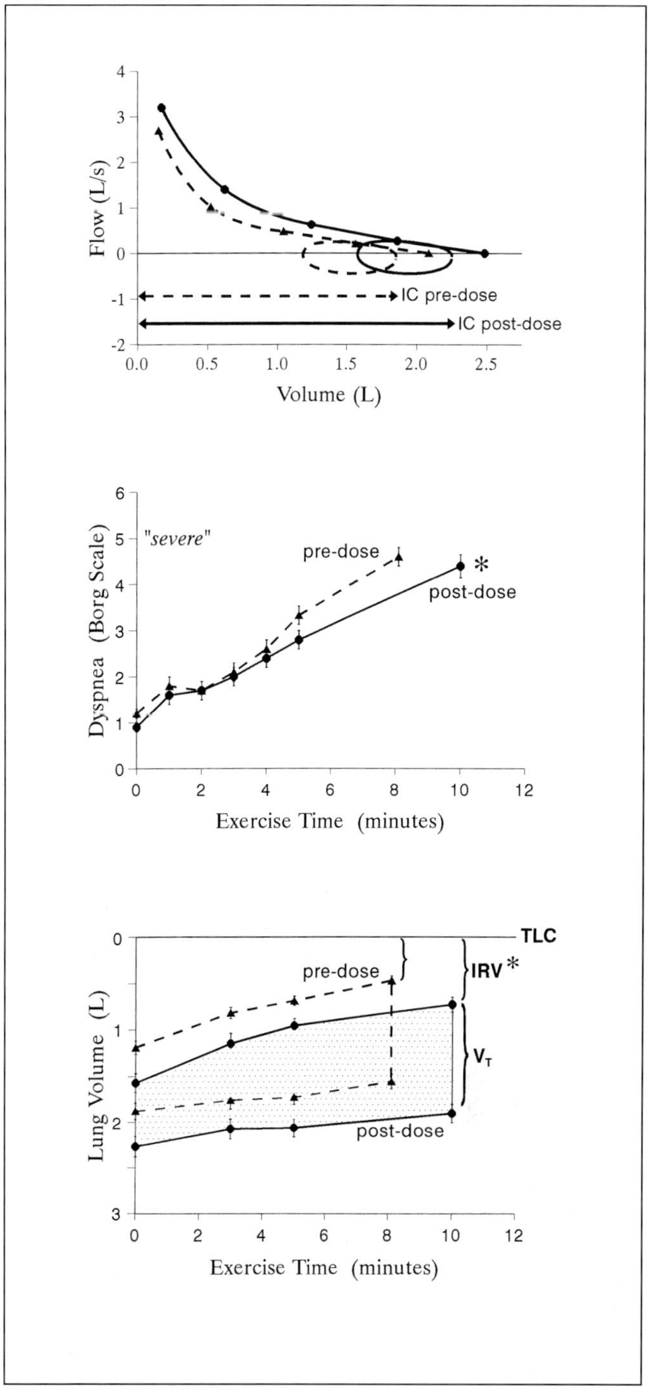

Fig. 7. Responses to bronchodilator therapy (nebulized ipratropium bromide, 500 μg) are shown. As postdose maximal expiratory flow-volume relationships improved, tidal flow-volume curves at rest can shift to the right, i.e. lung hyperinflation is reduced as reflected by an increased IC (top panel). Exertional dyspnea decreased significantly (* $p < 0.05$) in response to bronchodilator therapy (middle panel). Operational lung volumes improve in response to bronchodilator therapy, i.e. mechanical constraints on V_T expansion are reduced as IC and IRV are increased significantly (* $p < 0.05$) (lower panel). Adapted from O'Donnell et al. [58], with permission.

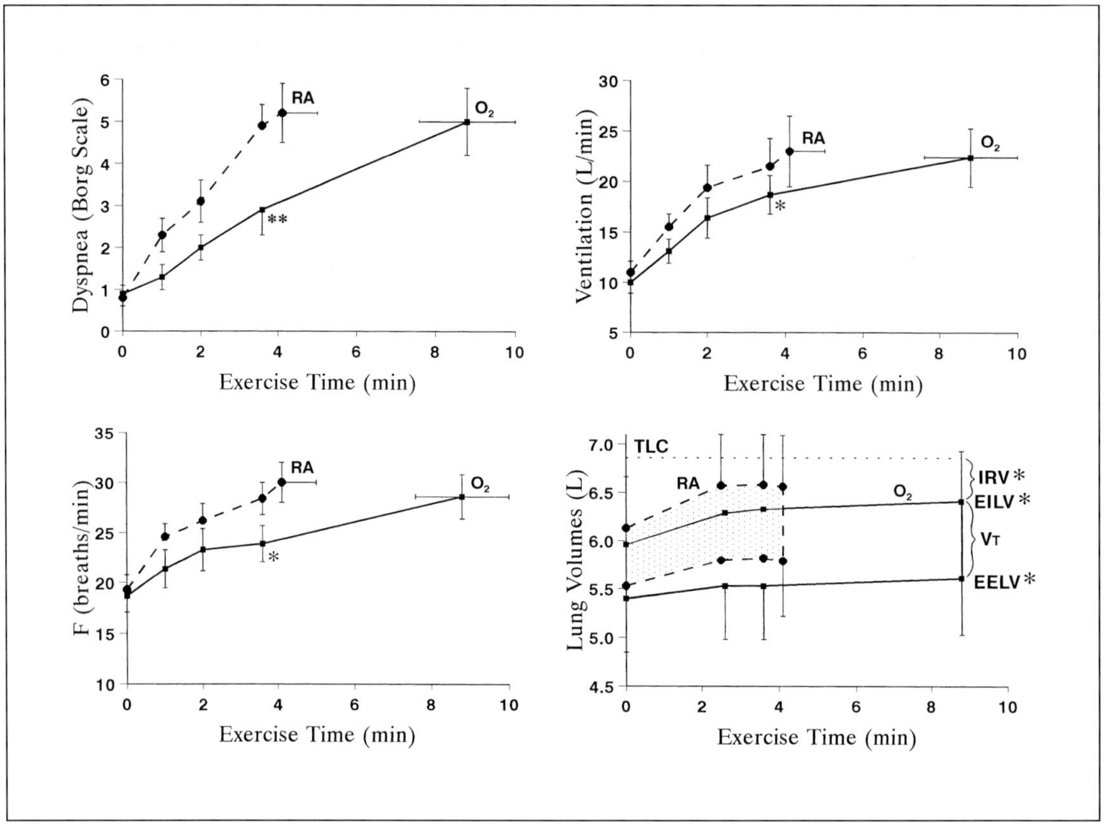

Fig. 8. Dyspnea, V_E, breathing frequency (F), and operating lung volumes plotted against time in patients randomized to room air (RA) or 60% oxygen. While breathing oxygen, there were significant increases in exercise endurance, with significant decreases in dyspnea, V_E, F, EELV (i.e. increased IC) and EILV (i.e. increased IRV) at isotime during exercise (* $p < 0.05$, ** $p < 0.01$). Adapted from O'Donnell et al. [92], with permission.

Conclusion

On the basis of extensive studies in COPD patients, we can conclude that ventilatory limitation contributes importantly, and often predominantly, to exercise limitation. Expiratory flow limitation is the hallmark of this heterogeneous condition and its most important consequence is resting hyperinflation and further dynamic hyperinflation during exercise, which accelerates ventilatory limitation, respiratory discomfort, and exercise termination. The recognition that DH is one factor contributing to reduced ventilatory capacity is potentially clinically important since this is at least partially reversible and can, therefore, be manipulated for the patient's benefit. Interventions that improve airway function and lung emptying (i.e. bronchodilators) will reduce operating lung volumes during exercise and delay the occurrence of critical ventilatory constraints, thus improving exercise endurance and symptoms. Similarly, interventions that reduce ventilatory demand (i.e. oxygen therapy) will also delay the rate of DH and its deleterious consequences in selected patients.

Reduced activity levels, as a result of dyspnea and cardioventilatory impairment, eventually lead to alterations in the structure and function of the peripheral muscles, which further curtail exercise capacity in a vicious cycle. Disuse atrophy, reduced oxygen delivery and/or blood perfusion to the active muscle, together with perceived leg discomfort, are all likely instrumental in contributing to exercise limitation. There is now good evidence that exercise reconditioning and strength training can partially reverse these abnormalities. Comprehensive management strategies that incorporate pharmacologic therapies and exercise training, can maximize exercise capabilities and thus, the health status of patients with advanced symptomatic disease.

References

1 Borg GAV: Psychophysical basis of perceived exertion. Med Sci Sports Exerc 1982;14:377–381.

2 Gift AG: Validation of a vertical visual analogue scale as a measure of clinical dyspnea. Rehab Nurs 1989;14:313–325.

3 Johnson BD, Weisman IM, Zeballos RJ, Beck KC: Emerging concepts in the evaluation of ventilatory limitation during exercise: The exercise tidal flow-volume loop. Chest 1999;116: 488–503.

4 O'Donnell DE, Revill S, Webb KA: Dynamic hyperinflation and exercise intolerance in COPD. Am J Respir Crit Care Med, 2001;164: in press.

5 Grimby G, Bunn J, Mead J: Relative contribution of rib cage and abdomen to ventilation during exercise. J Appl Physiol 1968;24:159–166.

6 Potter WA, Olafson S, Hyatt RE: Ventilatory mechanics and expiratory flow limitation during exercise in patients with obstructive lung disease. J Clin Invest 1971;50:910–919.

7 Dodd DS, Brancatisano T, Engel LA: Chest wall mechanics during exercise in patients with severe chronic airway obstruction. Am Rev Respir Dis 1984;129:33–38.

8 Stubbing DG, Pengelly LD, Morse JLC, Jones NL: Pulmonary mechanics during exercise in subjects with chronic airflow obstruction. J Appl Physiol 1980;49:511–515.

9 Henke KG, Sharratt M, Peglow DF, Dempsey JA: Regulation of end-expiratory lung volume during exercise. J Appl Physiol 1988;64:135–146.

10 Lind F, Hesser CM: Breathing pattern and lung volumes during exercise. Acta Physiol Scand 1984;120:123–19.

11 Druz WS, Sharp JT: Activity of respiratory muscles in upright and recumbent humans. J Appl Physiol 1981;41:1522–1561.

12 O'Donnell DE, Lam M, Webb KA: Measurement of symptoms, lung hyperinflation and endurance during exercise in chronic obstructive pulmonary disease. Am J Respir Crit Care Med 1998;158:1557–1565.

13 Hyatt RE: Expiratory flow limitation. J Appl Physiol 1983;55:1–8.

14 Eltayara L, Becklake MR, Volta CA, Milic-Emili J: Relationship between chronic dyspnea and expiratory flow limitation in patients with chronic obstructive pulmonary disease. Am J Respir Crit Care Med 1996;154:1726–1734.

15 O'Donnell DE, Sanii R, Anthonisen NR, Younes M: Effect of dynamic airway compression on breathing pattern and respiratory sensation in severe chronic obstructive pulmonary disease. Am Rev Respir Dis 1987;135:912–918.

16 O'Donnell DE, Sanii R, Anthonisen NR, Younes M: Expiratory resistive loading in patients with severe chronic airflow limitation: An evaluation of ventilatory mechanics and compensatory responses. Am Rev Respir Dis 1987;136:102–107.

17 Gandevia B, Hugh-Jones P: Terminology of measurements of ventilatory capacity. Thorax 1957;1:290–293.

18 Dillard TA, Piantadosi S, Rajagopal KR: Determinants of maximum exercise capacity in patients with chronic airflow obstruction. Chest 1989;96:267–271.

19 O'Donnell DE, Bain DJ, Webb KA: Factors contributing to relief of exertional breathlessness during hyperoxia in chronic airflow limitation. Am J Respir Crit Care Med 1997;155: 530–535.

20 O'Donnell DE, Sanii R, Younes M: Improvements in exercise endurance in patients with chronic airflow limitation using CPAP. Am Rev Respir Dis 1988;138:1510–1514.

21 Richardson RS, Sheldon J, Poole DC, Hopkins SR, Ries AL, Wagner PD: Evidence of skeletal muscle metabolic reserve during whole body exercise in patients with chronic obstructive pulmonary disease. Am J Respir Crit Care Med 1999;159:881–885

22 Pride NB, Macklem PT: Lung mechanics in disease; in Fishman AP (ed): Handbook of Physiology, sect 3, vol III, part 2: The Respiratory System. Bethesda, American Physiological Society, 1986, pp 659–692.

23 Younes M: Determinants of thoracic excursions during exercise; in Whipp BJ, Wasserman K (eds): Lung Biology in Health and Disease, vol 42: Exercise, Pulmonary Physiology and Pathophysiology. New York, Marcel Dekker, 1991, pp 1–65.

24 Johnson BD, Dempsey JA: Demand vs. capacity in the aging pulmonary system; in Holloszy JO (ed): Exercise and Sports Science Reviews. Baltimore, Williams & Wilkins, 1991, pp 171–210.

25 Johnson BD, Reddan DF, Pegelow KC, Seow KC, Dempsey JA: Flow limitation and regulation of functional residual capacity during exercise in a physically active aging population. Am Rev Respir Dis 1991;143:960–967.

26 Marin JM, Carrizo SJ, Gascon M, Sanchez A, Gallego BA, Celli BR: Inspiratory capacity, dynamic hyperinflation, breathlessness and exercise performance during the 6-minute-walk test in chronic obstructive pulmonary disease. Am J Respir Crit Care Med 2001;163:1395–1399.

27 O'Donnell DE, Webb KA: Breathlessness in patients with severe chronic airflow limitation: Physiologic correlates. Chest 1992;102:824–831.

28 Sinderby C, Spahija J, Beck J, Kaminski D, Yan S, Comtois N, Sliwinski P: Diaphragm activation during exercise in chronic obstructive pulmonary disease. Am J Respir Crit Care Med 2001;163:1637–1641.

29 Tantucci C, Duguet A, Similowski T, Zelter M, Derenne JP, Milic-Emili J: Effect of salbutamol on dynamic hyperinflation in chronic obstructive pulmonary disease patients. Eur Respir J 1998;12:799–804.

30 Diaz O, Villafranco C, Ghezzo H, Borzone G, Leiva A, Milic-Emili J, Lisboa C: Exercise tolerance in COPD patients with and without tidal expiratory flow limitation at rest. Eur Respir J 2000;16:269–275.

31 Levison H, Cherniack RM: Ventilatory cost of exercise in chronic obstructive pulmonary disease. J Appl Physiol 1968:25:21–27.

32 Niance V, Yernault JC, de Troyer A: Intrinsic PEEP in patients with chronic obstructive pulmonary disease. Am Rev Respir Dis 1993;148: 1037–1042.

33 Lougheed MD, Webb KA, O'Donnell DE: Breathlessness during induced lung hyperinflation in asthma: The role of the inspiratory threshold load. Am J Respir Crit Care Med 1995;152:911–920.

34 Leblanc P, Summers E, Inman MD, Jones NL, Campbell EJ, Killian KJ: Inspiratory muscles during exercise: A problem of supply and demand. J Appl Physiol 1988;64:2482–2489.

35 O'Donnell DE, Chau LKL, Bertley JC, Webb KA: Qualitative aspects of exertional breathlessness in chronic airflow limitation: Pathophysiologic mechanisms. Am J Respir Crit Care Med 1997;155:109–115.

36 Rochester DF, Braun NMT: Determinants of maximal inspiratory pressure in chronic obstructive pulmonary disease. Am Rev Respir Dis 1970;132:42–47.

37 Killian KJ, Jones NL: Respiratory muscles and dyspnea. Clin Chest Med 1988;9:237–248.

38 O'Donnell DE, Webb KA: Exertional breathlessness in patients with chronic airflow limitation: The role of hyperinflation. Am Rev Respir Dis 1993;148:1351–1357.

39 Meek PM, Schwartzstein RMS, Adams L, Altose MD, Breslin EH, Carrieri-Kohlman V, Gift A, Hanley MV, Harver A, Jones PW, Killian K, Knobel A, Lareau S, Mahler DA, O'Donnell DE, Steele B, Stuhlbarg M, Title M: Dyspnea mechanism, assessment and management: A consensus statement (American Thoracic Society). Am J Respir Crit Care Med 1999;159:321–340.

40 O'Donnell DE: Exertional breathlessness in chronic respiratory disease; in Mahler DA (ed): Lung Biology in Health and Disease, vol III: Dyspnea. New York, Marcel Dekker, 1998, pp 97–147.

41 Killian KJ, Campbell EJM: Dyspnea; in Roussos C, Macklem PT (eds): Lung Biology in Health and Disease, vol 29 (part B): The Thorax. New York, Marcel Dekker, 1985, pp 787–828.

42 Altose M, Cherniack N, Fishman AP: Respiratory sensations and dyspnea: Perspectives. J Appl Physiol 1985;58:1051–1054.

43 Chen Z, Eldridge FL, Wagner PG: Respiratory associated rhythmic firing of midbrain neurones in cats: Relation to level of respiratory drive. J Appl Physiol 1991;437:305–325.

44 Chen Z, Eldridge FL, Wagner PG: Respiratory-associated thalamic activity is related to level of respiratory drive. Respir Physiol 1992;90: 99–113.

45 Davenport PW, Friedman WA, Thompson FJ, Franzen O: Respiratory-related cortical potentials evoked by inspiratory occlusion in humans. J Appl Physiol 1986;60:1843–1948.
46 Gandevia SC, Macefield G: Projection of low threshold afferents from human intercostal muscles to the cerebral cortex. Respir Physiol 1989;77:203–214.
47 Homma I, Kanamara A, Sibuya M: Proprioceptive chest wall afferents and the effect on respiratory sensation; in Von Euler C, Katz-Salamon M (eds): Respiratory Psychophysiology. New York, Stockton Press, 1988, pp 161–166.
48 Banzett RB, Lansing RW, Reid MB, Adams L, Brown R. 'Air hunger' arising from increased PCO_2 in mechanically ventilated quadriplegics. Respir Physiol 1989;76:53–68.
49 Altose MD, Syed I, Shoos L: Effects of chest wall vibration on the intensity of dyspnea during constrained breathing. Proc Int Union Physiol Sci 1989;17:288.
50 Matthews PBC: Where does Sherrington's 'muscular sense' originate: Muscles, joints, corollary discharge? Ann Rev Neurosci 1982;5: 189–218.
51 Roland PE, Ladegaard-Pederson HA: A quantitative analysis of sensation of tension and kinaesthesia in man: Evidence for peripherally originating muscular sense and a sense of effort. Brain 1977;100:671–692.
52 Noble MIM, Eisele JH, Trenchard D, Guz A: Effect of selective peripheral nerve blocks on respiratory sensations; in Porter R (ed): Breathing: Hering-Breyer Symposium. London, Churchill, 1970, pp 233–246.
53 Zechman FR Jr, Wiley RL: Afferent inputs to breathing: Respiratory sensation; in Fishman AP (ed): Handbook of Physiology, sect 3, vol II, part 2: The Respiratory System. Bethesda, American Physiology Society, 1986, pp 449–74.
54 Banzett RB, Dempsey JA, O'Donnell DE, Wamboldt MZ: Symptom perception and respiratory sensation in asthma. Am J Respir Crit Care Med 2000;162:1178–1182.
55 Kukorelli T, Namenyi J, Adam G: Visceral afferent projection areas in the cortex representation of the carotid sinus receptor area. Acta Physiol Acad Sci 1969;36:261–263.
56 Belman MJ, Botnick WC, Shin JW: Inhaled bronchodilators reduce dynamic hyperinflation during exercise in patients with chronic obstructive pulmonary disease. Am J Respir Crit Care Med 1996;153:967–975.
57 Chrystyn H, Mulley BA, Peake MD: Dose response relation to oral theophylline in severe chronic obstructive airways disease. BMJ 1988;297:1506–1510.
58 O'Donnell DE, Lam M, Webb KA: Spirometric correlates of improvement in exercise performance after anticholinergic therapy in COPD. Am J Respir Crit Care Med 1999;160:542–549.
59 Martinez FJ, Montes de Oca M, Whyte RI, Stetz J, Gay SE, Celli BR: Lung-volume reduction improves dyspnea, dynamic hyperinflation and respiratory muscle function. Am J Respir Crit Care Med 1997;155:1984–1990.
60 Laghi F, Jurban A, Topeli A, Fahey PH, Garrity F Jr, Archids JM, DePinto DJ, Edwards LC, Tobin MJ: Effect of lung volume reduction surgery on neuromechanical coupling of the diaphgram. Am J Respir Crit Care Med 1998; 157:475–483.
61 O'Donnell DE, Bertley J, Webb KA, Conlan AA: Mechanisms of relief of exertional breathlessness following unilateral bullectomy and lung volume reduction surgery in advanced chronic airflow limitation. Chest 1996:110:18–27.
62 Petrof BJ, Calderini E, Gottfried SB: Effect of CPAP on respiratory effort and dyspnea during exercise in severe COPD. J Appl Physiol 1990; 69:178–188.
63 Barbara JA, Roca J, Ramirez J, Wagner PD, Usetti P, Rodriquez-Roisin R: Gas exchange during exercise in mild chronic obstructive pulmonary disease. Am Rev Respir Dis 1991;144: 520–525.
64 Dantzker DR, D'Alonzo GE: The effect of exercise on pulmonary gas exchange in patients with severe chronic obstructive pulmonary disease. Am Rev Respir Dis 1986;134:1135–1139.
65 Dillard TA, Piantadosi S, Rajagopal KR: Prediction of ventilation at maximal exercise in chronic airflow obstruction. Am Rev Respir Dis 1985;132:230–235.
66 O'Donnell DE, McGuire M, Samis L, Webb KA: Effects of general exercise training on ventilatory and peripheral muscle strength and endurance in chronic airflow limitation. Am J Respir Crit Care Med 1998;157:1489–1497.
67 Begin P, Grassino A: Inspiratory muscle dysfunction and chronic hypercapnia in chronic obstructive pulmonary disease. Am Rev Respir Dis 1991;143:905–912.
68 Borrows B, Earle RH: Course and prognosis of chronic obstructive lung disease: A prospective study of 200 patients. N Engl J Med 1969;280: 397–404.
69 Altose MD, McCauley WC, Kelsen SG, Cherniack NS: Effects of hypercapnia and inspiratory flow-resistive loading on respiratory activity in chronic airways obstruction. J Clin Invest 1977;59:500–507.
70 Light RW, Mahutte CK, Brown SE: Etiology of carbon dioxide retention at rest and during exercise in chronic airflow obstruction. Chest 1988;94:61–67.
71 DeTroyer A, Leeper JB, McKenzie D, Gandevia S: Neural drive to the diaphragm in patients with severe COPD. Am J Respir Crit Care Med 1993;155:1335–1340.
72 Sorli J, Grassino A, Lorange G, Milic-Emili J: Control of breathing in patients with chronic obstructive lung disease. Clin Sci Mol Med 1978;54:296–304.
73 Moutain R, Zwillich C, Weil J: Hypoventilation in obstructive lung disease: The role of familial factors. N Engl J Med 1978;298:521–525.
74 Montes de Oca M, Celli BR: Mouth occlusion pressure, CO_2 response and hypercapnia in severe obstructive pulmonary disease. Eur Respir J 1998;12:666–671.
75 Scano G, Spinelli A, Duranti R, Gorini M, Gigliotti F, Goti P, Milic-Emili J: Carbon dioxide responsiveness in COPD patients with and without hypercapnia. Eur Respir J 1995;8:78–85.
76 Montes de Oca M, Celli B: Respiratory muscle recruitment and exercise performance in eucapnic and hypercapnic severe chronic obstructive pulmonary disease. Am J Respir Crit Care Med 2000;61:880–885.
77 O'Donnell DE, D'Arsigny C, Webb KA: Mechanisms of exercise-induced hypercapnia in advanced COPD. Am J Respir Crit Care Med 2001;63:A21.
78 O'Donnell DE, McGuire M, Samis L, Webb KA: The impact of exercise reconditioning on breathlessness in severe chronic airflow limitation. Am J Respir Crit Care Med 1995;152: 2005–2013.
79 Light RW, Muro JR, Sato RI, Stansbury DW, Fischer CE, Brown SE: Effects of oral morphine on breathlessness and exercise tolerance in patients with chronic obstructive pulmonary disease. Am Rev Respir Dis 1989;139:126–133.
80 Bye PT, Esau SA, Levy Levy RO, Shiner RJ, Macklem PT, Martin JG, Pardy RL: Ventilatory muscle function during exercise in air and oxygen in patients with chronic airflow limitation. Am Rev Respir Dis 1985;32:236–240.
81 Grassino A, Gross D, Macklem PT, Roussos C, Zagelbaum G: Inspiratory muscle fatigue as a factor limiting exercise. Bull Eur Pathophysiol Respir 1979;15:105–111.
82 Kyroussis D, Polkey MK, Keilty SEJ, Mills GH, Hamnegard CH, Moxham J, Green M: Exhaustive exercise shows inspiratory muscle relaxation rate in chronic obstructive pulmonary disease. Am J Respir Crit Care Med 1996; 53:787–793.
83 Polkey MI, Kyroussis D, Mills GH, Hamnegard C, Keilty SEJ, Green M, Moxham J: Inspiratory pressure support reduces slowing of inspiratory muscle relaxation rate during exhaustive treadmill walking in severe COPD. Am J Respir Crit Care Med 1996;154:1146–1150.
84 Similowski T, Yan S, Gauthier AP, Macklem PT, Bellemere F: Contractile properties of the human diaphragm during chronic hyperinflation. N Engl J Med 1991;325:917–923.
85 Orozco-Levi M, Gea J, Lloreta JL, Felez M, Minguella J, Serano S, Broquetas JM: Subcellular adaptation of the human diaphragm in chronic obstructive pulmonary disease. Eur Respir J 1999;13:371–378.
86 Levine S, Kaiser L, Leferovich J, Tikunov B: Cellular adaptations in the diaphgram in chronic obstructive pulmonary disease. N Engl J Med 1997;337:1799–1806.
87 Mercadier JJ, Schwartz K, Schiaffino S, Wisnewsky C, Ausoni S, Heimburger M, Marrash R, Pariente R, Aubier M: Myosin heavy chain gene expression changes in the diaphragm of patients with chronic lung hyperinflation. Am J Physiol 1988:274:L527–L534.
88 Smith K, Cook D, Guyatt GH, Madhoven J, Oxman AD: Respiratory muscle training in chronic airflow obstruction. Am Rev Respir Dis 1992;145:533–539.

89 Harver A, Mahler DA, Daubenspeck JA: Targeted inspiratory muscle training improves respiratory muscle function and reduces dyspnea in chronic obstructive pulmonary disease. Ann Intern Med 1989;111:117–124.
90 Kim J, Larson J, Covey M, Vitalo C, Alex C, Patel M: Inspiratory muscle training in patients with chronic obstructive pulmonary disease. Nurs Res 1993;42:356–362.
91 Lisboa C, Munoz V, Beroiza T, Leiva A, Cruz E: Inspiratory muscle training in chronic airflow limitation: Comparison of two different training loads with a threshold device. Eur Respir J 1994;7:1266–1274.
92 O'Donnell DE, D'Arsigny C, Webb KA: Effects of hyperoxia on ventilatory limitation during exercise in advanced chronic obstructive pulmonary disease. Am J Respir Crit Care Med 2001;163:892–898.
93 Webb KA, D'Arsigny C, O'Donnell DE: Exercise response to added oxygen in patients with COPD and variable gas exchange abnormalities. Am Rev Respir Crit Care Med 2001;163: A169.
94 O'Donnell DE, D'Arsigny C, Hollingworth EN, Webb KA.: Oxygen reduces dynamic hyperinflation and improves exercise performance in hypoxic patients with COPD. Am J Respir Crit Care Med 2000;161:A753.
95 Kyroussis D, Polkey MI, Hammegard G-H, Mills GH, Green M, Moxham J: Respiratory muscle activity in patients with COPD walking to exhaustion with and without pressure support. Eur Respir J 2000;15:649–655.
96 Mador MJ, Kufel TJ, Pineda LA, Sharma GK: Diaphragmatic fatigue and high intensity exercise in patients with chronic obstructive pulmonary disease. Am J Respir Crit Care Med 2000;161:118–123.
97 Roussos C, Macklem PT: The respiratory muscles. N Engl J Med 1982;307:786–797.
98 Leaver DG, Pride NB: Flow volume curves and expiratory pressures during exercise in patients with chronic airflow obstruction. Scand J Respir Dis 1971;42(suppl):23–27.
99 Kayser B, Sliwinski P, Yan S, Tobias M, Macklem PT: Respiratory effort sensation during exercise with induced expiratory flow limitation in healthy humans. J Appl Physiol 1997;83:936–947.
100 Gosker HR, Wouters EF, Van der Vusse GJ, Schols AM: Skeletal muscle dysfunction in chronic obstructive pulmonary disease and chronic heart failure: Underlying mechanisms and therapy perspectives. Am J Clin Nutr 2000;71:1033–1047.
101 Casaburi R: Skeletal muscle dysfunction in chronic obstructive pulmonary disease. Med Sci Sports Exerc 2001;33(suppl 7):S662–S670.
102 Killian KJ, Leblanc P, Martin DH, Summers E, Jones NL, Campbell EJM: Exercise capacity and ventilatory, circulatory and symptom limitation in patients with chronic airflow limitation. Am Rev Respir Dis 1992;146: 935–940.
103 Hamilton AL, Killian KJ, Summers L, Jones NL: Symptom intensity and subjective limitation to exercise in patients with cardiorespiratory disorders. Chest 1996;110:1255–1263.
104 O'Donnell DE, Webb KA: Exercise reconditioning in patients with chronic airflow limitation; in Torg JS, Shepherd RJ (eds): Current Therapy in Sports Medicine, ed 3. St. Louis, Mosby Year Book, 1995, pp 678–684.
105 Bernard S, Leblanc P, Whittom F, Carrier G, Jobin J, Belleau R, Maltais F: Peripheral muscle weakness in patients with chronic obstructive pulmonary disease. Am J Respir Crit Care Med 1998;158;629–634.
106 Wilson DO, Rogers RM, Wright EC, Anthonisen NR: Body weight in chronic obstructive pulmonary disease: The National Institutes of Health intermittent positive pressure breathing trial. Am Rev Respir Dis 1989;139:1435–1438.
107 Gosselink R, Trooster T, Decramer M: Peripheral muscle weakness contributes to exercise limitation in COPD. Am J Respir Crit Care Med 1996;153:976–980.
108 Whittom F, Jobin J, Simard PM, Leblanc P, Simard C, Bernard S, Belleau R, Maltais F: Histochemical and morphological characteristics of the vastus lateralis muscle in patients with chronic obstructive pulmonary disease. Med Sci Sports Exerc 1998;30:1467–1474.
109 Jakobsson P, Jorfeldt L, Henriksson J: Metabolic enzyme activity in the quadriceps femoris muscle in patients with severe chronic obstructive pulmonary disease. Am J Respir Crit Care Med 1995;151:374–377.
110 Jobin J, Maltais F, Doyon JF, Leblanc P, Simard PM, Simard AA, Simard C: Chronic obstructive pulmonary disease: Capillarity and fiber-type characteristics of skeletal muscle. J Cardiopul Rehab 1998;18:432–437.
111 Casaburi R: Deconditioning; in Fishman AP (ed): Lung Biology in Health and Disease: Pulmonary Rehabilitation. New York, Marcel Dekker, 1996, pp 213–230.
112 Casaburi R: Exercise training in chronic obstructive lung disease; in Casaburi R, Petty TL (eds): Principles and Practice of Pulmonary Rehabilitation. Philadelphia, Saunders 1993, pp 204–224.
113 Cooper CB: Determining the role of exercise in patients with chronic obstructive pulmonary disease. Med Sci Sports Exerc 1995;27: 147–157.
114 Casaburi R, Porszasz J, Burns MR, Carithers ER, Chang RSY, Cooper CB: Physiologic benefits of exercise training in rehabilitation of patients with severe chronic obstructive pulmonary disease. Am J Respir Crit Care Med 1997;115:1541–1551.
115 Wilson JR, Martin JL, Schwartz D, Ferraro N: Exercise intolerance in patients with chronic heart failure: Role of impaired nutritive flow to skeletal muscle. Circulation 1984; 69:1079–1087.
116 Green HR: Myofibrillar composition and mechanical function in mammalian skeletal muscle; in Shepard RJ (ed): Sports Science Reviews. Champaign, Human Kinetic Publishers, 1992, pp 43–64.
117 Semple PD, Bestall GH, Watson WS, Hume R: Hypothalamic-pituitary dysfunction in respiratory hypoxia. Thorax 1981;36:605–609.
118 Semple PD, Bestall GH, Watson WS, Hume R: Serum testosterone depression associated with hypoxia in respiratory failure. Clin Sci 1989;58:105–106.
119 Semple PD, Watson WS, Bestall GH, Bethel MIF, Grant JK, Hume R: Diet, absorption, and hormone studies in relation to body weight in obstructive airways disease. Thorax 1979;34:783–788.
120 Takabatake N, Nakamura H, Mingmihaba O, Inage M, Inoue S, Kagaya S, Yamaki M, Tomoike H: A novel pathophysiologic phenomenon in cachexic patients with chronic obstructive pulmonary disease. Am J Respir Crit Car Med 2001;163:1314–1319.
121 Heunks KMA, Vina J, Van Herwaarden CLA, Folgering MTM, Gimeno A, Dekhuizen PNR: Xanthine oxidase is involved in exercise-induced oxidative stress in chronic obstructive pulmonary disease. Am J Physiol 1999;277:R1697–R1704.
122 Vina J, Severa E, Acensi M, Sastre J, Pallardo JS, Ferrero JS, Garcia-de-la-Asuncion J, Anton V, Marin J: Exercise causes blood glutathione oxidation in chronic obstructive pulmonary disease and prevention by O_2 therapy. J Appl Physiol 1996;2199–2202.
123 Casaburi R, Patessio A, Ioli F, Zanaboni S, Donner CF, Wasserman K: Reduction in exercise lactic acidosis and ventilation as a result of exercise training in obstructive lung disease. Am Rev Respir Dis 1991;143:9–18.
124 Maltais F, Leblanc P, Simard C, Jobin J, Berube C, Bruneau J, Carrier L, Belleau R: Skeletal muscle adaptation to endurance training in patients with chronic obstructive pulmonary disease. Am J Respir Crit Care Med 1996;154:442–447.
125 Casaburi R, Porszasz J, Burns MR, Carithers ER, Chang RSY, Cooper CB: Physiologic benefits of exercise training in rehabilitation of patients with severe chronic obstructive pulmonary disease. Am J Respir Crit Care Med 1997;155:1541–1551.
126 Bernard S, Whittom F, Leblanc P, Jobin J, Belleau R, Berube C, Carrier G, Maltais F: Aerobic and strength training in patients with chronic obstructive pulmonary disease. Am J Respir Crit Care Med 1999;159:896–901.
127 Kochakian CD, Stettner CE: Effect of testosterone propionate and grown hormone on weight and composition of body and organs of the mouse. Am J Physiol 1948;155:255–265.
128 Simon M, Leblanc P, Jobin J, Desmeules M, Sullivan MJ, Maltais F: Limitation of lower limb and VO_2 during cycling exercise in COPD patients. J Appl Physiol 2001;190: 1013–1019.
129 Harms GA, Babcock MA, McClaren SR, Pegelow DF, Nickele GA, Nelson WB, Dempsey JA: Respiratory muscle work compromises leg blood flow during maximal exercise. J Appl Physiol 1997;82:1573–1583.

130 Light RW, Mintz WM, Linden GS, Brown SE: Hemodynamics of patients with severe chronic obstructive pulmonary disease during progressive upright exercise. Am Rev Respir Dis 1984;130:391–395.
131 Mahler DA, Brent BN, Loke J, Zaret BL, Matthay RA: Right ventricular performance and central hemodynamics during upright exercise in patients with chronic obstructive pulmonary disease. Am Rev Respir Dis 1984; 130:722–729.
132 Oswald-Mammosser M, Apprill M, Bachez P, Ehrhart M, Weitzenblum E: Pulmonary hemodynamics in chronic obstructive pulmonary disease of the emphysematous type. Respiration 1991;58:304–310.
133 Magee F, Wright JL, Wiggs BR, Pare PD, Hogg JC: Pulmonary vascular structure and function in chronic obstructive pulmonary disease. Thorax 1988;43:183–189.
134 Agusti AGN, Barbera JA, Roca J, Wagner PD, Guitart R, Rodriguez-Roisin R: Hypoxic pulmonary vasoconstriction and gas exchange during exercise in chronic obstructive pulmonary disease. Chest 1990;97:268–275.
135 Matthay RA, Berger HJ, Davies RA, Loke J, Mahler DA, Gottschalk A, Zaret BL: Right and left ventricular exercise performance in chronic obstructive pulmonary disease: Radionuclide assessment. Ann Intern Med 1980;93:234–239.
136 Vizza CD, Lynch JP, Ochoa LL, Richardson G, Trulock EP: Right and left ventricular dysfunction in patients with severe pulmonary disease. Chest 1998;113:576–583.
137 Morrison DA, Adock K, Collins CM, Goldman S, Caldwell JH, Schwartz MI: Right ventricular dysfunction and the exercise limitation of chronic obstructive pulmonary disease. J Am Coll Cardiol 1987;9:1219–1229.
138 Dimopoulou I, Tsintzas OK, Daganou M, Cokkinos DV, Tzelepis GE: Contribution of lung function to exercise capacity in patients with chronic heart failure. Respiration 1999; 66:144–149.
139 Koskolou MD, Calbet JA, Radegran G, Roach RC: Hypoxia and the cardiovascular response to dynamic knee-extensor exercise. Am J Physiol 1997;272:H2655–2663.
140 Montes de Oca M, Rassulo J, Celli BR: Respiratory muscle and cardiopulmonary function during exercise in very severe COPD. Am J Respir Crit Care Med 1996;154:1284–1289.
141 Spence DPS, Hay JG, Pearson MG, Calverley PMA: Oxygen desaturation and breathlessness during corridor walking in chronic obstructive lung disease: Effect of oxitropium bromide. Thorax 1993;48:1145–1150.
142 Hay JG, Stone P, Carter J, Church S, Eyre-Brook A, Pearson M, Woodcock A, Calverley PMA: Bronchodilator reversibility, exercise performance and breathlessness in stable chronic obstructive pulmonary disease. Eur Respir J 1992;5:659–664.
143 Mahler DA, Mathay RA, Synder PE, Wells CK, Loke J: Sustained release theophylline reduces dyspnea in non-reversible obstructive airways disease. Am Rev Respir Dis 1985; 131:22–25.
144 Papiris S, Galavotti V, Sturani C: Effects of beta agonists on breathlessness and exercise tolerance in patients with chronic obstructive pulmonary disease. Respiration 1986;49: 101–108.
145 Oga T, Nishimura K, Tsukino M, Hajiro T, Ideda A, Izumi T: The effects of oxitropium bromide on exercise performance in patients with stable chronic obstructive pulmonary disease: A comparison of three different exercise tests. Am J Respir Crit Care Med 2000; 161:1897–1901.
146 O'Donnell DE, Forkert L, Webb KA: Evaluation of bronchodilator responses in patients with 'irreversible' emphysema. Eur Respir J 2001;in press.
147 O'Donnell DE: Assessment of bronchodilator efficacy in symptomatic COPD: Is spirometry useful? Chest 2000;117:S42–S47.
148 Chronos N, Adams L, Guz A: Effect of hyperoxia and hypoxia on exercise-induced breathlessness in normal subjects. Clin Sci 1988;74:531–537.
149 Lane R, Cockcroft A, Adams L, Guz A: Arterial oxygen saturation and breathlessness in patients with chronic obstructive airways disease. Clin Sci 1987;72:693–698.
150 Woodcock AA, Gross ER, Geddes DM: Oxygen relieves breathlessness in 'pink puffers'. Lancet 1981;i:907–909.
151 Stein DA, Bradley BL, Miller W: Mechanisms of oxygen effects on exercise in patients with chronic obstructive pulmonary disease. Chest 1982;81:6–10.
152 Libby DM, Biscoe WA, King TKC: Relief of hypoxia-related bronchoconstriction by breathing 30 percent oxygen. Am Rev Respir Dis 1981;123:171–175.
153 Dean NC, Brown JK, Himelman RB, Doherty JJ, Gold WM, Stuhlbarg MS: Oxygen may improve dyspnea and endurance in patients with chronic obstructive pulmonary disease and only mild hypoxemia. Am Rev Respir Dis 1992;148:941–945.
154 O'Donnell DE: Ventilatory limitations in chronic obstructive pulmonary disease. Med Sci Sports Exerc 2001;33(suppl 7):S647–S655.

Denis E. O'Donnell, MD, FRCP(I), FRCP(C)
Division of Respiratory and Critical Care Medicine
102 Stuart Street
Kingston, Ont. K7L 2V6 (Canada)
Tel. +1 613 548 2339, Fax +1 613 549 1459
E-Mail odonnell@post.queensu.ca

Weisman IM, Zeballos RJ (eds): Clinical Exercise Testing.
Prog Respir Res. Basel, Karger, 2002, vol 32, pp 159–172

The Importance of Exercise Training in Pulmonary Rehabilitation

Bartolome R. Celli

Pulmonary and Critical Care Division, St. Elizabeth's Medical Center, and
Tufts University School of Medicine, Boston, Mass., USA

Summary

Patients suffering from chronic respiratory diseases decrease their overall physical activity, because any form of exercise will often result in worsening dyspnea. The progressive deconditioning associated with inactivity initiates a vicious cycle where dyspnea increases, at ever lower physical demands. With time, the patients will also adopt a breathing pattern (usually fast and shallow) that is detrimental to overall gas exchange, which may in turn worsen their symptoms. In general, physical reconditioning is a broad therapeutic concept that has unfortunately been equated with simple lower extremity exercise training. In this chapter, I shall review the current knowledge regarding reconditioning in much broader terms. The effect and role of leg and arm training will be critically analyzed and practical recommendations will be given. Because I also believe it to be important, I shall review the concept of breathing retraining in its broad definition. A word of caution must be raised. The data which forms the basis of our current knowledge in terms of reconditioning, has been obtained from patients with intrinsic lung disease, such as emphysema, bronchitis, bronchiectasis, cystic fibrosis and acute respiratory failure. Very little is known about reconditioning in patients with pure 'pump failure', such as those with degenerative neuromuscular diseases. There is every reason to believe that, in these patients, physical exercise may worsen rather than improve their overall function and sensation of well being. On the other hand, pure breathing retraining, such as slow deep breathing, could have a more universal application as long as extra loads are not placed on already weakened and dysfunctional respiratory muscles. As will be reviewed in this chapter, patients with symptomatic 'pump failure' may benefit more from ventilatory assistance and resting than from further training. This chapter is organized with this in mind.

Physical Reconditioning

General Principles

The short- and long-term effects of systematic exercise conditioning has been the subject of extensive investigation and are addressed in detail in the chapter by Troosters T. et al., pp 60–71. However, I shall briefly review the topic as an introduction to the application of these concepts to patients with respiratory disease. In normal individuals, participation in an exercise-training program results in several objective changes: (1) there is increased maximal oxygen uptake, primarily due to increases in blood volume, hemoglobin and heart stroke volume with improvement in the peripheral utilization of oxygen; (2) with specific training there is increase in muscular strength and endurance, primarily, resulting from enlargement of muscle fibers and improved blood and energy supply; (3) better muscle coordination; (4) change in body composition with increased muscle mass and loss of adipose tissue, and (5) improved sensation of well-being. In patients with obstruction to airflow, participation in a similar program will result in different outcomes depending on the severity of the obstruction. Patients with mild-to-moderate disease will, as a rule, manifest the same findings as normals whereas, as we shall discuss later, patients with the severe form will be able to increase exercise endurance and improve their sensation of well-being with little if any increase in the maximal oxygen uptake. Very little is known regarding outcomes different from the specific effects of training on exercise performance in these patients. Similarly, once an effect has been shown, there has been little systematic information regarding the effect of maintenance programs on any of the outcomes, including exercise performance.

In patients with COPD, tolerance to exercise is decreased. The most important factors thought to contribute to this limitation of exercise in patients with COPD are: (1) alterations in pulmonary mechanics; (2) abnormal gas exchange; (3) dysfunction of the respiratory muscles; (4) alterations in cardiac performance; (5) malnutrition, and (6) development of dyspnea. Other factors deserve to be mentioned but are less well characterized. They include: active smoking, abnormal peripheral muscle function and polycythemia. Although the most severe patients cannot exercise to the levels where the training effect is thought to occur (above anaerobic threshold), a large body of evidence supports exercise training as a beneficial therapeutic tool useful in helping these patients achieve their full potential.

Physiologic Adaptation to Training

There are several principles that apply to exercise training, and we must understand them in the context of prescribing exercise to patients with severe pulmonary problems. They are: (1) specificity of training; (2) intensity and duration of the exercise load, and (3) detraining effect.

(1) Specificity of training. This principle is based on the observations that programs can be tailored to achieve specific goals and that the training of muscles or muscle groups is beneficial only to the trained muscle.

Utilization of high resistance, low repetition stimulus increases muscle strength (weight lifting), whereas low resistance, high repetition routines increase muscle endurance. Strength training is achieved by increasing myofibrils in certain muscle fibers whereas endurance training increases the number of capillaries and mitochondrial content in the trained muscles.

The training is specific to the trained muscle. Clausen et al. [1] trained subjects in their arms and legs and observed that the decreased heart rate observed for arm muscle training could not be transferred to the leg group and vice versa. Davies and Sargeant [2] showed that if training was completed for one leg, the beneficial effect could not be transferred to exercise involving the untrained leg. Belman and Kendregan [3] confirmed these findings in patients with COPD. They examined the effect of 6 weeks of training in 8 patients who only trained their arms and 7 patients who only trained their legs. They observed improved exercise only for the exercise for which the patients trained. Interestingly, they failed to see any changes in muscle enzyme content of biopsies taken before and after the exercise training program [3].

(2) Intensity, frequency and duration of the exercise load. These factors profoundly affect the degree of the training effect. Athletes will usually train at maximal or near maximal levels in order to rapidly achieve the desired effects. On the other hand, middle age nonathletes may require less intense exercise. Siegel et al. [4] showed that training sessions of 30 min close to 3 times a week for 15 weeks significantly improved maximal oxygen uptake if the heart rate was raised over 80% of the predicted maximal rate. In patients with chronic lung disease, the issue of exercise intensity and duration has been studied by different authors, as we shall review later, but it would appear that the larger the number of sessions and the more intense (as a function of maximal performance), the better the results.

In their work, Belman and Kendregan [3] exercised patients at 30% of maximal and after 6 weeks of 4 times weekly training where the load was increased as tolerated, they observed significant improvement in endurance time in 9 of the 15 patients. It is possible that the relatively low training level (30% of maximal) may help explain why 6 of their patients failed to increase the endurance time. In contrast, Niederman et al. [5] started the exercise at 50% of maximal cycle ergometer level and increased its intensity on a weekly basis and observed endurance improvement in most patients. In a very interesting study, Clark et al. [6] randomized 16 patients with COPD to a control group and 32 other patients to a daily training program lasting 12 weeks. The patients had moderate airflow obstruction (FEV_1 of 1.7 ± 0.3 liters). Training of the patients included isotonic endurance exercises of upper and lower extremity, and isokinetic muscle strength. After the 12 weeks, the patients in the exercise group improved their exercise endurance without worsening of dyspnea. The patients also increased their walked distance. This study is important because it raised the question whether moderate intensity strength training may induce beneficial changes similar or additive to those already described for classical endurance training.

Other authors have used higher starting exercise levels and have achieved a better endurance effect [7–11].

The best study in this regard is that of Casaburi et al. [11] who studied 19 patients with moderate COPD (mean ± SD FEV_1 of 1.8 ± 0.53 liters) who could achieve anaerobic threshold, before and after randomly assigned training at low intensity (50% of maximal) or high intensity (80% of maximal) exercise. The authors showed that the high intensity training program was more effective than the low intensity one. They also observed a decrease in ventilatory requirement for exercise after training, that was proportional to the drop in lactate at a given work rate. Using a different study design, Puente-Maestu et al. [12] randomized 35 patients with COPD (FEV_1 of 1.09 ± 0.17 liters) to either supervised training on a treadmill or to self-monitored walking program. Both groups trained four times a week. As expected, the intensity of training was different for the two groups (35 ± 10 vs. 70 ± 22 W). The mean endurance time at submaximal workload (70% of maximal pretraining workload) increased more in the supervised group when compared with the usual care one.

It seems that training is achieved if the intensity of exercise is higher than of minimal, and that the intensity of training can be increased as tolerated. In other words, any exercise is better than none, and indeed good results have been shown even for patients with minimal exercise performance when tested [9, 12]. However, more exercise induces larger changes [11, 12].

The number of exercise sessions is also a matter of debate [3, 13]. As shown in table 1, in general as the number of sessions is increased, so is the change in observed endurance time. Since stopping the exercise results in a loss of the training effect, the optimal plan should involve an intense training phase and a maintenance phase. This latter part is very difficult to implement and results in the frequently observed failure to maintain and preserve the beneficial effects achieved through the training. Unfortunately, there is no study in any respiratory disease that has addressed this important issue.

(3) Detraining effect. This principle is based on observations that the effect achieved by training is lost after the exercise is stopped. Saltin et al. [14] showed that bed rest in normal subjects resulted in a significant decrease in maximal oxygen uptake within 21 days of resting. It took between 10 and 50 days for the values to return to those seen before resting. Keens et al. [15] examined ventilatory muscle endurance after training in normal subjects who had undergone ventilatory muscle training. Within 1 month of having stopped training, the subjects had lost the training effect that they had achieved. Therefore, it seems important to continue to train, but the minimum practical and effective timing of maintenance training remains to be determined.

Table 1. Number of sessions of exercise in these studies that summarized the improvement in exercise endurance

Author	Sessions	Endurance change, %
Belman	45	50
Epstein	19	30
Make	12	12

Our exercise program is based on the data and concepts developed above. Patients are exercised at 70% of the maximal work achieved in a test day. This work is increased on a weekly basis as tolerated by the patient. We aim to complete 24 sessions. This is achieved in the outpatient setting by sessions held three times weekly. In contrast, the program may be completed quicker if the patient is in the hospital, because the sessions are completed on a daily basis. Each session lasts 30 min if tolerated by the patient, otherwise it is begun as tolerated by the patient and no further load is provided until the patient can complete the 30 min of the session. A close communication exists between the person in charge of the training and the rehabilitation planning team. In those settings where metabolic measurements are not possible, the use of the perception of dyspnea using a Borg visual analog scale can substitute a target work rate. This has been shown in a study of 15 patients by Horowitz et al. [16]. It is appealing to use dyspnea and not heart rate as the target to train patients with lung disease, as breathlessness constitutes their most important complaint.

Lower Extremity Exercise

A large number of studies have shown that the inclusion of leg exercise in the training of patients with lung disease is beneficial [18–21]. Cockcroft et al. [22] randomized 39 dyspneic patients younger than 70 years and not on oxygen to a treatment group that spent 6 weeks in a rehabilitation center, where they underwent gradual endurance exercise training, and a control group that received medical care but was given no special advice to exercise. The control group served as such for 4 months and was then admitted to the rehabilitation center for 6 weeks. Just like the treated patients, they were instructed

Table 2. Controlled studies of rehabilitation with exercise in patients with COPD

Author	Patients	Duration	Results
Cockroft	18 T	daily, 16 weeks	↑ 12 MW, VO_2
	16 C	–	no change
Sinclair	17 T	daily, 40 weeks	↑ FVC, ↑ 12 MW
	16 C	–	no change
O'Donnell	23 T	daily, 8 weeks	↑ FVC, ↑ 12 MW ↓ dyspnea
	13 C	–	no change
Reardon	10 T	2 ×/week, 6 weeks	↓ dyspnea
	10 C	–	no change
Ries	57 T	daily, 8 weeks	↑ exercise capacity ↓ dyspnea ↑ self efficacy
	62 C	daily, 8 weeks education	no change
Wijkstra	28 T	daily, 12 weeks at home	↑ exercise capacity ↑ quality of life
	15 C	–	no change
Goldstein	45 T	daily, 24 weeks	↑ 6MWD VO_2 ↓ dyspnea, ↓ S.O.B.
	44 C	none, 24 weeks	no change
Guell	30 T	daily, 12 weeks	↑ 6MWD ↓ dyspnea, ↑ QoL
	30 C	usual care	no change

T = Treated; C = controls; 12 MW = 12-min walk distance; 6MWD = 6-min walk distance; FVC = forced vital capacity; VO_2 = peak oxygen uptake.

to exercise at home afterward. Both groups were similar at baseline. After rehabilitation, only 2 of the 16 control patients manifested improvement in dyspnea and cough, whereas 16 of the 18 patients included in the treatment group manifested improvement in these symptoms. More importantly, the treated patients showed significant improvement in the 12-min walk and in the peak oxygen uptake when compared with the controls. In a different setting, Sinclair and Ingram [33] randomized 33 patients with chronic bronchitis and dyspnea to two groups. The 17 patients in the treatment group exercised by climbing up and down on two 24-cm steps twice daily. The exercise time was increased to tolerance. The patients exercised at home and were evaluated by the treatment team weekly. The control group did not exercise but were all reassessed after 6 months. There were no changes in the degree of airflow obstruction in either group. Similarly, there was no improvement in strength of the quadriceps, the minute ventilation and heart rate. In contrast, the 12-min walk test significantly increased in the patients that were trained. These two studies are particularly important in that they were well designed and used randomization in the assignment of patients to the specific treatment groups. O'Donnell et al. [24] compared breathlessness, 6-min walking distance and cycle ergometer work, between two age-matched groups of patients with moderate COPD. The endurance exercise trained group (n = 23) achieved significant reduction in dyspnea scores, and increased the distance walked as well as the cycle ergometry work, when compared to the control group (n = 13). This trial is important in that it not only documented increased endurance, but for the first time evaluated the patient's perception of dyspnea which is the most problematic symptom and the one leading to physical limitation.

Since those initial studies, several randomized trials have documented the beneficial effect of lower extremity exercise [25–27]. Perhaps the most important one is the study by Ries et al. [27]. In this study, 119 patients were randomized to an education support group (n = 62) or to a similar educational program with the addition of 3 times weekly walking exercise for 8 weeks (n = 57). At 2 months and still seen at 4, 6 and 12 months, the patient who exercised manifested increased exercise endurance, less dyspnea with exercise and with activity of daily living and statistically not significant increase in survival. More recently, Guell et al. [28] randomized 60 patients with moderate degree of COPD (FEV_1 of 35 ± 14% predicted) to either usual care without supervised exercise or pulmonary rehabilitation. Pulmonary rehabilitation included 3 months of five 30-min sessions every week of cycle ergometry, starting at 50% of the maximal load achieved during a baseline evaluation. The workload was progressively increased as tolerated. After 2 years, the 30 patients randomized to exercise not only manifested significant favorable differences compared with usual care in the distance walked over 6 min, but also in dyspnea and in the emotion component of the disease-specific Chronic Respiratory Questionnaire. These landmark studies have established the pivotal role of exercise in the proven benefit of pulmonary rehabilitation. The results of the most important studies are summarized in table 2.

Numerous studies using patients as their own controls have shown similar results, with significant increases in exercise endurance. The mechanism by which this improvement occurs remains a matter of debate. Several studies, including those of Paez et al. [21] and Mohsenifar et al. [7] have demonstrated a decrease in heart rate at a similar work level, a hallmark of a training effect for the specific exercise. This is perhaps related to a decrease in exercise lactate level as suggested by Woolf and Suero [29]. More recent evidence in support of a training effect is provided by the study of Casaburi et al. [11]. In their group of trained patients with COPD, they showed a reduction in exercise lactic acidosis and ventilation after patients were trained. Furthermore, the reduction was proportional to the intensity of the training. There was a 12% decrease in the lactic acidosis rise in patients trained with the low work rate (50% of maximum) and 32% decrease in the ones trained with the high work rate (80% of maximum). In both groups there were significant decreases in heart rate after training. Other studies have failed to document either an increase in maximum O_2 uptake, a decrease in heart rate or lactate at similar work level. The most important study in this group is the one by Belman and Kendregan [3] which failed to show a decrease in heart rate at the same workload as represented by the VO_2. These authors went further and analyzed muscle biopsies oxidative enzyme content before and after training. They observed no change in this parameter. Interestingly, 9 of the treated patients improved their exercise endurance. As stated previously, it is possible that this study used too low a training effort since training was started at 30% of the maximum achieved during their testing. That this may be so is supported by two studies from one same group [30, 31]. They first showed that muscle biopsies from the legs of patients with COPD had decreased content of oxidative enzymes in their mitochondria [30]. Subsequently, and extremely important for those that believe in the physiologic training, the mitochondrial enzymatic content significantly increased after exercise training [31]. In that same group of patients they also documented a delay of onset of the lactase threshold after training.

The evidence therefore indicates that patients with COPD can be trained to a level that produces physiologic changes consistent with improved muscle performance.

Two studies addressed the issue of whether patients with the most severe COPD can undergo exercise training. The reason for the question relates to the fact that many patients with the most severe COPD do not exercise to the intensity required to reach anaerobic threshold or to train the cardiovascular system. Niederman et al. [5] exercised 33 patients with different degrees of COPD (FEV_1 ranging from 0.33 to 3.82 l). When they evaluated the response to training, there was no correlation between the degree of obstruction and the observed improvement. In other words, the patients with very low FEV_1 were as likely to improve as the patients with high FEV_1. Similarly, ZuWallack et al. [10] evaluated 50 patients with COPD (FEV_1 range from 0.38 to 3.24 l) before and after exercise training. They observed an inverse relationship between the baseline 12-min walk distance and VO_2 and the improvement. They concluded that patients with poor performance on either the 12-min walking distance or maximal exercise test are not necessarily poor candidates for an exercise program. Couser et al. [32] evaluated whether age could be a factor limiting exercise training. In a large cohort of patients, the authors noted that endurance, as measured by the 6-min walked distance, increased in a similar proportion after exercise training in older (>75 years) compared with younger (<75 years) patients. From this data, it seems prudent to conclude that any patient capable of undergoing leg exercise endurance training will benefit from a program that includes leg exercise.

As to the type of exercise training to be prescribed and the testing modality, again different studies have used different training techniques. Most studies include walking both as a measurement of exercise tolerance and of the training program. The classic 6- or 12-min walk (6 or 12 MWD) where the distance walked over 6 or 12 min is recorded is very good for patients with moderate-to-severe COPD but may not be taxing enough for patients with a lesser degree of airflow obstruction [33]. In at least one study, the 12 MWD has been shown to predict survival. We have evaluated stair climbing and shown that the peak oxygen uptake can be estimated from the number of steps climbed during a symptom-limited test [34]. Several studies have used treadmill testing and/or step testing even though the training has been done with the patient walking. Oxygen uptake is higher for stair climbing or treadmill testing than for the more commonly used leg ergometry presumably because the former uses more body muscles than leg cycling. Leg ergometry has become very popular in its use as a testing device and has been the training apparatus for most recent studies. It is certainly smaller than the treadmill and with relatively inexpensive units in the market, it is possible to place several together and train groups of patients simultaneously.

All the studies quoted relied on either in-hospital or out-patient hospital training. Very little information exists regarding implementation of such programs at home. In an unique report, O'Hara et al. [35] enrolled 14 patients with moderate COPD (FEV_1 of 1.17 ± 0.76 l) in a home exercise program. The authors randomized the patients to daily walking while carrying a light weight

Table 3. Training method for leg exercise

1	Train at 60–70% of maximal work capacity*
2	Increase work every 5th session as tolerated
3	Monitor: dyspnea heart rate
4	Increase work after 20–30 min of submaximal targeted work is achieved
5	Aim for 24 sessions

* Work capacity as determined by an exercise test, not necessarily by evaluating heart rate (see text for discussion).

backpack (2.6 ± 0.5 kg) or the same backpacking regime with additional weight lifting and strength limb exercises. These included wrist curl, arms curls, partial leg squats, calf raises and supine dumbbell press. The initial load was 4.3 ± 0.9 kg and was increased weekly by 1.2 ± 0.5 kg for 6 weeks to reach 10.4 ± 2.6 kg by the last week. The weight lifters performed 10 repetitions three times avoiding dyspnea, breatholding and fatigue for a total time of 30 min daily. Patients documented their exercises in a diary. Health care personnel visited the patients on a weekly basis. After training, all weight lifters had reduced their minute ventilation during bicycle ergometry, when compared with controls. Furthermore, the weight-trained patients showed a 16% increase in exercise endurance. This study suggests that exercise training can be achieved at home with relatively inexpensive programs, with the beneficial consequence of no hospital visits and in the comfort of a home. This initial report is supported by recent data that supervised exercise at home achieves the same outcomes as that obtained in the hospitals [36].

In our pulmonary rehabilitation program, we complete testing in an electrically braked ergometer while the training is done in mechanically controlled ergometers, either as an out-patient or as an in-patient depending on the patient's condition. Table 3 practically describes how we train our patients. The program may be tailored to each individual and to the available training equipment.

Upper Extremity Exercise

As stated before, most of our knowledge about exercise conditioning in patients undergoing rehabilitation is derived from programs emphasizing leg training. This is unfortunate, because the performance of many everyday tasks requires not only the hands, but also the concerted action of other muscle groups that partake in upper torso and arm positioning. Some of the muscles of the upper torso and shoulder girdle serve a dual function (respiratory and postural). Muscles such as the upper and lower trapezius, latissimus dorsi, serratus anterior, subclavius, pectoralis minor and major possess a thoracic and an extrathoracic anchoring point. Depending on the anchoring point they may help position the arms or shoulder or if given an extra thoracic fulcrum (such as fixing the arms in a supported position) they may exert a pulling force on the rib cage. We have shown that in patients with chronic airflow obstruction, as severity worsens, the diaphragm loses its force-generating capacity and the muscles of the rib cage become more important in the generation of inspiratory pressures [37]. When patients perform unsupported arm exercise, some of the shoulder girdle muscles have to decrease their participation in ventilation and if the task involves complex purposeful arm movements, the pattern of ventilation may be affected. Tangri and Wolf [38] used a pneumobelt to study breathing patterns in 7 patients with COPD while they performed simple activities of daily living such as tying their shoes and brushing their teeth. The patients developed an irregular and rapid pattern of breathing with the arm exercise. After the exercise, the patients breathed faster and deeper, which according to the authors was done to restore the blood gases to normal. We have explored the ventilatory response to unsupported arm exercise and compared it with the response to leg exercise in patients with severe chronic lung disease [39]. Arm exercise resulted in a dyssynchronous thoracoabdominal excursion that was not solely due to diaphragmatic fatigue. The dyspnea that was reported by the patients was associated with a dyssynchronous breathing pattern. We concluded that unsupported arm exercise could shift work to the diaphragm and in some way lead to dyssynchrony. To test this hypothesis, we have used pleural pressure (Ppl) versus gastric pressure (Pg) plots (with a gastric and endoesophageal balloon) and evaluated the changes as well as the ventilatory response to unsupported arm exercise and compared it to leg cycle ergometry in normal subjects and patients with airflow obstruction [40, 41]. We documented increased diaphragmatic pressure excursion with arm exercise and alterations in the pattern of pressure generation with more contribution by the diaphragm and abdominal muscles of respiration and less contribution by the inspiratory muscles of the rib cage.

Our knowledge of ventilatory response to arm exercise was based on arm cycle ergometry. It is known that at a given work load in normal subjects arm cranking is more demanding than leg cycling as shown by higher VO_2, V_E, heart rate, blood pressure and lactate production [42–44].

At maximal effort, however, VO_2, V_E, cardiac output and lactate levels are lower during arm than leg cycle ergometry [45, 46]. Very little is known about the metabolic and ventilatory cost of simple arm elevation. Some recent reports underscore the importance of arm position in ventilation. Banzett et al. [47] showed that arms bracing increases the capacity to sustain maximal ventilation when compared to lifting the elbows from the braced position. Others have shown a decrease in the maximum attainable workload and increases in oxygen uptake and ventilation at any given workload when normal subjects exercised with their arms elevated [48, 49]. We evaluated the metabolic and respiratory consequence of simple arm elevation in patients with COPD [50]. Elevation of the arms to 90° in front of them results in a significant increase in VO_2 and VCO_2. There were concomitant increases in heart rate and V_E. When ventilatory muscle recruitment patterns were evaluated with the use of continuous recording of Pg and Ppl, there was a shift in the contribution to ventilation by the different muscle groups, toward increased diaphragmatic and abdominal muscle use. The observations suggest that if we trained the arms to perform more work or if we decreased the ventilatory requirement for the same work, we should improve the patient's capacity to perform arm activity.

There are several studies that have utilized both arm and leg training and have shown that the addition of arm training results in improved performance and that the improved performance is for the most part task specific. In their study, Belman and Kendregan [3] showed a significant increase in arm exercise endurance after exercise training. Lake et al. [51] randomized patients to arm exercise, leg exercise and arm and leg exercise. There were increases for arm ergometry in the arm group, for leg ergometry in the leg group and increased improvement in sensation of well-being when both exercises were combined. Ries et al. [52] studied the effect of two forms of arm exercise: gravity-resistance and modified proprioceptive neuromuscular facilitation and compared them with no arm exercise in a group of 45 patients with COPD who were involved in a comprehensive, multidisciplinary pulmonary rehabilitation program. Even though only 20 patients completed the program, they showed improved performance on tests that were specific for the training. The patients reported a decrease in the fatigue in all tests performed. It is worth pointing out that in the study of Keens et al. [15], a group of patients with cystic fibrosis underwent upper extremity training consisting of swimming and canoeing for 1.5 h daily. At the end of 6 weeks, there was increased upper extremity endurance, but, most importantly, there was an increase in maximal sustainable ventilatory capacity that was similar to that obtained with ventilatory muscle training. This suggests that ventilatory muscles could be trained by using an arm exercise training program.

Because simple arm elevation results in a significant increase in V_E, VO_2 and VCO_2, we studied 14 patients with COPD before and after 8 weeks of 3 times weekly 20-min sessions of unsupported arm and leg exercise as part of a comprehensive rehabilitation program. In this study, we wanted to test whether arm training decreases ventilatory requirement for arm activity. After training, there was a 35% decrease in the rise of VO_2 and VCO_2 brought about by arm elevation. This was associated with a significant decrease in V_E [53]. Because the patients also trained their legs, we could not conclude that the improvement was due to the arm exercise. To answer this question, we have recently completed a study of 26 patients with COPD that were randomized to either unsupported arm training (11 patients) or resistance breathing training (14 patients). After 24 sessions, arm endurance increased only for the unsupported arm training group and not for resistance breathing. Interestingly, maximal inspiratory pressure increased significantly for both groups, indicating that by training the arms, we could be inducing ventilatory muscle training for those muscles of the rib cage that hinge on the shoulder girdle [54].

Based on the information available, we include arm exercise in our rehabilitation program. As seen in table 4 and 5, the methods for supported and unsupported arm vary in their implementation. Arm ergometry is performed for 20 min per session. We start at 60% of the maximal work achieved in the exercise test. The work is increased weekly as tolerated. Dyspnea and heart rate are monitored. Maximal work capacity is defined as the watts that the patient is capable of achieving. If the patient's limiting symptom is dyspnea at minimal work, we exercise him at 60% of the work that makes him stop. In the most severe patients, the heart rate is unreliable since they may be tachycardic even at rest and may not show any significant increase with exercise. In these patients, dyspnea may be a more reliable index to follow. In contrast, unsupported arm exercise training is achieved by having the patient lift a dowel (750 g in weight) to shoulder level at the same rhythm as the patient's breathing rate. The sequence is repeated for 2 min with a 2-min resting period. The exercises are repeated for 30 min. Dyspnea and heart rate are then monitored. The load is increased by 250 g weekly as tolerated. We aim to complete 24 sessions. Martinez et al. [55] compared unsupported arm

Table 4. Training methods for supported (ergometry) arm exercise training

1	Train at 50–60% of maximal work capacity*
2	Increase work every 5th session as tolerated
3	Monitor: dyspnea heart rate
4	Train for as long as tolerated up to 30 min

* Work capacity as determined by an exercise test, not necessarily by evaluating heart rate (see text for discussion).

Table 5. Method for unsupported arm training

1	Dowl (weight = 750 g)
2	Lift to shoulder level for 2 min; rate equal to breathing rate
3	Rest for 2 min
4	Repeat sequence as tolerated for up to 32 min
5	Monitor: dyspnea heart rate
6	Increase weight (250 g) every 5th session as tolerated

training with arm ergometry training in a randomized clinical trial. Total endurance time improved significantly for both groups, but unsupported arm training decreased oxygen uptake at the same workload when compared to arm cranking training. They concluded that arm exercise against gravity may be more effective in training patients for activities that resemble those used during daily living.

An increasing body of evidence (table 6) indicates that upper extremity exercise training results in improved performance for arm activities. There also is a drop in the ventilatory requirements for similar upper extremity activities. All this should result in an improvement in the capacity of the patients to perform activities of daily living.

Conclusion

This first section reviewed the physiological correlates of exercise training and addressed the specific training of legs and arms. A critical review of the literature indicates that exercise conditioning that includes leg and arm training, improves exercise performance and seems to have physiological explanations different from simple dys-

Table 6. Controlled studies of arm exercise in patients with chronic obstructive lung disease

Authors	Patients	Duration	Course and type	Results
Keens	7 arms 4 VMT 4 control	1.5 h q.d. 4 weeks 15 min q.d. 4 weeks –	swimming/canoeing VMT sham	↑ VMT (56%) ↑ VME(52%) ↑ VME (22%)
Belman	8 arms 7 legs	20 min 4 ×/week 20 min 4×/week 6 weeks	arm ergometry cycle ergometry	↑ arm cycle, no ↑ PFT ↑ leg cycle, no ↑ PFT
Lake	6 arms 6 leg 7 arms and legs	1 h 3×/week 8 weeks 1 h 8 weeks 1 h 3×/week	several types walking combined	no change PI_{max} VME no change PI_{max} VME no change PI_{max} VME
Ries	8 gravity resistance arms 9 neuromuscular facilitation 11 controls	15 min q.d. 6 weeks 15 min q.d. 6 weeks –	low resistance, high repitition weight lifts 6 weeks walk	↑ arm endurance ↓ dyspnea ↑ arm endurance ↓ dyspnea no change
Epstein	13 arm 10 VMT	30 min q.d. 8 weeks 30 min q.d. 8 weeks	UAE VMT	↓ VO_2 and VE for arm elevation ↑ PI_{max} ↑ PI_{max} and VME

VMT = Ventilatory muscle training; VME = ventilatory muscle endurance; PFT = pulmonary function tests; PI_{max} = maximal inspiratory pressure.

pnea desensitization. The practical aspects of implementation of an exercise program within the context of pulmonary rehabilitation are reviewed. They are reachable by anyone interested in them and result in a rewarding component of any program.

Respiratory Muscles and Breathing Training

It was Leith and Bradley [56] who first demonstrated that, like their skeletal counterparts, the respiratory muscles of normal individuals could be specifically trained to improve their strength or their endurance. Subsequent to that observation, multiple studies have shown that a training response will occur if there is enough of a stimulus. An increase in inspiratory muscle strength (and perhaps endurance) should result in improved respiratory muscle function by decreasing the ratio of the pressure required to breath or P_i and the maximal pressure that the respiratory system can generate or Pi_{max} (P_I/PI_{max}). This ratio, which represents the effort required to complete each breath, as a function of the force reserve, has been shown to be the most important determinant for the development of fatigue in loaded respiratory muscles [57]. Since reduced inspiratory muscle strength is evident in patients with COPD, considerable efforts have been made to define the role of respiratory muscle training in these patients.

Ventilatory Muscle Strength and Endurance Training

Strength Training

To achieve this goal a high-intensity, low-frequency stimulus is needed. Inspiratory muscles are trained by inspiratory maneuvers being performed against a closed glottis or shutter. Several studies have shown an increase in maximal inspiratory pressures when the respiratory muscles have been specifically trained for strength. Lecoq et al. [58] studied 9 patients (some of whom had COPD) and after 4 weeks showed a 50% increase in PI_{max}. Reid et al. [59] observed a 53% increase in Pi_{max} in 6 COPD patients after 5 weeks of training [55]. Both groups noticed a smaller but significant increase in expiratory muscle pressure. The clinical importance of strength training for the respiratory muscles has not been explored and, although theoretically important (decreasing P_I/PI_{max}), it has not been shown to play a clinical role. It is nevertheless important to point out that respiratory muscle strength has been shown to increase as a by-product of the endurance training achieved with the use of resistive loads. It is then possible that some of the observed benefits reported after endurance training may relate to the increased strength.

Endurance Training

This is achieved by low-intensity, high-frequency training programs. The programs that have been used are of 3 types: flow resistive loading, threshold loading, and voluntary isocapneic hyperpnea.

Flow Resistive and Threshold Loading

In flow resistive training, the load has consisted mainly of decreasing inspiratory breathing hole size. The load will increase provided that frequency, tidal volume and inspiratory time are held constant. Although most studies in patients with COPD have shown an improvement in the time that a given respiratory load can be maintained (ventilatory muscle endurance), the results have to be interpreted with caution since it has been shown that endurance can be influenced and actually increased with changes in the pattern of breathing. Threshold loading has been employed and has been shown to result in some muscle training. This is done by assuring that at least the inspired pressure is high enough to ensure training, independent of inspiratory flow rate. Although breathing pattern is important (inspiratory time or T_I and respiratory rate), it is not as critically important. Many studies have not been controlled and it is very difficult to interpret the results as a product of the training. The controlled studies summarized in table 7 have shown an increase in the endurance time that the ventilatory muscles could tolerate a known load, some of them have shown a significant increase in strength [60–68] and a decrease in dyspnea to inspiratory load and exercise [54, 66]. In the studies where systemic exercise performance was evaluated, there was a minimal increase in walking distance [60–62, 67–70]. In a recent study, Weiner et al. [70] randomized 36 COPD patients to 3 groups. Group 1 received specific ventilatory muscle threshold training (VMT) combined with general exercise reconditioning. Group 2 received exercise training alone while group 3 received no training. VM training improved VM strength and endurance (as is already known), but patients treated with the combination of exercise and VMT manifested a significant increase in exercise tolerance when compared with those who only exercised. In a companion article, the same group reported that asthmatic patients treated with VM training not only increased strength but also showed an improvement in asthma symptoms, hospitalizations, emergency department visits, school or work absenteeism and medication consumption [71]. Lisboa et al. [69] have shown

Table 7. Controlled trials of ventilatory muscle resistive training in COPD

Author	Patients	Type	Frequency	Duration	Results
Pardy	9	RB	BID	8 weeks	↑ ET, ↑ 12 MW
	8	PT	3×/week	8 weeks	no change
Larson	10	RB	QD 30% PI_{max}	8 weeks 30 min	↑ PI_{max}, ↑ ET ↑ 12 MW
	12	RB	QD 15% PI_{max}	8 weeks 30 min	no ↑ in PI, end time or 12 MW
Harver	10	RB	BID	8 weeks 15 min	↑ PI_{max}
	9	sham	BID	8 weeks 15 min	no change
Belman	8	RB	QD	6 weeks	↑ ET, 30 min, ↑ PI_{max}
	9	RB	QD	6 weeks	30 min
Chen	7	RB	QD	4 weeks	↑ ET (30 min)
	6	sham	QD	4 weeks	no change (30 min)
Bjerre	14	RB	QD	6 weeks 45 min	↑ ET no exercise
	14	sham	QD	6 weeks 45 min	no change
Falk	12	RB	QD	12 months	↑ ET (45 min) no exercise change
	15	sham	QD	12 months	no change
Noseda	12	RB	QD	8 weeks	↑ ET (30 min)
	13	breathing exercises	QD	8 weeks	no change
Jones	7	RB	QD	10 weeks	↑ EE (30 min)
	6	sham	QD	10 weeks	↑ EE
	8	exercise	QD	10 weeks	↑ EE
Weiner	12	RB + exercise	QD	3 months	↑↑ exercise, ↑ PI_{max}
	12	exercise	QD	3 months	↑ exercise
	12	control	none	3 months	no change
Lisboa	10	RB 12% PI_{max}	QD	5 weeks	no change
	10	RB 30% Pi_{max}	QD	5 weeks	↑ Pi_{max}, ↑ ET ↓ dyspnea

RB = Resistive breathing; PT = physical therapy; ET = endurance time for loaded breathing; PI_{max} = maximal inspiratory pressure; BID = twice daily; QD = once daily; EE = leg exercise endurance.

that VMT at 30% of Pi_{max} seem to not only increase leg ergometry endurance, but also improve baseline dyspnea score and breathlessness with exercise.

From the data obtained, it is clear that VMT with resistive breathing results in improved VM strength and endurance. In COPD, it is not clear whether this effort results in decreased morbidity or mortality, or offers any clinical advantage that makes it worth the effort. In many of the studies, compliance was low with up to 50% of patients failing to complete the studies. On the other hand, if confirmed by others, the studies by Weiner et al. [71] and Lisboa et al. [69] suggest that this form of treatment for certain patients should be further explored.

Ventilatory Isocapneic Hyperpnea

This is a training method by which patients maintain high levels of ventilation over time (15 min, 2 or 3 times daily). The oxygen and carbon dioxide are kept constant in the breathing circuit. The results of an uncontrolled study showed that after 6 weeks of training, the patients with COPD not only increased their maximal sustained ventilatory capacity but also increased arm and leg exercise performance [72]. Two controlled studies [73, 74] (table 8) also reported increases in MSVC in COPD in patients trained for 6 weeks, but their exercise endurance was not better than the improvement observed in the control group.

It seems that respiratory muscle training results in increased strength and capacity of the muscles to endure a respiratory load. There is debate as to whether it also results in improved exercise performance or in performance of activities of daily living. From the respiratory muscle factors that may contribute to ventilatory limitation in COPD, it seems logical to predict that increases in strength and endurance should help respiratory muscle function but this is perhaps only important in the capacity of the patients to handle inspiratory loads, for example in acute exacerbations of their disease. It is less likely that ventilatory muscle training will greatly impact on systemic exercise performance.

Table 8. Controlled trials of ventilatory isocapneic hyperpnea in patients with COPD

Authors	Patients	Type	Frequency	Duration	Results
Ries	5	VIH	45 min	6 weeks	↑ MSVC ↑ exercise
	7	Walking	45 min	6 weeks	↑ exercise
Levine	15	VIH	15 min	6 weeks	↑ MSVC ↑ exercise ↑ ADL
	17	IPPB	15 min	6 weeks	↑ ADL ↑ exercise

VIH = Ventilatory isocapneic hyperpnea; MSVC = maximal sustainable ventilatory capacity; ADL = activities of daily living; IPPB = intermittent positive pressure breathing.

Ventilatory Muscle Training in the Patient in Intensive Care

Very little objective data exist that allow a valid conclusion for this important question. It is apparent that as soon as a patient is left to breathe on his own (as during any form of weaning), the respiratory muscles are being retrained. Unconsciously, we have been using this methodology when we placed patients on T-piece or low synchronized mandatory intermittent ventilation (SIMV), but we have not analyzed results in terms of this being a training method. More often, we think of training in terms of the addition of an external load above and beyond spontaneous respiration. There is very little experience in patients who have or are recovering from ventilatory failure. Belman [75] reported improvement in 2 patients. In a larger but still uncontrolled study, Aldrich et al. [76] recruited 30 patients with stable chronic respiratory failure for at least 3 weeks who failed repeated weaning attempts. Patients with active infections or unstable cardiovascular, renal or endocrine problems were not included. The authors also excluded patients with gross malnutrition (albumin <2.5 g/dl) and/or neuromuscular disease. The patients were intermittently trained by having them breathe through one inspiratory resistor while the patients spontaneously breathed or were supported 2–8 breaths per minute with synchronized mandatory ventilation (SIMV). In these patients maximal inspiratory pressure or P_{Imax} improved from -37 ± 15 to -46 ± 15 cm H_2O while vital capacity increased from 561 ± 325 to 901 ± 480 ml. Of the 30 patients, 12 were weaned after 10–46 days of training (40% success). Because it is uncontrolled and used a selected group of patients, these findings may not apply to most patients recovering from respiratory failure, and the success rate is not much different from those reported in weaning facilities that have not used VMT [77]. In spite of these encouraging reports, before ventilatory muscle training can be recommended as a form of treatment for patients with respiratory failure, more vigorous studies need to be completed.

Finally, it is important to state that ventilatory muscle training, specially with resistive or threshold loading, may be deleterious. It has been shown that breathing at high P_I/P_{Imax} or prolonged T_I/T_{tot} may induce muscle fatigue [78]. In patients with COPD, fatigue may precipitate ventilatory failure because the muscles of ventilation cannot be rested, as is customary in the training of peripheral muscles in athletes. Increased P_I is an intrinsic part of VMT, hence it is possible that if an intense enough program is enforced, fatigue may actually be precipitated.

Breathing Retraining

There are other less conventional forms of training that are open to critical review but that are conceptually solid and may offer new avenues of treatment. As we have seen, the ventilated patient has a high ventilatory drive. As a matter of fact, it has been shown that patients who failed a ventilator weaning trial, manifest higher drive than those patients who successfully weaned. Although limited, we shall review the available data.

Table 9. Work of breathing, exercise endurance and maximal transdiaphragmatic pressure before and after pulmonary rehabilitation

	Endurance time, s	∫ Pesdt cm $H_2O \cdot min^{-1}$	Pdi_{max} cm H_2O
Pre-rehab	434	288	48
Post-rehab	512*	219*	52

F Pesdt = Work of breathing as estimated by the pressure time index calculated from continuous recording of endoesophageal pressure (Ppl); Pdi_{max} = maximal transdiaphragmatic pressure.

* $p < 0.05$.

Biofeedback. In a relatively large study, Holliday and Hyers [79] studied 40 patients after at least 7 days of mechanical ventilation. They were randomized to conventional weaning or weaning with the use of electromyographic feedback training using the frontalis signal as indicative of tension and to induce relaxation. They also used surface EMG of intercostals and diaphragm as indicators of respiratory muscle activity. Using feedback signals to encourage relaxation and larger tidal volumes, there were differences between treated and untreated patients. The results indicate a reduction in mean ventilator days for the biofeedback group. Tidal volume and mean inspiratory flow increased significantly for this group. The increase was also significant when corrected by diaphragmatic EMG amplitude, which was interpreted as improved diaphragmatic efficiency. The authors concluded that breathing retraining resulted in a more efficient breathing pattern which in turn decreased dyspnea and anxiety and allowed for quicker weaning time in the treated patients [79]. We have studied some of these factors. Work of breathing, as determined by the pressure time integral of the excursions of the continuously recorded P_{pl}, was measured before and after rehabilitation in 16 patients with COPD. In these patients, there were no changes in pulmonary functions but there was a significant decrease in the pressure time index at the exercise isotime after rehabilitation (table 9). This drop was mostly due to a decrease in respiratory frequency [80]. Finally, retraining in breathing techniques or pursed lip breathing that decreases breathing frequency has been shown to result in increases in tidal volume oxygen saturation and decreases in dyspnea.

In the previously referred work by Epstein et al. [81] from our lab, analysis of the many factors that may have contributed to improved exercise endurance for upper extremity exercise after upper extremity training the most striking was a drop in VT/TI at exercise isotime. We believe this may represent better coordination of the respiratory muscles.

Yoga. There are other ways to alter ventilatory patterns to more effective ones. Yoga is a philosophical doctrine that includes control of posture and voluntary control of breathing. The latter includes slow deep breaths with apnea at end of inspiration and expiration and/or utilization of rapid abdominal maneuvers. The breathing rate may be brought down to 4–6 breaths per minute. Stanescu et al. [82] compared the breathing patterns of 8 well-trained yoga practitioners with 8 controls matched for sex, age and height. The yoga group had a pattern of breathing characterized by ample tidal volume and slow breathing frequency. They also had a lower ventilatory response to CO_2 rebreathing. The mechanism by which this seems to concur is not clear. They include habituation to chronic overstimulation of stretch receptors. Again, it is possible that since ventilation is automatically controlled by structures in the upper medulla and brain stem and voluntarily by the cortex, sustained slow deep breathing may become a 'learned' reflex. Whatever the mechanism, this may have applications. Tandon [83] studied patients with CAO trained in yoga breathing and compared them with controls. The patients better controlled dyspnea and improved their exercise tolerance.

Postural Changes. It is known that musculoskeletal tone and contraction may be determined by habitual positioning. Over the last few years, increasing attention has been given to the voluntary inhibition of those patterns. This has been particularly useful for artists. Recently, Austin et al. [84] demonstrated improved peak expiratory flow rate, maximal voluntary ventilation and maximal inspiratory and expiratory pressures in normal subjects who underwent lessons in proprioceptive musculoskeletal education compared to controls. This lessons per se have not been systematically evaluated in patients with lung disease but breathing retraining (pursed lip breathing and diaphragmatic breathing) constitutes a form of therapy that resembles the above-discussed techniques.

Pursed Lip Breathing. Indeed, pursed lip breathing results in slowing of the breathing rate with increases in tidal volume. As Roa et al. [85] showed in our laboratory, PLB will result in a shift in the pattern of recruitment of the ventilatory muscles from one that is predominantly diaphragmatic to one that recruits more the accessory muscles of the rib cage and abdominal muscles of exhalation. Perhaps this shift may contribute to the relief dyspnea that has been reported by patients when this breathing technique is adopted. Patients on ventilators cannot purse lip breath but it has been shown that the administration of respiratory retard or positive end expiratory pressure improves oxygenation, decreases respiratory rate, augments ventilation and improves work of breathing in weaning patients. PLB and PEEP may have similar physiologic effects and make the former therapy indicated once the latter has been discontinued.

In summary, there are more unresolved questions than absolute facts in the area of training and respiratory muscle function. A wealth of information remains to be gained if systematic scientific analysis is applied to answer many of the questions we have addressed in this review. It is rewarding to see that widespread interest in applied respiratory physiology has begun to produce results that may benefit the large number of patients suffering from disabling respiratory diseases and for whom there are no other viable therapeutic options. There is every reason to believe that all of us involved in direct patient care will be able to apply relatively simple programs that will enhance their quality of life.

References

1 Clausen JP, Clausen K, Rasmussen B, Trap-Jensen J: Central and peripheral circulatory changes after training of the arms or legs. Am J Physiol 1973;225:675–682.

2 Davis CT, Sargeant AJ: Effects of training on the physiological responses to one and two legged work. J Appl Physiol 1975;38:377–381.

3 Belman MJ, Kendregan BA: Exercise training fails to increase skeletal muscle enzymes in patients with chronic obstructive pulmonary disease. Am Rev Respir Dis 1981;123:256–261.

4 Siegel W, Blonquist G, Mitchell JH: Effects of a quantitated physical training program on middle-aged sedentary man. Circulation 1970;41:19–29.

5 Niederman MS, Clemente PH, Fein A, et al: Benefits of a multidisciplinary pulmonary rehabilitation program. Improvements are independent of lung function. Chest 1991;99:798–804.

6 Clark CJ, Cochrane E, Mackay E: Low intensity peripheral muscle conditioning improves exercise tolerance and breathlessness in COPD. Eur Repir J 1996;9:2590–2596.

7 Mohsenifar Z, Horak D, Brown H, Koerner SK: Sensitive indices of improvement in a pulmonary rehabilitation program. Chest 1983;83:189–192.

8 Holle RH, Williams DB, Vandree JC, Starks GL, Schoene RB: Increased muscle efficiency and sustained benefits in an outpatient community hospital-based pulmonary rehabilitation program. Chest 1988;94:1161–1168.

9 Zack M, Palange A: Oxygen supplemented exercise of ventilatory and nonventilatory muscles in pulmonary rehabilitation. Chest 1985;88:669–675.

10 ZuWallack RL, Patel K, Reardon JZ, Clark BA, Normandin EA: Predictors of improvement in the 12-minute walking distance following a six-week outpatient pulmonary rehabilitation program. Chest 1991;99:805–808.

11 Casaburi R, Patessio A, Ioli F, Zanabouri S, Donner C, Wasserman K: Reductions in exercise lactic acidosis and ventilation as a result of exercise training in patients with obstructive lung disease. Am Rev Respir Dis 1991;143:9–18.

12 Puente-Maestu L, Sanz M, Sanz P, Ruiz de Ona JM, Rodriguez-Hermosa JL, Whipp B: Effects of two types of training on pulmonary and cardiac responses to moderate exercise in patients with COPD. Eur Respir J 2000;15:1026–1032.

13 Make BJ, Buchholz J: Exercise training in COPD patients improves cardiac function. Am Rev Respir Dis 1991;143:80A.

14 Saltin B, Blomquist G, Mitchell JH, et al: Response to exercise after bed rest and training. Circulation 1968;38:1–78.

15 Keens TG, Krastins IR, Wannamaker EM, Levinson H, Crozier DN, Bryan AC: Ventilatory muscle endurance training in normal subjects and patients with cystic fibrosis. Am Rev Respir Dis 1977;116:853–860.

16 Horowitz MB, Littenberg B, Mahler D: Dyspnea ratings for prescribing exercise intensity in patients with COPD. Chest 1997;109:1169–1175.

17 Moser KM, Bokinsky GC, Savage RT, et al: Results of comprehensive rehabilitation programs. Arch Int Med 1980;140:1596–1601.

18 Beaumont A, Cockcroft A, Guz A: A self-paced treadmill walking test for breathless patients. Thorax 1985;40:459–464.

19 Christie D: Physical training in chronic obstructive lung disease. Br Med J 1968;2:150–151.

20 Hughes RL, Davidson R: Limitations of exercise reconditioning in COPD. Chest 1983;83:241–249.

21 Paez PN, Phillipson EA, Mosangkay M, et al: The physiologic basis of training patients with emphysema. Am Rev Respir Dis 1967;95:944–953.

22 Cockcroft AE, Saunders MJ, Berry G: Randomized controlled trial of rehabilitation in chronic respiratory disability. Thorax 1981;36:200–203.

23 Sinclair DJ, Ingram CG: Controlled trial of supervised exercise training in chronic bronchitis. Br Med J 1980;1:519–521.

24 O'Donnell DE, Webb HA, McGuire MA: Older patients with COPD: Benefits of exercise training. Geriatrics 1993;48:59–66.

25 Goldstein RS, Gork EH, Stubing D, et al: Randomized trial of respiratory rehabilitation. Lancet 1994;344:1394–1398.

26 Reardon J, Awad E, Normandin E, et al: The effect of comprehensive outpatient pulmonary rehabilitation on dyspnea. Chest 1994;105:1046–1048.

27 Ries AZ, Kaplan R, Linberg T, et al: Effects of pulmonary rehabilitation on physiologic and psychosocial outcomes in patients with chronic obstructive pulmonary disease. Ann Intern Med 1995;122:823–827.

28 Guell R, Casan P, Belda J, Sangenis P, Morante F, Guyatt G, Sanchis J: Long-term effects of outpatient rehabilitation in COPD. Chest 2000;117:976–983.

29 Woolf CR, Suero JT: Alterations in lung mechanics and gas exchange following training in chronic obstructive lung disease. Chest 1969;55:37–44.

30 Maltais F, Simard A, Simard J, Jobin J, Desgagnes P, and LeBlanc P: Oxidative capacity of the skeletal muscle and lactic acid kinetics during exercise in normal subjects and in patients with COPD. Am J Respir Crit Care Med 1995;153:288–293.

31 Maltais F, Leblanc P, Simard C, et al: Skeletal muscle adaptation to endurance training in patients with chronic obstructive pulmonary disease. Am J Respir Crit Care Med 1996;154:442–447.

32 Couser J, Guthmann R, Hamadeh M, Kane CS: Pulmonary Rehabilitation improves exercise capacity in older elderly patients with COPD. Chest 1995;107:730–734.

33 McGavin CR, Gupta SP, McHardy GJ: Twelve minute walking test for assessing disability in chronic bronchitis. Br Med J 1976;i:822–823.

34 Pollock M, Roa J, Benditt J, Celli BR: Stair climbing (SC) predicts maximal oxygen uptake in patients with chronic airflow obstruction. Chest 1993;104;1378–1383.

35 O'Hara WJ, Lasachuk BP, Matheson P, Renahan MC: Schloter DS, Lilker ES: Weight training and backpacking in chronic obstructive pulmonary disease. Respir Care 1984;29:1202–1210.

36 Wykstra PJ, Van Altens R, Kran J, et al: Quality of life in patients with chronic obstructive pulmonary disease improves after rehabilitation in house. Eur Respir J 1994;7:269–274.

37 Martinez FJ, Couser J, Celli BR: Factors that determine ventilatory muscle recruitment in patients with chronic airflow obstruction. Am Rev Respir Dis 1990;142:276–282.
38 Tangri S, Woolf CR: The breathing pattern in chronic obstructive lung disease, during the performance of some common daily activities. Chest 1973;63:126–127.
39 Celli BR, Rassulo J, Make B: Dyssynchronous breathing associated with arm but not leg exercise in patients with COPD. N Engl J Med 1968;314:1485–1490.
40 Criner GJ, Celli BR: Effect of unsupported arm exercise on ventilatory muscle recruitment in patients with severe chronic airflow obstruction. Am Rev Respir Dis 1988;138:856–867.
41 Celli BR, Criner GJ, Rassulo J: Ventilatory muscle recruitment during unsupported arm exercise in normal subjects. J Appl Physiol 1988;64:1936–1941.
42 Bobbert AC: Physiological comparison of three types of ergometry. J Appl Physiol 1960;15: 1007–1014.
43 Davis JA, Vodak P, Wilmore JH, Vodak J, Kwitz P: Anaerobic threshold and maximal power for three modes of exercise. J Appl Physiol 1976;41:549–550.
44 Steinberg J, Astrand PO, Ekblom B, Royce J, Sattin P: Hemodynamic response to work with different muscle groups, sitting and supine. J Appl Physiol 1967;22:61–70.
45 Reybrouck T, Heigenhouser GF, Faulkner JA: Limitations to maximum oxygen uptake in arm, leg and combined arm-leg ergometry. J Appl Physiol 1975;38:774–779.
46 Martin TW, Zeballos RJ, Weisman IM: Gas exchange during maximal upper extremity exercise. Chest 1991;99:420–425.
47 Banzett R, Topulus G, Leith D, Natios C: Bracing arms increases the capacity for sustained hyperpnea. Am Rev Respir Dis 1988;138:106–109.
48 Maestro L, Dolmage T, Avendano MA, Goldstein R: Influence of arm position in ventilation during incremental exercise in healthy individuals. Chest 1990;98:113(S).
49 Dolmage TE, Maestro L, Avendano M, Goldstein RS: The ventilatory response to arm elevation of patients with chronic obstructive pulmonary disease. Chest 1993;104:1097–1100.
50 Martinez FJ, Couser J, Celli BR: Factors influencing ventilatory muscle recruitment in patients with chronic airflow obstruction. Am Rev Respir Dis 1990;142:276–282.
51 Lake FR, Hendersen K, Briffa T, et al: Upper limb and lower limb exercise training in patients with chronic airflow obstruction. Chest 1990;97:1077–1082.
52 Ries AL, Ellis B, Hawkins RW: Upper extremity exercise training in chronic obstructive pulmonary disease. Chest 1988;93:688–692.
53 Couser J, Martinez F, Celli B: Pulmonary rehabilitation that include arm exercise, reduces metabolic and ventilatory requirements for simple arm elevation. Chest 1993;103:37–38.
54 Epstein S, Breslin E, Roa J, Celli B: Impact of unsupported arm training (AT) and ventilatory muscle training (VMT) on the metabolic and ventilatory consequences of unsupported arm elevation (UAE) and exercise (UAEx) in patients with chronic airflow obstruction. Am Rev Respir Dis 1991;143:81A.
55 Martinez FJ, Vogel PD, DuPont DN, et al: Supported arm exercise vs. unsupported arm exercise in the rehabilitation of patients with chronic airflow obstruction. Chest 1993;103: 1397–2002.
56 Leith DE, Bradley M: Ventilatory muscle strength and endurance training. J Appl Physiol 1976;4:508–516.
57 Roussos CH, Macklem PT: The respiratory muscles. N Engl J Med 1982;307:786–797.
58 Lecog A, Delhez L, Janssens S, et al: Reentrainement de la fonction motrice ventilatoire chez des insuffisants respiratoire chroniques. Acta Tuberc Pneumol Belg 1970;61:63–69.
59 Reid WD, Warren CP: Ventilatory muscle strength and endurance training in elderly subjects and patients with chronic airflow limitation: A pilot study. Physio Canada 1984;36: 305–311.
60 Pardy R, Livingston R, Despas P, et al: Inspiratory muscle training compared with physiotherapy in patients with chronic airflow limitation. Am Rev Respir Dis 1981;123:421–425.
61 Larson JL, Kim MJ, Sharp JT: Inspiratory muscle training with a pressure threshold breathing device in patients with chronic obstructive pulmonary disease. Am Rev Respir Dis 1988;138:689–696.
62 Harver A, Mahler D, Daubenspeck J: Targeted inspiratory muscle training improves respiratory muscle function and reduces dyspnea in patients with chronic obstructive pulmonary disease. Ann Int Med 1989;111:117–124.
63 Belman M, Shadmehr R: Targeted resistive ventilatory muscle training in chronic obstructive pulmonary disease. J Appl Physiol 1988; 65:2726–2735.
64 Chen H, Dukes R, Martin B: Inspiratory muscle training in patients with chronic obstructive pulmonary disease. Thorax 1985 131:251–255.
65 Bjerre-Jempsen K, Secher N, Kok-Jensen A: Inspiratory resistance training in severe chronic obstructive pulmonary disease. Eur J Respir Dis 1981;62:405–411.
66 Falk P, Eriksen AM, Kolliker K, et al: Relieving dyspnea with an inexpensive and simple method in patients with severe chronic airflow limitation. Eur J Respir Dis 1985;66:181–186.
67 Noseda A, Carpiaux J, Vandeput N, et al: Resistive inspiratory muscle training and exercise performance in COPD patients: A comparative study with conventional breathing retraining. Bull Eur Physiopathol Respir 1987; 23:457–463.
68 Jones DT, Thomson RA, Sears MR: Physical exercise and resistive breathing training in severe chronic airways obstruction. Are they effective? Eur J Respir Dis 1985;67:159–166.
69 Lisboa C, Munoz V, Beroiza T, et al: Inspiratory muscle training in chronic airflow limitation: Comparison of two different training loads with a threshold device. Eur Respir J 1994;7:1266–1270.
70 Weiner P, Azyad Y, Ganan R: Inspiratory muscle training, combined with general exercise reconditioning in patients with COPD. Chest 1992;102:1351–1356.
71 Weiner P, Azyad Y, Ganam R, Weiner M: Inspiratory muscle training in asthma. Chest 1992;102:1357–1361.
72 Belman M, Mittman C: Ventilatory muscle training improves exercise capacity in chronic obstructive pulmonary disease patients. Am Rev Respir Dis 1980;121:273–280.
73 Ries AL, Moser KM: Comparison of isocapneic hyperventilation and walking exercise training at home in pulmonary rehabilitation. Chest 1986;90:285–289.
74 Levine S, Weiser P, Gillen J: Evaluation of a ventilatory muscle endurance training program in the rehabilitation of patients with chronic obstructive pulmonary disease. Am Rev Respir Dis 1986;133:400–406.
75 Belman MJ: Respiratory failure treated by ventilatory muscle training (VMT): A report of two cases. Eur J Respir Dis 1981;62:391–393.
76 Aldrich TK, Karpel JP, Uhrlass RM, et al: Weaning from mechanical ventilation: Adjunctive use of inspiratory muscle resistive training. Crit Care 1989;17:143–147.
77 Scheinhorn DJ, Ho C: Avoiding home mechanical ventilation; the regional weaning center. Proc Int Conf Pulm. Rehab and Home Vent, 1991, vol 3, p A35.
78 Bellemare F, Grassino A: Evaluation of diaphragmatic fatigue. J Appl Physiol 1982;53: 1196–1206.
79 Holliday J, Hyers T: The reduction of weaning time from mechanical ventilation using tidal volume and relaxation biofeedback. Am Rev Respir Dis 1990 141:1214–1220.
80 Benditt J, Pollock M, Breslin E, Celli B: Comprehensive pulmonary rehabilitation decreases the work of breathing during leg cycle ergometry in patients with severe chronic airflow obstruction (CAO). Am Rev Respir Dis 1990; 141:A509.
81 Epstein S, Celli B, Martinez F, Couser J, Roa J, Pollock M, Benditt J: Arm training reduces the VO_2 and VE cost of unsupported arm exercise and elevation in chronic obstructive pulmonary disease. J Cardiopulmonary Rehabil 1997;17:171–177.
82 Stanescu D, Nemery B, Veriter C, Marechal C: Pattern of breathing and ventilatory response to CO_2 in subjects practicing hatha-yoga. J Appl Physiol 1981;51:1625–1629.
83 Tandon M: Adjunct treatment with yoga in chronic severe airways obstruction. Thorax 1980;33:514–517.
84 Austin J, Pullin G: Improved respiratory function after lessons in the Alexander technique of musculoskeletal education. Am Rev Respir Dis 1984;129:A275.
85 Roa J, Epstein S, Breslin E, Shannon T, Celli B: Work of breathing and ventilatory muscle recruitment during pursed lip breathing. Am Rev Respir Dis 1991;143:A77.

Bartolome R. Celli, MD
Chief of Pulmonary and Critical Care
St. Elizabeth's Medical Center
736 Cambridge St., Boston, MA 02135 (USA)
Tel. +1 617 789 2554, Fax +1 617 752 7756
E-Mail bcelli@cchcs.org

Weisman IM, Zeballos RJ (eds): Clinical Exercise Testing.
Prog Respir Res. Basel, Karger, 2002, vol 32, pp 173–185

Functional Evaluation in Lung Volume Reduction Surgery

Frank C. Sciurba Sanjay A. Patel

Division of Pulmonary and Critical Care Medicine, University of Pittsburgh, Pa., USA

Summary

Lung volume reduction surgery (LVRS) remains a controversial intervention for patients with advanced emphysema due to the inconsistent outcome and poorly defined selection criteria. In selected patients, LVRS can elicit significant functional improvements and partial reversal of the pathophysiologic cascade has been observed. Improvements in lung elastic recoil and more appropriate resizing of the lung relative to the chest wall translate into improved inspiratory and expiratory airflow with less dynamic hyperinflation during exercise. Further improvements in gas exchange are attributed to improved regional V-Q matching and increases in mixed venous oxygen saturation. Improvements in cardiovascular and peripheral muscle function may complement the pulmonary effects to even further impact on exercise performance. Parameters derived from exercise testing may contribute significantly to outcome and risk stratification since they integrate the functional impact of complex changes in many interrelated physiologic domains. Results from the ongoing NETT should clarify many of these unresolved issues.

Lung Volume Reduction Surgery Background

Nearly 8 years after its reintroduction, lung volume reduction surgery (LVRS) remains a highly controversial intervention for patients with advanced emphysema [Cooper et al., 1995; Sciurba, 1997; Utz et al, 1998; Drazen, 2001]. Various surgical approaches have included unilateral stapling and laser techniques; however, a bilateral stapling approach involving resection of 20–30% of the diseased lung through either a thoracoscopic or median sternotomy incision has resulted in the greatest degree of spirometric improvement [McKenna et al., 1996; Kotloff et al., 1996; Cooper et al., 1996]. While short-term results of this procedure have been promising, yielding improvements in FEV_1 of 27–96%, its widespread acceptance has been tempered for several reasons:

(a) In most reported series, follow-up rates beyond 3–6 months are low. Thus, results may be overly optimistic, since those who did not return for follow-up may have poorer outcomes than those who did [Health Technology Assessment, 1996].

(b) The mortality rate in general practice appeared to be considerably higher than the 3–10% rate reported in the literature [Keenan et al., 1996; Mckenna et al., 1996; Cooper et al., 1996; Miller et al., 1996]. A report issued by the Center for Health Care Technology determined the 3- to 12-month postoperative mortality rate using the objective social security death index for all Medicare recipients who were billed for the procedure to be in the 14–23% range [Health Technology Assessment, 1996].

(c) The mean values of functional improvement reported in the literature make it impossible to distinguish a response due to a large proportion of patients with clinically significant improvements from one due to a small number of patients with disproportionately large improvements.

(d) Current selection criteria have failed to consistently distinguish patients with acceptable risk of morbidity and mortality or those with a likelihood of physiologic response to the intervention.

(e) Commonly reported simple physiologic outcome parameters such as FEV_1 may not reflect true functional improvement following LVRS, which potentially has opposing effects on pulmonary mechanics and vasculature. Integrative functional measurements such as exercise testing are more likely to reflect true physiologic improvements, but have only been reported as short term results in small subsets of patients.

(f) The interpretation of long-term functional and mortality data in non-randomized trials is dependent on comparisons to historical controls. Depending on the center, only 20–40% of patients referred for evaluation are ultimately accepted for surgery; such preselection creates a subgroup which is not easily compared to existing populations in the literature.

(g) Randomized controlled trials in the literature only report short term data and were too small to identify baseline characteristics predictive of response [Criner et al., 1999; Geddes et al., 2000; Pompeo et al., 2000].

Such gaps in the existing literature are being addressed by the National Emphysema Treatment Trial (NETT) [The National Emphysema Treatment Trial Research Group, 1999]. This multicenter trial is a cooperative effort of the National Institutes of Health and the Agency for Medicare and Medicaid (formerly the Health Care Financing Administration). In this trial, subjects are randomized to either maximal medical therapy including formal pulmonary rehabilitation or LVRS with pulmonary rehabilitation. The primary outcome parameters are mortality and maximal exercise watts measured during symptom-limited incremental cycle ergometry. 1,100 patients from 17 centers have been randomized into this trial as of October 2001. A subgroup, representing 14% of subjects randomized, has been identified as having excessive postoperative mortality and will be discussed below [NETT Research Group, 2001]. Ongoing data collection and analysis should identify predictors of long-term functional exercise responses and mortality in the remaining 86% of subjects. It is anticipated that preoperative parameters identifying a disproportionately low risk group will eventually also be defined.

Rationale for the Use of Exercise Testing in the Evaluation of LVRS

Various physiologic parameters, including expiratory flow rate, end-expiratory lung volume, pulmonary vascular resistance, gas exchange and peripheral muscle conditioning can be affected independently and may even respond in contradictory directions after LVRS. No single physiologic attribute adequately reflects the clinical response to LVRS. Thus, the primary outcome parameter following LVRS should be able to represent this complexity of physiologic changes in an integrated fashion. While subjective questionnaires assessing symptoms or health-related quality of life may loosely perform this function, we will restrict the discussion to exercise testing.

Various investigators have used the 6-min walk test (6MWT) or maximal incremental cardiopulmonary exercise testing (CPX) as tools to evaluate LVRS response. Although most studies have used 6MWT for functional assessment, walk distance correlates modestly, at best, with measures of dyspnea, quality of life or other objective functional measures such as CPX [Leyenson et al., 2000; Ferguson et al., 1998]. Keller et al. [1997] reported that of exercise measures, V_E/MVV best correlated with reductions in dyspnea and that 6MWT was not a correlate. Similarly, another study found that improvement in maximum oxygen consumption (VO_2), but not 6MWT, correlated with improvement in dyspnea ($r^2 = 0.59$, $p < 0.01$) and quality of life measures of physical function (SF-36) ($r^2 = 0.31$) [Ferguson et al., 1998].

The LVRS experience at our institution suggests that improvements in spirometry and lung volumes account for much more of the variability ($r^2 = 0.42$) in exercise watts response, but much less of the variability in 6MWT response ($r^2 = 0.21$), in optimal multiple regression models. Thus, CPX may reflect true physiologic improvements better than 6MWT and may be a more meaningful outcome parameter for LVRS.

Physiological Response to Lung Volume Reduction Surgery

Elucidation of the basic physiologic mechanisms of improvement following LVRS not only enhances the scientific validity of the surgery, but may enable us to identify and optimize selection criteria which predict those changes. In this regard, cardiopulmonary exercise performance, in addition to reflecting the integrated effects of changes in multiple underlying mechanisms, can further elucidate the mechanisms of improvement after LVRS.

Lung and Chest Wall Mechanics during Rest and Exertion

The early hypothesis of Brantigan suggested that LVRS, as was reported in the 1960s, results in partial res-

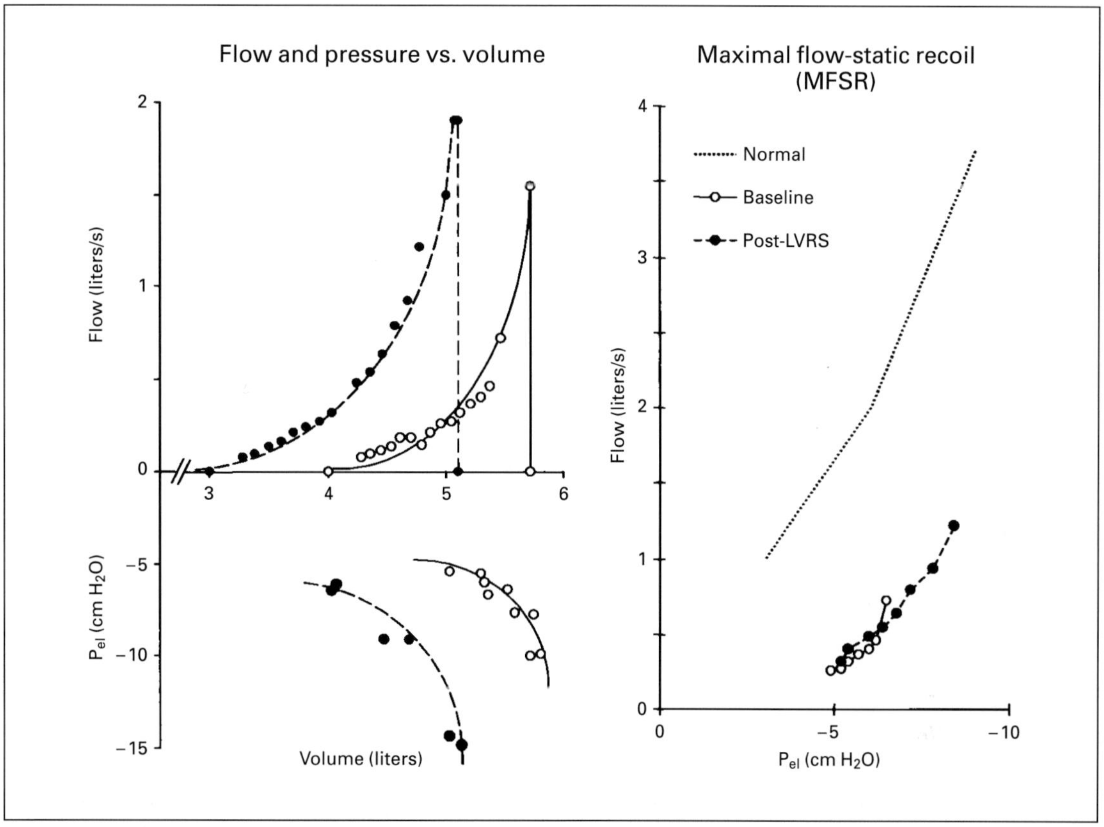

Fig. 1. Left panel: Static recoil (P_{el})-volume and flow-volume relationships for a 58-year-old man before (open circles) and after (closed circles) bilateral LVRS are shown. Note the higher flows and shift to lower lung volumes in the flow-volume loop. Right panel: Maximal flow-static recoil (MFSR) curve is plotted by matching iso-volume values for flow and P_{el} from the plots on the left. The MFSR curve suggests the improvement in flow is almost entirely attributable to increased lung recoil.

toration of the diminished lung elastic recoil pressure found in advanced emphysema. Experiments at that time documenting improved airway conductance/volume relationship following this procedure also attributed these improvements to renewed tethering of the airways in association with changes in lung recoil [Rogers et al., 1968]. Lung resection, on the other hand, in the form of lobectomy for carcinoma, while reducing lung volume, did not elicit similar changes in conductance because of simultaneous removal of large conducting airways.

More recent reports have documented an increase in maximal static recoil pressure (P_{el}-max) and the coefficient of retraction (P_{el}-max/TLC) after LVRS, further supporting Brantigan's hypothesis. In one series of 20 consecutive patients, the coefficient of retraction increased from 1.3 ± 0.6 to 1.8 ± 0.8 cm H_2O 3 months following either unilateral or bilateral LVRS [Sciurba, 1996]. This change reflects an improvement in the effective driving pressure generating expiratory flow, and should result in proportional improvements in air flow at all lung volumes and consequent reductions in lung hyperinflation. While the change in elastic recoil measurements did not significantly correlate with degree of functional improvement, there was a significantly greater improvement in walking distance in the 16 patients with improved P_{el} (+146 ft) compared to the 4 patients without improvement (–102 ft).

A subsequent study evaluating the bilateral procedure has confirmed improvements in maximal lung recoil pressure. Conductance of the upstream airway segment (maximal flow/P_{el}) was also analyzed and improved significantly in this group [Gelb et al., 1996b]. Flow from maximal expiratory maneuvers was compared to the static recoil pressure curves at constant volume (MFSR plot) using the techniques of Black and Hyatt [Black et al., 1972] (fig. 1). Inspection of the MFSR curves in this paper reveals 9 of

12 patients with very little shift or change in slope of the MFSR line but, rather, extension of the pre-operative line to higher recoil pressures and thus higher flows. These findings confirm that the increased expiratory flow rates in this series were largely related to improvements in lung elastic recoil. Interestingly, 3 patients, in addition to improving P_{el}, had significant increases in slope and upward shifts in the MFSR line, suggesting improved airway conductance independent of global improvements in lung elastic recoil (fig. 1). This small subset of patients demonstrating a marked shift in the MFSR slope following surgery may represent patients with significant re-expansion of regionally compressed airways.

Thus 'volume reduction' is, in part, due to more complete expiratory flow attributable to a global increase in lung elastic recoil. On the other hand, regions of lung 'heterogeneity' are often specifically targeted which have such long time constants that they simply act as space, occupying residual volume. Resection of these extremely slow lung units (in contrast to units with more average time constants, as is likely with diffuse emphysema) should reduce lung volume disproportionately to and possibly independently of increases in global lung elastic recoil. This concept is highlighted in an elegant model by Fessler and Permutt [1998] which, in essence, attributes the improvements following LVRS to a more appropriate resizing of the lung to the chest wall. In this model, the dominant impact of LVRS lies in the relatively greater reduction in RV compared to TLC, and a consequent increase in VC. In their model, this increase in VC is the dominant factor effecting an increase in FEV_1. This is in accordance with the minimal change in the FEV_1/FVC ratio observed in most patients following LVRS. This model exemplifies the importance of elucidating mechanisms, as it predicts that the best responders to LVRS will be those with the highest pre-operative RV/TLC, a finding which has been subsequently confirmed [Patel et al., 2001; Ingenito et al., 2001; Flaherty et al., 2001].

While the changes in lung mechanics discussed above represent the primary mechanical effects of LVRS, the consequent 'volume reduction' may secondarily elicit considerable improvement in inspiratory muscle function as well. A less hyperinflated chest wall returns to a more compliant region of its pressure-volume curve and reduces the work of the respiratory muscles [Gelb et al., 1996a]. Partial normalization of the end-expiratory diaphragmatic curvature and restoration of the normal bucket handle configuration of the rib cage further contribute to restoration of respiratory muscle efficiency [Lando et al., 1999; Bellemare et al., 2001].

Accordingly, significant increases in maximal inspiratory pressure and trans-diaphragmatic pressure (P_{di}) of 25–50% have been documented following LVRS [Teschler et al., 1996; Sciurba, 1997; Laghi et al., 1998; Criner et al., 1998]. Other reports have provided evidence that intrinsic positive end-expiratory pressure may decrease following LVRS, further decreasing the oxygen cost of breathing [Gelb et al., 1996a, Sciurba et al., 1996a, b; Lahrmann et al., 1999; Tschernko et al., 1997]. Improved neuro-mechanical coupling of the diaphragm, as indicated by increases in twitch P_{di} with phrenic nerve stimulation, have also been documented following LVRS [Laghi et al., 1998, Criner et al., 1998].

In summary, changes in resting pulmonary mechanics and diaphragmatic function translate into improved airflow with less hyperinflation during exertion. Figure 2 illustrates the impact of LVRS on minute ventilation and respiratory timing following LVRS during exercise which has been found by many investigators [Sciurba, 1997, Benditt et al., 1997b, Martinez et al., 1997; Tschernko et al., 1997; Keller et al., 1997; Criner et al., 1999; Ferguson et al., 1998; Stammberger et al., 1998]. At iso-workloads patients have a slower respiratory rate with significantly greater tidal volumes and associated improved inspiratory flow rates. This results in significantly lower Borg dyspnea ratings at equivalent workloads. At maximal exertion, respiratory rate is similar before and after surgery, but tidal volume and minute ventilation are significantly increased. The improved tidal volumes observed may be due to a reduction in dynamic hyperinflation associated with the significantly greater inspiratory and expiratory flow rates. Furthermore, the changes in diaphragm function described above result in relatively greater contributions of the diaphragm to tidal breathing at rest and during exertion (fig. 3), and correlate with improvements in exercise performance [Benditt et al., 1997b; Martinez et al., 1997; Laghi et al., 1998].

Impact of LVRS on Resting and Exercise Gas Exchange

While resting and exercise arterial oxygenation has been shown to improve following bilateral LVRS, the improvement is variable [Christensen et al., 1999] and the precise mechanisms of improvement are unclear. Potential mechanisms include global increases in alveolar ventilation, regional improvements in V/Q matching due to local re-expansion of less diseased but previously poorly ventilated lung, and improved mixed venous saturation secondary to improved right or left heart function.

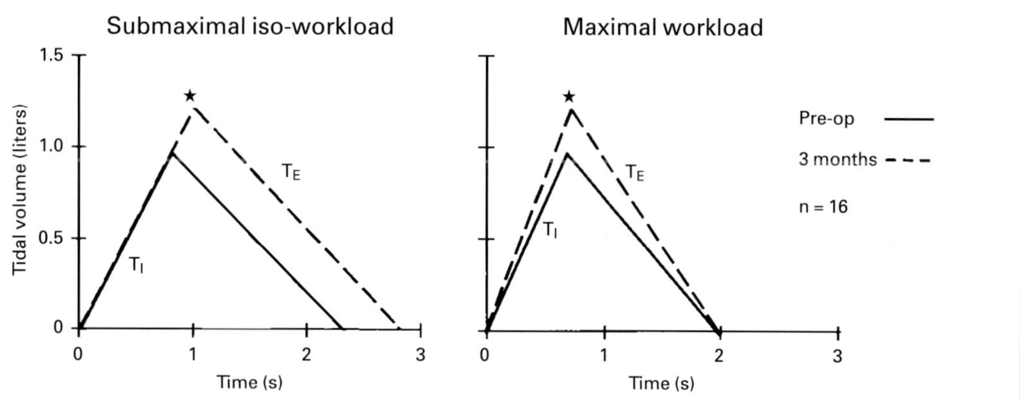

	Pre-op		3 months	Pre-op		3 months
V_E (liters/min)	25.9 ± 6.20	→	27.0 ± 7.2	30.3 ± 8.90	→	37.4 ± 10.20*
T_I/T_{total}	0.41 ± 0.01	→	0.41 ± 0.01	0.35 ± 0.01	→	0.36 ± 0.01
V_T/T_I (liters/s)	1.22 ± 0.06	→	1.22 ± 0.06	1.46 ± 0.10	→	1.75 ± 0.10*
Borg resp	4.67 ± 2.74	→	1.84 ± 1.98*	6.40 ± 2.64	→	5.34 ± 3.21

*$p < 0.001$

Fig. 2. Effect of LVRS on minute volume (V_E), tidal volume (V_T), inspiratory-expiratory ratios in 16 patients during incremental cycle ergometry before (solid lines) and 3 months after (dashed lines) LVRS. Left panel: Postoperatively, at iso-workloads, patients demonstrate a slower respiratory rate (longer respiratory cycle duration) with greater tidal volume and greater inspiratory flow rates (V_T/T_I) in association with lower Borg dyspnea ratings. Right panel: At maximal exercise, respiratory rate is similar after LVRS, but V_E and V_T are significantly increased, in association with lower Borg dyspnea ratings despite higher levels of work achieved. Adapted from Sciurba [1997].

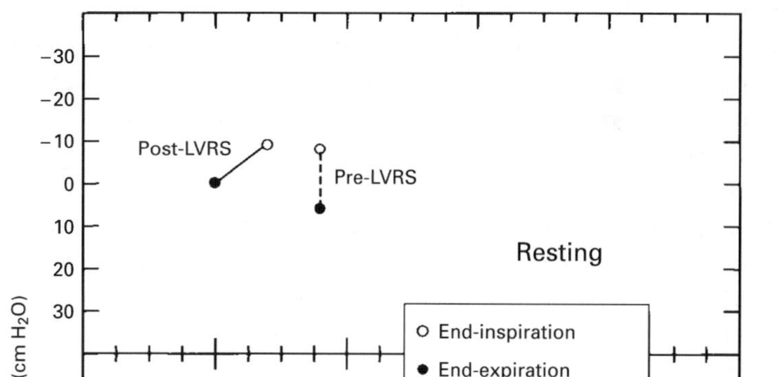

Fig. 3. Gastric pressure (P_{ga}) vs. esophageal pressure (P_{es}) at rest and isowatt exercise, before (dashed lines) and after LVRS (solid lines). The pressure changes reflect the dramatic reduction in P_{ga} at end expiration during exertion following LVRS thought to be related to excessive activation of the abdominal muscles of expiration associated with severe COPD. Adapted from Benditt et al. [1997].

The significant improvement in resting arterial $PaCO_2$ described in most series may be the result of improved alveolar ventilation due to improved pulmonary mechanics, but reductions in dead space ventilation from removal of partially ventilated bullae and increases in capillary flow to high V/Q areas are likely mechanisms as well.

After LVRS, arterial PaO_2 is higher during isowatt exertion, but there may be no significant differences at maximal exertion. Similarly, resting and exercise $PaCO_2$ decreases due to both an increase in alveolar ventilation and reduction in proportion of dead space ventilation [Sciurba et al., 1996a; Ferguson et al., 1998; Keller et al., 1997].

Pulmonary Vascular Function at Rest and with Exertion

The great majority of research on LVRS has been directed at the pulmonary mechanical effects of the surgery. But very little attention has been directed at its potential impact on pulmonary vascular function, which may independently influence exercise tolerance and survival. On the one hand, resection of perfused lung could further decrease vascular reserve. On the other hand, a decrease in vascular resistance may occur through recruitment of vessels in re-expanding lung tissue or through improved elastic recoil, which may increase radial traction on extraalveolar vessels.

Significant increases in right-ventricular fractional area of contraction have been reported following LVRS using echocardiographic techniques, suggesting improvements in pulmonary vascular function [Sciurba et al., 1996b]. Furthermore, reduced end-expiratory esophageal pressure, and hence pericardial pressure, may improve right- and left-ventricular filling and cardiac output. LVRS-mediated reductions in exercise-induced dynamic hyperinflation [Martinez et al., 1997; O'Donnell et al., 1996] may diminish rises in intrathoracic pressure and, therefore, pulmonary vascular resistance elevations during exertion.

However, hemodynamic studies on patients before and after LVRS show mixed results. This is not surprising given the potentially opposing effects described. Some reports, including one study evaluating patients with more diffuse disease, raise concern about postoperative increases in pulmonary vascular resistance both at rest and with exertion [Weg et al., 1999; Haniuda et al., 2000]. Conversely, another study revealed a reduction in heart rate at iso-workloads following LVRS and thus increased oxygen pulse [Benditt et al., 1997a], suggesting that cardiovascular function improves on average following LVRS. However, two studies found no effect on pulmonary artery pressure after LVRS [Thurnheer et al., 1998; Oswald-Mammosser et al., 1998].

It is clear, however, from the above studies that individual patients may demonstrate deterioration in pulmonary vascular function. Unfortunately, at present, preoperative identification of these individuals is not possible. Furthermore, it is likely that such effects would impact negatively on exercise performance independently of observed pulmonary mechanical improvements. Further research including results of the NETT should clarify these issues.

Peripheral Muscle Conditioning

Another potentially important mechanism of improvement is facilitation of cardiovascular and peripheral muscle training, enabled by improvements in pulmonary mechanical factors. Significant increases in thigh muscle cross-sectional area and patient weight occur following LVRS, and these changes correlate with improvements in 6MWT and DLCO [Donahoe et al., 1996; Christensen et al., 1999].

Following LVRS, patients may have profound residual deconditioning from chronic inactivity. With a successful surgical outcome, this deconditioning may become the limiting factor to exertion if ventilatory mechanical limitation no longer exists (fig. 4). The extent to which these severely deconditioned and potentially myopathic patients can recover following aggressive rehabilitation is uncertain. It is likely, however, that the magnitude of improvements in functional exercise tolerance lags behind the improvements in pulmonary mechanics following LVRS, as the elimination of the mechanical ventilatory limitation re-enables peripheral muscle training potential. Furthermore, if this occurs, exercise function may be maintained above pre-operative levels, even while pulmonary function parameters decline [Flaherty et al., 2001].

Clinical Utility of Exercise Testing

Assessing the Response to LVRS

LVRS has improved pulmonary function [Cooper et al., 1996], exercise capacity [Keller et al., 1997; Martinez et al., 1997; Benditt et al., 1997a; Ferguson et al., 1998; Criner et al., 1999], dyspnea [Sciurba et al., 1996b; Martinez et al., 1997] and quality of life [Moy et al., 1999; Leyenson et al., 2000] in selected emphysema patients. Its impact on long-term mortality will not be known until the results of the NETT are available [The NETT Research

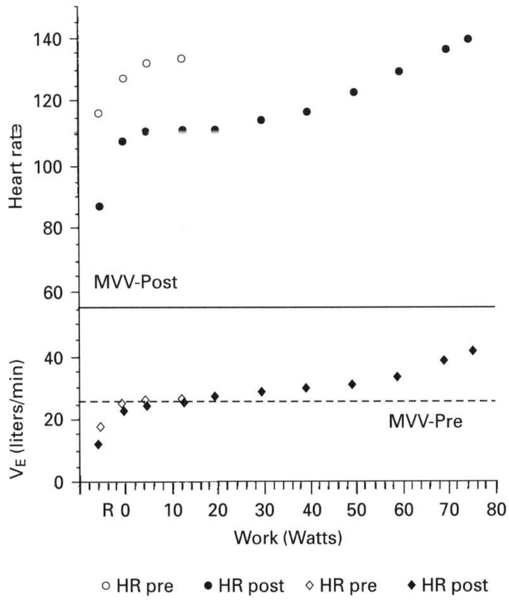

	Pre-op	Pos-op
Peak VO_2 ml/kg/min	9.4	15.5
V_D/V_{Tmax}	0.45	0.39
PCO_{2max} (mm Hg)	42	37
ΔBE_{max}	–0.9	–3.4
PO_2 (13 W) (mm Hg)	51	0

Fig. 4. Typical exercise response following LVRS. Pre-operative ventilatory limitation is suggested by the minute ventilation (V_E) (open diamonds) at peak exercise approching the pre-operative maximal voluntary ventilation (MVV) (dashed line), causing termination of exercise at only 13 watts. Following LVRS (black diamonds), the V_E at maximal exertion no longer approaches the improved MVV (solid line). Instead, increased heart rate and base excess at maximal exercise (ΔBE max) suggest that exercise limitation due to cardiovascular or muscular deconditioning are now unmasked.

Group, 1996]. Most studies have noted modest correlations at best between improvements in pulmonary function measures and dyspnea and quality of life [Moy et al., 1999; Leyenson et al., 2000] or measures of functional capacity. As such, more meaningful measures of improvement, such as 6MWT or CPX, are commonly reported outcomes.

Improvement in Walk Distance. While consistent improvements in 6MWT have been reported, few studies report detailed methodology of their walk testing. Given that 6MWT is highly dependent upon methodologic factors [Sciurba and Slivka, 1998], results among centers are difficult to generalize. A representative subset of studies reporting 6MWT changes after LVRS are summarized in table 1. Clearly, there is wide variability in baseline values between centers and in the response to surgery, with mean short term improvements ranging from 11 to 51% for unilateral surgery and from 12 to 57% for bilateral surgery. This variability highlights the impact of differing selection criteria, incomplete follow-up, and the uncontrolled design of most published reports.

Studies suggest that this short term improvement in walk distance is maintained at 12 [Gelb et al., 2001], 18 [Cordova et al., 1997] and 36 [Flaherty et al., 2001] months of follow-up. Analysis of the LVRS experience at our institution, however, suggests that initial improvements (896–1,020 ft) may not be durable (decreasing back to 889 ft at 2 years) (fig. 5).

Three randomized trials have assessed improvement in walk testing after LVRS as compared to pulmonary rehabilitation control arms. Pompeo et al. [2001] demonstrated 2.1 times greater improvement in 6MWT (180 vs. 85 ft) after LVRS as compared to 6 weeks of comprehensive pulmonary rehabilitation. Similarly, Criner et al. [2000] reported 3 times greater 6MWT increase (305 vs. 102 ft) following LVRS as compared to 12 weeks of rehabilitation. However, their study had a significant number of medical- to surgical-arm crossovers (13 of 18) and an intent-to-treat analysis did not reach statistical significance. Geddes et al. [2000], using the related shuttle-walk test, also reported greater improvements in walk distance with LVRS as compared to 6 weeks of pulmonary rehabil-

Table 1. Studies evaluating 6-min walk distance following LVRS

A Non-randomized studies

Author	n	Follow up months	6MWT pre-op, ft	6MWT post-LVRS, ft	Δ6MW %	Surgical approach
Short term studies						
Sciurba, 1996	20	3	819±284	916±286	11	unilateral
Miller, 1996	40	3	1,020	1,250	23	33 bilateral +
		6		1,600	57	7 unilateral
Keenan, 1996	40	3	784±51	894±49	14	unilateral
Cooper 1996	101	6	1,125	1,311	17	bilateral MS
Kotloff, 1996	46	6	999±241	1,181±287	18	bilateral MS
	26	6	969±305	1,244±331	28	bilateral VATS
Bingisser, 1996	20	3	1,624*	2,257*	39	bilateral VATS
Argenziano, 1997	66	3	590±360	888±360	51	unilateral advanced disease
Keller, 1997	25	4.2	934±297	1,071±241	15	unilateral
Ferguson, 1998	18	4	1,081±109	1,273±101	18	bilateral MS
Date, 1998	33	3	1,184±46	1,407±52	19	bilateral MS
Shade, 1999	33	3–6	948±298	1,128±269	19	bilateral MS
Sciurba, unpubl. data	56	3	862±279	968±316	12	unilateral
	55	3	863±258	1,006±253	17	bilateral
Longer term studies						
Cordova, 1997	26	6	824±374	1,115±276	35	treadmill CPX
	12	12		1,269±269	54	bilateral MS
	6	18		1,187±253	44	
Gelb, 2001	12	6	823±374	1,269±269	54	
		12		1,187±253	44	
Flaherty, 2001	69	12	871	1,326	52	all bilateral
	51	24		1,371	57	
	34	36		1,390	60	
Sciurba, unpubl. data	32	3	896±208	1,020±216	14	11 bilateral +
		24		889±254	NS	16 unilateral

B Randomized studies

Author	n	Follow up months	Δ6MWT (medical arm)	Δ6MWT (LVRS arm)	p value	Comments
Criner, 1999	28	3	+85	+180	0.001	significant with crossovers analyzed
Geddes, 2000	24	6	−66±66**	164±131**	0.02	shuttle walk test;
		12	−246±66**	72±299**	0.05	compared to baseline
Pompeo, 2000	55	6	±102	±305	<0.0002	17 bilateral + 13 unilateral

* 12-min walk test. ** Estimated from figures.
All improvements in Δ6MW reached statistical significance except as noted.

itation and further documented sustained differences at 1 year.

Improvement in Cardiopulmonary Exercise Test Parameters. Improvements in CPX parameters are also reported following LVRS (table 2). Short-term increases in maximal workload at 3–6 months have ranged from 20 to 69% and increases in peak VO_2 have ranged from 3.4 to 30%. Unfortunately, there are limited data documenting the durability of these functional improvements. Two studies, though small in size, do suggest that at least a sub-

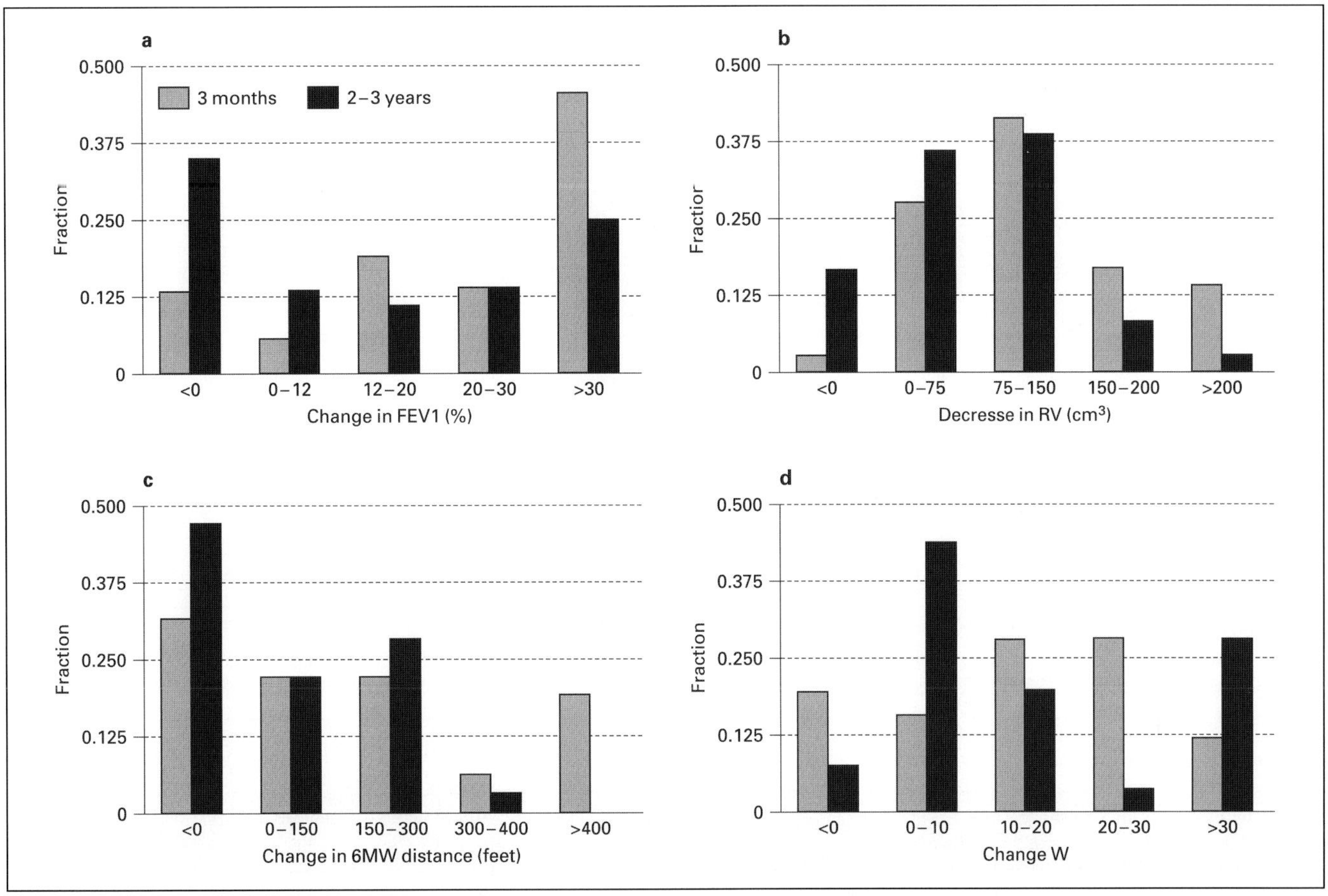

Fig. 5. Short- and long-term response to LVRS. Note the heterogeneity of short and long term response to LVRS. This highlights the fact that simple mean values reported in many studies do not reflect the most probable response of any individual. Although a subset of patients exhibit dramatic short-term improvements in FEV_1 (**a**, n = 36), RV (**b**, n = 36), 6-min walk testing (6MWT) (**c**, n = 32), and exercise watts (**d**, n = 27), a far fewer number maintain these responses at 2–3 years. From Sciurba [unpubl. data].

set of patients maintain these improvements in peak VO_2 (12–35% from baseline) at 1 year [Cordova et al., 1997] and further [Gelb et al., 2001]. Likewise, at our institution, long-term follow-up of 27 subjects reveals sustained improvements in maximal watts (52% greater than baseline) at a mean follow-up of 24.8 months.

Two small randomized trials have demonstrated greater improvement in CPX parameters after LVRS compared to pulmonary rehabilitation controls. Criner et al. [1999] demonstrated significant differences in VO_2 response, but only if a large number of medical- to surgical-arm crossover subjects (13 of 18) were analyzed with the LVRS group. An intent-to-treat analysis failed to reach statistical significance. More recently, a larger study by Pompeo et al. [2001] more clearly demonstrated a greater benefit in incremental treadmill exercise parameters after LVRS as compared to a control group undergoing 6 weeks of pulmonary rehabilitation. However, subjects in that study did not undergo pulmonary rehabilitation prior to randomization, making it difficult to discriminate improvements due to LVRS from those simply related to pulmonary rehabilitation.

While maximal VO_2 is generally considered a more accurate indicator of aerobic fitness than maximal workload, there are theoretical reasons that this may not be the case in LVRS. One would anticipate that after LVRS, decreases in respiratory muscle work would decrease respiratory muscle oxygen consumption. As a result, improvements in maximal oxygen consumption of exercising skeletal muscle may be masked due to a significant decrease in oxygen consumption of the working respiratory muscles. This is essentially a reversal the respiratory

Table 2. Studies evaluating maximal exercise response following LVRS

A Non-randomized Studies

Author	n	Follow up months	VO_2, pre-op ml/kg/min	VO_2, post-LVRS ml/kg/min	ΔVO_2 %	Work, W pre-op	Work, W post-LVRS	ΔW	Surgical approach
Short term studies									
Bingisser, 1996	20	3	10.0±2.5	13.0±2.3	30	31±12	47±14	52	bilateral VATS
Keller, 1997	25	4.2	9.7±2.0	11.8±3.0	27	37±19	52±21	41	unilateral
Benditt, 1997	21	3	+0.16 l/min		25	+17.5		46	bilateral MS
Ferguson, 1998	18	4	0.73 l/min	0.76 l/min	3.4	40	48	20	bilateral MS
Stammberger, 1998	40	3	10.0±0.4	12.8±0.3	28	34.3±2	48.9±2.4	43	bilateral VATS
Shade, 1999	33	3–6	0.82±0.21 l/min	0.91±0.2 l/min	11				bilateral MS
Rogers, 2000	21	3				26±23	44±27	69	bilateral
Sciurba, unpublished	45	3	10.9±1.9	11.8±2.8	8	20.2±30.0	30.6±24.6	51	unilateral
	32	3	11.3±2.1	12.4±2.5	10	25.2±22.0	42.3±24.6	68	bilateral
Longer term studies									
Cordova, 1997	10	12	12.6±3.9	14.1±3.5	12				treadmill CPX bilateral MS
Gelb, 2001	3	60	5.53	7.47	35				
Sciurba, unpublished	27	3	11.6±2.1	12.8±2.9		26.9±24.2	44.4±25.8	65	11 bilateral +
		24.8		11.9±2.4			40.8±28.1	52	16 unilateral

B Randomized Studies

Author	n	Follow up months	ΔVO_2 (medical)	ΔVO_2 (LVRS)	p value	ΔWork (medical)	ΔWork (LVRS)	Comments
Criner, 1999	28	3	+0.7 ml/kg/min	+1.9 ml/kg/min	<0.01			analyzed with crossovers
Pompeo, 2000	55	6				+0.48* (60%)	+1.52* (223%)	treadmill CPX

* Bruce class (incremental treadmill test, Bruce protocol).

muscle 'steal syndrome' initially described by Dempsey et al. [1990].

Unfortunately, differences in exercise responses across institutions may be more reflective of a lack of standardization of the exercise protocol than of differences in patient outcome. For example, the absence of unloaded pedaling prior to incrementation may result in disproportionate changes in workload relative to maximal VO_2. The resulting variability may decrease the power of a study to determine a change. Likewise, differences in rate of workload incrementation and whether or not supplemental oxygen is administered can independently affect the exercise outcome parameters. Such interinstitutional differences have broad implications if parameters are to be generalized and used as selection criteria at other institutions.

Predicting LVRS Outcomes

As discussed, it is uncertain which outcome measures (e.g. spirometry, 6-min walk distance, maximal watts, dyspnea, quality of life) most meaningfully measures response to LVRS. This is an important question since different outcomes may have differing preoperative predictors. For example, predictors of short-term response may differ from those of a long-term response, and predictors of spirometric improvement may differ from predictors of functional response. Nonetheless, studies evaluating the predictive role of various physiologic and functional measures are reviewed here.

Preoperative Pulmonary Function Assessment. Pulmonary function testing has typically been used to identify optimal candidates for LVRS. Some authors have suggested that patients with a very low FEV_1 have an unacceptable risk to benefit ratio [Fujita and Barnes, 1996]. However, many reports have demonstrated acceptable morbidity, mortality, and short-term spirometric response in patients with FEV_1 <500 cm^3 [McKenna et al., 1997; Argenziano et al., 1996; Eugene et al., 1997]. Theoretical work [Fessler and Permutt, 1998] (discussed previously) suggesting a predictive role for RV/TLC, is supported by reports of greater improvements in dyspnea [Kurosawa et al., 1997], spirometry [Flaherty et al., 2001; Patel et al., 2001] and quality of life [Butler et al., 1997] in patients with greater preoperative RV/TLC. More involved physiologic measures such as inspiratory lung resistance [Ingenito et al., 1998], mean airway resistance and intrinsic PEEP [Tschernko et al., 1999] have also been associated with spirometric response.

Early reports suggesting greater mortality in patients with a lower DLCO [Keenan et al., 1996; Hazelrigg et al., 1996] have recently been corroborated in an early report of the NETT, which found subjects with an FEV_1 <20% of predicted and either a DLCO ≤20% of predicted or homogeneous emphysema by computed tomography, suffered greater surgical mortality [NETT Research Group, 2001].

Preoperative Functional Assessment. A limited number of studies have evaluated the predictive role of preoperative 6 MWT. One study found that patients dying after laser LVRS had lower 6 MWT (356 vs. 714 ft) when compared to survivors [Hazelrigg et al., 1996]. Similarly, another study reported that patients (n = 47) with either 6 MWT <200 m or resting $PaCO_2$ >45 were more likely to experience an unacceptable postoperative outcome (6 months mortality or length of stay >3 weeks) (p = 0.0025) [Szekely et al., 1997]. However, other studies have not found 6MWT to be a predictor of mortality or morbidity [Glasspole et al., 2000].

Preoperative assessment using CPX is less well studied. Maximal VO_2 was not a good correlate of short-term improvement in VO_2 after surgery [Stammberger et al., 1998]. Likewise, maximal VO_2 was not significantly different between short term survivors and nonsurvivors (0.66 vs. 0.51 liters/min, p = NS) in another study [Szekely, 1997]. However, the role of CPX in predicting long-term functional outcomes or long-term survival after LVRS has not been reported.

As such, we recently reviewed the LVRS experience at our institution. 126 subjects completed preoperative CPX and another 44 subjects were deemed too ill to undergo CPX or rapidly desaturated on room air (group I). Baseline pO_2 <55 mm Hg, pCO_2 >45 mm Hg, age >70, FEV_1 <20% of predicted and DLCO ≤20% of predicted were univariate predictors of long-term survival. The survival of group I (n = 44) was worse than those able to maintain 0–25 W (n = 81) (p = 0.08). Furthermore, those capable of greater than 25 W (n = 45) had the best survival (p = 0.02). An age- and sex-adjusted multivariate Cox proportional hazards model revealed that pO_2 <55 mm Hg (hazard ratio (HR) = 2.0, p = 0.1), FEV_1 <20% of predicted (HR = 2.0, p = 0.04) and inability to maintain 25 W during CPX (HR = 1.9, p = 0.03) were independent predictors of long-term survival. Thus, CPX may independently predict long-term survival after LVRS and may have value in preoperative risk stratification.

Preoperative stratification of CPX results into cardiovascular and ventilatory limited subgroups may also add insights into postoperative functional changes, although there is no published data available. Intuitively, LVRS, which has its greatest impact on pulmonary mechanics, should be less effective in improving functional capacity in individuals who approach a cardiovascular limitation.

Conclusions

LVRS can elicit significant functional improvements and partial reversal of the pathophysiologic cascade present in many patients with emphysema. On the other hand, many questions remain unresolved. Most importantly, these relate to the long-term efficacy of the procedure relative to a matched control group, and to optimizing patient selection criteria. CPX and, to a lesser extent, 6MWT, may be the best outcome and risk stratification parameters since they integrate the functional impact of complex changes in many interrelated physiologic domains. Results from the ongoing NETT should clarify many of these unresolved issues.

References

Argenziano M, Moazami N, Thomashow B, et al: Extended indications for lung volume reduction surgery in advanced emphysema. Ann Thorac Surg 1996;62:1588–1597.

Argenziano M, Thomashow B, Jellen PA, et al: Functional comparison of unilateral versus bilateral lung volume reduction surgery. Ann Thorac Surg 1997;64:321–327.

Benditt JO, Lewis S, Wood DE, Klima L, Albert RK: Lung volume reduction surgery improves maximal O_2 consumption, maximal minute ventilation O_2 pulse, and dead space-to-tidal volume ratio during leg cycle ergometry. AJRCCM 1997;156:561–566.

Benditt JO, Wood DE, McCool FD, et al: Changes in breathing and ventilatory muscle recruitment patterns induced by lung volume reduction surgery. AJRCCM 1997;55:279–284.

Bellemare JF, Cordeau MP, Leblanc P, Bellemare F: Thoracic dimensions at maximum lung inflation in normal subjects and in patients with obstructive and restrictive lung diseases. Chest 2001;119:376–386.

Bingisser R, Zollinger A, Hauser M, et al: Bilateral volume reduction surgery for diffuse pulmonary emphysema by video-assisted thoracoscopy. J Thorac Cardiovasc Surg 1996;112:875–882.

Black LF, Hyatt RE, Stubbs SE: Mechanisms of expiratory airflow limitation in chronic obstructive pulmonary disease associated with alpha-1 antitrypsin deficiency. ARRD 1972;105: 891.

Brenner M, McKenna RJ, Chen JC, et al: Survival following bilateral staple lung volume reduction surgery for emphysema. Chest 1999;115: 390–396.

Butler C, Benditt J, Lewis S, et al: Improvement in quality of life correlates with changes in lung volume and exercise function but not with air flow limitation of dyspnea. AJRCCM 1997; 155(suppl):A795.

Christensen PJ. Paine R 3rd, Curtis JL, et al: Weight gain after lung volume reduction surgery is not correlated with improvement in pulmonary mechanics. Chest 1999;116:1601–1607.

Cooper JD, Patterson GA, Sundaresan RS, et al: Results of 150 consecutive bilateral lung volume reduction procedures in patients with severe emphysema. J Thorac Cardiovasc Surg 1996;112:1319–1330.

Cooper JD, Trulock AN, Triantafillou G, et al: Bilateral pneumectomy (volume reduction) for chronic obstructive pulmonary disease. J Thorac Cardiovasc Surg 1995;109:106–119.

Cordova F, O'Brien G, Furukawa A, et al: Stability of improvements in exercise performance and quality of life following lung volume reduction surgery in severe COPD. Chest 1997;112:907–915.

Criner GJ, Cordova FC, Furukawa S, et al: Prospective randomized trial comparing bilateral lung volume reduction surgery to pulmonary rehabilitation in severe COPD. AJRCCM 1999;160:2018–2027.

Criner G, Cordova FC, Leyenson V, et al: Effect of lung volume reduction surgery on diaphragm strength. AJRCCM 1998;157:1578–1585.

Date H, Goto K, Souda R, et al: Bilateral lung volume reduction surgery via median sternotomy for severe pulmonary emphysema. Ann Thorac Surg 1998;65:939–42.

Dempsey JA, Johnson BD, Saupe KW: Adaptations and limitations in the pulmonary system during exercise. Chest 1990;97(3S):81S–87S.

Donahoe MP, Landreneau R, Sciurba FC, et al: The effect of volume reduction surgery on body composition in patients with end-stage emphysema. J Respir Crit Care Med 1996;153:451.

Drazen JM: Surgery for emphysema – not for everyone (letter). NEJM 2001;345:1126–1127.

Eugene J, Dajee A, Kayaleh R, et al: Reduction pneumoplasty for patients with a forced expired volume in 1 second of 500 milliliters or less. Ann Thorac Surg 1997;63:186–192.

Ferguson GT, Fernandez E, Zamora MR, et al: Improved exercise performance following lung volume reduction surgery for emphysema. AJRCCM 1998;157:1195–1203.

Fessler HE, Permutt S: Lung volume reduction surgery and airflow limitation. AJRCCM 1998; 157:715–722.

Flaherty KR, Kazerooni EA, Curtis JL, et al: Short-term and long-term outcomes after bilateral lung volume reduction surgery: Prediction by quantitative CT. Chest 2001;119:1337–1346.

Fujita RA, Barnes GB: Morbidity and mortality after thoracoscopic pneumonoplasty. Ann Thorac Surg 1996;62:251–257.

Geddes D, Davies M, Koyama H, et al: Effect of lung volume reduction surgery in patients with severe emphysema. NEJM 2000;343:239–245.

Gelb AF, McKenna RJ, Brenner M, et al: Contributions of lung and chest wall mechanics following emphysema resection. Chest 1996a;110: 11–17.

Gelb AF, McKenna RJ, Brenner M, et al: Lung function 5 yr after lung volume reduction surgery for emphysema. AJRCCM 2001;163: 1562–1566.

Gelb AF, Zamel N, McKenna RJ, Brenner M: Mechanism of short-term improvement in lung function after emphysema resection. AJRCCM 1996b;154:945–951.

Glasspole IN, Gabbay E, Smith JA, et al: Predictors of perioperative morbidity and mortality in lung volume reduction surgery. Ann Thorac Surg 2000;69:1711–1716.

Haniuda M., Kubo K, Fujimoto K, et al: Different effects of lung volume reduction surgery and lobectomy on pulmonary circulation. Ann Surg 2000;231:119–125.

Hazelrigg S, Boley T, Henkle J, et al: Thoracoscopic laser bullectomy: A prospective study with three month results. J Thorac Cardiovasc Surg 1996;112:319–327.

Health Technology Assessment: Lung volume reduction surgery for end-stage chronic obstructive pulmonary disease; in Holohan TV, Handelsman H (eds): Center for Health Care Technology. Agency for Health Care Policy and Research, 1996.

Ingenito EP, Evans RB, Loring SH, et al: Relation between pre-operative inspiratory lung resistance and the outcome of lung volume reduction surgery for emphysema. NEJM 1998;338: 1181–1185.

Ingenito EP, Loring SH, Moy ML, et al: Comparison of physiological and radiological screening for lung volume reduction surgery. AJRCCM 2001;163:1068–1073.

Keller CA, Ruppel G, Hibbett A, Osterloh J, Naunheim KS: Thoracoscopic lung volume reduction surgery reduces dyspnea and improves exercise capacity in patients with emphysema. AJRCCM 1997;156:60–67.

Keenan RJ, Landreneau RJ, Sciurba FC, et al: Unilateral thoracoscopic surgical approach for diffuse emphysema. J Thorac Cardiovasc Surg 1996;111:308–316.

Kesten S, Elpern E, Warren W and Szidon P: Loss of pulmonary function gains after lung volume reduction surgery. J Heart Lung Transplant 1998;18:266–268.

Kotloff RM, Tino G, Bavaria JE, et al: Bilateral lung volume reduction surgery for advanced emphysema. Chest 1996;110:1399–1406.

Kurosawa H, Hida W, Kikuchi Y, et al: Hyperinflation estimated by residual volume can predict benefit of lung volume reduction surgery in patients with emphysema. AJRCCM 1997; 155(suppl):A605.

Lahrmann H, Wild M, Wanke T, et al: Neural drive to the diaphragm after lung volume reduction surgery. Chest 1999;116:1593–1600.

Laghi F, Jubran A, Topeli A, et al: Effect of lung volume reduction surgery on neuromechanical coupling of the diaphragm. AJRCCM 1998; 157:475–483.

Lando Y, Boiselle P, Shade D, et al: Effect of lung volume reduction surgery on bony thorax configuration in severe COPD. Chest 1999;116: 30–39.

Leyenson V, Furukawa S, Kuzma AM, et al: Correlation of changes in quality of life after lung volume reduction surgery with changes in lung function, exercise, and gas exchange. Chest 2000;118:728–735.

Martinez FJ, Montes de Oca M, Whyte RI, et al: Lung-volume reduction improves dyspnea, dynamic hyperinflation, and respiratory muscle function. AJRCCM 1997;155:1984–1990.

McKenna RJ, Brenner M, Fischel RJ, Gelb AF: Should lung volume reduction for emphysema be unilateral or bilateral? J Thorac Cardiovasc Surg 1996;112:1331–1339.

McKenna RJ, Brenner M, Fischel RJ, et al: Patient selection criteria for lung volume reduction surgery. J Thorac Cardiovasc Surg 1997;114: 957–964.

Miller JI, Lee RB, Mansour KA: Lung volume reduction surgery: Lessons learned. Ann Thorac Surg 1996;61:1464–1469.

Moy M, Ingenito EP, Mentzer SJ, et al: Health-related quality of life improves following pulmonary rehabilitation and lung volume reduction surgery. Chest 1999;115:383–389.

The National Emphysema Treatment Trial Research Group: Rationale and Design of the National Emphysema Treatment Trial: A prospective randomized trial of lung volume reduction surgery. Chest 1999;116:1750–1761.
The National Emphysema Treatment Trial Research Group: Patients at high risk of death after lung volume reduction surgery. NEJM 2001;345:1075–1083.
O'Donnell DE, Webb KA, Bertley JC, et al: Mechanisms of relief of exertional breathlessness following unilateral bullectomy and lung volume reduction surgery in emphysema. Chest 1996; 110:18–27.
Oswald-Mammosser M, Kessler R, Massard G, et al: Effect of lung volume reduction surgery on gas exchange and pulmonary hemodynamics at rest and during exercise. AJRCCM 1998;158: 1020–1025.
Patel SA, Sciurba FC, Slivka WA, et al: Pre-operative inspiratory conductance complements rv/tlc in predicting response to lung volume reduction surgery. AJRCCM 2001;163:A486.
Pompeo E, Marino M, Nofroni I, et al: Reduction pneumoplasty versus respiratory rehabilitation in severe emphysema: A randomized study. Ann Thorac Surg 2000;70:948–954.
Rogers RM, Coxson HO, Sciurba FC, et al: Preoperative severity of emphysema predictive of improvement after lung volume reduction surgery: Use of CT morphometry. Chest 2000; 118:1240–1247.
Rogers RM, DuBois AB, Blakemore WS: Effect of removal of bullae on airway conductance volume ratios. J Clin Invest 1968;47:2569.
Sciurba FC: Early and long term functional outcomes following lung volume reduction surgery. Clin Chest Med 1997;18:259–276.
Sciurba FC, Keenan RJ, Harris SP, et al: Exercise gas exchange response to unilateral and bilateral lung reduction surgery for diffuse emphysema. Chest 1996a;110(4):56S.
Sciurba FC, Rogers RM, Keenan RJ, Slivka WA, Gorscan JE, Ferson PF, Holbert M, Brown ML, Landreneau RJ: Improvement in pulmonary function and elastic recoil after lung-reduction surgery for diffuse emphysema. NEJM 1996b;334:1095–1099.
Sciurba FC, Slivka WA: Six-minute walk testing. Semin Resp Crit Care Med 1998;19:383–392.
Shade D, Cordova F, Lando Y, et al: Relationship between resting hypercapnia and physiologic parameters before and after lung volume reduction surgery in severe chronic obstructive pulmonary disease. AJRCCM 1999;159:1405–1411.
Stammberger U, Bloch K, Thurnheer R, et al: Exercise performance and gas exchange after bilateral video assisted thoracoscopic lung volume reduction for severe emphysema. Eur Resp J 1998;12:785–792.
Szekely LA, Oelberg DA, et al: preoperative predictors of operative morbidity and mortality in COPD patients undergoing bilateral lung volume reduction surgery. Chest 1997;111:550–558.
Teschler H, Stamatis G, el-Raouf Farhat AA, et al: Effect of surgical lung volume reduction on respiratory muscle function in pulmonary emphysema. Eur Respir J 1996;9:1779–1784.
Tschernko EM, Kritzinger M, et al: Lung volume reduction surgery: Preoperative functional predictors for postoperative outcome. Anesth Analgesia 1999;88:28–33.
Tschernko EM, Wisser E, Wanke T, et al: Changes in ventilatory mechanics and diaphragm function after lung volume reduction surgery in patients with COPD. Thorax 1997;52:545–550.
Thurnheer R, Bingisser, R, Stammberger U, et al: Effect of lung volume reduction surgery on pulmonary hemodynamics in severe pulmonary emphysema. Eur J Cardiothorac Surg 1998;13: 253–258.
Utz JP, Hubmayr RD, Deschamps C: Lung volume reduction surgery for emphysema: Out on a limb without a NETT. Mayo Clin Proc 1998; 73:552–566.
Weg IL, Rossoff L, McKeon K, et al: Development of pulmonary hypertension after lung volume reduction surgery. AJRCCM 1999;159:552–556.

Frank Sciurba, MD
Division of Pulmonary and Critical Care Medicine
Suite 1117 Kaufmann Bldg.
3471 5th Ave, Pittsburgh, PA 15213 (USA)
Tel. +1 412 648 6494, Fax +1 412 648 6495
E-Mail sciurbafc@msx.upmc.edu

Weisman IM, Zeballos RJ (eds): Clinical Exercise Testing.
Prog Respir Res. Basel, Karger, 2002, vol 32, pp 186–199

Cardiorespiratory Responses during Exercise in Interstitial Lung Disease

Bharath S. Krishnan[a] Darcy D. Marciniuk[b]

[a]Faculty of Physical Activity Studies, University of Regina, Saskatchewan, and
[b]Division of Respiratory Medicine, University of Saskatchewan, Royal University Hospital, Saskatoon, Saskatchewan, Canada

Summary

Clinical exercise testing has increasingly become an available and essential tool both in the understanding of the pathophysiology of disease and in the assessment of treatment of disease and disability. The integrative cardiopulmonary approach to exercise testing and interpretation has led to CPET being used in a variety of clinical settings as well as in recovery from disease and surgery. While currently the utility of integrative CPET in the diagnosis of unexplained dyspnea and exercise intolerance and in the assessment of impairment and disability due to specific disease is evident, future studies are required to standardize the conduct of CPET and interpretation of data and thus improve the discriminatory ability of CPET in cardiopulmonary disease and its management.

The term interstitial lung disease (ILD) describes a diverse group of parenchymal disorders that are chiefly characterized by a reduction in lung volume and lung compliance, and an increase in lung recoil pressure at a given absolute lung volume [1, 2]. While ILD is commonly idiopathic in nature ('idiopathic pulmonary fibrosis', IPF), many diseases such as collagen vascular disorders, connective tissue diseases, drug-induced reactions, and diseases secondary to occupational or environmental exposures, have been shown to cause or be associated with ILD [3, 4]. While their underlying etiology may differ, these disorders present with common clinical, radiographic and pathophysiological characteristics. Although the progressive parenchymal degeneration results in increasing ventilatory and circulatory impairment [5], the large functional reserve of the respiratory system ensures that these patients initially remain largely asymptomatic at rest. Accordingly, most patients with ILD present clinically with a history of insidious onset of exertional dyspnea. By imposing an increasing demand on their intrinsic structural and functional reserves, physical activity typically elicits clinical symptoms and therefore, exercise testing is useful in the assessment of abnormal function and disability in patients with ILD.

This chapter will focus primarily on recent research into the mechanisms underlying exercise limitation and advances made in cardiopulmonary exercise testing (CPET) in the diagnosis and management of ILD. As cardiopulmonary limitations to exercise caused by diseases producing a restrictive lung defect due primarily to involvement of the chest wall, pleura and respiratory muscles have been reviewed recently [4], they will not be discussed in this report. The reader is referred to appropriate literature [6–9] and to 'Normal Responses and Limitations to Exercise' [elsewhere in this volume] for a detailed understanding and interpretation of the physiological responses to exercise in both health and disease. Finally, comprehensive recent reviews of exercise pathophysiology in ILD [10, 11], exercise testing and interpretation in ILD [12], recent advances in pulmonary function testing

Table 1. Factors contributing to exercise limitation in ILD

1	Gas exchange impairment
2	Dynamic ventilatory mechanics
3	Dyspnea
4	Other factors
	Respiratory muscles
	Cardiac factors
	Lactic Acidosis
	Reduced fitness levels
	Other factors (e.g. peripheral vascular disease, motivation)

[13], and emerging concepts in the assessment of exercise ventilatory limitation [14] should be consulted for a better understanding and application of CPET in clinical practice in general, and specifically in management of the patient with ILD. In order to facilitate a better understanding of the exercise responses in patients with ILD, CPET data from ILD patients will be compared with normal healthy young adults throughout this review.

Pathophysiology of Exercise Limitation in ILD

Some of the known factors that contribute to exercise limitation in patients with ILD are summarized in table 1. Most ILD patients demonstrate an impairment of maximal exercise ability and sub-maximal exercise endurance; compared with age- and sex-matched normal subjects, both maximal oxygen uptake ($\dot{V}O_2max$) and maximal work rate ($\dot{W}max$) are significantly reduced in ILD [15–18]. This reduction in aerobic capacity has been shown to be related to resting pulmonary function and can be appropriately used to assess disability in patients with ILD [10, 11]. While many resting lung function measurements such as forced expiratory volume in one second (FEV_1, %predicted), total lung capacity (%predicted), diffusion capacity for carbon monoxide (DLCO, %predicted), have been shown to correlate significantly with $\dot{V}O_2max$, (%predicted) [5, 16], results of routine pulmonary function testing alone cannot be used meaningfully either in the prediction or in the quantification of exercise responses or disability [15, 19, 20]. It has also been shown that many ILD patients with normal resting pulmonary function have abnormal exercise responses [5], thus reinforcing the utility of CPET in the early diagnosis of ILD.

While many studies have demonstrated the effect of the different abnormalities on exercise limitation in ILD, the precise role each of these factors contributes to exercise intolerance in these patients is not fully understood. The following is a summary of some of the underlying pathophysiological mechanisms that have been shown to be associated with exercise limitation in ILD patients.

Gas Exchange Impairment

Of the factors listed (table 1), abnormal gas exchange during exercise appears to be a major factor in exercise limitation in ILD patients. The manifestations of compromised gas exchange include significant arterial hypoxemia, widening of the alveolar-arterial O_2 gradient ($PAO_2 - PaO_2$) and a reduction in lung diffusing capacity. While there appears to be no clear relationship between resting PaO_2 and disease severity [21], most patients with significant disease demonstrate O_2 desaturation and a widening of $PAO_2 - PaO_2$ during exercise [22–25]. These changes have been attributed to the increasing ventilation of poorly perfused air spaces resulting in an increase in physiological dead space (VD/VT), thus adding to the ventilatory requirements of exercise [5]. Indeed, ventilation/perfusion ($\dot{V}/\dot{Q}$) inequalities and shunting have been shown to account for over 60% of the increased (A – a) O_2 gradient, while impaired O_2 diffusion contributes the remainder to arterial hypoxemia during exercise in ILD [5]. Furthermore, both high (↑VD/VT, ↑$P(a\text{-}ET)CO_2$) and low (↓PaO_2, ↑$PAO_2 - PaO_2$) $\dot{V}/\dot{Q}$ ratios have been shown to be present during exercise in a significant proportion of patients (65%) with ILD, and peak $\dot{V}O_2$ has been shown to correlate with the high $\dot{V}/\dot{Q}$ ratios [5]. As the pulmonary vascular derangements accompanying ILD result in two types of $\dot{V}/\dot{Q}$ abnormalities, viz. high $\dot{V}/\dot{Q}$, characterized by a high VD/VT associated with destruction of the pulmonary capillary bed, and/or a low $\dot{V}/\dot{Q}$ due to the shunt effect (increased intact capillary transit times), arterial blood-gas measurements combined with the calculation of VD/VT are therefore often necessary to fully understand the nature and degree of gas exchange abnormalities and the resultant exercise limitation [5, 11].

Other factors such as diffusion limitation [23, 25–27], and a low mixed venous PO_2 [28] have also been shown to contribute to the increased $PAO_2 - PaO_2$ during exercise. While most patients with ILD demonstrate a reduced diffusing capacity for carbon monoxide (DLCO) [29], and the degree of O_2 desaturation during exercise has been shown to correlate significantly with DLCO measured at rest [30], the predictive value of resting DLCO in arterial O_2 desaturation during exercise has nevertheless been questioned [31–33]. However, as resting DLCO has been shown to significantly correlate with $\dot{V}O_2max$ and $\dot{W}max$ in ILD [34, 35], and has been shown to be associated with a widening of $PAO_2 - PaO_2$ during exercise, a reduced DLCO does have a prognostic value in the degree of arterial hypoxemia ILD patients exhibit during exercise. Arterial hypoxemia during exercise may result in a reduced O_2 delivery to both exercising muscles [24, 36] and the heart [37], all of which can contribute to exercise impairment in patients with significant ILD. Furthermore, the marked improvement in exercise endurance and gas exchange that is seen with supplemental O_2 breathing during exercise [15, 38], suggests that arterial hypoxemia and consequently reduced O_2 delivery to exercising muscles is a significant factor in exercise limitation in patients with ILD.

Dynamic Ventilatory Mechanics

Most of the alterations in respiratory mechanics in ILD (reduction in lung volumes and capacities, increased elastic recoil at functional residual capacity, FRC) are as a result of changes in the pressure-volume characteristics of the respiratory system [1, 3, 39]. These changes have an adverse functional impact on the demand/capacity relationships in the respiratory system and its ability to adapt to the increasing ventilatory demands of exercise. Thus, the increased ventilatory ($\dot{V}I$) response during submaximal exercise [16, 40] combined with a reduced ventilatory reserve (maximum voluntary ventilation, MVV) [7] due to altered respiratory mechanics in patients with ILD, results in a significant increase in $\dot{V}I$/MVV ratios during exercise. While the estimation of MVV (from forced expiratory volume in 1 s, FEV_1*35) is imprecise [41], it is not uncommon for the $\dot{V}I$/MVV ratio to approach 1 in ILD patients during exercise [42].

As the increased lung recoil at FRC results in a reduction of the expiratory reserve volume (ERV) [1, 39], the increase in tidal volume (VT) during exercise from ERV is significantly constrained and thus occurs from an encroachment on the inspiratory reserve volume (IRV) [42]. These constraints on exercise VT result in ILD patients adopting a rapid, shallow breathing pattern to meet the increasing ventilatory demands of exercise [16, 18] and these patterns of breathing have been shown to correlate well with disease severity [43, 44]. While $\dot{V}I$, at lower levels of exercise, is achieved by a combination of increases in VT and breathing frequency (f), further increases in $\dot{V}I$ at higher work rates are due to increases in f alone [18, 42]. The lung volume constraints on exercise $\dot{V}T$ ($\downarrow$ERV, $\uparrow$VT/inspiratory capacity (IC) ratio) result in significantly increased mechanical constraints on exercise $\dot{V}I$ in patients with ILD. Furthermore, the rapid and shallow breathing pattern at a higher lung volume ($\uparrow$EILV/TLC), results in increased elastic work of the inspiratory muscles and may contribute to the marked dyspnea that ILD patients report during exercise.

Dyspnea

While exertional dyspnea is a common and disabling symptom in cardio-respiratory disease [45], it is usually the presenting symptom in most patients with ILD [3]. Most patients with ILD ascribe exercise termination to the dyspnea that they experience during and at peak exercise, some patients may stop exercise due to increasing leg fatigue [42, 46, 47]. While dyspnea, considered independently, may be a nondiscriminatory symptom in cardio-respiratory disease [48] and while its etiology in patients with ILD may be multifactorial [45], the results of several studies do suggest that exertional dyspnea may be pathognomonic of ILD and its severity. For example, it has been shown that valid dyspnea scores [49] correlate significantly with exercise endurance [46], DLCO and impaired gas exchange [49] and arterial hypoxemia [15] in exercising ILD patients. The dyspnea experienced during exercise has been found to be related significantly to the increased ventilatory effort and inspiratory muscle work [42, 45]. More recently, O'Donnell et al. [50] have demonstrated that while dyspnea intensity and inspiratory effort at peak exercise in ILD patients were similar to those from age-matched normal subjects, the qualitative perception of dyspnea was clearly attributable to (and correlated with) indices of altered respiratory mechanics. Specifically, this study showed that dyspnea scores were related to increased inspiratory muscle effort (measured as esophageal pressure) and that the resting VT/IC ratio (an index of VT constraint) in patients with ILD correlated significantly with the dyspnea-$\dot{V}O_2$ slope, suggesting that dyspnea and the perception of its severity is an important determinant of exercise limitation in patients with ILD.

Other Factors

Respiratory muscle function has been shown to be compromised in patients with significant ILD. While it has not been clearly shown whether maximal inspiratory pressures measured at rest are reduced in patients with ILD [50–52], recent data to suggest that inspiratory pressures (as %max) increased significantly during exercise in ILD patients [50]. This increase in inspiratory muscle work is used to overcome the increase in elastance associated with the rapid shallow breathing at high lung volumes during exercise [1, 39]. The lack of any change in EELV further reduces inspiratory muscle reserve and may contribute to their fatigue [42, 53]. The role of hypoxemia in causing inspiratory muscle fatigue has been questioned [54–56]. Respiratory muscle fatigue, if it occurs, has been shown to result in a rapid shallow breathing pattern [57]. However, the lack of any differences between breathing pattern at peak exercise and during recovery [58] and the lack of effect of supplemental O_2 on exercise breathing pattern [38, 59] suggest that inspiratory muscle fatigue, if present, was not due to arterial hypoxemia or possibly be an important factor in exercise limitation in patients with ILD.

While cardiovascular dysfunction has long been shown to be associated with the increased morbidity and mortality of patients with ILD [60–62], its role in exercise limitation in ILD patients has not been studied extensively. Patients with ILD usually show an elevated heart rate (HR) at rest and in response to exercise [16], which is thought to be associated with reduced stroke volume [36, 43, 63], ECG abnormalities [64] and abnormal right- and left-ventricular function [63, 65]. Cardiovascular function during exercise may be adversely affected by altered respiratory mechanics in ILD patients. The increased inspiratory intrapleural pressure at TLC often seen in ILD [1, 39] may impede left-ventricular filling and or increase left-ventricular afterload [66, 67]. Exercise-induced hypoxemia may also adversely affect myocardial function during exercise. Hypoxia has been shown to increase heart rate in humans [68, 69], possibly due to its stimulatory effect on circulating catecholamines [70]. It has also been suggested that supplemental O_2 breathing may improve exercise performance in hypoxemic patients by relieving myocardial ischemia [37].

Pulmonary hypertension is a common clinical finding [71, 72] and right ventricular hypertrophy is a universal finding at autopsy [73] in patients with ILD. Most patients with ILD develop significant pulmonary hypertension during exercise [72, 74–76], and this has been attributed to both the parenchymal degeneration [36, 71, 72, 75] and the high intrathoracic pressures caused by abnormal respiratory mechanics [72]. Furthermore, pulmonary hypertension has been shown to be significantly correlated with hypoxemia during exercise [72, 75], that which has been postulated to aggravate pulmonary hypertension at rest and increase morbidity in patients with ILD [36, 71, 75]. We have shown that while supplemental O_2 breathing improves exercise endurance, it also results in a lower HR trend during exercise in ILD patients [38]. It was also shown that hypoxemia played a more important role than abnormal respiratory mechanics in exercise limitation in ILD [59]. It has recently been suggested that gas exchange abnormalities secondary to the pathophysiology of the pulmonary circulation and circulatory dysfunction, are perhaps the most important factors in limiting exercise in patients with ILD [5].

Disease-Specific Differences in Exercise Responses

There have been few studies that have compared exercise responses in different forms of ILD, but the available data suggests that important differences exist amongst the various diseases that cause ILD. Patients with IPF demonstrate greater exercise impairment (with $\dot{V}I$/MVV ratios of 80%) compared to patients with sarcoidosis ($\dot{V}I$/MVV ratio <60%) suggesting that the latter group of patients have a greater ventilatory reserve at peak exercise [43]. This study also showed that many patients with sarcoidosis ascribed exercise cessation to leg fatigue and not dyspnea, suggesting that factors other than ventilatory limitation may have contributed to exercise termination in the sarcoidosis patients. Other studies of sarcoidosis [63, 65] or scleroderma [77] suggest that cardiac factors may predominate in exercise limitation in these patients. A recent study [78] suggests peripheral muscle dysfunction, not ventilatory or gas exchange impairment, contributes significantly to reduced exercise tolerance in patients with systemic lupus erythematosis. Differences in the degree of gas exchange impairment and arterial hypoxemia during exercise have also been demonstrated between patients with sarcoidosis/asbestosis and IPF [24, 79]. Patients with IPF often show an increased $PAO_2 - PaO_2$ and increased O_2 desaturation compared to patients with ILD caused by other diseases [31, 79]. While the results of these studies underscore important differences in exercise responses between IPF and ILD (due to other causes), it is not clear whether these differences are related to the severity of the underlying disease process, to the severity of the underlying restrictive defect, or both [10].

While it is evident that many factors are involved in exercise impairment in patients with ILD, the specific roles of each of these factors and others (table 1) continues to be examined. For example, the role of lactic acidosis and the effects of its prevention by supplemental O_2 breathing on the ventilatory response and exercise performance in patients with ILD will need to be addressed. It is also important to consider that many patients with ILD may be exercise intolerant because of poor physical fitness or the lack of motivation, rather than the effects of the disease per se. In this instance, the results of CPET would enable the clinician to accurately determine the factor(s) contributing to the patient's exercise limitation, and appropriately manage their symptoms and disease.

Table 2. Indications for CPET in ILD

1	Objective assessment of symptoms
2	Assessment of severity of disease
3	Assessment of factors contributing to exercise limitation
4	Assessment/titration of oxygen therapy
5	Prescription of an exercise training program
6	Disability assessment

Indications for CPET in ILD

Many ILD patients present initially with a history of insidious onset of exertional dyspnea. While there is a progressive decline in lung structure and function in these patients, the large functional reserve in the respiratory system ensures that these patients remain mostly asymptomatic at rest. Physical exercise imposes an increasing demand on respiratory reserves and is thus an effective method of eliciting symptoms as well as in the assessment of abnormal function and disability. CPET also aids in the objective assessment of the degree of functional limitation that accompanies physical effort in patients with diagnosed ILD and that limitation which may neither be predicted by, nor correlate with, the indicators of pulmonary derangement measured at rest [31, 33]. As table 2 indicates, in patients with altered pulmonary function at rest, CPET is useful in the objective assessment and the differential diagnosis of the causes of effort intolerance and dyspnea, both of which can be due to cardiac and/or respiratory disease [9, 45, 48, 80]. CPET also helps in the better understanding of the severity of the disease process and may help the clinician to relate the severity of reported symptoms with indices of disease severity [31]. The role of some of the other factors (table 1) and co-existent disease (or lack of fitness) in exercise intolerance in a specific ILD patient can be better understood by exercise testing. As resting measurements of SaO_2 do not reliably predict the degree of exercise-induced hypoxemia [79] and as supplemental O_2 breathing has been shown to increase exercise endurance [15, 38] and improve myocardial function [37], CPET is necessary for both the titration of and the assessment of the effectiveness of O_2 therapy. The impact of physical reconditioning on muscle strength and endurance, functional capacity and quality of life in patients with ILD participating in cardiopulmonary rehabilitation programs has not been studied adequately. While some studies suggest that while cardiopulmonary rehabilitation resulted in no improvement in resting pulmonary function, the 6-min walking distance improved significantly [81] and many patients report the benefits of participating in an exercise training program. However, comprehensive CPET is usually required before enrolment in such programs and enables the clinician to both ensure patients' safety as well as objectively assess the benefits of these programs. The role of CPET in documenting the presence and assessment of the severity of impairment and disability in patients with ILD caused by occupational exposures is well established [82, 83]. Table 2, while by no means an exhaustive list, serves as a simple guide to highlight the more common indications for CPET in patients with ILD.

Cardiopulmonary Exercise Testing and Interpretation in ILD

This section deals with the specific responses and their interpretation in patients with ILD during cardiopulmonary exercise testing. Key details of exercise protocols, equipment, data collection and interpretation are also summarized. The data presented were collected in our laboratory over the years and have been published previously [38, 42, 84]. Data from healthy young subjects are also presented in order to facilitate the better understanding of key exercise responses in patients. For more detailed information, the reader is urged to refer to other reports on clinical exercise testing in ILD [10], integrated cardiopulmonary exercise testing and interpretation [6, 8], and physiological principles of exercise testing [7, 9].

Exercise Testing Protocol and Techniques of Measurement

The two commonly used test protocols in our laboratory are: (1) symptom-limited maximal incremental exercise test, and (2) constant work rate exercise test. For the maximal test, work load increments (10–25 watts/min) are chosen based on the expected peak work rate (max) and the ability of the patient to sustain exercise for at least 8–10 min such that meaningful data can be collected for analysis. Constant submaximal work rate (~60–75% $\dot{W}max$) protocols, though not commonly employed, are better than the step test and the 6-min walk test and may be useful in assessing the effects of therapy or interventions.

Cycle ergometer exercise is usually preferable to treadmill exercise as: (1) it is more economical; (2) it provides a more accurate measure of external work rate, and (3) patients feel familiarized and more secure during maximal exercise when seated than when running on a treadmill. Whatever the choice of equipment (cycle ergometer or treadmill) in a particular clinical laboratory, it is crucial to ensure its periodic calibration so that reliable, accurate, reproducible and clinically relevant data can be collected and interpreted. We have shown previously that such measures result in a high reproducibility (coefficient of variation ~ 5%) of both submaximal and peak exercise data in patients with ILD (even in those who had not previously performed cycle ergometer exercise) [17]. It is important to take this variability into consideration when conducting and interpreting exercise tests in patients with ILD.

While exercise testing in a physician-supervised setting is considered relatively safe [9], it is important to consider that the risk of serious morbidity or mortality in ILD patients during exercise is quite low (1 in 10,000) with deaths reported only in patients with known or suspected cardiac disease [85]. Precautionary measures such as a normal pre-exercise resting 12-lead ECG (to exclude arrhythmias and/or significant ischemia), an experienced attendant physician equipped with facilities for cardiopulmonary resuscitation, contribute to the reduction of risk significantly [86]. Furthermore, ECG monitoring throughout exercise and after (during the warm down period) is mandatory. While patients should be encouraged to exercise to their symptom-limited maximum, they should be given unambiguous instructions to stop exercise immediately if they develop any chest pain, dizziness or other symptoms of significant discomfort. The attending physician should also stop the exercise test if the patient develops any of the known and accepted indications for exercise stoppage [9]. Upon completion of the exercise test, patients should be monitored for at least 10–15 min more (both ECG and SaO_2 monitoring) and should be reassessed by the physician before being allowed to leave the laboratory [86]. Informed written consent must be obtained from all patients before any exercise testing is undertaken.

Useful Measurements during CPET

Table 3 summarizes some of the routinely available and easy to measure variables using current computerized exercise testing systems. In most cases, respired airflow (inspired and expired), O_2 and CO_2 concentrations, ECG and SaO_2 signals are acquired and digitized both for storage and off-line data analysis of derived variables. These include: (1) O_2 uptake ($\dot{V}O_2$); (2) CO_2 output ($\dot{V}CO_2$); (3) respiratory exchange ratio (R = $\dot{V}CO_2/\dot{V}O_2$); (4) end-tidal CO_2 tension ($PETCO_2$); (5) heart rate (HR); (6) arterial O_2 saturation (SaO_2); (7) tidal volume (VT), and (8) breathing frequency (f) and minute ventilation ($\dot{V}I$). Other variables such as dead space ventilation (VD/VT) and ventilatory cost of O_2 uptake and CO_2 output ($\dot{V}I/\dot{V}O_2$, $\dot{V}I/\dot{V}CO_2$) can also be derived from the above data. However, it is important to note that arterial blood-gas measurements are required for accurate assessments of VD/VT [87]. Borg scores (dyspnea and leg fatigue) are recorded at rest, during exercise and especially at end exercise in our laboratory. Subjects are carefully instructed about the usage of Borg scores before exercise commences. Inspiratory capacity (IC) maneuvers at rest, during and at end exercise are also recorded when tidal flow volume loops need to be analyzed for the assessment of operating lung volumes and ventilatory mechanics during exercise. Finger-tip pulse oximetry is most commonly used for the measurement of SaO_2 in our laboratory, as it is an effective and a non-invasive measure of arterial O_2 saturation [88]. While it is possible that pulse-oximetry may overestimate true SaO_2 at high work rates and at low work rates in people with a darker complexion [89] and the validity of SaO_2 measurements using ear oximetry may be questionable [89, 90], pulse oximetry remains an effective, simple and noninvasive method of measuring SaO_2 during exercise [91]. Furthermore, pulse oximetry data have been shown to correlate well with simultaneous blood-gas measurements especially when trends in SaO_2 (not absolute values in a clinically relevant range) are required [88, 91]. However, as shown before [5, 11], invasive techniques

Table 3. Useful measurements during CPET in ILD

Measured variables
Respiratory flow and volume (pneumotachograph)
Mean-expired and end-tidal PO_2 and PCO_2 (mass spectrometer/gas analyzer)
Arterial O_2 saturation (pulse oximeter)
Heart rate (ECG electrodes)
Work rate (cycle ergometer)
Inspiratory capacity (IC) at rest, during and at end exercise
Borg scores (dyspnea and leg fatigue)
Derived variables
Oxygen uptake ($\dot{V}O_2$)
Carbon dioxide output ($\dot{V}CO_2$)
Respiratory exchange ratio (R = $\dot{V}CO_2/\dot{V}O_2$)
Minute ventilation ($\dot{V}_I$)
Ventilatory equivalents for O_2 and CO_2 ($\dot{V}I/\dot{V}O_2$, $\dot{V}I/\dot{V}CO_2$)
Tidal volume (VT)
Respiratory frequency (f)
VD/VT – Dead space ventilation (from arterial blood gas measurements)
End-expiratory (EELV) and end-inspiratory (EILV) lung volumes
Exercise tidal flow-volume loops

(measurement of arterial blood gases, $PAO_2 - PaO_2$, VD/VT) are sometimes necessary in the accurate assessment of both the nature and degree of gas exchange impairment during exercise in some patients with ILD.

Interpretation of Exercise Test Results

Characteristic responses to exercise testing that are demonstrated by patients with ILD are listed in table 4. As the interpretation of results of exercise testing in cardiopulmonary disease is a complex process, the reader is urged to consult additional literature on this topic [6–8, 10, 12]. Briefly, it is important to remember that no set of responses to exercise is invariable in any one disease state (e.g. O_2 desaturation may occur in patients with chronic airflow limitation or pulmonary vascular disease). Furthermore, it must be considered that the results of exercise testing in a patient with ILD may be influenced by a second disease process such as ischemic heart disease or other connective tissue disorders that may cause muscle weakness. These factors as well as others such as poor physical fitness and/or malingering may also contribute to exercise limitation in patients with ILD. The attending physician would therefore have to consider the results of exercise testing within the context of all other relevant clinical information (history, physical examination, chest film, pulmonary function, etc.) for appropriate and effective interpretation.

The guidelines for proper interpretation of cardiopulmonary exercise testing in general include: (1) How limited is the patient? (2) What factors contribute to exercise limitation? (3) What are the abnormal patterns that are elicited? (4) Which clinical disorder(s) may result in these patterns? It is also important to ensure that the exercise test was maximal. The criteria for a maximal exercise test are discussed elsewhere [6, 12]. Commonly demonstrated patterns of response to maximal exercise testing in ILD patients are summarized in table 4 and include: (1) reduction in peak $\dot{V}O_2$ and $\dot{W}$max; (2) significant O_2 desaturation during and at end exercise; (3) reduction in peak heart rate; (4) reduction in peak $\dot{V}$I that approaches (or sometimes exceeds) maximum voluntary ventilation (MVV) calculated from FEV_1 (MVV = FEV_1*35); (5) unchanged $PaCO_2$ during exercise; (6) a rapid (↑f) and shallow (↓VT) breathing pattern, and (7) high VD/VT ratios. These patterns of response are fairly similar among various disease processes that cause ILD [11, 24, 34, 43, 78, 92, 93]. However, notable differences in ventilatory mechanics and degree of O_2 desaturation have been demonstrated in patients with ILD and these seem related to both the underlying pathology and disease severity.

Table 4. Characteristic responses during CPET in ILD

Reduced peak $\dot{V}O_2$ and $\dot{W}$max
Lower maximal heart rate
Arterial O_2 desaturation during and at end exercise
Higher $\dot{V}$I at submaximal work rates
Reduced peak $\dot{V}$I
High f, low VT at submaximal work rates
Normal peak VT/VC ratio
Higher peak $\dot{V}$I/FEV_1*35 ratio
High VD/VT ratios
Unchanged $PaCO_2$ during exercise

Results of Pulmonary Function Testing and CPET (Normals vs. ILD)

Table 5 summarizes the results of pulmonary function testing and maximal incremental exercise testing in both ILD patients and healthy young subjects [38, 84]. Wherever possible, data have been presented as % predicted values. The ILD patients demonstrate a significant reduction in both absolute and relative lung volumes and capacities and a significant reduction in DLCO (<50% pred). There was no evidence of airflow limitation in these patients (FEV_1/FVC ~ 80%). The data suggest that the exercise tests were maximal (note the significant O_2 desaturation at end exercise) and that there is clear evidence of exercise limitation in these ILD patients (see earlier). Figure 1a–h illustrates the temporal course of some key variables during exercise testing in both patients with ILD and healthy subjects. It is evident from figure 1a that patients with ILD stopped exercise at a much lower peak $\dot{V}O_2$ (56% pred) and a lower peak heart rate (80% pred). However, the heart rate response at a given metabolic rate was significantly higher in the ILD patients compared to healthy subjects. This phenomenon of an increased heart rate response to exercise in patients with significant ILD is possibly secondary to a reduction in stroke volume that apparently worsens with an increase in disease severity [26, 43, 94].

The most commonly observed phenomenon in ILD patients during exercise is arterial O_2 desaturation and is shown in figure 1b. While SaO_2 in healthy subjects remains mostly stable throughout and till end exercise, it falls significantly (Δ ~ 5%) throughout exercise in patients with ILD, reaching its nadir at peak exercise (SaO_2 has frequently been shown to fall to 85%, or lower). However, as discussed earlier, while arterial O_2 desaturation during exercise is typical of ILD patients, it is by no means specific to ILD and may occur with exercise in oth-

Table 5. Results of pulmonary function testing and CPET (Normals vs. ILD) [38, 84]

Variable	Normals	ILD
Age, years	21 ± 2	49 ± 15
n	9 (4 m, 5 f)	7 (6 m, 1 f)
TLC, liters	5.73 ± 1.09 (99% pred)	4.60 ± 0.25 (70% pred)
VC, liters	4.79 ± 0.91 (104% pred)	3.22 + 0.27 (70% pred)
FEV_1, liters	3.84 ± 0.69 (97% pred)	2.55 ± 0.24 (74% pred)
DLCO, %pred	89 ± 9	48 ± 7
FEV_1/FVC, %	86 ± 3	79 ± 2
Peak $\dot{V}O_2$, liters/min	2.82 ± 0.88 (98% pred)	1.32 ± 0.05 (56% pred)
$\dot{W}$max, watts	209 ± 68 (99% pred)	106 ± 14 (55% pred)
Peak heart rate	186 ± 11 (95% pred)	143 ± 4 (80% pred)
Peak $\dot{V}I$, liters/min	106 ± 44	63 ± 6
Peak $\dot{V}I$, %FEV_1*35	76 ± 22	75 ± 25
Peak VT/VC, %	53 ± 8	57 ± 13
SaO_2 (end exercise, %)	95 ± 2	84 ± 2

er disease states [58, 91]. The relationship between $\dot{V}CO_2$ and $\dot{V}O_2$ is shown in figure 1c. Also shown is the line of identity which corresponds to an R = 1, levels above which increased R values imply a change to anaerobic metabolism. While it is an imprecise technique for the assessment of metabolic acidosis or the lactate threshold, the $\dot{V}CO_2$ – $\dot{V}O_2$ relationship allows a quick and noninvasive estimate of the anaerobic threshold [95]. It is also important to remember that changes in anaerobic threshold may be nonspecific and may be affected by specific disease states, therapeutic interventions, including supplemental O_2 breathing [38].

Figure 1d describes the relationship between $\dot{V}O_2$ and $PaCO_2$ (derived from $PETCO_2$) [9]. $PETCO_2$ represents a noninvasive estimate of $PaCO_2$ and can be measured by most commercially available exercise testing systems. While $PETCO_2$ has been shown to correlate well with actual $PaCO_2$, its utility is only as an estimate (not a measure) of $PaCO_2$. The data show that normal subjects tend to regulate their $PaCO_2$ at ~ 40 mm Hg during exercise, until the onset of metabolic acidosis and the compensatory increase in ventilation, cause a fall in arterial PCO_2. The measurement of $PETCO_2$ (or estimated $PaCO_2$) in ILD patients during exercise has only limited diagnostic value as it has been shown that $PaCO_2$ remains stable and unchanged (from resting values) during exercise in patients with ILD [10]. However, the stability of the $PaCO_2$ throughout and at peak exercise implies that there was no increase in alveolar ventilation in the patients with ILD (compared to normal subjects).

The ventilatory response to exercise and the maximal predicted values for $\dot{V}I$ (from MVV = FEV_1*35) in both groups are shown in figure 1e. While peak $\dot{V}I$ is reduced significantly in patients with ILD (compared to healthy subjects), both groups achieved over 75% of peak predicted $\dot{V}I$ at end exercise. Furthermore, the increased ventilatory response during submaximal exercise is typical of patients with ILD and is further described in figure 1f as $\dot{V}I/\dot{V}CO_2$. This variable normally falls early in exercise and increases later during heavy exercise with the development of metabolic acidosis and hyperventilation. Normal subjects have a $\dot{V}I/\dot{V}CO_2$ ratio of 25–35 during exercise and the elevated $\dot{V}I/\dot{V}CO_2$ ratio in the ILD patients implies that there was an increase in dead space ventilation (VD/VT), with little or no increase in alveolar ventilation (stable $PaCO_2$; fig. 1d).

Figures 1f and 1g describe the differences in pattern of breathing at various ventilatory levels between the healthy subjects and ILD patients. In both groups, the initial increase in $\dot{V}I$ at lower levels of $\dot{V}I$ is achieved by a combination of increases in VT and f. At higher $\dot{V}I$ levels increases in f predominate in contributing to the increase in $\dot{V}I$ as VT gradually becomes asymptotic. The increase in f is consequent to a decrease in both inspiratory and expiratory durations [10, 52]. As suggested earlier, patients with ILD adopt a rapid (↑f) and shallow (↓VT) breathing pattern at any given level of ventilation compared to healthy subjects. It must noted here that while the ratio VT_{max} to VC has been suggested as being different in patients with ILD, it appears to have little or limited diagnostic value [10], as similar ratios (VT/VC

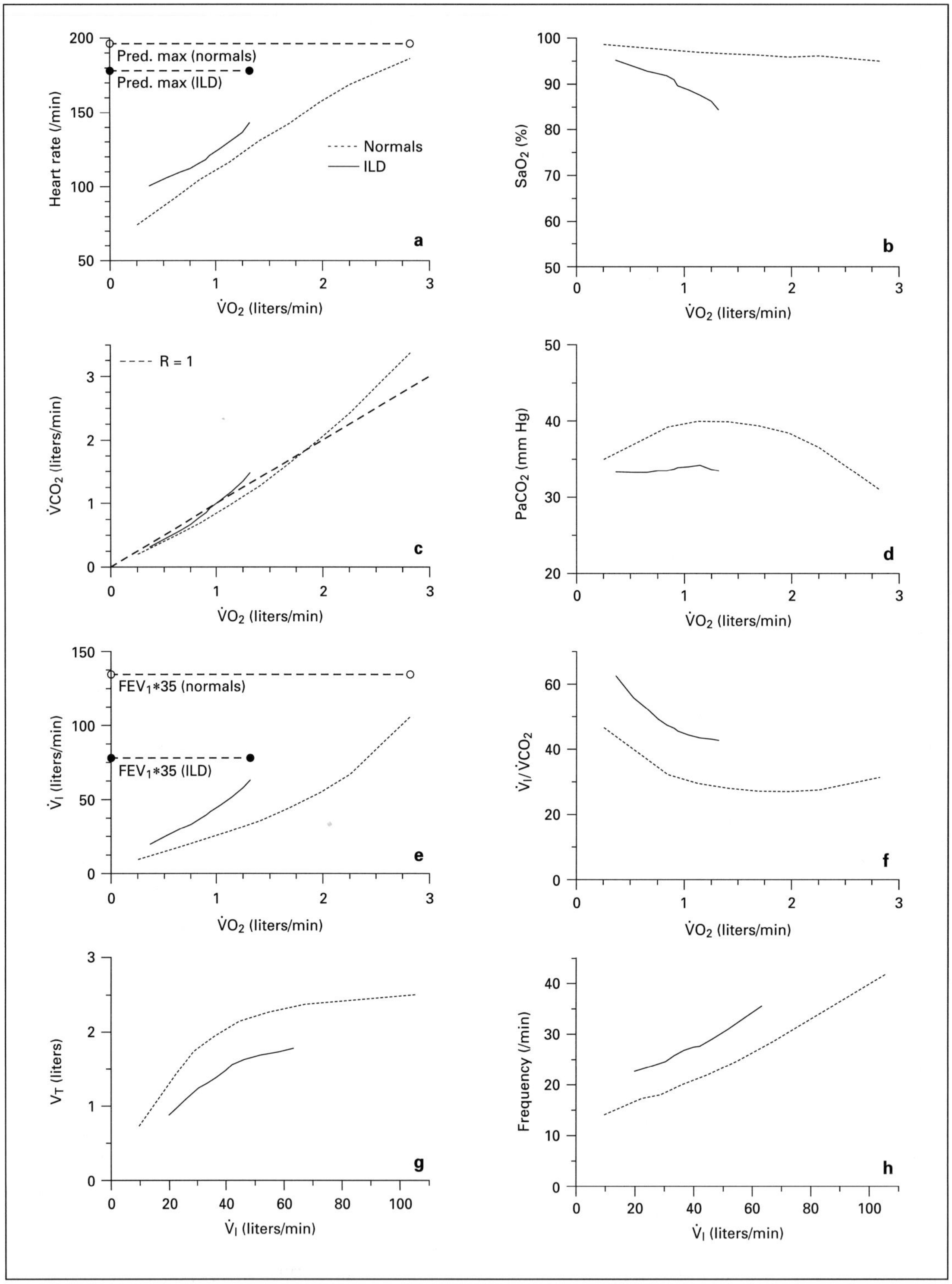

Fig. 1. Results of exercise testing compared between healthy subjects (dashed lines, open circles) and patients with ILD (solid lines, closed circles) (see table 5 for more details) [38, 84]. $\dot{V}O_2$ = Oxygen uptake; SaO_2 = arterial O_2 saturation; $\dot{V}CO_2$ = CO_2 output; $PaCO_2$ = arterial CO_2 tension; $\dot{V}I$ = minute ventilation; VT = tidal volume.

~ 55%) have been found in healthy subjects and in patients with ILD, chronic airflow limitation or congestive cardiac failure [58, 96].

The abnormal respiratory mechanics results in a significantly reduced maximal voluntary ventilation (MVV) or ventilatory reserve ($\dot{V}I$/MVV) in patients with ILD [7, 16]. The combination of an increased $\dot{V}I$ at submaximal work rates and the reduction in MVV results in the increase of the ventilatory demand/capacity ($\dot{V}I$/MVV) ratio during exercise. It is not uncommon for $\dot{V}I$/MVV to exceed 0.8 in many patients with significant ILD or $\dot{V}I$/MVV to approach 1 in patients with severe ILD during exercise [18], resulting in significant ventilatory constraints on exercise performance. Traditionally the assessment of the degree of ventilatory constraint has been based on estimation of the ventilatory reserve or how close to MVV (or its estimate) does peak $\dot{V}I$ get during exercise. Ventilatory reserve is dependent on numerous factors [14], chief among which are: (1) the maximal flow-volume envelope (which is further dependent on age, sex, body size, muscle function, genetic makeup, aging and disease); (2) airway function (bronchodilatation or bronchoconstriction) during exercise, and (3) the lung volumes at which tidal breathing occurs relative to total lung capacity and residual volume (the limits of end-inspiratory and end-expiratory lung volumes). It follows that breathing at low lung volumes (near RV) the shape of the maximal flow volume envelope limits the available ventilatory reserve which can be further compromised by an increase in chest wall stiffness. Breathing at higher lung volumes (near TLC), while contributing to a greater ventilatory reserve, does result in increasing elastic loads on the inspiratory muscles and therefore the work of breathing. Even a visual analysis of the appropriately placed (within the maximal loop) exercise tidal flow-volume loops can provide valuable insights into the role of respiratory mechanics and respiratory muscle energetics in their contribution to ventilatory limits on exercise performance. The estimation of ventilatory reserve based on FEV_1 on the other hand neither provides any detailed information on breathing strategy, nor account for the increasing inspiratory and expiratory flow constraints during exercise.

More recently, newer techniques that can quantify mechanical ventilatory constraints during exercise have been developed, although these have not yet been validated for clinical use [42, 97, 98]. Briefly, these techniques calculate a theoretical maximum ventilatory capacity (MVC) which is based on the maximal available inspiratory and expiratory airflows (from the maximal flow-volume loops) over the range of tidal breathing from measured exercise EELV. The term $\dot{V}E_{cap}$ had originally been used to describe such a measure of ventilatory capacity which is independent of volitional effort and accounts for changes in dynamic airway function during exercise. Thus, if there is no flow limitation (i.e. tidal expiratory flow does not meet (or exceed) maximal available airflow throughout expiration), maximal ventilatory capacity (MVC = $\dot{V}E_{cap}$) is an effective measure of the ventilatory reserve for a given breathing pattern at any lung volume [41, 42]. More details on this technique and its superiority over the MVV (FEV_1*35) method, in the assessment of ventilatory reserve in a wide range of subjects during exercise, have been published recently [14]. The results of analyses of mechanical constraints on exercise performance based on exercise flow-volume relationships in patients with ILD are now presented in figures 2 and 3.

Exercise Tidal Flow-Volume Relationships (Normals vs. ILD)

Figure 2 illustrates flow-volume relationships during exercise in both healthy subjects [84] and in patients with ILD [42]. Data shown are maximal expiratory and inspiratory loops and tidal loops at rest and at different exercise intensities (50 and 100% $\dot{V}O_2$max in healthy subjects during incremental exercise and at 40, 70 and 90% $\dot{V}O_2$max in ILD patients performing constant work-rate exercise). The data show that with increasing exercise intensity, both healthy subjects and patients with ILD are able to increase inspiratory and expiratory flows and show no evidence of expiratory flow limitation during exercise. While these increases in flows are possible even with a significant fall in EELV (from resting values) in healthy subjects, the patients with ILD show no change in EELV from resting values during exercise. This is as a result of the marked reduction in expiratory reserve volume with ILD [1, 39], with increases in exercise VT possible only from the inspiratory reserve volume (↑EILV). It has been suggested that any possible fall in EELV could have been affected by hypoxemia which has shown to affect resting lung volume and respiratory mechanics [42, 99]. The increase in ventilation was thus more dependent on an increase in breathing frequency (and increased flows) in these patients. While these patients, as a group, do not show evidence of expiratory flow limitation, our study [42] showed that significant expiratory flow limitation, high EILV/TLC and VT/VC ratios were present in those subjects who stopped exercise due to dyspnea. In contrast there was no flow limitation in patients who stopped exercise due to leg fatigue. Interestingly, the patients with

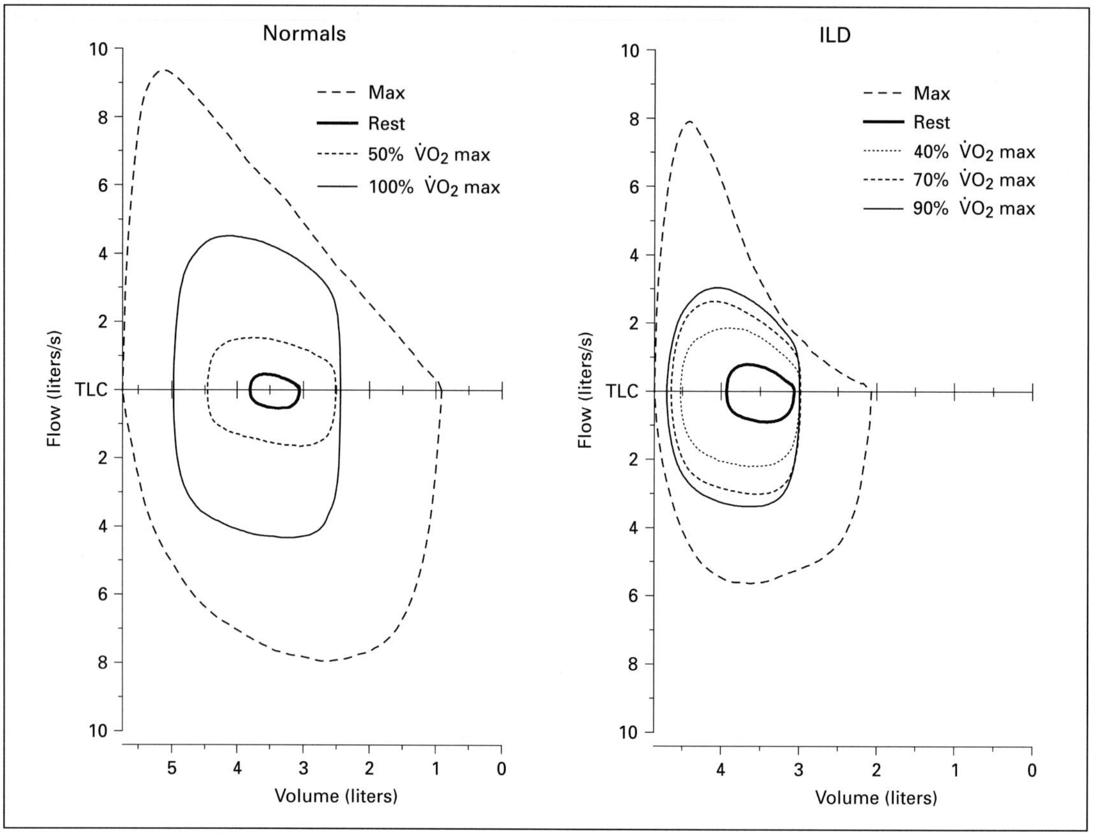
Normals
ILD
Max
Rest
50% V̇O2 max
100% V̇O2 max
40% V̇O2 max
70% V̇O2 max
90% V̇O2 max
Flow (liters/s)
TLC
Volume (liters)

2

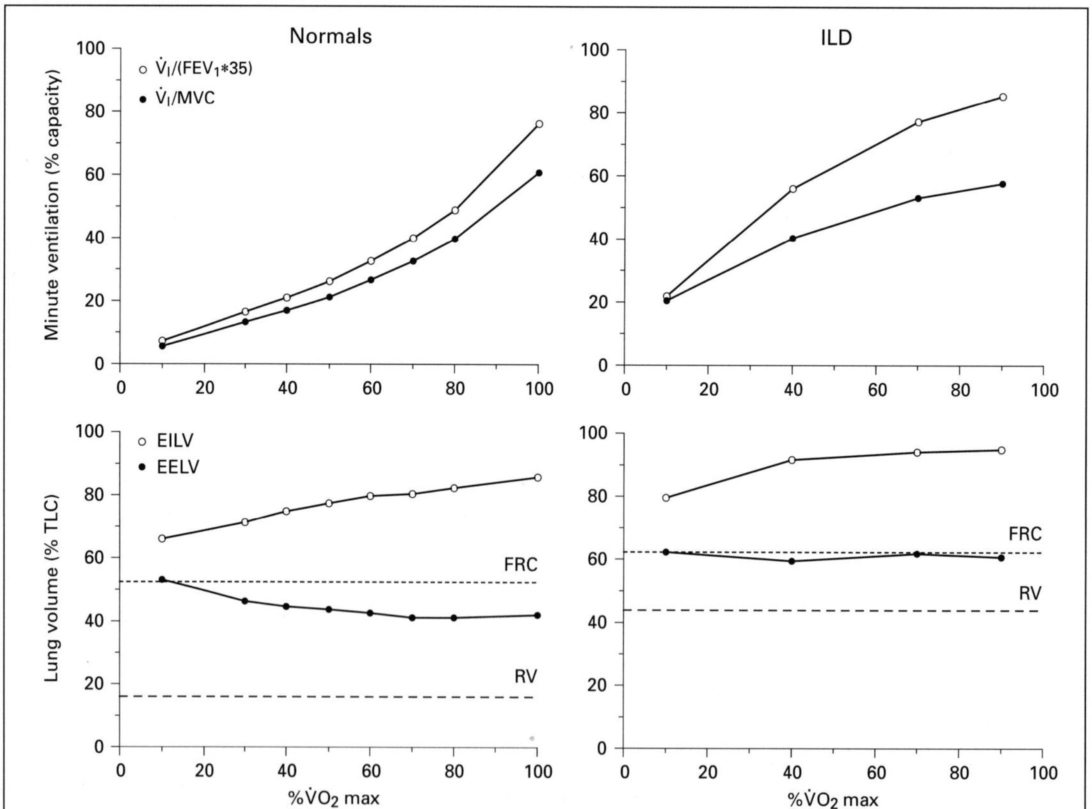
Normals
ILD
V̇I/(FEV1*35)
V̇I/MVC
Minute ventilation (% capacity)
EILV
EELV
FRC
RV
Lung volume (% TLC)
%V̇O2 max

3

the most mechanical constraints (flow limitation and ↑EELV) had the least O_2 desaturation but higher dyspnea scores. These data combined with improved exercise performance with supplemental O_2 breathing [38] imply that while expiratory flow limitation may occur in some ILD patients and may contribute to the dyspnea of exercise, it is arterial hypoxemia and not respiratory mechanics that plays a predominant role in exercise limitation in patients with ILD.

Ventilatory Mechanics and Lung Volumes during Exercise (Normals vs. ILD)

Figure 3 summarizes the comparisons between the two techniques (MVV and MVC) used in the estimation of ventilatory capacity during exercise in both healthy subjects and patients with ILD. It is evident that even in healthy subjects the ventilatory demand/capacity ratio is higher when MVV (FEV_1*35) is used as an index of ventilatory reserve, although these differences are small at low exercise intensities. However, in patients with ILD, the $\dot{V}I$/MVV ratio is significantly greater at all exercise intensities. It has been shown previously that MVC (estimated from flow-volume loops and breathing pattern) is significantly greater than MVV (FEV_1*35) in patients with ILD [42]. Figure 3 emphasizes the fact that MVV thus significantly underestimates potential ventilatory reserve at least in patients with ILD during exercise. In contrast, the $\dot{V}I$/MVC data (peak <60%) suggest that a significant potential for increasing ventilation exists in these patients during exercise. Figure 3 also describes differences in breathing pattern (i.e. tidal volume changes) during exercise between healthy subjects and patients with ILD. While VT in healthy subjects increases as a result of changes in both EILV and EELV, it remains constant in patients with ILD. Furthermore, as EELV does not change significantly during exercise (from resting values), patients with ILD are required to breathe at higher lung volumes (EILV >90%) throughout exercise resulting in a significant increase in respiratory muscle work and dyspnea [50], both of which contribute significantly to exercise limitation in these patients.

Fig. 2. Maximal (long-dashed lines) and tidal flow volume loops at rest (thick solid lines) and during exercise at different intensities in healthy subjects (50% VO_2max = medium-dashed line and 100% $\dot{V}O_2$max = solid line) and in patients with ILD (40% $\dot{V}O_2$max = small-dashed line, 70% $\dot{V}O_2$max = medium-dashed line and 90% $\dot{V}O_2$max = solid line) [42, 84]. $\dot{V}O_2$max = Maximal O_2 uptake.

Fig. 3. Comparison of ventilatory constraints and lung volumes during exercise in healthy subjects (open circles) and patients with ILD (closed circles) [42, 84]. $\dot{V}I$ = Minute ventilation; FEV_1 = forced expiratory volume in 1 s; MVC = maximal ventilatory capacity; EILV = end-inspiratory lung volume; EELV = end-expiratory lung volume; FRC = functional residual capacity; RV = residual volume; TLC = total lung capacity.

Impact of CPET on Patient Management in ILD

As exertional dyspnea and exercise intolerance are perhaps the most important common clinical presentations of ILD, clinical management should include measures that alleviate dyspnea as well as improve exercise capacity, both of which have a direct and immediate impact on the daily lives of these patients. Primarily, CPET provides the clinician an objective method of assessment of the effects of the specific abnormalities caused by the disease, as well as assess the effectiveness of treatment of specific disease and its symptoms in these patients. O_2 therapy, sufficient to prevent arterial O_2 desaturation has been shown to improve exercise performance in ILD [15, 38] and remains the mainstay of management of patients with severe ILD. Newer modalities of treatment of exertional dyspnea that have been tested and include inhaled morphine [100] or anesthetic [101] aerosols, have shown no effects on exertional dyspnea, ventilatory response to exercise or exercise capacity. The effects of inhaled nitric oxide (NO) on pulmonary hypertension has also been studied and it has been shown that while inhaled NO (without supplemental O_2) causes a significant fall in mean pulmonary artery pressure and pulmonary vascular resistance, PaO_2 does not improve [102]. It has also been shown that ILD patients have lower levels of intrinsic NO and also fail to show any increase in NO production during exercise [103]. Thus, it is evident that CPET has an important role to play in clinical decision making, individual patient management and on the assessment of the effectiveness of specific therapeutic modalities and physical rehabilitation in patients with ILD.

Acknowledgments

The research that was discussed in this report was supported by operating grants from the Medical Research Council of Canada, the Heart and Stroke Foundation of Canada, the Saskatchewan Lung Association and the Saskatchewan Health Research Board. The authors wish to express their appreciation to Mr. R. Clemens who has ably assisted with the research and with the preparation of the manuscript.

References

1 Pride NB, Macklem PT: Lung Mechanics in Disease; in: Fishman AP, Macklem PT, Mead J (eds): Handbook of Physiology: The Respiratory System, Mechanics of Breathing. Baltimore, Williams & Wilkins, 1986, vol 2, pp 659–692.
2 Baydur A: Pulmonary physiology in interstitial lung disease: Recent developments in diagnostic and prognostic implications. Curr Opin Pulm Med 1996;2:370–375.
3 Schwarz MI: Clinical overview of interstitial lung disease; in Manning S (ed): Interstitial Lung Disease. St. Louis, Mosby-Year Book, 1993, pp 1–22.
4 Hsia CC: Cardiopulmonary limitations to exercise in restrictive lung disease. Med Sci Sports Exerc 1999;31:S28–32.
5 Hansen JE, Wasserman K: Pathophysiology of activity limitation in patients with interstitial lung disease. Chest 1996;109:1566–1576.
6 Younes M: Interpretation of clinical exercise testing in respiratory disease. Clin Chest Med 1984;5:189–206.
7 Wasserman K, Hansen JE, Sue DY, Whipp BJ, Casaburi R: Principles of Exercise Testing and Interpretation. Philadelphia, Lea & Febiger, 1994.
8 Weisman IM, Zeballos RJ: An integrated approach to the interpretation of cardiopulmonary exercise testing. Clin Chest Med 1994;15: 421–445.
9 Jones NL: Clinical Exercise Testing. Philadelphia, Saunders, 1997.
10 Marciniuk DD, Gallagher CG: Clinical exercise testing in interstitial lung disease. Clin Chest Med 1994;15:287–303.
11 Markovitz GH, Cooper CB: Exercise and interstitial lung disease. Curr Opin Pulm Med 1998; 4:272–280.
12 Harris-Eze AO, Marciniuk DD: The role of exercise testing in interstitial lung disease. Clin Pulm Med 1995;2:213–220.
13 Johnson BD, Beck KC, Zeballos RJ, Weisman IM: Advances in pulmonary laboratory testing. Chest 1999;116:1377–1387.
14 Johnson BD, Weisman IM, Zeballos RJ, Beck KC: Emerging concepts in the evaluation of ventilatory limitation during exercise: The exercise tidal flow-volume loop. Chest 1999;116: 488–503.
15 Bye PT, Anderson SD, Woolcock AJ, Young IH, Alison JA: Bicycle endurance performance of patients with interstitial lung disease breathing air and oxygen. Am Rev Respir Dis 1982; 126:1005–1012.
16 Burdon JG, Killian KJ, Jones NL: Pattern of breathing during exercise in patients with interstitial lung disease. Thorax 1983;38:778–784.
17 Marciniuk DD, Watts RE, Gallagher CG: Reproducibility of incremental maximal cycle ergometer testing in patients with restrictive lung disease. Thorax 1993;48:894–898.
18 Marciniuk DD, Watts RE, Gallagher CG: Dead space loading and exercise limitation in patients with interstitial lung disease. Chest 1994;105:183–189.
19 Epler GR, Saber FA, Gaensler EA: Determination of severe impairment (disability) in interstitial lung disease. Am Rev Respir Dis 1980; 121:647–659.
20 Cotes JE, Zejda J, King B: Lung function impairment as a guide to exercise limitation in work-related lung disorders. Am Rev Respir Dis 1988;137:1089–1093.
21 Javaheri S, Sicilian L: Lung function, breathing pattern, and gas exchange in interstitial lung disease. Thorax 1992;47:93–97.
22 Kelley MA, Daniele RP: Exercise testing in interstitial lung disease. Clin Chest Med 1984; 5:145–156.
23 Jernudd-Wilhelmsson Y, Hornblad Y, Hedenstierna G: Ventilation-perfusion relationships in interstitial lung disease. Eur J Respir Dis 1986;68:39–49.
24 Agusti AG, Roca J, Rodriguez-Roisin R, Xaubet A, Agusti-Vidal A: Different patterns of gas exchange response to exercise in asbestosis and idiopathic pulmonary fibrosis. Eur Respir J 1988;1:510–516.
25 Agusti AG, Roca J, Gea J, Wagner PD, Xaubet A, Rodriguez-Roisin R: Mechanisms of gas-exchange impairment in idiopathic pulmonary fibrosis. Am Rev Respir Dis 1991;143:219–225.
26 Hughes JM, Lockwood DN, Jones HA, Clark RJ: DLCO/Q and diffusion limitation at rest and on exercise in patients with interstitial fibrosis. Respir Physiol 1991;83:155–166.
27 Agusti C, Xaubet A, Agusti AG, Roca J, Ramirez J, Rodriguez-Roisin R: Clinical and functional assessment of patients with idiopathic pulmonary fibrosis: Results of a 3-year follow-up. Eur Respir J 1994;7:643–650.
28 Wagner PD: Ventilation-perfusion matching during exercise. Chest 1992;101:192S–198S.
29 Crystal RG, Fulmer JD, Roberts WC, Moss ML, Line BR, Reynolds HY: Idiopathic pulmonary fibrosis: Clinical, histologic, radiographic, physiologic, scintigraphic, cytologic, and biochemical aspects. Ann Intern Med 1976;85:769–788.
30 Nordenfelt I, Svensson G: The transfer factor (diffusing capacity) as a predictor of hypoxaemia during exercise in restrictive and chronic obstructive pulmonary disease. Clin Physiol 1987;7:423–430.
31 Risk C, Epler GR, Gaensler EA: Exercise alveolar-arterial oxygen pressure difference in interstitial lung disease. Chest 1984;85:69–74.
32 Kelley MA, Panettieri RA Jr, Krupinski AV: Resting single-breath diffusing capacity as a screening test for exercise-induced hypoxemia. Am J Med 1986;80:807–812.
33 Bradvik I, Wollmer P, Blom-Bulow B, Albrechtsson U, Jonson B: Lung mechanics and gas exchange during exercise in pulmonary sarcoidosis. Chest 1991;99:572–578.
34 Crausman RS, Jennings CA, Tuder RM, Ackerson LM, Irvin CG, King TE Jr: Pulmonary histiocytosis X: Pulmonary function and exercise pathophysiology. Am J Respir Crit Care Med 1996;153:426–435.
35 Hansen JE, Wasserman K: Exercise testing in patients with interstitial lung disease. Chest 1998;113:1148–1149.
36 Bush A, Busst CM: Cardiovascular function at rest and on exercise in patients with cryptogenic fibrosing alveolitis. Thorax 1988;43:276–283.
37 Morrison DA, Stovall JR: Increased exercise capacity in hypoxemic patients after long-term oxygen therapy. Chest 1992;102:542–550.
38 Harris-Eze AO, Sridhar G, Clemens RE, Gallagher CG, Marciniuk DD: Oxygen improves maximal exercise performance in interstitial lung disease. Am J Respir Crit Care Med 1994; 150:1616–1622.
39 Warren CP, Tse KS, Cherniack RM: Mechanical properties of the lung in extrinsic allergic alveolitis. Thorax 1978;33:315–321.
40 Hansen JE, Sue DY, Wasserman K: Predicted values for clinical exercise testing. Am Rev Respir Dis 1984;129:S49–55.
41 Gallagher CG: Exercise and chronic obstructive pulmonary disease. Med Clin North Am 1990;74:619–641.
42 Marciniuk DD, Sridhar G, Clemens RE, Zintel TA, Gallagher CG: Lung volumes and expiratory flow limitation during exercise in interstitial lung disease. J Appl Physiol 1994;77:963–973.
43 Spiro SG, Dowdeswell IR, Clark TJ: An analysis of submaximal exercise responses in patients with sarcoidosis and fibrosing alveolitis. Br J Dis Chest 1981;75:169–180.
44 Renzi G, Milic-Emili J, Grassino AE: The pattern of breathing in diffuse lung fibrosis. Bull Eur Physiopathol Respir 1982;18:461–472.
45 Leblanc P, Bowie DM, Summers E, Jones NL, Killian KJ: Breathlessness and exercise in patients with cardiorespiratory disease. Am Rev Respir Dis 1986;133:21–25.
46 Young IH, Daviskas E, Keena VA: Effect of low dose nebulised morphine on exercise endurance in patients with chronic lung disease. Thorax 1989;44:387–390.
47 Rampulla C, Baiocchi S, Dacosto E, Ambrosino N: Dyspnea on exercise: Pathophysiologic mechanisms. Chest 1992;101:248S–252S.
48 Mahler DA, Harver A, Lentine T, Scott JA, Beck K, Schwartzstein RM: Descriptors of breathlessness in cardiorespiratory diseases. Am J Respir Crit Care Med 1996;154:1357–1363.
49 Mahler DA, Harver A, Rosiello R, Daubenspeck JA: Measurement of respiratory sensation in interstitial lung disease: Evaluation of clinical dyspnea ratings and magnitude scaling. Chest 1989;96:767–771.
50 O'Donnell DE, Chau LK, Webb KA: Qualitative aspects of exertional dyspnea in patients with interstitial lung disease. J Appl Physiol 1998;84:2000–2009.
51 De Troyer A, Yernault JC: Inspiratory muscle force in normal subjects and patients with interstitial lung disease. Thorax 1980;35:92–100.
52 DiMarco AF, Kelsen SG, Cherniack NS, Gothe B: Occlusion pressure and breathing pattern in patients with interstitial lung disease. Am Rev Respir Dis 1983;127:425–430.
53 Fitting JW: Respiratory muscle fatigue limiting physical exercise? Eur Respir J 1991;4:103–108.
54 Ameredes BT, Clanton TL: Hyperoxia and moderate hypoxia fail to affect inspiratory muscle fatigue in humans. J Appl Physiol 1989; 66:894–900.
55 Moxham J: Respiratory muscle fatigue: Mechanisms, evaluation and therapy. Br J Anaesth 1990;65:43–53.

56 NHLBI Workshop Summary: Respiratory muscle fatigue. Report of the Respiratory Muscle Fatigue Workshop Group. Am Rev Respir Dis 1990;142:474–480.
57 Gallagher CG, Hof VI, Younes M: Effect of inspiratory muscle fatigue on breathing pattern. J Appl Physiol 1985;59:1152–1158.
58 Gallagher CG, Younes M: Breathing pattern during and after maximal exercise in patients with chronic obstructive lung disease, interstitial lung disease, and cardiac disease, and in normal subjects. Am Rev Respir Dis 1986;133:581–586.
59 Harris-Eze AO, Sridhar G, Clemens RE, Zintel TA, Gallagher CG, Marciniuk DD: Role of hypoxemia and pulmonary mechanics in exercise limitation in interstitial lung disease. Am J Respir Crit Care Med 1996;154:994–1001.
60 Roberts WC, McAllister HA Jr, Ferrans VJ: Sarcoidosis of the heart. A clinicopathologic study of 35 necropsy patients (group 1) and review of 78 previously described necropsy patients (group 11). Am J Med 1977;63:86–108.
61 Silverman KJ, Hutchins GM, Bulkley BH: Cardiac sarcoid: A clinicopathologic study of 84 unselected patients with systemic sarcoidosis. Circulation 1978;58:1204–1211.
62 Fleming HA: Sarcoid heart disease. Br Med J (Clin Res Ed) 1986;292:1095 1096.
63 Gibbons WJ, Levy RD, Nava S, et al: Subclinical cardiac dysfunction in sarcoidosis. Chest 1991;100:44–50.
64 Shah NS, Velury S, Mascarenhas D, Spodick DH: Electrocardiographic features of restrictive pulmonary disease, and comparison with those of obstructive pulmonary disease. Am J Cardiol 1992;70:394–395.
65 Baughman RP, Gerson M, Bosken CH: Right and left ventricular function at rest and with exercise in patients with sarcoidosis. Chest 1984;85:301–306.
66 Pinsky MR: Effects of changing intrathoracic pressure on the normal and failing heart; in Lenfant C, Scharf SM, Cassidy SS (eds): Lung Biology in Health and Disease, Heart-Lung Interactions in Health and Disease. New York, Marcel Dekker, 1989, vol 42, pp 839–878.
67 Rodarte JR, Rehder K: Dynamics of Respiration; in Fishman AP, Macklem PT, Mead J (eds): Handbook of Physiology: The Respiratory System, Mechanics of Breathing. Baltimore, Williams & Wilkins, 1986, vol 2, pp 131–144.
68 Welch HG: Effects of hypoxia and hyperoxia on human performance. Exerc Sport Sci Rev 1987;15:191–221.
69 Miyamoto K, Nishimura M, Akiyama Y, Yamamoto H, Kishi F, Kawakami Y: Augmented heart rate response to hypoxia in patients with chronic obstructive pulmonary disease. Am Rev Respir Dis 1992;145:1384–1388.
70 Davidson D, Stalcup SA, Mellins RB: Systemic hemodynamics affecting cardiac output during hypocapnic and hypercapnic hypoxia. J Appl Physiol 1986;60:1230–1236.
71 Enson Y, Thomas HM 3rd, Bosken CH, et al: Pulmonary hypertension in interstitial lung disease: Relation of vascular resistance to abnormal lung structure. Trans Assoc Am Physicians 1975;88:248–255.
72 Hawrylkiewicz I, Izdebska-Makosa Z, Grebska E, Zielinski J: Pulmonary haemodynamics at rest and on exercise in patients with idiopathic pulmonary fibrosis. Bull Eur Physiopathol Respir 1982;18:403–410.
73 Packe GE, Cayton RM, Edwards CW: Comparison of right ventricular size at necropsy in interstitial pulmonary fibrosis and in chronic bronchitis and emphysema. Thorax 1980;40:712.
74 Widimsky J, Riedel M, Stanek V: Central haemodynamics during exercise in patients with restrictive pulmonary disease. Bull Eur Physiopathol Respir 1977;13:369–379.
75 Weitzenblum E, Ehrhart M, Rasaholinjanahary J, Hirth C: Pulmonary hemodynamics in idiopathic pulmonary fibrosis and other interstitial pulmonary diseases. Respiration 1983;44:118–127.
76 Agusti AG, Rodriguez-Roisin R: Effect of pulmonary hypertension on gas exchange. Eur Respir J 1993;6:1371–1377.
77 Follansbee WP, Curtiss EI, Medsger TA Jr, Owens GR, Steen VD, Rodnan GP: Myocardial function and perfusion in the CREST syndrome variant of progressive systemic sclerosis: Exercise radionuclide evaluation and comparison with diffuse scleroderma. Am J Med 1984;77:489–496.
78 Forte S, Carlone S, Vaccaro F, et al: Pulmonary gas exchange and exercise capacity in patients with systemic lupus erythematosus. J Rheumatol 1999;26:2591–2594.
79 Keogh BA, Lakatos E, Price D, Crystal RG: Importance of the lower respiratory tract in oxygen transfer: Exercise testing in patients with interstitial and destructive lung disease. Am Rev Respir Dis 1984;129:S76–80.
80 Mahler DA, Horowitz MB: Clinical evaluation of exertional dyspnea. Clin Chest Med 1994;15:259–269.
81 Foster S, Thomas HM 3rd: Pulmonary rehabilitation in lung disease other than chronic obstructive pulmonary disease. Am Rev Respir Dis 1990;141:601–604.
82 Sue DY, Wasserman K: Impact of integrative cardiopulmonary exercise testing on clinical decision making. Chest 1991;99:981–992.
83 Sue DY: Exercise testing in the evaluation of impairment and disability. Clin Chest Med 1994;15:369–387.
84 Krishnan B, Clemens RE, Laframboise K, Nagpal A, Marciniuk DD: Does the ventilatory response limit exercise performance in the normal aged? Am J Resp Crit Care Med 1999;159:A418.
85 Rochmis P, Blackburn H: Exercise tests: A survey of procedures, safety, and litigation experience in approximately 170,000 tests. JAMA 1971;217:1061–1066.
86 AARC Clinical Practice Guidelin: Exercise testing for evaluation of hypoxemia and/or desaturation. American Association for Respiratory Care. Respir Care 1992;37:907–912.
87 Lewis DA, Sietsema KE, Casaburi R, Sue DY: Inaccuracy of noninvasive estimates of VD/VT in clinical exercise testing. Chest 1994;106:1476–1480.
88 Martin D, Powers S, Cicale M, Collop N, Huang D, Criswell D: Validity of pulse oximery during exercise in elite endurance athletes. J Appl Physiol 1992;72:455–458.
89 Zeballos RJ, Weisman IM: Reliability of noninvasive oximetry in black subjects during exercise and hypoxia. Am Rev Respir Dis 1991;144:1240–1244.
90 Hansen JE, Casaburi R: Validity of ear oximetry in clinical exercise testing. Chest 1987;91:333–337.
91 Escourrou PJ, Delaperche MF, Visseaux A: Reliability of pulse oximetry during exercise in pulmonary patients. Chest 1990;97:635–638.
92 Miller A, Bhuptani A, Sloane MF, Brown LK, Teirstein AS: Cardiorespiratory responses to incremental exercise in patients with asbestos-related pleural thickening and normal or slightly abnormal lung function. Chest 1993;103:1045–1050.
93 Karetzky M, McDonough M: Exercise and resting pulmonary function in sarcoidosis. Sarcoidosis Vasc Diffuse Lung Dis 1996;13:43–49.
94 Fischbein A, Luo JC, Solomon SJ, Horowitz S, Hailoo W, Miller A: Clinical findings among hard metal workers. Br J Ind Med 1992;49:17–24.
95 Beaver WL, Wasserman K, Whipp BJ: A new method for detecting anaerobic threshold by gas exchange. J Appl Physiol 1986;60:2020–2027.
96 Gowda K, Zintel T, McParland C, Orchard R, Gallagher CG: Diagnostic value of maximal exercise tidal volume. Chest 1990;98:1351–1354.
97 Babb TG, Viggiano R, Hurley B, Staats B, Rodarte JR: Effect of mild-to-moderate airflow limitation on exercise capacity. J Appl Physiol 1991;70:223–230.
98 Johnson BD, Scanlon PD, Beck KC: Regulation of ventilatory capacity during exercise in asthmatics. J Appl Physiol 1995;79:892–901.
99 Garfinkel F, Fitzgerald RS: The effect of hyperoxia, hypoxia and hypercapnia on FRC and occlusion pressure in human subjects. Respir Physiol 1978;33:241–250.
100 Harris-Eze AO, Sridhar G, Clemens RE, Zintel TA, Gallagher CG, Marciniuk DD: Low-dose nebulized morphine does not improve exercise in interstitial lung disease. Am J Respir Crit Care Med 1995;152:1940–1945.
101 Winning AJ, Hamilton RD, Guz A: Ventilation and breathlessness on maximal exercise in patients with interstitial lung disease after local anaesthetic aerosol inhalation. Clin Sci (Colch) 1988;74:275–281.
102 Yoshida M, Taguchi O, Gabazza EC, et al: The effect of low-dose inhalation of nitric oxide in patients with pulmonary fibrosis. Eur Respir J 1997;10:2051–2054.
103 Riley MS, Porszasz J, Miranda J, Engelen MP, Brundage B, Wasserman K: Exhaled nitric oxide during exercise in primary pulmonary hypertension and pulmonary fibrosis. Chest 1997;111:44–50.

Bharath S. Krishnan, MBBS, PhD
Faculty of Physical Activity Studies
University of Regina, 3737 Wascana Parkway
Regina, Saskatchewan S4S 0A2 (Canada)
Tel. +1 306 585 4370, Fax +1 306 585 4854
E-Mail bharath.krishnan@uregina.ca

Weisman IM, Zeballos RJ (eds): Clinical Exercise Testing.
Prog Respir Res. Basel, Karger, 2002, vol 32, pp 200–204

Role of Cardiopulmonary Exercise Testing in Patients with Pulmonary Vascular Disease

David M. Systrom Barbara A. Cockrill Charles A. Hales

Pulmonary and Critical Care Unit, Medical Services, Massachusetts General Hospital and Harvard Medical School, Boston, Mass., USA

Summary

Making the diagnosis of early and mild pulmonary hypertension through measurements performed on the patient at rest is notoriously difficult. Most such patients present with dyspnea or fatigue of unknown origin, which are classic indications for cardiopulmonary exercise testing (CPET). Noninvasive CPET abnormalities suggestive of pulmonary hypertension include low $\dot{V}O_2$max, early anaerobic threshold, inefficient ventilation and arterial O_2 desaturation. For the patient with relatively severe, established precapillary pulmonary vascular disease, CPET can also be used safely to predict survival and to follow natural history or response to treatment.

Introduction

This chapter will discuss the pathophysiology of the exercise limit in pulmonary arterial hypertension (PHTN) and its detection by cardiopulmonary exercise testing (CPET). The exercise responses in COPD, interstitial lung disease, congestive heart failure and the use of CPET in lung transplantation and other thoracic surgical techniques are discussed elsewhere.

Pulmonary Hypertension

PHTN can be defined as a mean pulmonary artery pressure (PAP) at rest of greater than 25 mm Hg or more than 30 mm Hg with exercise. PHTN can occur due to increased cardiac output (Q_T), pulmonary capillary wedge pressure (PCWP) or pulmonary vascular resistance (PVR). The PHTN associated with high output states is generally mild and of little clinical relevance unless there is a coexisting intrinsic abnormality of the pulmonary circulation. Left-ventricular (LV) systolic dysfunction is frequent cause of PHTN and influences exercise capacity [1]. LV diastolic dysfunction is more likely to be associated with dynamic exercise-induced PHTN. These forms of pulmonary venous hypertension, deserve mention because they are associated with inefficient ventilation during CPET [2] and may be confused with precapillary disease. The detection and evaluation of diseases manifested by increased PVR is the subject of the present chapter.

Secondary Precapillary PHTN

Precapillary PHTN may be primary (PPH) or secondary to a known disease process, but both forms have varying degrees of pulmonary artery vasoconstriction and remodeling in common. Secondary PHTN may be a coincidental feature of a disease that predominately affects the airways or lung interstitium or it may be largely responsible for the patient's pathologic and clinical presentation. For instance, many patients with COPD are more limited by lung mechanics [3] than by mild [4, 5] secondary PHTN which has little bearing on exercise tolerance. When the disease is advanced, however, the pulmonary vascular component may compromise aerobic capacity [6] and influence survival [7, 8]. Patients with interstitial lung disease tend to present earlier than those with COPD with clinical and CPET features of pulmonary vascular disease [9, 10]. Other secondary causes of PHTN (table 1) not associated with significant obstruction or restriction are quite similar pathologically and clinically to PPH and for simplicity they will be discussed together. Early diagnosis of secondary PHTN is critical as withdrawal of the offending drug or treatment of the underlying cause may avoid progressive PHTN with its attendant morbidity and mortality.

Primary Pulmonary Hypertension

PPH is by definition a disease of uncertain etiology characterized by a sustained elevation of PAP without demonstrable cause [11, 12] after a comprehensive medical work-up [13]. The early and correct diagnosis of PPH is also increasingly important given the development of increasingly effective medical therapies [14–22] and because of the long wait at most transplant centers for a donor lung [23].

While history, physical exam and laboratory work up may suggest secondary forms of PHTN, the diagnosis of PPH is much more difficult [13]. Signs and symptoms related to PHTN are insensitive and nonspecific, as are tests of resting pulmonary function [24] and gas exchange [25]. Transthoracic Doppler echocardiography has recently evolved as a screening test of choice. Advantages include its noninvasive nature, ability to exclude secondary left ventricular causes and quantification of PHTN as well as RV size and function. Disadvantages, however, include the fact that the clinician must consider cardiac causes of exercise intolerance in a young patient in ordering the test and underestimation of PAP in certain patients [26]. Perhaps even more important, some symptomatic patients appear to have only mild PHTN at rest or none, but with the stress of exercise (which makes echocardiography technically difficult) dynamic PHTN is elicited [25, 27]. If dynamic PHTN represent early and more treatable disease [5, 28], a screening test done solely at rest may be inappropriately insensitive.

Table 1. Secondary pulmonary vasculopathies

Sleep disordered breathing [50]
Connective tissue disease [9]
HIV infection [51]
Chronic thromboembolic disease [52]
Portopulmonary hypertension [53]
Drugs [54]

Normal Pulmonary Circulatory Response to Exercise

The normal pulmonary circulation, even in the elderly, is a compliant structure able to receive a 5-fold increase in blood flow with only a minimal pressure rise. Right-sided pressures do increase during incremental exercise [29, 30], but at peak exercise RAP should be in the low teens, mean PAP <30 mm Hg and PCWP <20 mm Hg [29, 30]. Changes in PCW and RA pressure are linearly related. For each 1 mm Hg rise of RA pressure, PCW pressure rises 1.4 mm Hg [29]. A markedly increased or decreased slope of this relation suggests disproportionate left- or right-ventricular dysfunction, respectively.

The increase in pressure gradient across the pulmonary vascular bed during exercise is less than the increase in cardiac output and pulmonary vascular resistance (PVR) therefore falls. This deviation from the classic Ohm-resistor pressure-flow relationship is due to both passive and active recruitment and distention of the pulmonary capillary bed [29, 30]. Reeves et al. [30] found that in young healthy subjects, the upper limit of a normal PVR_{max} is 56 $dyn \cdot s \cdot cm^{-5}$ (0.7 Wood units). Granath et al. [31] studied 27 healthy older men (age 71 $\pm$ 6 SD years) and found an upper 95% confidence interval for PVR_{max} of 120 $dyn \cdot s \cdot cm^{-5}$ (1.5 Wood units).

At peak exercise in the normal human, rapid red cell transit time through the pulmonary capillary presents a challenge to oxygen loading. Increased alveolar PO_2, improved matching of ventilation and perfusion in the upright lung, recruitment of a structurally intact alveolar capillary surface area and reduction of venous admixture prevent arterial O_2 desaturation at high cardiac output, with the exception of the rare elite endurance athlete [32, 33].

Ventilation, which is tightly linked to $\dot{V}CO_2$ throughout incremental exercise, becomes more efficient if pulmonary circulatory structure and function are normal. A

Table 2. Abnormal pulmonary vascular response to incremental exercise

PAP > 30 mm Hg [11, 12, 40]
PVR > 1.5 Wood units [31]
$\dot{Q}t$ < 80% predicted
PCWP/RAP slope < 1.4 [29]
RAP > 14 mm Hg [29]
RVEF < 0.45 [55]

Table 3. CPET characteristics of PHTN*

Decreased $\dot{V}O_2$max
Decreased AT
Increased $\dot{V}_E/\dot{V}CO_2$ slope and absolute value at AT
Hyperventilation during submaximal exercise
Blunted V_D/V_T fall
Arterial O_2 desaturation or widened $P(A\text{-}a)O_2$

* See ref [34, 35, 41] for normal values.

decrease in alveolar dead space occurs as part of pulmonary vascular distention and recruitment, especially at the apices of the upright lung. This and normal augmentation of V_T decrease physiologic V_D/V_T to <0.3 at peak exercise. The $\dot{V}_E/\dot{V}CO_2$ falls as a result to <37 at the ventilatory threshold [34], though this normal response is dependent on age and gender [35].

Abnormal Pulmonary Circulatory Response to Exercise

Direct measurement of pulmonary hemodynamics at rest or as part of CPET (table 2) gives insight into the pathogenesis of symptoms, can confirm the diagnosis of PHTN, quantify disease severity, help with prognostication and guide therapy. In PHTN, pulmonary vasoconstriction and structural remodeling limit the stroke volume response to CPET through increased right heart afterload [34]. When the right ventricle dilates chronically or dynamically during exercise, ventricular interdependence decreases LV compliance and diastolic filling.

In patients with PHTN, a first pass radionuclide heart scan may show a compromised rise in RVEF and normal LVEF [36], blunted left-ventricular end-diastolic volume response, SV and $\dot{Q}t_{max}$ [37] <80% predicted [for calculation, see ref. 6]. CPET done with a right heart catheter in place will reveal an abnormal rise in right atrial and mean pulmonary artery pressures [38] (table 2) with a relatively normal PCWP. The combination of increased pressure gradient across the pulmonary vascular bed and inadequate cardiac output leads to a blunted fall of PVR.

Although right heart catheterization is a critical step in the confirmation, grading and treatment of PHTN, its attendant risks [39, 40] suggest the need for an alternative screening test that is noninvasive, safe, reproducible and sensitive.

Diagnosis of PHTN by CPET

The pitfalls in the diagnosis of early and mild PHTN noted above have provided impetus for CPET interpretation algorithms based on patterns of change of multiple physiologic responses to exercise [41–43] (table 3). Most patients with PPH present with dyspnea or fatigue of unknown origin [11, 12, 34], which are classic indications for CPET [41].

By the time the patient is symptomatic, $\dot{V}O_2$max is usually significantly reduced, though well described cases of significant PHTN have been described with surprising well-preserved overall aerobic capacity [39]. A depressed maximum O_2 uptake is related to decreased maximal cardiac output (discussed above) and arterial O_2 desaturation. Inadequate O_2 delivery is associated with a low ventilatory and lactate 'anaerobic' thresholds (AT) [34].

Ventilation in patients with PHTN is excessive [44], but because the maximum voluntary ventilation is usually near-normal, relatively normal breathing reserve at peak exercise is most often found [34]. Inefficient ventilation during incremental exercise, usually denoted by an increased slope of the linear phase of $\dot{V}_E/\dot{V}CO_2$ or its absolute value at the ventilatory threshold however, is a characteristic of both arterial [34] and venous [2] PHTN. The importance of $\dot{V}_E/\dot{V}CO_2$ is explained by its inverse relationship to arterial $PaCO_2$ and physiologic dead space to tidal volume ratio: $\dot{V}_E/\dot{V}CO_2 = k/(PaCO_2\ (1 - V_D/V_T))$. Failure of normal pulmonary vascular distention and recruitment during exercise in PPH creates underperfused, ventilated lung units, increasing V_D/V_T and the ventilatory requirement of exercise. Hyperventilation during submaximal exercise is also seen in PPH and likely related to hypoxemic stimulation of arterial chemoreceptors and stimulation of pulmonary circulatory mechanoreceptors [45]. Thus, the combined influence of two invasively measured variables, V_D/V_T and $PaCO_2$, makes the noninvasive $\dot{V}_E/\dot{V}CO_2$ a potentially powerful marker of the abnormal pulmonary vasculature.

Arterial O_2 desaturation and/or exaggerated widening of the $P(A\text{-}a)O_2$ with exercise is thought to be a gas exchange feature that distinguishes pulmonary arterial from venous hypertension [41]. In precapillary disease, abnormally widened $P(A\text{-}a)O_2$ is due both to $\dot{V}/\dot{Q}$ mismatching and a diffusion defect induced by a rapid red cell transit time through a poorly compliant and recruitable pulmonary circulation. Occasionally, a sudden fall in arterial oxygen saturation heralds the opening of a patent foramen ovale and increased right to left shunting due to elevation of right atrial pressure [41].

Grading PHTN Severity and Therapeutic Response by CPET

In PPH, CPET parameters of aerobic function and gas exchange such as $\dot{V}O_2$max, AT, $\dot{V}_E/\dot{V}CO_2$ slope and absolute value at AT correlate with NYHA classification [34]. $\dot{V}O_2$max and AT also correlate with resting pulmonary hemodynamics [34]. In one recent study which employed micromanometer tipped pulmonary artery catheters during CPET, ventilatory equivalents were correlated with pulmonary hemodynamics [38]. $\dot{V}O_2$max correlates with survival in chronic thromboembolic pulmonary hypertension [26]. In established PPH, the 6 minute walk also predicts survival [8, 46].

An increasing number of studies have utilized the 6 min walk or CPET to follow patients with established PPH and its response to therapy [16, 22, 47–49]. Iwase and colleagues [49] recently described the temporal pattern of recovery of CPET parameters following pulmonary thromboendarterectomy for chronic thromboembolic PHTN. Interestingly, ventilatory efficiency returned toward normal during the first postoperative month and correlated with improved PVR. $\dot{V}O_2$max, likely reflecting whole body effects of chronic disease, took longer to recover [49].

Conclusions

Cardiopulmonary exercise testing is a useful tool for the detection of pulmonary vascular disease, especially in the patient with dyspnea or fatigue of unknown origin. CPET characteristics of PHTN include abnormal $\dot{V}O_2$max, early AT, inefficient ventilation and arterial O_2 desaturation. For the PPH patient with relatively severe, established disease, CPET can be performed safely [34], and used to stratify survival and to follow natural history or response to treatment.

Acknowledgments

Dr. Systrom is supported by NHLBI 1K24 HLO4022-02. Dr. Hales is supported by NIH HL39150-13 and HL63982-02.

References

1 Koelling TM, Kirmse M, Di Salvo TG, Dec GW, Zapol WM, Semigran MJ: Inhaled nitric oxide improves exercise capacity in patients with severe heart failure and right ventricular dysfunction. Am J Cardiol 1998;81:1494–1497.

2 Kleber FX, Vietzke G, Wernecke KD, Bauer U, Opitz C, Wensel R, Sperfeld A, Glaser S: Impairment of ventilatory efficiency in heart failure: prognostic impact. Circulation 2000; 101:2803–2809.

3 Medoff BD, Oelberg DA, Kanarek DJ, Systrom DM: Breathing reserve at the lactate threshold to differentiate a pulmonary mechanical from cardiovascular limit to exercise. Chest 1998; 113:913–918.

4 Stevens D, Sharma K, Szidon P, Rich S, McLaughlin V, Kesten S: Severe pulmonary hypertension associated with COPD. Ann Transplant 2000;5:8–12.

5 Kessler R, Faller M, Weitzenblum E, Chaouat A, Aykut A, Ducolone A, Ehrhart M, Oswald-Mammosser M: 'Natural history' of pulmonary hypertension in a series of 131 patients with chronic obstructive lung disease. Am J Respir Crit Care Med 2001;164:219–224.

6 Oelberg DA, Kacmarek RM, Pappagianopoulos PP, Ginns LC, Systrom DM: Ventilatory and cardiovascular responses to inspired He-O_2 during exercise in chronic obstructive pulmonary disease. Am J Respir Crit Care Med 1998;158:1876–1882.

7 Pierson DJ: Pathophysiology and clinical effects of chronic hypoxia. Respir Care 2000;45: 39–51; discussion 51–3.

8 Stricker H, Domenighetti G, Popov W, Speich R, Nicod L, Aubert JD, Soler M: Severe pulmonary hypertension: Data from the Swiss Registry. Swiss Med Wkly 2001;131:346–350.

9 Hsia CC: Cardiopulmonary limitations to exercise in restrictive lung disease. Med Sci Sports Exerc 1999;31:S28–32.

10 Orfanos SE, Psevdi E, Stratigis N, Langleben D, Catravas JD, Kyriakidis M, Moutsopoulos HM, Roussos C, Vlachoyiannopoulos PG: Pulmonary capillary endothelial dysfunction in early systemic sclerosis. Arthritis Rheum 2001; 44:902–911.

11 Rubin LJ: Primary pulmonary hypertension. N Engl J Med 1997;336:111–117.

12 Gaine SP, Rubin LJ: Primary pulmonary hypertension. Lancet 1998;352:719–725.

13 McGoon M: The assessment of pulmonary hypertension. Clin Chest Med 2001;22:493–508.

14 Galie N, Manes A, Branzi A: Medical therapy of pulmonary hypertension: The prostacyclins. Clin Chest Med 2001;22:529–537.

15 Naeije R, Vachiery J-L: Medical therapy of pulmonary hypertension. Clin Chest Med 2001; 22:517–527.

16 Machherndl S, Kneussl M, Baumgartner H, Schneider B, Petkov V, Schenk P, Lang IM: Long-term treatment of pulmonary hypertension with aerosolized iloprost. Eur Respir J 2001;17:8–13.

17 Naeije R, Vachiery JL: Medical therapy of pulmonary hypertension: Conventional therapies. Clin Chest Med 2001;22:517–527.
18 Nagaya N, Uematsu M, Oya H, Sato N, Sakamaki F, Kyotani S, Ueno K, Nakanishi N, Yamagishi M, Miyatake K: Short-term oral administration of *L*-arginine improves hemodynamics and exercise capacity in patients with precapillary pulmonary hypertension. Am J Respir Crit Care Med 2001;163:887–891.
19 Nauser TD, Stites SW: Diagnosis and treatment of pulmonary hypertension. Am Fam Physician 2001;63:1789–1798.
20 Rubin LJ, Mendoza J, Hood H, McGoon M, Barst R, Williams WB, Diehl JH, Crow J, Long W: Treatment of primary pulmonary hypertension with continuous intravenous prostacyclin (epoprostenol): Results of a randomized trial. Ann Intern Med 1990;112:485–491.
21 Stricker H, Domenighetti G, Fiori G, Mombelli G: Sustained improvement of performance and haemodynamics with long-term aerosolised prostacyclin therapy in severe pulmonary hypertension. Schweiz Med Wochenschr 1999; 129:923–927.
22 Wax D, Garofano R, Barst RJ: Effects of long-term infusion of prostacyclin on exercise performance in patients with primary pulmonary hypertension. Chest 1999;116:914–920.
23 Trulock E: Lung transplantation for primary pulmonary hypertension. Clin Chest Med 2001;22:583–593.
24 Moser K, Auger W, Fedullo P: Chronic thromboembolic pulmonary hypertension: Clinical picture and surgical treatment. Eur Respir J 1992;5:334–342.
25 Mohsenifar Z, Tashkin ED, Levy SE, Bjerke RD, Clements PJ, Furst D: Lack of sensitivity of measurements of V_D/V_T at rest and during exercise in detection of hemodynamically significant pulmonary vascular abnormalities in collagen vascular disease. Am Rev Respir Dis 1981;123:508–512.
26 Lewczuk J, Piszko P, Jagas J, Porada A, Wojciak S, Sobkowicz B, Wrabec K: Prognostic factors in medically treated patients with chronic pulmonary embolism. Chest 2001;119:818–823.
27 Mohsenifar Z, Taskin DP, Wolfe JD, Genovese M: Abnormal responses of wasted ventilation fraction (V_D/V_T) during exercise in patients with pulmonary vascular abnormalities. Respiration 1983;44:44–49.
28 Kullo I, Tajik A, McGoon M: Unexplained mild pulmonary hypertension detected by Doppler echocardiography: Clinical profile and follow-up of 29 patients. Circulation 1998;98: I-615.
29 Reeves JT, Groves BM, Cymerman A, et al: Operation Everest II: Cardiac filling pressures during cycle exercise at sea level. Respir Physiol 1990;80:147–154.
30 Reeves JT, Moon RE, Grover RF, et al: Increased wedge pressure facilitates decreased lung vascular resistance during upright exercise. Chest 1988;93(suppl):97S–99S.
31 Granath A, Strandell T: Circulation in healthy old men, studied by right heart catheterization at rest and during exercise in supine and sitting position. Act Med Scand 1964;176:425–446.
32 Hopkins SR, Schoene RB, Henderson WR, Spragg RG, Martin TR, West JB: Intense exercise impairs the integrity of the pulmonary blood-gas barrier in elite athletes. Am J Respir Crit Care Med 1997;155:1090–1094.
33 Dempsey JA, Johnson BD, Saupe KW: Adaptations and limitations in the pulmonary system during exercise. Chest 1990;97(suppl): 81S–87S.
34 Sun XG, Hansen JE, Oudiz RJ, Wasserman K: Exercise pathophysiology in patients with primary pulmonary hypertension. Circulation 2001;104:429–435.
35 Habedank D, Reindl I, Vietzke G, Bauer U, Sperfeld A, Glaser S, Wernecke KD, Kleber FX: Ventilatory efficiency and exercise tolerance in 101 healthy volunteers. Eur J Appl Physiol Occup Physiol 1998;77:421–426.
36 Matthay RA, Arroliga AC, Wiedemann HP, Schulman DS, Mahler DA: Right ventricular function at rest and during exercise in chronic obstructive pulmonary disease. Chest 1992; 101:255S–262S.
37 Maroni JM, Oelberg DA, Pappagianopoulos P, Boucher CA, Systrom DM: Maximum cardiac output during incremental exercise by first-pass radionuclide ventriculography. Chest 1998;114:457–461.
38 Raeside DA, Smith A, Brown A, Patel KR, Madhok R, Cleland J, Peacock AJ: Pulmonary artery pressure measurement during exercise testing in patients with suspected pulmonary hypertension. Eur Respir J 2000;16:282–287.
39 Rhodes J, Barst R, Garofano R, Thoele D, Gersony W: Hemodynamic correlates of exercise function in patients with primary pulmonary hypertension. J Am Coll Cardiol 1991;18: 1738–1744.
40 Rich S, Dantzker DR, Ayres SM, Bergofsky EH, Brundage BH, Detre KM, Fishman AP, Goldring RM, Groves BM, Koerner SK, et al: Primary pulmonary hypertension: A national prospective study. Ann Intern Med 1987;107: 216–223.
41 Wasserman K, Hansen JE, Sue DY, Casaburi R, Whipp BJ: Principles of Exercise Testing and Interpretation. Baltimore, Lippincott, Williams & Wilkins, 1999, pp 173–174.
42 Weisman IM, Zeballos RJ: An integrated approach to the interpretation of cardiopulmonary exercise testing. Clin Chest Med 1994;15: 421–445.
43 Eschenbacher WL, Mannina A: An algorithm for the interpretation of cardiopulmonary exercise tests. Chest 1990;97:263–267.
44 Theodore J, Robin ED, Morris AJR, Burke CM, Jamieson SW, Van Kessel A, Stinson EB, Shumway NE: Augmented ventilatory response to exercise in pulmonary hypertension. Chest 1986;89:39–44.
45 Jones PW, Huszczuk A, Wasserman K: Cardiac output as a controller of ventilation through changes in right ventricular load. J Appl Physiol 1982;53:218–224.
46 Miyamoto S, Nagaya N, Satoh T, Kyotani S, Sakamaki F, Fujita M, Nakanishi N, Miyatake K: Clinical correlates and prognostic significance of six-minute walk test in patients with primary pulmonary hypertension: Comparison with cardiopulmonary exercise testing. Am J Respir Crit Care Med 2000;161:487–492.
47 Barst RJ, Rubin LJ, McGoon MD, Caldwell EJ, Long WA, Levy PS: Survival in primary pulmonary hypertension with long-term continuous intravenous prostacyclin. Ann Intern Med 1994;121:409–415.
48 Channick RN, Simonneau G, Sitbon O, Robbins IM, Frost A, Tapson VF, Badesch DB, Roux S, Rainisio M, Bodin F, Rubin LJ: Effects of the dual endothelin-receptor antagonist bosentan in patients with pulmonary hypertension: A randomised placebo-controlled study. Lancet 2001;358:1119–1123.
49 Iwase T, Nagaya N, Ando M, Satoh T, Sakamaki F, Kyotani S, Takaki H, Goto Y, Ohkita Y, Uematsu M, Nakanishi N, Miyatake K: Acute and chronic effects of surgical thromboendarterectomy on exercise capacity and ventilatory efficiency in patients with chronic thromboembolic pulmonary hypertension. Heart 2001;86: 188–192.
50 Bady E, Achkar A, Pascal S, Orvoen-Frija E, Laaban JP: Pulmonary arterial hypertension in patients with sleep apnoea syndrome. Thorax 2000;55:934–939.
51 Mehta NJ, Khan IA, Mehta RN, Sepkowitz DA: HIV-Related pulmonary hypertension: Analytic review of 131 cases. Chest 2000;118: 1133–1141.
52 Fedullo P, Auger W, Channick R, Kerr K, Rubin L: Chronic thromboembolic pulmonary hypertension. Clin Chest Med 2001;22:561–581.
53 Krowka MJ, McGoon MD: Portopulmonary hypertension: The next step. Chest 1997;112: 869–870.
54 Abenhaim L, Moride Y, Brenot F, Rich S, Benichou J, Kurz X, Higenbottam T, Oakley C, Wouters E, Aubier M, Simonneau G, Begaud B: Appetite-suppressant drugs and the risk of primary pulmonary hypertension. International Primary Pulmonary Hypertension Study Group. N Engl J Med 1996;335:609–616.
55 Brent BN, Mahler D, Matthay RA, Berger HJ, Zaret BL: Noninvasive diagnosis of pulmonary arterial hypertension in chronic obstructive pulmonary disease: Right ventricular ejection fraction at rest. Am J Cardiol 1984;53:1349–1353.

David M. Systrom, MD
Pulmonary and Critical Care Unit
Medical Services
Massachusetts General Hospital and
Harvard Medical School
Fruit Street, Bigelow 952
Boston, MA 02114 (USA)
Tel. +1 617 726 3734, Fax +1 617 724 6954
E-Mail dsystrom@partners.org

Weisman IM, Zeballos RJ (eds): Clinical Exercise Testing.
Prog Respir Res. Basel, Karger, 2002, vol 32, pp 205–216

Asthma and Exercise

Ricardo A. Tan Sheldon L. Spector

California Allergy and Asthma Medical Group, Inc., Palmdale, Calif., USA

Summary

Exercise-induced asthma (EIA) is characterized by transient airway obstruction after strenuous exertion. Methacholine and histamine challenge testing may be done to confirm suspected asthma but a negative response does not rule out EIA. Exercise testing on a treadmill or cycle ergometer or hyperventilation testing is needed to rule out EIA. Prevention is the main objective in managing EIA. Nonpharmacologic measures include warming up, covering the mouth and nose in cold weather, and warming down after exercise. Inhaled β-agonists are the medications of choice for EIA prophylaxis. Inhaled cromolyn or nedocromil and antileukotriene agents may also be effective. Education regarding the nature and management of EIA is important not only for asthmatics but also their families and coaches. With the proper precautions and workout techniques, there is no limit to what persons with asthma can achieve in sports.

Introduction

Exercise-induced asthma (EIA), also referred to as exercise-induced airway narrowing or exercise-induced bronchospasm (EIB), is defined as acute airway narrowing occurring after strenuous exertion. Exercise and hyperventilation have long been observed to be significant triggers of bronchial obstruction in chronic asthma. Some asthmatics exhibit symptoms only after exercise with no other triggers. EIA occurs in 40–90% of asthmatics [1, 2] and in 6–13% of the general population [3]. The presence of atopy is strongly associated with EIA [4]. Up to 40% of patients with allergic rhinitis have EIA. In children and young adults, EIA is especially significant as their early exposure to sports can be affected by this problem [5]. For athletic individuals, asthma symptoms induced only by exertion can be sufficiently limiting. As more athletes with asthma compete and succeed at the highest levels of performance, it is important to be familiar with the nature and therapy of exercise-induced asthma so that we can encourage our patients to continue an active life in a safe and healthy manner.

Pathophysiology

The pathogenesis of exercise-induced asthma is not clearly defined. However, there are physiologic events about which there is general agreement. Inhalation of large volumes of dry, cold air during exercise leads to loss of heat and water from the bronchial mucosa leading to airway cooling and drying. Numerous studies have documented the importance of (1) the amount of ventilation, and (2) the temperature of inspired air in producing airway obstruction [6, 7]. The larger the amount of ventilation and the colder the air inspired, the greater the severity of airway narrowing. Warm, humidified air diminishes the degree of bronchospasm. It is important to note that despite these general observations, EIA can still occur even when exercise is done in a warm environment [8].

Table 1. Clinical features of EIA

Requires 3–8 min of exercise at 80% or more of maximal heart rate
Peak symptoms occur at 8–15 min after exercise
Spontaneous recovery within 60 min
Refractory period of up to 4 h after exercise
Bronchospasm provoked faster by dry and cold air

There are two prominent theories about how airway cooling leads to bronchoconstriction. EIA is believed to involve (a) mucosal drying and increased osmolarity stimulating mast cell degranulation [9] and/or (b) rapid airway rewarming causing vascular congestion, increased permeability and edema leading to obstruction [10]. A combination of these two mechanisms is more likely at work in EIA.

The first theory proposes that the increase in osmolarity in the airway mucosa produced by airway drying and cooling stimulates the release of inflammatory mediators from mast cells, including histamine and leukotrienes, that cause bronchoconstriction [9, 11]. The efficacy of the mast cell stabilizers (cromolyn and nedocromil) and anti-leukotriene agents in preventing EIA support this mechanism.

In the other proposed mechanism, airway cooling does not cause bronchoconstriction directly. Rather, it is the rapid rewarming of the airways after exercise that leads to bronchoconstriction. Proponents of this mechanism believe that with rapid rewarming, there is a 'vascular phenomenon' of reactive hyperemia with sudden blood flow and vascular permeability leading to edema and airway obstruction [10]. The greater the difference between the airway temperature during and after exercise, the greater the severity of obstruction. The observation that inhaling warm air after exercise worsens the bronchoconstriction while cold air lessens it appears to support this theory [12].

The observed high prevalence of EIA and bronchial hyperresponsiveness (BHR) in elite athletes has led some investigators to question whether the milder exercise-induced narrowing seen in elite athletes is truly EIA or a separate condition caused by airway injury from factors such as repetitive high-intensity exertion [13].

EIA generally does not manifest during the exercise activity but afterwards. In fact, there is bronchodilation during exercise and this is most likely due to sympathetic stimulation from catecholamines such as epinephrine [14]. Some persons may complain of symptoms during exercise but studies show that this is often due to preexisting obstruction or poor conditioning rather than true exercise-induced bronchoconstriction [15].

Clinical Features

Exercise-induced asthma is usually preceded by at least 3–8 min of exercise. Bronchospasm and/or symptoms of chest tightness, cough, wheezing and dyspnea start soon after the end of exercise and peak in about 8–15 min [16]. There is spontaneous recovery within 60 min after the exercise ends (table 1). A late phase response has been described occurring 4–6 h after exercise in some patients [17]. Other studies have failed to demonstrate this response and there is controversy regarding whether a late phase response to exercise exists or whether the observed changes are due to fluctuations in the underlying asthma [18]. Although EIA has traditionally been observed only after exercise, newer studies suggest that bronchospasm may occur during exercise, especially during prolonged exertion.

If the person attempts to exercise again after the symptoms subside, he will experience less symptoms the second time. This has been referred to as the refractory period. The duration of this period has been observed by different authors to be anywhere from 40 min to up to 3 h. Some authors believe 'refractory period' is inaccurate since the person is refractory only to exercise but not to other stimuli such as allergens [15]. Depletion of catecholamines has been proposed as a mechanism for this phenomenon. When indomethacin, a prostaglandin inhibitor is given during an exercise challenge, the refractory period appears to be eliminated implying that prostaglandins also released during exercise may play a protective role [19].

Diagnosis

In patients with clear-cut symptoms of chest tightness, wheezing, dyspnea or cough after exercise, the history and a physical examination while symptomatic can usually provide a diagnosis of EIA. In persons with nonspecific respiratory symptoms and no history of asthma, diagnostic tests may be necessary. Spirometry should first be done to check for airway obstruction as manifested by a decreased forced expiratory volume in one second (FEV_1) and/or peak expiratory flow rate (PEFR). Significant improvement in pulmonary function after using an inhaled β-agonist confirms the diagnosis of asthma.

Vocal cord dysfunction is an important differential diagnosis for asthma. It is caused by abnormal adduction of the vocal cords leading to episodic choking or shortness of breath. A flow-volume loop obtained during spirometry when a patient has symptoms will show a characteristic flattened inspiratory portion [20]. Direct laryngoscopy can also visualize the characteristic changes in the vocal cords.

Testing for nonspecific bronchial hyperreactivity by bronchial challenge is often used to diagnose asthma if spirometry does not demonstrate any airway obstruction or reversibility after bronchodilator intake. Spirometry will often be abnormal only during symptomatic periods. Methacholine is the most commonly used bronchoconstrictor agent used for challenges. A positive methacholine challenge can confirm the presence of asthma. However, a negative challenge does not rule out EIA, especially in mild asthmatics with no other triggers. In these patients, an exercise challenge may be needed to diagnose EIA [21]. Persons presumed to have EIA but who do not respond to β-agonist or cromolyn prophylaxis may also need to be reevaluated with an exercise test. Differential diagnoses for exercise-associated symptoms include poor conditioning, cardiac disorders and chronic obstructive pulmonary disease.

Methacholine Challenge Testing

Bronchoprovocation or bronchial challenge testing with inhaled bronchoconstrictor agents such as methacholine and histamine in a controlled setting and measuring their response by pulmonary function testing is used to evaluate nonspecific BHR. This procedure is most commonly used to confirm the presence of asthma in patients with atypical symptoms such as chronic cough without wheezing or dyspnea. It is also used to monitor the response of airway inflammation to therapy. Challenges with exercise, inhaled cold air and inhaled nonionic aerosols can also detect nonspecific BHR. Leukotrienes, prostaglandins and adenosine are also used as bronchoprovocation agents in research studies.

Methacholine and histamine are the two most widely employed bronchoconstrictor agents for challenges. The responses elicited are usually short-lived and therefore ideal for testing. Methacholine is generally preferred over histamine. Histamine has a tendency to produce tachyphylaxis with repeated challenges and is associated with side effects such as headache and tachycardia. Responsiveness to these bronchoconstrictor agents correlates well with asthma severity.

In general, challenge testing should be done when the subject's airway responsiveness is as close to baseline as possible. The subjects' baseline FEV_1 should be at least 70% of predicted. Symptomatic asthma or other pulmonary conditions may be contraindications to the procedure. Anxiety or anticipation may influence the bronchial response so it is important to reassure the patient that there is no 'correct' response to the test and that there may be an increase, decrease or no change in lung function. Circadian rhythms may also play a role in the response to challenge but no specific recommendations on the best time for testing are available at this time. Challenges should not be performed after recent allergen exposure, exercise, exposure to pollutants and during ongoing or recent viral infections, all of which can increase airway hyperresponsiveness and affect test results. Coffee, chocolate, cola drinks and smoking should be avoided at least 6 h prior to the challenge. Short acting β-agonist agents, short-acting theophylline preparations, α-adrenergic agents and cromolyn sodium should be stopped at least 8 h before testing. Anticholinergic agents, long-acting β-agonists, long-acting theophylline preparations and leukotriene modifiers should be stopped at least 24 h prior to the challenge. Antihistamines should be avoided for 48 h or longer depending on their half-life. Nedocromil should be withheld for 48 h [22]. The American Thoracic Society Guidelines for Methacholine and Exercise Testing do not require withholding of systemic or inhaled steroids prior to challenges as they do not block the bronchoconstriction induced by methacholine or histamine. Bronchial challenges done in patients already on corticosteroids are usually done for research purposes to follow changes in BHR. However, systemic and inhaled steroids may decrease chronic BHR and may be withheld depending on the purpose of the challenge [14, 22].

Several standard protocols for bronchial challenges can be used [23–26]. The ATS Guidelines recommends modified versions of the (a) two minute tidal breathing protocol [26], or (b) the five breath dosing protocol [24]. The latter is more widely used and is described here (table 2).

A baseline spirometry is done prior to the challenge. A control dose is then administered with 5 breaths of a saline solution control. A fall of 15% or more in the FEV_1 following saline inhalation is a contraindication to continuing the bronchial challenge. The starting concentration considered safe for methacholine or histamine is usually less than 0.1 mg/ml (table 3). The subject is given 5 breaths of each progressively higher concentration of methacholine or histamine. Spirometry is performed after each set of 5 breaths. The challenge is stopped as soon as

Table 2. Sequence of 5 breath dosing protocol for methacholine challenge [22]

1	Perform baseline spirometry and record baseline vital signs; FEV_1 should be at least 70% of predicted for challenge to proceed
2	Administer 5 breaths of saline control solution; do spirometry at 30 and 90 s after the last breath; the best FEV_1 after saline inhalation is used as the reference point for $PC_{20}FEV_1$. If FEV_1 falls 15% or more from baseline, stop challenge and treat subject with nebulized β-agonist treatment; otherwise, proceed to step 3
3	Administer 5 breaths of most dilute concentration (usually less than 0.1 mg/ml); do spirometry 30 and 90 s after last breath; subject may do 2–4 efforts within 3 min
4	Repeat step 3 with progressively higher concentration of methacholine; stop challenge when subject FEV_1 falls 20% or more, or after highest concentration of methacholine has been given (usually 16 mg/ml)
5	$PC_{20}FEV_1$ (concentration in mg/ml required to drop subject's FEV_1 by 20% from reference FEV_1 after saline control) is computed; A $PC_{20}FEV_1$ of 8 mg/ml or less is most widely considered a positive challenge

Table 3. Suggested dilution schedule for methacholine using 5-breath dosimeter protocol [22]

	Add NaCl ml	Dilution mg/ml
100 mg (powdered)	6.25	A 16
3 ml of dilution A	9	B 4
3 ml of dilution B	9	C 1
3 ml of dilution C	9	D 0.25
3 ml of dilution D	9	E 0.0625

the FEV_1 drops by 20% or more. The response to provocation is most commonly measured by the concentration (mg/ml) of methacholine or histamine required to decrease the subject's FEV_1 by 20% from the baseline saline control (PC_{20} FEV_1). An alternative measure is the cumulative dose (in micromoles or breath units) required for a FEV_1 fall of 20% (PD_{20} FEV1). Each breath unit is equivalent to one breath of a 1 mg/ml concentration [27].

A $PC_{20}FEV_1$ of 8 mg/ml or less of methacholine or histamine will be seen in 85–100% of asthmatics and is generally used as the cut-off value for a positive challenge [23, 28]. Less than 5% of normal patients will have a 20% fall in FEV_1 after 5 inhalations of the usual maximal concentration of histamine (10 mg/ml) and methacholine (25 mg/ml) [24].

Exercise Testing

Exercise testing can be utilized for detection of nonspecific BHR and confirming the diagnosis of asthma but a methacholine challenge is usually easier to perform for this purpose. A negative methacholine challenge does not rule out exercise-induced asthma and exercise testing is indicated to specifically diagnose bronchoconstriction induced by exercise. It is also indicated to determine the severity and response to treatment of known EIA.

General Considerations

Precautions and required washout of medications are generally the same as those for the methacholine challenge.

A careful history and physical exam should be done prior to considering exercise testing for suspected asthma. Contraindications to bronchial exercise testing include a history of angina pectoris, proven myocardial infarction or clinically significant valvular disease [29]. An ECG and chest X-ray should be done to detect any cardiac abnormalities. A stress ECG, and in some situations arterial blood gases may be required, especially in subjects over 35 years old with cardiac risk factors such as hypertension, obesity or diabetes [30, 31].

In exercise testing, it is essential that the subject not exercise for at least 4 h before the challenge. This is important to avoid the refractory period that can occur for up to 4 h after exercise in subjects with EIA [32].

The temperature and humidity of inhaled air are factors that can affect the occurrence and severity of EIA and these should be controlled during the challenge [33]. To maximize conditions for induction of EIA, this is best done by having the subject inhale dry, cool compressed air that is less than 25 °C and with less than 10 mg/l water content through a mouthpiece. A less controlled but acceptable alternative is to perform the challenge in an air-conditioned room with a temperature less than 25 °C and humidity less than 50% [22]. A noseclip is used to prevent nasal breathing, which has been shown to have a beneficial effect in EIA by decreasing water loss [34]. Mouth breathing alone, which is associated with increased water loss, increases the likelihood of EIA.

Exercise Protocol

Different protocols have been proposed to standardize exercise testing. Although there is no one standardized protocol recommended at this time, the American Thoracic Society has formulated guidelines for the different aspects of the exercise challenge [22]. The American Academy of Allergy Bronchopovocation Committee also formulated guidelines in 1979 that are still followed today [31].

A baseline spirometry is performed prior to the challenge. Various pulmonary function values have been studied in exercise, including peak expiratory flow rate (PEFR), forced expiratory flow (FEF_{25-75}), forced vital capacity (FVC), forced expiratory volume in 1 s (FEV_1) and specific airway conductance (SG_{aw}) [35]. For exercise testing, FEV_1 is the preferred measure of pulmonary function. The best of three acceptable efforts is used as the baseline value [36].

The treadmill and cycle ergometer are the most commonly used equipment in exercise protocols with each having both advantages and disadvantages. Bronchoconstriction is easier to provoke with the treadmill due to a faster increase in minute ventilation [37]. Walking or running on the treadmill may be easier for some subjects having difficulty with the coordination needed for cycling. However, the work rate on the treadmill can be harder to accurately measure because of variables such as the subject's weight [38]. In contrast, the work rate achieved on the cycle ergometer is affected by fewer variables and can easily be determined accurately [22]. Cycling is the preferred alternative for subjects who are unable to walk briskly or run due to problems such as weakness or arthritis. Another advantage of the cycle ergometer is the lack of requirement to adjust variables such as speed and incline. Many investigators feel that although treadmill running appears to elicit more bronchoconstriction, the cycle ergometer is easier to use and can identify most patients with EIA readily if done properly [39].

Treadmill Testing

The treadmill is the most commonly used equipment for performing the exercise challenge (table 4). Electrocardiographic monitoring with an oscilloscope or video screen for cardiac rhythm and heart rate is usually integrated into most treadmill equipment used for clinical testing. Cardiac rhythm should be monitored continuously throughout the test in real time. Care must be taken to tape down the ECG electrodes to keep them from falling off sweaty skin. Areas of the chest where the electrodes are placed may be shaved to facilitate attachment of electrodes. Pulse oximetry may also be measured. Blood pressure should be periodically checked during and after the challenge preferably with automatically inflating arm cuffs.

Table 4. General sequence of treadmill exercise challenge (summarized from American Thoracic Society [22]).

1	Baseline spirometry done for preexercise FEV_1
2	Treadmill speed and grade increased progressively to bring heart rate to 80–90% of maximum age-adjusted predicted value ideally within 2–3 min
3	Subject should exercise at target heart rate for at least 4 min. Some authors prefer between 5 and 8 min
4	Testing should be stopped for significant adverse chest symptoms, severe dyspnea, appearance of new ECG abnormalities, fall in blood pressure or any other adverse signs or symptoms
5	After testing stopped, heart rate and ECG should be monitored for at least 3 additional minutes
6	Spirometry is performed 5, 10, 15, 20 and 30 min postexercise
7	A fall of 10% from the pre-exercise FEV_1 is generally considered abnormal; a 15% drop is required for diagnosis by some practitioners
8	Continue checking spirometry even if FEV_1 fall is diagnostic before 30 min in order to determine nadir or lowest FEV_1 which correlates with EIA severity
9	Serial post-exercise spirometry may be stopped if 2 consecutive FEV_1 values after the nadir show improvement
10	Administer inhaled β-agonist treatment as needed to bring FEV_1 back to within 10% of pre-exercise value

The amount of exercise-induced work or stress that will be used in the challenge can be quantified in terms of heart rate and/or oxygen consumption (ml/min) if the latter is measured during the challenge. Obviously, factors such as the subject's age, weight and level of aerobic fitness will affect these values. In general, however, a work level that increases the heart rate to more than 90% or more of the maximum predicted values for age or the oxygen consumption to 30–40 ml/kg are considered an adequate stimulus for EIA [31]. Other protocols consider a target heart rate of 80% of the maximum predicted adequate [22]. Continuous monitoring of the subject's heart rate rather than ventilation is preferred and more practical. The subject's maximum predicted heart rate is determined from tables based on age [40] (table 5). The target heart rate for the subject during the challenge is 80–90% of the maximum predicted.

The target heart rate can be reached in different ways. Protocols have ranged from those that aim to raise the heart rate incrementally over 15–25 min to those that raise it rapidly to the target in 1–2 min [30]. A stepped approach that increases work in 3 stages is tolerated by most age groups and is commonly followed [31]. Whatever the protocol used, the ATS recommends that the target heart rate should be reached in 2–3 min and maintained at a steady state for at least 4 min with the total duration of the challenge at 6–8 min. The rationale for this recommendation is that a long warm-up period can induce a refractory period while extended exercise at the target heart rate may actually diminish bronchoconstriction [22, 41]. However, many authors prefer protocols, including the stepped protocol often used in research studies, with a longer total duration that has a warm-up period of 4 min and a steady state period of 5–8 min [30]. This preference is based on the observation that at least 5 min of exercise at the target heart rate is needed in many subjects, especially athletic fit ones, to provoke EIA.

Table 5. Average age-specific heart rates

Age years	Maximum heart rate/min	Maximum heart rate/min				
		95%	90%	85%	80%	75%
5	206	196	185	175	165	155
10	202	192	182	172	162	152
15	198	188	178	168	158	149
20	194	184	175	165	155	146
25	191	181	172	162	153	143
30	187	178	168	159	150	140
35	183	174	165	156	146	137
40	180	171	162	153	144	135
45	176	167	158	150	141	132
50	172	163	155	146	138	129
55	169	161	152	144	135	127
60	165	157	149	140	132	124
65	161	153	145	137	129	121
70	157	149	141	133	126	118
75	154	146	139	131	123	116
80	150	143	135	128	120	113
85	146	139	131	124	117	110
90	143	136	129	122	114	107

Maximum heart rate (y) derived from linear regression equation $y = 209.2 - 0.74x$, where x is age in years. Note that predicted maximum heart rate has a standard deviation of approximately ± 10 bpm. From Johnson and Buskirk [40].

The speed and incline (grade) of the treadmill are raised to produce progressive increases in the heart rate. Table 6 shows a suggested stepwise guide with the speed and incline expected to induce the desired heart rate at each stage. Nomograms based on studies of previous challenges are helpful in planning the treadmill settings for speed and incline before starting the challenge (fig. 1). The speed is based on subject height while the incline is based on age.

The subject should have comfortable clothing and running shoes on for the procedure. The subject is instructed to stand on the treadmill and hold on lightly to the rails as the treadmill starts to move. He or she then takes long, slow steps and lets go of the railing when a comfortable balance and rhythm is achieved. The speed and incline are then increased until the subject is running or walking fast. Subject should be instructed not to hold on to the railing while running since this will lessen the work effort.

The challenge should be stopped if there any cardiovascular or severe asthma symptoms develop. A physician or technician trained in cardiopulmonary resuscitation should administer the challenge with emergency equipment readily available. Indications for terminating the challenge include excessive fatigue or dyspnea, a drop in blood pressure, angina-like symptoms with or without ECG changes, ataxia, premature ventricular beats (more

Table 6. Stepped protocol with suggested speed and incline settings [31]

Step	Duration min	Target heart rate	Treadmill	
			rate	incline
I	2	50% predicted maximum*	2.5 mph	0%
II	2	70% predicted maximum	2/3 target conditions by height**	determined by age**
III	5–8	90% predicted maximum	target conditions by height	determined by age

* Predicted maximum age-adjusted heart rate from table 7.
** Target exercise of treadmill rate and incline from figure 1.

than 25% of beats or 10/min) or ventricular tachycardia, widening of the QRS complex, supraventricular tachycardia and rate-dependent heart block [29].

After exercise, the heart rate and ECG should be monitored for up to 3 min [30]. The subject's FEV_1 is measured in the sitting position at 5, 10, 15, 20 and 30 min postexercise. A fall of 10% from the preexercise value is considered abnormal while some investigators require a 15% drop for a diagnosis of EIA [22]. As long as the patient is stable, spirometry measurements should be continued even after the FEV_1 has dropped by 15% in order to determine the nadir or lowest point and assess the severity of EIA. If 2 subsequent FEV_1 measurements after the nadir show improvement, the measurements may be stopped. A nebulized β-agonist treatment can be administered if the subject's FEV_1 does not return spontaneously to within 10% of the preexercise value [22].

Cycle Ergometer

The cycle ergometer is easier for many patients to use, especially young children and older subjects. It has been generally considered less 'asthmagenic' than the treadmill [30] but many investigators now consider it just as effective in bronchial provocation when the target workload is achieved [38].

Monitoring of vital signs is easier with cycling since the subject is moving less. A target heart rate or ventilation is set prior to the challenge in the same manner as with the treadmill. A target work rate that will induce the target heart rate or ventilation can then be calculated and used to adjust the ergometer. As with treadmill testing, the ATS recommends that the target work intensity as measured by heart rate or ventilation should be sustained for at least 4 min [22] while other practitioners prefer to maintain it for 5–8 min.

Hyperventilation

The amount of ventilation is the ultimate determinant leading to EIA and this can be achieved by either exercise or hyperventilation [42]. Eucapnic voluntary hyperventilation (EVH) is therefore a valid alternative test for EIA. It requires more equipment but is ideal for patients who are unable to perform physical exercise. The subject breathes through a valve box with a pump set to a specific minute ventilation. A reservoir balloon is attached to the valve box and the patient breathes with enough force to prevent deflation of the balloon. The subject inhales a mixture of cooled room air with a low concentration of carbon dioxide to prevent hypocapnia which has a bronchoconstrictive effect. A simplified system using a compressed gas mixture containing 5% carbon dioxide can also be used [43]. The aim is usually to achieve approximately 60–70% of maximum voluntary ventilation. Dosing schedules differing in target minute ventilation and duration have been recommended [44]. A fall of 10% in the FEV_1 is also considered suggestive of asthma while other authors require a 15% fall for diagnosis [16].

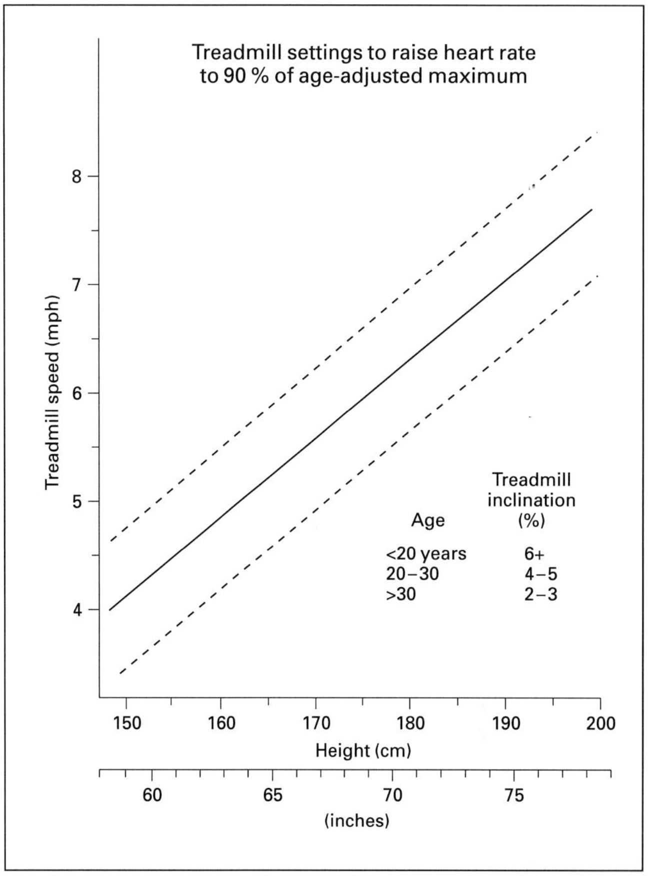

Fig. 1. Treadmill settings for speed and incline. From Eggleston et al. [31].

Comparison of Bronchial Provocation Challenges

Challenges with bronchoconstrictor agents such as methacholine and histamine produce direct constriction of bronchial smooth muscle in susceptible subjects with BHR. On the other hand, exercise and hyperventilation challenges induce bronchospasm in asthmatics by a sequence of inflammatory events. Since other mediators such as leukotrienes are likely released in EIA, a negative methacholine or histamine challenge does not rule out EIA. When utilized for the detection of BHR in a study of

Table 7. Nonpharmacologic measures for EIA

Warm up for at least 10 min before actual exercise
Cover mouth and nose with scarf or surgical mask during cold weather
Exercise in warm, humidified environments if possible
Warm down or gradually lower the intensity of exercise

patients with unexplained dyspnea, the exercise challenge was of low clinical utility when compared to the methacholine challenge [45].

The treadmill and cycle ergometer are probably both equally effective in provoking EIA when performed properly. Isocapnic ventilation is the alternative if exercise testing cannot be done. More comparative studies need to be done to determine the comparative usefulness of these different modes in EIA diagnosis.

Exercise challenges using minimum or no equipment have been studied for screening large populations such as students and schoolchildren. Free range running can be used but safety concerns limit its use [46].

Therapy

Prevention is the primary mode of therapy for EIA. There are non-pharmacologic and pharmacologic measures that can be taken to prevent or lessen the symptoms of EIA.

Nonpharmacologic Therapy (table 7)

Important factors affecting the intensity of EIA are the person's underlying baseline bronchial reactivity and level of conditioning as well as the amount of ventilation and air temperature during exercise. The first two factors depend on previous levels of asthma control and general fitness while the latter two depend on the nature and environment of the exertion.

An asthmatic's bronchial reactivity is increased with repeated exposure to allergens such as animal dander, pollen, dust mites and mold. Recurrent viral infections can also lead to increased bronchial reactivity. Avoidance measures and environmental control to minimize allergen exposure is essential for good asthma control. Bronchial hyperresponsiveness and the response to exercise can be diminished by maintenance anti-inflammatory therapy with medications such as inhaled steroids and antileukotrienes [47].

Good conditioning and aerobic fitness is also important in lessening EIA. Asthmatics should not be discouraged from exercising. Persons who exercise regularly do not have the rapid and abrupt increases in minute ventilation that are more likely to stimulate EIA.

Whether or not physical training improves BHR and pulmonary function remains unclear. While some studies report no improvement in EIA severity with training programs, there are several studies that do [48–50]. In one study, a 25% improvement in the severity of EIA was observed with a training program [49]. Most authors believe that a regular regimen of moderate exercise tailored to a patient's asthma severity should be prescribed for its physical, social and emotional benefits [51]. Walking or jogging are good initial activities. Swimming is often recommended as an ideal sport for asthmatics as the warm, humidified air around the pool lowers the occurrence of EIA.

Sports and EIA

Athletes in general have a 35% incidence of EIA [46]. A survey of US athletes in the 1998 Winter Olympics surprisingly showed that 43% had a previous diagnosis of asthma [52]. Early recognition of patients at risk for EIA is a first step towards diagnosis and preventive treatment. In a study involving 238 male high school varsity football players, a significant rate of previously undiagnosed EIA was observed and associated with risk factors including a history of wheezing, residence in a poverty area, race and remote history of asthma. This study suggested that a simple screening 1 mile outdoor run may identify individuals at risk [46].

The amount of ventilation in exercise is directly related to the intensity of the activity. It is the increase in ventilation produced by exercise and not the kind of exercise that is crucial in EIA. This means that any exercise can lead to EIA if it is done hard enough or long enough to increase the amount of air being inhaled. In fact, hyperventilation maneuvers can be used in some instances instead of an exercise challenge to diagnose EIA. The intensity of the exercise is important because it is directly proportional to the amount of ventilation. Vigorous activities such as basketball or soccer can cause more severe attacks than less vigorous ones like baseball.

Cool and dry air worsens airway cooling causing more symptoms. Running in warm days cause less problems than the same activity during cold days. Figure skaters and hockey players who have asthma are more prone to EIA in their particular sports because of the cold environment. The incidence of exercise-induced bronchospasm in competitive figure skaters has been found in several studies to be up to 30–35% [53, 54]. One study suggests that it may be helpful to screen for EIA in aspiring figure skaters so that education and preventive measures can be done [54]. Covering the nose and mouth with a scarf or surgical mask when exercising in cold weather has been found to lessen EIA by warming inhaled air [55]. Swimming has been recommended to many asthmatics because the warm, humidified air around the swimming pool allows more active exertion without triggering asthma.

As mentioned earlier, a refractory period occurs up to several hours after recovery from EIA. Athletes with asthma can take advantage of this by always warming up prior to vigorous exertion. This warm-up period induces a refractory period during which there are less asthma symptoms with the actual exercise [56]. A warm-up period of 10 min is usually adequate [57]. Runners can warm up by running repeated short sprints [58]. Gradual increase in intensity of exercise as opposed to rapid increases is also beneficial [11]. Warming down or slowly lessening the intensity of exercise instead of stopping abruptly can also make EIA less severe. This may make airway rewarming and the resultant vascular dilation and edema more gradual and less intense [10].

Education on the nature of EIA and how to control it with or without medications needs to be given to asthmatics as well as family members and coaches. Today, there is no reason for asthma to be a restricting factor in sports. Many well-known athletes have asthma, including Dennis Rodman and Jackie Joyner-Kersee. Nancy Hogshead, the Olympic swimmer gives the athlete's perspective on asthma in her book, Asthma and Exercise [59].

Pharmacologic Therapy (table 8)

Inhaled β-agonists are the medications of choice for prophylaxis of EIA. If given 15 min to an hour before exercise, short-acting β-agonists such as albuterol (Ventolin™) and terbutaline (Brethaire™) can prevent symptoms. Long-acting inhaled β-agonists such as salmeterol (Serevent™) have a slower onset of action, act for 12 h at a time and should be taken at least 1–2 h before exercise [60]. Formoterol (Foradil™), a new rapid-acting β-agonist with a long duration of action (up to 12 h) may be ideal for use just before exercise. Albuterol, terbutaline, salmeterol and salmeterol/ipatropium (Combivent™) are the only inhaled β-agonists allowed by the US and International Olympic Committees (table 9). The National Collegiate Athletic Association (NCAA), on the other hand, allows all inhaled β-agonists [21].

Table 8. Pharmacologic agents

First-line
Inhaled β-agonists
Inhaled cromolyn and nedocromil
Additional agents
Antileukotriene agents
Calcium channel blockers
Oral β-agonists
α-Agonists
Theophylline
Inhaled anticholinergic agents (e.g. ipatropium bromide)
Newer agents
Inhaled heparin
Inhaled furosemide

Table 9. Asthma drugs in the Olympics [from The United States Anti-Doping Agency (USADA) Guide to Prohibited Classes of Substances and Prohibited Methods of Doping. Updated December 2000]

Allowed
Albuterol*
Terbutaline*
Salmeterol*
Salmeterol/ipratropium*
Cromolyn/nedocromil
Aminophylline/theophylline
Ipratropium
Antileukotrienes
All inhaled and nasal corticosteroids
Banned
All inhaled β-agonists not listed above
All oral and injectable β-agonists
All systemic corticosteroids

* Written notification of asthma and/or exercise-induced asthma by a respiratory or team physician is necessary and must be provided to USADA and the Relevant Medical Authority prior to competition.

The next most commonly used prophylactic agents for EIA are the inhaled mast cell stabilizers cromolyn and nedocromil. When used 10–20 min before exercise, they have been found to block or attenuate EIA. Cromolyn and nedocromil are approved for use by the US and International Olympic committees. When compared with inhaled β-agonists, cromolyn is not as effective in preventing EIA [61].

The antileukotrienes are currently recommended mainly for chronic asthma therapy but have both been shown to diminish bronchospasm in exercise challenge studies [62]. The two types of antileukotrienes are leukotriene receptor antagonists, e.g. zafirlukast (Accolate™) or montelukast (Singulair™), and 5-lipoxygenase inhibitors (e.g. zileuton (Zyflo™). In one study, standard single doses of montelukast, zafirlukast and zileuton were as effective as salmeterol in attenuating EIA. Zileuton had a shorter duration of action (up to 4 h) while montelukast, zafirlukast and salmeterol were protective for up to 8 h [63]. When compared in the long-term treatment of EIA over 8 weeks, montelukast and salmeterol were both found to be effective but salmeterol lost much of its protective effect after 4 and 8 weeks of use [64].

Other agents which may be added include inhaled anticholinergic agents, theophylline, calcium channel blockers, antihistamines, α-agonists and oral β-agonists [65]. These agents have shown varying protection against EIA in different studies and may not be as effective if used alone.

The widely used anticoagulant heparin,when given in the inhaled form, has been shown in at least one study to be more effective than cromolyn in preventing EIA. Its mechanism of action is not clear but is thought to be due to inhibition of mast cell release [66]. Another widely used drug, the diuretic furosemide, when given in the inhaled form, has been shown in several studies to inhibit EIA in children and adults [67, 68]. Further studies in larger groups are needed to confirm the effectiveness in preventing EIA.

Pharmacologic treatment after the symptoms of EIA have started is identical to treatment of asthma symptoms from other triggers. Appropriate anti-inflammatory treatment of underlying chronic persistent asthma with inhaled steroids and other medications will decrease the incidence of exercise-induced bronchospasm.

Conclusions

Exercise-induced asthma (EIA) is characterized by transient airway obstruction occurring after strenuous exertion. A fall of 15% or more in the FEV_1 after exercise is diagnostic while a 10% drop is already considered abnormal. Inhalation of large volumes of dry, cold air during exercise leads to loss of heat and water from the bronchial mucosa and airway cooling and drying. Proposed mechanisms for bronchoconstriction include (a) mucosal drying and increased osmolarity stimulating mast cell degranulation, and (b) rapid airway rewarming after exercise causing vascular congestion, increased permeability and edema leading to obstruction. EIA symptoms start after exercise, peak 8–15 min postexercise and spontaneously resolve in about 60 min. A refractory period lasts up to 3 h after recovery, during which repeat exercise causes less bronchospasm. The amount of ventilation and the temperature of inspired air are important factors in determining the severity of EIA. Greater ventilation and cold,dry air increase the risk for EIA.

Methacholine and histamine challenge testing may be done to detect nonspecific BHR to confirm suspected asthma but a negative response does not rule out EIA. Exercise or hyperventilation testing is needed to rule out EIA. The treadmill and cycle ergometer are the preferred modes of exercise testing. Both have advantages and disadvantages but are appropriate diagnostic tools for EIA diagnosis when performed properly. Hyperventilation testing is an alternative for those unable to do exercise testing.

Prevention is the main objective in managing EIA. Nonpharmacologic measures include warming up prior to vigorous exertion, covering the mouth and nose in cold weather, exercising in warm, humidified environments if possible and warming down after exercise. Aerobic fitness and good control of baseline bronchial reactivity also help diminish the effects of EIA.

Inhaled β-agonists are the medications of choice for EIA prophylaxis. Inhaled cromolyn or nedocromil may also be used. Antileukotriene agents have been shown to diminish EIA after single doses and with chronic usage without loss of protection. If inhaled β-agonists or cromolyn are not adequate for prophylaxis, additional agents can be considered including antileukotrienes, anticholinergic agents [such as ipatropium bromide (Atrovent™)], theophylline, calcium channel blockers, a-agonists, antihistamines and oral β-agonists. Newer agents under study include inhaled heparin and inhaled furosemide.

Education regarding the nature and management of EIA is important not only for asthmatics but also their families and coaches. With the proper precautions and workout techniques, there is no limit to what persons with asthma can achieve in sports.

References

1 Bardagi S, Agudo A, Gonzalez CA, Romero PV: Prevalence of exercise-induced narrowing in schoolchildren from a Mediterranean town. Am Rev Resp Dis 1993;147:1112–1115.

2 Karjalainen J: Exercise response in 404 young men with asthma: No evidence for a late asthmatic reaction. Thorax 1991;46:100–104.

3 Milgrom H, Taussig LM: Keeping children with exercise-induced asthma active. Pediatrics 1999;104:38.

4 Helenius IJ, Tikkanen HO, Haahtela T: Occurence of exercise induced bronchospasm in elite runners: Dependence on atopy and exposure to cold air and pollen. Br J Sports Med 1998;32:125–129.

5 Afrasiabi R, Spector SL: Exercise-induced asthma: It needn't sideline your patients. Phys Sportsmed 1991;19:49–62.

6 Strauss RH, McFadden ER Jr, Ingram RH Jr, Jaeger JJ: Enhancement of exercise-induced asthma by cold air. N Engl J Med 1977;297:743–747.

7 Deal EC Jr, McFadden ER Jr, Ingram RH Jr, Strauss RH, Jaeger JJ: Role of respiratory heat exchange in production of exercise-induced asthma. J Appl Physiol 1979;46:467–475.

8 Anderson SD, Schoeffel RE, Black JL, Daviskas E: Airway cooling as the stimulus to exercise-induced asthma: A reevaluation. Eur J Respir Dis 1985;67:20–30.

9 Sheppard D, Eschenbacher WL: Respiratory water loss as a stimulus to exercise-induced bronchoconstriction asthma. J Allergy Clin immunol 1984;73:640–642.

10 McFadden ER Jr: Exercise-induced airway obstruction. Clin Chest Med 1995;16:671–682.

11 Spector SL: Update on exercise-induced asthma. Ann Allergy 1993;71:571–577.

12 McFadden ER Jr, Lenner KA, Strohl KP: Postexertional airway rewarming and thermally-induced asthma. J Clin Invest 1986;78:18–25.

13 Anderson SD, Holzer K: Exercise-induced asthma: Is it the right diagnosis in elite athletes? J Allergy Clin Immunol 2000;106:419–428.

14 Spector SL: Allergen inhalation challenges; in Spector SL (ed): Provocative Testing in Clinical Practice. New York, Marcel Dekker, 1995, pp 325–368.

15 McFadden ER Jr, Gilbert IA: Exercise-induced asthma. N Engl J Med 1994;330:1362–1367.

16 Godfrey S: Bronchial challenge by exercise or hyperventilation; in Spector SL (ed): Provocative Challenge Procedures: Background and Methodology. Mount Kisco, Futura, 1989, pp 365–394.

17 Boulet LP, Legris C, Turcotte H, et al: Prevalence and characteristics of late asthmatic response to exercise. J Allergy Clin Immunol 1987;80:655.

18 Peroni DG, Boner AL: Exercise-induced asthma: Is there space for late-phase reactions? Eur Resp J 1996;9:1335–1338.

19 O'Byrne PM, Jones JL: Effect of indomethacin on exercise-induced bronchoconstriction and refractoriness after exercise. Am Rev Respir Dis 1986;134:69–72.

20 McFadden ER, Zawadski DK: Vocal cord dysfunction masquerading as exercise induced asthma: A physiologic cause for choking during athletic activities. Am J Resp Crit Care Med 1996;153:942–947.

21 Nastasi KJ, Heinly TL, Blaiss MS: Exercise-induced asthma and the athlete. J Asthma 1995;32:249–257.

22 American Thoracic Society: Guidelines for methacholine and exercise challenge testing 1999. Am J Respir Crit Care Med 2000;141:309–329.

23 Cockcroft DW, Killian DN, Mellon JJ, Hargreave FE: Bronchial reactivity to inhaled histamine: A method and clinical survey. Clin Allergy 1977;7:235.

24 Chai H, Farr RS, Froehlich LA, Mathison DA, McLean JA, Rosenthal RR, Sheffer AL, Spector SL, Townley RG: Standardization of bronchial inhalation challenge procedures. J Allergy Clin Immunol 1975;56:323–327.

25 Yan K, Salome CM, Woolcock AJ: Rapid method for measurement of bronchial responsiveness. Thorax 1983;38:760–765.

26 Juniper EF, Cockcroft DW, Hargreave FE: Tidal breathing method. In Histamine and Methachioline Inhalation Tests: Laboratory Procedure and Standardization, ed. 2. Lund, Astra Draco AB, Lund, 1994.

27 Fish JE: Bronchial challenge testing; in Middleton E Jr, et al (eds): Allergy: Principles and Practice, ed. 4. St Louis, Mosby, 1993, pp 613–627.

28 Hopp RJ, Bewtra AK, Nair NM et al: Specificity and sensitivity of methacholine inhalation challenge in normal and asthmatic children. J Allergy Clin Immunol 1984;74:154.

29 Trautlein JJ: Risk factors in exercise testing. J Allergy Clin Immunol 1979;64:625–626.

30 Cropp GJA: The exercise provocation test: Standardization of procedures and evaluation of response. JACI 1979;64:627–633.

31 Eggleston PA, Rosenthal RR, Anderson SD, Anderson R, et al: Guidelines for the methodology of exercise challenge testing of asthmatics. JACI 1979;64:642–645.

32 Edmunds AT, Tooley M, Godfrey S: The refractory period after exercise-induced asthma: Its duration and relation to severity of exercise. Am Rev Resp Dis 1978;117:247–254.

33 Anderson SD, Schoeffel RE, Follet R, et al: Sensitivity to heat and water loss at rest and during exercise in asthmatic patients. Eur J Resp Dis 1982;63:459–471.

34 Shturman-Elistein R, Zeballos RJ, Buckley JM, et al: The beneficial effect of nasal breathing on exercise-induced bronchoconstriction. Am Rev Resp Dis 1978;118:65–73.

35 Cropp GJA: Relative sensitivity of different pulmonary function tests in the evaluation of exercise-induced asthma. Pediatrics 1975;56 (suppl):860.

36 American Thoracic Society: Standardization of spirometry: 1994 update. Am J Resp Crit Care Med 1995;152:1107–1136.

37 Anderson SD, Connolly NM, Godfrey S: Comparison of bronchoconstriction induced by cycling and running. Thorax 1971;26:396–401.

38 Souhrada JF, Souhrada M: Provocative challenge by exercise or hyperventilation; in Spector SL (ed): Provocation Testing in Clinical Practice. New York, Marcel Dekker, 1995, pp 425–449.

39 McFadden ER: Exercise-induced airway narrowing; in Middleton E (ed): Allergy: Principles and Practice, ed 5. Mosby, New York, 1998, pp 953–962.

40 Johnson WR, Buskirk ER (eds): Science and Medicine of Exercise and Sports, ed 2. New York, Harper & Row, 1974, p 125.

41 Silverman M, Anderson SD: Standardization of exercise tests in asthmatic children. Arch Dis Child 1972;47:882–889.

42 Zeballos RJ, Shturman-Ellstein R, McNally JF Jr, Hirsch JE, Souhrada JF: The role of hyperventilation in exercise-induced bronchoconstriction. Am Rev Resp Dis 1978;118:877–884.

43 Phillips YY, Jaeger JJ, Laube BL, Rosenthal RR: Eucapnic voluntary hyperventilation of compressed gas mixture. Am Rev Resp Dis 1985;131:31–35.

44 Argyros GJ, Roach JM, Hurwitz KM, Eliasson AH, Phillips YY: Eucapnic voluntary hyperventilation as a bronchoprovocation technique: Development of a standardized dosing schedule in asthmatics. Chest 1996;109:1520–1524.

45 Zeballos RJ, Weisman IM, Connery SM, Bradley JP: Standard treadmill vs incremental cycle ergometry in the evaluation of airway hyperreactivity in unexplained dyspnea. Am J Resp Crit Care Med 1999;159:A419.

46 Kukafka DS, Lang DM, Porer S, Rogers J, Ciccolella D, Polansky M, D'Alonzo GE Jr: Exercise-induced bronchospasm in high school athletes via a free running test: Incidence and epidemiology. Chest 1998;114:1613–1622.

47 Freezer NJ, Croasdell H, Doull IJ, Holgate ST: Effect of regular inhaled beclomethasone on exercise and metacholine airway responses in schoolchildren with recurrent wheeze. Eur Resp J 1995;8:1488–1493.

48 Svenonius E, Kautto R, Arborelius M: Improvement after training of children with exercise-induced asthma. Acta Paediatr Scand 1983;72:23–30.

49 Henriksen JM, Nielsen TT: Effect of physical training on exercise-induced bronchoconstriction. Acta Paediatr Scand 1983;72:31–36.

50 Haas F, Pasierski S, Levine N, et al: Effect of aerobic training on forced expiratory airflow in exercising asthmatic humans. J Appl Physiol 1987;63:1230–1235.

51 Satta A: Exercise training in asthma. J Sports Med Phys Fitness 2000;40:277–283.

52 Weiler JM, Ryan EJ: Asthma in United States Olympic athletes who participated in the 1998 Olympic Winter Games. J Allergy Clin Immunol 2000;106:267–271.
53 Provost-Craig MA, Arbour KS, Sestili DC, Chabalko JJ, Ekinci E: The incidence of exercise-induced bronchospasm in competitive figure skaters. J Asthma 1996;33:67–71.
54 Mannix ET, Farber MO, Palange P, Galassetti P, Manfredi R: Exercise-induced asthma in figure skaters. Chest 1996;109:312–315.
55 Schacter EN, Lach E, Lee M: The protective effect of a cold weather mask on exercise-induced asthma. Ann Allergy 1981;46:12–16.
56 Reiff DB, Nozhat BC, Neil BP, Philip WI: The effect of prolonged submaximal warm-up exercise on exercise-induced asthma. Am Rev Respir Dis 1989;139:479–484.
57 Wright LA, Martin RJ: Nocturnal asthma and exercise-induced bronchospasm. Postgrad Med 1995;97:83–90.
58 Schnall RP, Landau LI: Protective effects of repeated short sprints in exercise-induced asthma. Thorax 1980;35:828–832.
59 Hogshead N, Couzens GS: Asthma and Exercise. New York, Henry Holt, 1990.
60 Schaanning J, Vilsik J, Henriksen AH, Bratten G: Efficacy and duration of salmeterol powder inhalation in protecting against exercise-induced bronchoconstriction. Ann Allergy Asthma Immunol 1996;76:57–60.
61 Rohr AS, Siegel SC, Katz RM, et al: A comparison of inhaled albuterol and cromolyn in the prophylaxis of exercise-induced bronchospasm. Ann Allergy 1987;59:107–109.
62 Makker HK, Lau LC, Thomson HW, Binks SM, Holgate ST: The protective effect of inhaled LTD_4 receptor antagonist ICI 204219 against exercise-induced asthma. Am Rev Respir Dis 1993;147:1413–1418.
63 Coreno A, Skowronski M, Kotaru C, McFadden ER: Comparative effects of along-acting beta-2-agonists, leukotriene receptor antagonists, and a 5-lipoxygenase inhibitor on EIA. JACI 2000;106:500–506.
64 Villaran C, O'Neill SJ, Helbling A, van Noord JA: Montelukast versus salmeterol in patients with asthma and exercise-induced bronchoconstriction. Montelukast/Salmeterol Exercise Study Group. J Allergy Clin Immunol 1999; 104:547–553.
65 Spector SL: Treatments of exercise-induced asthma other than B-agonists; in Weiler J (ed): Allergic and Respiratory Diseases in Sports Medicine. New York, Marcel Dekker, 1997.
66 Garrigo J, Danta I, Ahmed T: Time course of the protective effect of inhaled heparin on exercise-induced asthma. Am J Resp Crit Care Med 1996;153:1702–1707.
67 Novembre E, Frongia G, Lombardi E, Rest M, et al: The preventive effects and duration of action of two doses of inhaled furosemide on exercise-induced asthma in children. J Allergy Clin Immunol 1995;96:906–909.
68 Munyard P, Chung KF, Bush A: Inhaled furosemide and exercise-induced bronchoconstriction in children with asthma. Thorax 1995;50: 677–679.

Ricardo A. Tan, MD
California Allergy and Asthma
Medical Group, Inc.
11645 Wilshire Blvd., Suite 1090
Palmdale, CA 90025 (USA)
Tel. +1 310 966 9022, Fax +1 310 966 9042
E-Mail rtantan@aol.com

Weisman IM, Zeballos RJ (eds): Clinical Exercise Testing.
Prog Respir Res. Basel, Karger, 2002, vol 32, pp 217–230

Evaluation of Impairment and Disability: The Role of Cardiopulmonary Exercise Testing

Darryl Y. Sue

UCLA School of Medicine, Los Angeles, Calif., and Medical-Respiratory Intensive Care Unit and Associate Chair, Department of Medicine, Harbor-UCLA Medical Center, Torrance, Calif., USA

Summary

Cardiopulmonary exercise testing has a strong physiological basis and well-documented clinical rationale for impairment evaluation. Both determination and quantitation of impairment are enhanced by exercise testing, notably because of the inadequacy of resting pulmonary function tests to predict exercise capacity, and both over- and underestimation of work capacity have been found. Furthermore, exercise arterial blood gases are very sensitive tests for subtle lung disease. Exercise testing can be especially useful in those with co-existing disorders or unsuspected cardiovascular disorders. Exercise testing is not indicated in those who lack complaints of exertional dyspnea or fatigue, and those with severe respiratory impairment (ATS criteria for impairment by FEV_1 or DLCO) also do not require exercise testing. Cardiopulmonary exercise testing can provide objective determination of exercise capacity, increased sensitivity for pulmonary gas exchange abnormalities, and the ability to identify unsuspected or unanticipated non-pulmonary causes of impairment.

Introduction

Cardiopulmonary exercise testing has become well established as a clinical tool for evaluating patients in wide variety of clinical situations. For severe congestive heart failure, measurement of peak oxygen uptake ($\dot{V}O_2$) is the best discriminant for selection of patients to undergo heart transplantation, and many clinicians depend on exercise testing to determine postoperative risk in patients with marginal cardiopulmonary function. Finally, a primary role for exercise testing remains in the evaluation of patients with unexplained dyspnea or exercise intolerance. In such patients, common (ischemic heart disease, ventilatory limitation), unusual disorders (mitochondrial myopathies), and combined disorders may be suggested or confirmed.

The determination and quantification of impairment, not withstanding disability, can be complex, difficult, or contested, and objective measurements of functional capacity and its loss should be valuable adjuncts to other clinical information. Although it would appear that complaints about functional or work capacity could be ideally evaluated during actual exercise, integrative cardiopulmonary exercise testing has been characterized as expensive, unavailable, and difficult to perform [1–2]. Nevertheless, there are considerable data supporting the use of cardiopulmonary exercise testing in impairment evaluation, much of which demonstrate that estimation of exercise capacity from clinical and physiological measurements at rest is poor at best.

Not all assessment of impairment relates to occupational exposures, and not all determinations of disability are questions about the ability to perform a job [1]. However, the focus of this discussion is on determining impairment in patients with occupational disease. A standardized approach to all patients or claimants is impractical, even those with potential occupational diseases from

Table 1. Cardiopulmonary exercise testing: clinical questions compared to impairment/disability

Clinical question	Impairment/disability question	Physiological variables
Is maximum exercise capacity reduced compared to normal?	What is the maximum exercise capacity?	Peak $\dot{V}O_2$ compared to normal and expressed as ml/kg/min
Does impaired O_2 flow limit exercise capacity at submaximal work rates?	What is the maximum sustainable level of exercise?	$\dot{V}O_2$ at the lactic acidosis threshold; work rate at the lactic acidosis threshold
Does reduced ventilatory capacity limit maximum exercise?	How much reduction in ventilatory capacity is seen at maximum exercise?	Breathing reserve
How severe are pulmonary gas exchange abnormalities during exercise?	Is there evidence of subtle pulmonary gas exchange abnormalities that would indicate the presence of unsuspected lung disease?	Arterial blood gases (PaO_2), alveolar-arterial PO_2 difference, dead space/tidal volume ratio
Is exercise limited by cardiovascular factors, effort, or musculoskeletal problems?	Are there coexisting conditions that limit exercise outside of the lungs?	Heart rate and heart rate reserve, blood lactate during recovery, breathing reserve
	Can the subject perform exercise at a level and duration comparable to that of a specific job or occupation?	Estimate or measurement of task specific requirements ($\dot{V}O_2$)

exposure to the same injurious substance. For example, physicians sometimes seek to link a toxin or injurious substance to a disease in a causal sense. In others, the injury is established already but the extent of impairment or loss of capacity is in question. A variety of strategies, ranging from epidemiological to medical evaluation of an individual patient, have been used. Because the lungs are often the most heavily involved in a variety of occupations, interstitial lung disease, occupational asthma, chronic obstructive lung disease, lung cancer, and pleuropulmonary disorders are among the most common evaluated. However, the age of these subjects (many men) together with other factors simultaneously put them at risk for ischemic heart disease and congestive heart failure. The question that we should ask, therefore, is whether pulmonary function tests, including spirometry, lung volumes, and diffusing capacity for carbon monoxide, along with radiographic imaging, are sufficient to estimate exercise capacity and its reciprocal, impairment. Even at first glance, the answer should be no. That is, while pulmonary function tests at rest go a long way in quantifying the capacity of the respiratory system, they say nothing about the demand of exercise. Furthermore, none of these tests provide information about the cardiovascular system or the musculoskeletal capacity of the subject, or help determine either peak capacity or sustainable work rate. In theory, cardiopulmonary exercise testing would be ideal for the purpose of impairment evaluation, largely becomes it overcomes the limitations of resting studies, integrates information about all systems involved with exercise, is intrinsically quantitative, and provides measurements of both demand and capacity.

The integrative cardiopulmonary exercise test has two major components. There is an exercise stress given to the patient in the laboratory (usually treadmill or cycle ergometer) that is designed to reproduce the symptoms, if any, noted by the patient during exertion. Second, respired gas exchange and other data are collected during exercise that allow an assessment of work capacity and, importantly, the integrative function of the organ systems necessary to perform exercise. The questions asked in a typical clinical situation are designed to identify or confirm dysfunction of each of the various organ systems (table 1).

When the integrative cardiopulmonary exercise test is employed for evaluation of occupational disease, different questions may be appropriate (table 1). In a patient with known exposure to asbestos who has interstitial lung disease (asbestosis), reduced vital capacity, and an abnormal chest roentgenogram, the severity of the impairment rather than the presence of asbestosis may be in question. On occasion, this individual may be completely asymptomatic and have no complaints about exercise intolerance, yet be a claimant in an individual or group action related to occupational exposure. Often, a patient or claimant with complaints of exercise intolerance may have co-existing cardiopulmonary disease, obesity, disorders caused by smoking, poor conditioning, or other factors unrelated to the occupational exposure. Finally, a comparison of work capacity measured during the exercise test to the estimated rate of work being performed on a given job may help in determining disability as opposed to impairment.

Defining Impairment and Disability

This discussion cannot review in detail the definitions of impairment, disability, and fitness for work, and there are several comprehensive sources of this information [1–5]. However, it is important to distinguish impairment and disability. Impairment, as used in the United States, is considered to be decreased functional capacity on a medical basis. Impairment lends itself to being measurable, often in an objective manner. For example, the American Thoracic Society statement described impairment as '...purely a medical definition. Most impairments result from a functional abnormality, which may or may not be stable at the time the evaluation is made, and may be temporary or permanent' [3]. The American Medical Association (AMA) definition of impairment is similar: 'a loss, loss of use, or derangement of any body part, organ sytem, or organ function' [2]. Disability is a more global statement about the impact of identified impairment on the subject. Disability assessment requires social, economic, environmental, and other data. Disability was defined by the American Thoracic Society as 'a term that indicates the total effect of impairment on a patient's life. It is affected by such diverse factors as age, gender, education, economic and social environment, and energy requirements of the occupation' [3]. The AMA defines disability as 'an alteration of an individual's capacity to meet personal, social, or occupational demands or statutory or regulatory requirements because of an impairment' [2]. Physicians are tasked with identifying and measuring impairment but, although opinions are sought from physicians about a patient's disability, disability decisions are most often made through an administrative or other nonmedical system. An increasingly important concept is accommodation with respect to disability. The level and type of disability may change as the job requirement and environment change to accommodate an individual. At times, conflicts develop because some physicians are asked to act in the patient's best interest, while others represent the employer. World Health Organization definitions were different [6], for example. Impairment was defined as any loss or abnormality of psychological, physiological, or anatomical structure or function while disability was defined as any restriction or lack (resulting from impairment) of ability to perform an activity within the range considered normal for a human being. Thus, disability here is more similar to a global form of impairment. The WHO reserved the term handicap to represent the total effect of disability on the subject's life and work.

Harber and Fedoruk [7] point out a fundamental difference that physicians must keep in mind. The usual evaluation of a patient seeks to determine if the patient's function is abnormal; that is, sufficiently different (lower) than a normal population. Thus, a vital capacity that is below the 95% confidence limit for a sample of the same gender, height, and age would be interpreted as abnormal. For impairment evaluation, however, this is overly simplistic because it focuses on the amount of function lost, but does not address the level of function remaining.

Because cardiopulmonary exercise testing provides objective measurement of physiologic function, this form of testing clearly relates to assessing impairment rather than disability. Thus, physicians using exercise testing can make a statement about maximum or sustained exercise capacity, and whether and how much exercise capacity is limited. Furthermore, if findings warrant, information about abnormal physiologic function may be found, such as abnormal lung gas exchange. On the other hand, exercise testing helps in disability evaluation only so much as it provides information about impairment.

Physiological Basis for Cardiopulmonary Exercise Testing

The features of cardiopulmonary exercise testing that lend itself particularly well to the assessment of impairment include (1) objective measurements of work performance, albeit usually with a non-work related task; (2) measurements of physiological function of several organ systems, and (3) evidence that decision-making in the impairment process is improved.

Simple measurements of exercise capacity such as a timed walk, or treadmill or cycle exercise with electrocardiogram monitoring, do not require much equipment and may be useful in determining suitability for major surgery, risk stratification after myocardial infarction, or screening for ischemic heart disease in certain populations. However, impairment evaluation is often more subtle and requires more sophisticated methods. This is because claimants and subjects may have little or no impairment, few symptoms, and may not have a single disorder or abnormal organ system.

Integrative Cardiopulmonary Exercise Testing

Measurement of gas exchange during exercise, including oxygen uptake ($\dot{V}O_2$), carbon dioxide output ($\dot{V}CO_2$), heart rate, end-tidal PO_2 and PCO_2, and minute ventilation ($\dot{V}_E$) distinguishes integrative cardiopulmonary exercise testing from other kinds of exercise testing. Usually, pulse oximetry is used and, on occasion, arterial blood gases are very useful. Computer-controlled data collection using 'breath-by-breath' techniques are highly suitable during rapidly changing exercise stress, and commercial systems that incorporate gas analyzers, flow meters, and displays are readily available. Extensive discussion of interpretation of exercise gas exchange variables is provided in other references [8–11].

Exercise on a treadmill or cycle ergometer is performed because the leg muscles are able to generate a much larger work rate than the arms, and it is the physical work rate that creates the metabolic stress that tests the capacity of the heart, lungs, and circulation. The patient or subject performs a measured exercise stress while gas exchange measurements are made. Most often, the work rate being performed by the subject is increased incrementally every minute by increasing the resistance to pedaling a cycle ergometer or by increasing the slope or speed of the treadmill. The exercise protocol is planned in advance for the subject to reach a point of voluntary termination of exercise in 8–12 min. It is emphasized that this kind of testing depends on having the subject or patient exercise as much and as long as possible. The symptoms, if any, that stop exercise should be identified and recorded.

Exercise $\dot{V}O_2$ and Peak $\dot{V}O_2$

The question of whether a patient has normal exercise capacity (and therefore can perform work at this rate) is best answered by whether or not the peak $\dot{V}O_2$ during exercise is normal when compared to values found in normal subjects of the same gender, size, and age. If peak $\dot{V}O_2$ is normal in a given subject, this indicates that the functional capacities of the several organ systems needed to transport O_2 are normal. These include the respiratory system (lung gas transfer, pulmonary circulation, and ventilatory capacity), heart (heart rate and stroke volume), circulation (blood vessels and hemoglobin concentration), and ability of exercising muscles to take up and consume oxygen (sufficient muscle mass, normal oxidative metabolism, no musculoskeletal disorders). In contrast, the subject with a decreased peak $\dot{V}O_2$ is impaired by definition, and this finding triggers a search for the cause of decreased exercise capacity, with the goal of isolating the involved organ system and the mechanism of abnormality.

In assessing work capacity and cause of limitation, peak $\dot{V}O_2$ must not be designated as purely a pulmonary variable. For example, the quotient of $\dot{V}O_2$/heart rate is known as the oxygen-pulse (O_2-pulse) and, when measured at peak $\dot{V}O_2$, gives a non-invasive estimate of maximum cardiac stroke volume [10]. Similar, we can regard $\dot{V}O_2$ (and peak $\dot{V}O_2$) as equal to the product of cardiac output (Q) and the arterial-mixed venous O_2 content difference ($C[a\text{-}v]O_2$). Any limitation in the heart rate response (chronotropic incompetence, beta-blockade) or stroke volume response (cardiomyopathy, valvular heart disease) will cause a decrease in cardiac output. If, at peak exercise, arterial O_2 content is abnormally low, as seen in arterial hypoxemia, anemia, or carbon monoxide exposure, or mixed venous O_2 content is abnormally high, peak $\dot{V}O_2$ can be abnormally low.

Submaximal Exercise

Maximal exercise studies are essential in determining impairment because the exercise capacity, loss of capacity, and remaining capacity of the individual can be determined. But, submaximal measurements have a role in assessing work capacity, impairment, and disability as well. The increase in $\dot{V}O_2$ ($\Delta\dot{V}O_2$) per increase in work rate (ΔWR) during an exercise test in which work rate is increased linearly with time is related to the proportion of aerobic vs. anaerobic metabolism in the exercising muscles. A low $\Delta\dot{V}O_2/\Delta WR$ ratio means a greater proportion of anaerobic metabolism because of decreased oxygen availability to the exercising muscles [12–14]. This may be seen in those with heart or circulatory disorders, including pulmonary hypertension.

Lactic Acidosis Threshold and Sustained Exercise Capacity

The work rate at which there is a sustained appearance of blood lactate is important in assessing sustainable work capacity. During an incremental exercise test in a normal subject, lactic acid and lactate do not appear in the blood until the work rate exceeds some particular value for a subject doing that particular kind of work (e.g. leg cycling exercise). This lactate threshold, expressed as $\dot{V}O_2$, liters/min, is well below the peak $\dot{V}O_2$ in normals. Below this work rate, blood lactate is not different than at rest (<1–2 mEq/l); above this work rate, lactate is above this range and, if exercise at this level is continued, the lactate concentrations continues to rise. Lactate is the end product of anaerobic glycolysis, a metabolic pathway that produces energy from glucose or glycogen but requires no O_2. There is considerable evidence that the appearance of lactate during exercise indicates that an increasing proportion of energy production is produced from anaerobic metabolism in addition to energy produced from aerobic pathways, indicating that oxygen delivery to the exercising muscles is inadequate to meet fully the needs of oxidative metabolism [15–19]. Others have explained the appearance of lactate by other mechanisms, including decreased removal or metabolism of lactate or changes in the proportion of muscle fiber types participating in contraction. Regardless of the mechanism of physiologic mechanism of lactate appearance, the presence of increased blood lactate identifies a work rate above which sustained exercise cannot be performed. Below that work rate, a subject should be able to continue working at that rate indefinitely; above that work rate, the level of exercise cannot be sustained, and subjects are limited by progressive dyspnea or fatigue.

Clinically, patients with abnormally low capacity for oxygen delivery because of disorders of the lungs, heart, pulmonary or systemic circulation, or anemia during exercise develop lactate appearance at relatively low work rates, supporting the relationship between decreased oxygen delivery and likelihood of anaerobic metabolism. An estimate of the $\dot{V}O_2$ at which lactate appears in the blood can be made non-invasively by the finding of increasing amounts of CO_2 ($\dot{V}CO_2$) in the expired gas relative to the amount of oxygen taken up ($\dot{V}O_2$). The additional CO_2 is formed from reaction of lactic acid with bicarbonate, producing carbonic acid that dissociates into CO_2 and H_2O. In practice, this point can be found by either finding the point at which $\dot{V}CO_2$ increases more rapidly than $\dot{V}O_2$ during an incremental exercise test, or by identifying the point at which the additional CO_2 stimulates ventilation (increase in $\dot{V}_E$ and $\dot{V}_E/\dot{V}O_2$ relative to $\dot{V}_E/\dot{V}CO_2$) [20–22]. The $\dot{V}O_2$ where this occurs has been termed the anaerobic threshold or lactic acidosis threshold to distinguish this from the point at which blood lactate begins to accumulate.

Heart Rate Reserve and Breathing Reserve

In a subject with decreased peak $\dot{V}O_2$, the question of cardiac vs. respiratory limitation is frequently an issue. Heart rate reserve is the difference between predicted and actual maximum heart rate. A large heart rate reserve suggests that, at the time the subject stopped exercise, the limiting factor to further exercise was some organ system other than the heart. A large breathing reserve (maximum voluntary ventilation – maximum exercise $\dot{V}_E$) supports a limiting factor other than the ventilatory capacity. Not infrequently, both heart rate reserve and breathing reserve are high; in this situation, such things as peripheral vascular disease, myocardial ischemia, musculoskeletal disease, and lack of effort should be considered. A ventilatory limitation to exercise is also suggested when comparison to the maximum resting flow-volume loop for that patient is made [23, 24]. Both inspiratory and expiratory flows and tidal volume are superimposed onto the flow-volume loop; if they approach or reach the outer envelope, flow or ventilatory limitation is documented.

Pulmonary Gas Exchange and Efficiency of Ventilation

Pulmonary gas exchange efficiency and ventilation-perfusion mismatching are best assessed using arterial blood gases with calculation of alveolar-arterial PO_2 difference, arterial-end tidal PCO_2 difference, and dead space/tidal volume ratio. Arterial blood gases during exercise are among the most sensitive indicators of lung disease [25, 26], and these are likely to be earliest findings in patients with subtle or questionable interstitial lung disease or pulmonary vascular disease. Non-invasive measurements of ventilatory efficiency may be useful in those without arterial blood gases or as a screening tool. The ratio of minute ventilation to CO_2 output ($\dot{V}_E/\dot{V}CO_2$) in patients with congestive heart failure and pulmonary hypertension is an independent marker of severity of disease as well as correlating with other variables. Because $\dot{V}_E$ (BTPS)/$\dot{V}CO_2$ (STPD) is inversely proportional to alveolar PCO_2 and dead space/tidal volume ratio, a high ratio must mean either hyperventilation or high dead space/tidal volume ratio.

Physiologic Basis for Exercise Testing in Impairment Evaluation

Measurements that can be and usually are made during integrative cardiopulmonary exercise testing are shown in table 1, with each variable linked to specific questions about the function or dysfunction of an organ system. The potential features of integrative cardiopulmonary exercise testing that lend themselves particularly well to evaluation of impairment include: (1) objective measurement of maximum work capacity; (2) identification of the level of sustainable work rate; (3) clarification of cardiac compared to ventilatory limitation, and (4) high sensitivity for finding pulmonary gas exchange abnormalities compared to measurements made at rest.

In 1986, the American Thoracic Society statement on evaluation of impairment and disability secondary to

Table 2. American Thoracic Society (1986) recommendations for respiratory impairment

	FVC	FEV_1	FEV_1/FVC	DLCO
Normal	>80	>80	>75	>80
Mild	60–79	60–79	60–74	60–80
Moderate	50–59	40–59	40–59	40–59
Severe	<50	<40	<40	<40

Values are percentages of predicted value for each variable. FVC = Forced vital capacity; FEV_1 = forced expiratory volume in 1 s; DLCO = single-breath diffusing capacity for carbon monoxide. For impairment, any FVC, FEV_1, FEV_1/FVC, or DLCO in the mild, moderate, or severe impairment range defines the level of respiratory impairment.

respiratory disorders recommended a systematic evaluation process for the determination of impairment [3]. The statement was 'concerned primarily with impairments related to reduced lung function,' and presented a rating system for impairment from lung disease based on forced vital capacity (FVC), forced expiratory volume in 1 s (FEV_1), FEV_1/FVC, and single-breath diffusing capacity for carbon monoxide (DLCO) as shown in table 2. Thus, it was implied that there was a strong relationship between measurements made at rest (FEV_1 and DLCO) and measurements made during exercise (peak $\dot{V}O_2$ and work capacity). The authors concluded that the majority of subjects undergoing an evaluation for impairment would not require exercise testing, and resting pulmonary function provides sufficient information for accurate categorization of patients in terms of impairment.

It is important to review the basis for this conclusion and perhaps to consider if this recommendation is ideal for the population to be examined. First, can resting pulmonary function adequately predict peak $\dot{V}O_2$ and work capacity, especially in those with moderate decrease in lung function? Second, does an exercise test add to the accuracy of evaluation, notably in subjects for whom an exercise test might not otherwise be considered indicated?

Ventilatory Requirement during Exercise and Ventilatory Capacity

If exercise capacity is limited by shortness of breath, in most cases there is insufficient ventilatory capacity to meet the ventilatory requirement for the work being performed. The primary basis for potentially inaccurate prediction of maximum work capacity from resting pulmonary function (FEV_1) in patients with lung disease is that FEV_1 can only estimate ventilatory capacity but not ventilatory requirement. Ventilatory requirement is dependent on multiple variables as can be seen in the following formula relating minute ventilation ($\dot{V}_E$) to $\dot{V}O_2$:

$$\dot{V}_E = \dot{V}O_2 \times R \times 863/(PaCO_2 \times [1 - VD/VT])$$

where R is the gas exchange ratio (equal to the respiratory quotient in the steady-state), $PaCO_2$ is arterial partial pressure of CO_2, VD/VT is the dead-space/tidal volume ratio, and 863 adjusts for BTPS and STPD volumes and barometric pressure. If, on the cycle ergometer, there is a predictable relationship between $\dot{V}O_2$ and work rate (about 10 ml/min/W plus resting $\dot{V}O_2$ and $\dot{V}O_2$ of unloaded cycling) [10], then work rate can be substituted in this equation. However, rather than providing a prediction formula for exercise $\dot{V}_E$, this formula points out the pitfalls in trying to estimate how much ventilation an individual needs at a given work rate. Ventilatory requirement is inversely proportional to the efficiency of gas exchange (1 – VD/VT) and the ventilatory set point (PCO_2), and directly proportional to the gas exchange ratio and metabolic rate. The ventilatory set point is determined from a variety of factors, including genetic or familial chemosensitivity, metabolic acidosis or alkalosis, and degree of hypoxemia during exercise.

Ventilatory capacity (maximum exercise $\dot{V}_E$) is often predicted from FEV_1 [27, 28] or estimated from the maximum voluntary ventilation. The pattern of breathing (rate and tidal volume) varies between those with obstructive, interstitial restrictive, pleural restrictive, and other lung, heart, and chest wall disorders [24, 29]. Furthermore, inspiratory muscle fatigue is enhanced during exercise by hyperinflation, high airway resistance, and stiff lungs or chest wall; and fatigue during exercise cannot be anticipated from the FEV_1 determination.

Figure 1 incorporates estimates of ventilatory capacity superimposed on a range of ventilatory requirements (or demands) and demonstrates the range of peak $\dot{V}O_2$ (or work rate) that might be found for two hypothetical subjects having the same FEV_1. In this analysis, FEV_1 is used to predict maximum exercise minute ventilation ($\dot{V}_E$) by using two estimates of maximum minute ventilation from FEV_1 (7, 14). Panel a shows the two different maximum $\dot{V}_E$ values that would be predicted using 35 or 40 × FEV_1 = maximum $\dot{V}_E$. Next, in panel b, the dead space/tidal volume ratio (VD/VT) at maximum exercise ranges from about 0.12 to 0.30 at maximum exercise in normal subjects and may exceed 0.35 in those with ventilation-perfusion mismatching from lung disease. In this analysis, large

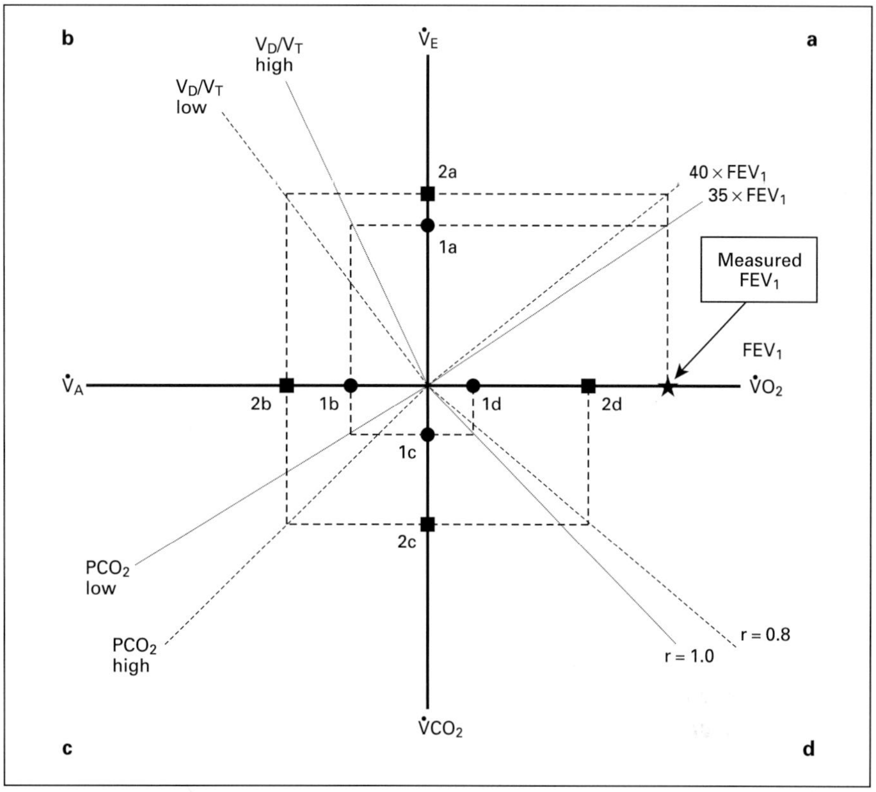

Fig. 1. Potential physiological basis for inaccuracy of predicting exercise capacity (maximum oxygen uptake, peak $\dot{V}O_2$) from lung function at rest (FEV_1) using a range of values to illustrate maximum differences. Maximum minute ventilation ($\dot{V}_E$) during exercise is assumed to be between 35 and 40 times FEV_1, so for a given FEV_1 (star), **a** shows the range of maximum $\dot{V}_E$ (1a and 2a). In **b**, for a range of dead space/tidal volume ratios (VD/VT), $\dot{V}_E$ can span a considerable range of alveolar ventilation ($\dot{V}_A$): points 1b and 2b. For a given alveolar ventilation, a greater CO_2 output ($\dot{V}CO_2$) can be eliminated at a higher than at a lower PCO_2 (1c and 2c). For different respiratory gas exchange ratios (R), a range of $\dot{V}O_2$ (1d–2d) for the different $\dot{V}CO_2$ is possible. Therefore, the same FEV_1 value in 2 different patients can be associated with a wide range of peak $\dot{V}O_2$ or work rates. This strongly suggests that maximum exercise capacity will be poorly predicted from FEV_1 alone. From Sue DY: Exercise testing in the evaluation of impairment and disability. Clin Chest Med 1994;15:369–387, with permission.

and small VD/VT values were chosen to illustrate the range of alveolar ventilation ($\dot{V}_E \times [1 - VD/VT]$) that may be seen. Considerable potential differences in $\dot{V}_A$ can be found. Although $\dot{V}_A$ is usually considered to determine PCO_2 at a given $\dot{V}CO_2$, in this example, the combination of $\dot{V}_A$ and PCO_2 values (high and low) shows the potential range of $\dot{V}CO_2$, (panel c). Finally, $\dot{V}O_2$ can be expressed as the quotient of $\dot{V}CO_2$ and R, the respiratory gas exchange ratio; the potential range of $\dot{V}O_2$ (and work rate) at maximum exercise can be determined (panel d). Therefore, the range of gas exchange disturbances in patients with lung disease has the potential of markedly dissociating any consistent relationship between FEV_1 and work capacity. In summary, this analysis shows that even if the ventilatory capacity of the respiratory system for ventilation is successfully predicted from resting FEV_1, the ventilatory requirement for a given level of work cannot be predicted from the FEV_1. Finally, although maximum exercise $\dot{V}_E$ is related to FEV_1 in most subjects, there are likely differences in this relationship between those with normal lung function, those with obstruction, patients with restrictive lung disease, and obese subjects [9, 10]. In summary, for resting pulmonary function to predict ideally exercise capacity, the requirements outlined in table 3 must be met.

Table 3. When is resting pulmonary function likely to predict exercise capacity?

Only when subjects or patients are ventilatory-limited during exercise
Metabolic rate increases in proportion to exercise work rate
Ventilatory requirement at a given metabolic rate is predictable ($\dot{V}_E/\dot{V}O_2$ or $\dot{V}_E/\dot{V}CO_2$)
Ventilatory response (CO_2 response) is predictable
Accurate measurement of pulmonary function at rest
Absence of cardiac disease (CHF, myocardial ischemia) during exercise

Can Exercise Performance Be Predicted Accurately from Resting Pulmonary Function?

Despite the physiological argument that anticipates inaccuracy in predicting exercise capacity from resting pulmonary function, clinical trials would be desirable to answer the question: Can resting lung function reliably estimate exercise performance?

Cotes et al. [30] tested the American Thoracic Society statement hypothesis [3] that exercise limitation could be predicted accurately from degree of lung function reduction, by using peak $\dot{V}O_2$ as the dependent variable in a stepwise multiple regression analysis to identify which variables significantly affected peak $\dot{V}O_2$, and how much of the variance (r^2) each of these variables could explain. A group of 157 men with a variety of suspected or known occupational lung disorders were studied, among whom there were diagnoses of coal workers' pneumoconiosis, silicosis, asbestosis, occupational asthma, and allergic alveolitis. All subjects had (1) FEV_1, FVC, or DLCO <80% of predicted, or FEV_1/FVC <75%; (2) limitation of exercise by dyspnea rather than chest pain, fatigue, or other reasons; (3) maximum $\dot{V}_E$ within 2 SD of the maximum $\dot{V}_E$ predicted from FEV_1. The latter criterion was meant to confirm that lack of breathing reserve was the essential cause of exercise termination; this would make it more likely that pulmonary function would predict exercise capacity. Results were expressed as fraction of total variance of peak $\dot{V}O_2$ (dependent variable) accounted for (r^2) by independent variables taken singly and stepwise. For single variables, variances were for FVC 15%, for FEV_1 20%, for FEV_1/FVC 8.4%, and for DLCO 25%. The combination of FEV_1 (or FVC and FEV_1/FVC) and DLCO could account for 29% of peak $\dot{V}O_2$ variance and 12–14% of peak $\dot{V}O_2$ expressed as % predicted. However, when FEV_1 (or FVC and FEV_1/FVC) was combined with exercise $\dot{V}_E$ (measured or extrapolated to the value at $\dot{V}O_2$ = 1 liter/min), these variables could account for 54% of the variance of peak $\dot{V}O_2$ and 44% of the variance in peak $\dot{V}O_2$, % predicted. The authors concluded that loss of exercise capacity was not accurately predicted from resting lung function indices alone, but the predictability of peak $\dot{V}O_2$ was enhanced by adding the result of $\dot{V}_E$ during submaximal exercise ($\dot{V}_E$ at $\dot{V}O_2$ = 1 liter/min). They commented that the assumption that a helpful and consistent relationship between resting pulmonary function and exercise capacity existed was based on a limited number of reports.

Using the ATS guidelines, Ortega et al. [31] also sought to determine the precision by which resting pulmonary function predicted exercise capacity, and especially how impairment and disability might be quantified. 78 stable men with chronic obstructive pulmonary disease (mean FEV_1 45%) were studied. Using ATS Guidelines to define severely impaired (FEV_1 <40% predicted, FVC <50% predicted, FEV_1/FVC <40%, or DLCO <40% predicted), 39 patients were classified in this category. Of these 39, peak $\dot{V}O_2$ in 23 (58.9%) was higher than 15 ml/kg/min; in 14 (35.9%), peak $\dot{V}O_2$ exceeded 60% of predicted. On the other hand, of the 39 who did not meet criteria for severe impairment, 8 (20.5%) had a peak $\dot{V}O_2$ <15 ml/kg/min and 13 (33.3%) had a peak $\dot{V}O_2$ <60% predicted. When their data are reported as likelihood ratios (LR), resting pulmonary function tests had an LR for peak $\dot{V}O_2$ <15 ml/kg/min of only 2.0 (sensitivity 41%, specificity 79.5%), the LR for peak $\dot{V}O_2$ <60% predicted was only 1.92 (sensitivity 64.1%, specificity 66.6%). There was a poor correlation of exercise capacity with FEV_1, FVC, lung volumes, and arterial blood gases at rest, with r^2 ranging from 0.05 to 0.28. The authors concluded that resting pulmonary function tests are not predictive of exercise performance in COPD, and that cardiopulmonary exercise testing is needed for accurate determination of impairment.

Other studies have had varied results in different lung disorders. In obstructive lung disease, Vyas et al. [32] found that in 14 patients with a mean FEV_1 of 29% of predicted, the peak $\dot{V}O_2$ could be predicted satisfactorily. The percentage of variance explained for peak $\dot{V}O_2$ was 78–82% using FEV_1 and VC. Pineda et al. [33] found that FEV_1 accounted for 56% of the variance in peak $\dot{V}O_2$. Jones et al. [34] found a correlation between work rate and severity of airway obstruction (r = 0.621) but this explained just 37% of the variance in work rate. Foglio et al. [35] examined the determinants of exercise performance in 105 patients with chronic airway obstruction. In the model they used, age was the major factor but residual volume and dyspnea scores explained the largest amount of the variance. Because the covariates together only accounted for 26–34% of the variance, they concluded that FEV_1 was an inconsistent predictor, and suggested the importance of performance evaluation in these patients.

Carlson et al. [36] reported that exercise tolerance in COPD patients was difficult to predict from measurements of lung function. In a group of 119 patients with a mean FEV_1 = 1.41 ± 0.64 liters, stepwise linear regression yielded a prediction formula for peak $\dot{V}O_2$ that had an r = 0.90 using DLCO, MVV, peak exercise VD/VT, and resting $\dot{V}_E$. This formula, although it could account for 81% of the variance, had two important limitations. This formula used exercise VD/VT, thereby including a variable measured during exercise to predict exercise capacity. Using only resting pulmonary function, the multiple regression had an r^2 = 74%. In addition, the 95% confidence limit for a given individual patient averaged about 36% of the mean peak $\dot{V}O_2$ (0.233 liters/min with mean peak $\dot{V}O_2$ = 1.25 ± 0.50 liters/min).

Exertional dyspnea was the most frequent reason for stopping exercise in patients with interstitial lung disease as reported by Rampulla et al. [37], being found in 62%. These patients were severely limited with a mean peak $\dot{V}O_2$ of 15.1 ml/kg/min. The severity of dyspnea correlated with peak $\dot{V}O_2$ but dyspnea in individual subjects was not well predicted from resting lung function. However, in 20 men with pulmonary fibrosis reported by Spiro et al. [38], the mean peak $\dot{V}O_2$ of 1.4 liters/min correlated well with resting FEV_1, VC, and TLC. The report of Hansen and Wasserman [39] also compared resting FEV_1 % predicted, TLC % predicted, DLCO % predicted, and resting PaO_2 with peak $\dot{V}O_2$ % predicted in 42 patients with interstitial lung disease and no other limiting factors. Predicted values were used to standardize patients of different gender, age, and size. The correlation coefficients (r) and % variance explained (r^2) were, for FEV_1 r = 0.498, 24.8%, for TLC 0.574, 32.9%, DLCO 0.764, 58.3%, and resting PaO_2 0.570, 32.5%. The authors concluded that ventilatory mechanics did not limit exercise capacity in the majority of patients with interstitial lung disease. In several studies, Marciniuk et al. [23, 40] provided more evidence that mechanical ventilatory limitation did not determine maximal exercise performance in interstitial lung disease, but arterial hypoxemia might contribute greatly. First, patients with interstitial lung disease did not usually reach the maximal flow-volume envelope at the end of exercise, suggesting that ventilatory reserve was present [23]. Second, supplemental oxygen breathing significantly increased exercise performance in 7 patients with interstitial disease [40]. The latter group had a mean peak $\dot{V}O_2$ of only 56 ± 13% predicted, but oxygen breathing led to a significant increase in peak minute ventilation, work rate, exercise duration, and peak $\dot{V}O_2$ (1.25 ± 0.21 liters/min vs. 1.39 ± 0.26 liters/min).

Correlation with peak $\dot{V}O_2$ has not been the only relationship sought. Non-invasive measurements have been used to identify patients with abnormal exercise arterial blood gases, but sensitivity is poor. For example, in 276 current or former shipyard workers, the predictive ability of DLCO to find abnormal arterial blood gases was examined [25]. Abnormal exercise blood gases were defined as $P(A\text{-}a)O_2 > 35$ mm Hg, arterial-end tidal PCO_2 difference ($P[a\text{-}ET]CO_2$) > 0 mm Hg, or VD/VT >0.30 at maximum exercise. A DLCO <80% predicted had only 22% sensitivity although 96% specificity (likelihood ratio = 5.5); the 95% confidence limit for normal DLCO was even less sensitive. 53 patients with idiopathic pulmonary fibrosis described by Keogh et al. [41] had arterial $PaO_2 > 80$ mm Hg at rest, but decreased PaO_2 and increased $P(A\text{-}a)O_2$ during exercise. These authors concluded that exercise-induced hypoxemia was best demonstrated during an exercise test because it was not predictable from resting PaO_2. Hansen and Wasserman found that DLCO predicted exercise limitation better than either lung volumes or FEV_1 [39] in 42 patients with interstitial lung disease.

Asbestosis and other occupational lung diseases may behave differently than other interstitial lung diseases such as idiopathic pulmonary fibrosis. One group [42] studied 9 age-matched patients with each disorder with comparable peak $\dot{V}O_2$ (pulmonary fibrosis 1.09 ± 0.27 liters/min; asbestosis 1.07 ± 0.37 liters/min). Resting lung function was similar. Among the pulmonary fibrosis group, arterial PO_2 fell more, $P(A\text{-}a)O_2$ was larger, and VD/VT was greater during exercise than those with asbestosis. In contrast, asbestosis patients and those with cryptogenic fibrosing alveolitis matched for comparable degrees of exercise-induced desaturation and peak $\dot{V}O_2$ (1.3–1.5 liters/min) had similar resting lung function, DLCO, and severity of chest X-ray abnormality scores [43]. Dyspnea scores correlated with exercise performance in 153 workers exposed to silica dust and 62 patients with silicosis in a study by Wang et al. [44], but a considerable proportion (30–56%) of each group reported more severe dyspnea by questionnaire than was verified during exercise testing. They concluded that objective physiological measures like exercise testing may be of value in dyspneic silica exposed subjects. Another confounding factor after asbestos exposure may be the influence of pleural thickening or plaques. In a study of 90 subjects with asbestos exposure for at least 1 year and more than 20 years since first exposure, asbestosis was defined as ILO profusion of 1/0 or greater [45]. Among those without parenchymal involvement, diffuse pleural thickening was associated with lower maximal work capacity, and more severe increase in $P(A\text{-}a)O_2$ and VD/VT at maximum exercise. The authors hypothesized that subtle asbestos-induced parenchymal disease was present.

Impairment from Nonventilatory Limitation during Exercise

One of the major potential reasons why resting pulmonary function may not be highly predictive of exercise performance is nonventilatory limitation during exercise. The best correlation of pulmonary function and exercise capacity will be seen in those who are limited by dyspnea from lung disease rather than fatigue, chest pain, musculoskeletal disorders, or exercise-induced asthma or heart failure. Rampulla et al. [37] found that of 66 consecutive patients with chronic lung disease (COPD and interstitial lung disease), only 42% stopped exercise due to dyspnea while others stopped because of fatigue (41%), cardiac limitation (12%), and other reasons. In our study of exercise testing in impairment evaluation [46], 138 had abnormally low exercise capacity, yet only 18% of these were limited by obstructive or restrictive lung disease, while 69% had a cardiovascular cause of exercise limitation. These subjects' exercise capacities would have been poorly estimated from FEV_1, VC, or DLCO. Of the 42 patients with interstitial lung disease reported by Hansen and Wasserman [39], peak $\dot{V}O_2$ correlated much better with measurements of circulatory status, such as the lactic acidosis threshold, the oxygen-pulse extrapolated to predicted heart rate, and the ratio of $\dot{V}O_2$ to work rate, than with ventilatory or gas exchange variables. Because the severity of circulatory dysfunction correlated with the severity of lung impairment (loss of lung volume, abnormal gas transfer index, and dead space/tidal volume ratio), the pulmonary circulation was implicated in these patients rather than the heart or systemic circulation. Neder et al. [47] recently reported predictive values for exercise testing in normal subjects, using a randomly selected sample of 120 sedentary individuals from a pool of more than 8,000 subjects. Although the intent of the study was to establish another set of normal predictive values, their data provide evidence for potential success of predicting cardiovascular and ventilatory variables from resting data. For example, peak $\dot{V}O_2$ was fairly well predicted from age, size, activity score, and leisure time score, with coefficients explaining 70–90% of the variance. But ventilatory variables were much less predictable. Predicted maximum $\dot{V}_E$ when gender, age, and size were included as variables had r^2 values of only 0.379 (men) and 0.536 (women). There were similar r^2 values for $\dot{V}_E$/MVV, respiratory frequency, and tidal volume, as well as for heart rate and lactic acidosis threshold.

In summary, there is a limited physiological basis for predicting exercise capacity from resting pulmonary function in patients with lung disease, and non-ventilatory limitation is even harder to predict. Evidence supporting this concept comes from a number of studies demonstrating the poor predictive value of such variables as FVC, FEV_1, and DLCO. These results show, not surprisingly, that accurate determination of exercise capacity is best performed by actually performing an exercise test.

Cardiopulmonary Exercise Testing in the Assessment of Impairment and Disability

Cardiopulmonary exercise testing in impairment evaluation has been called 'difficult to perform, more expensive, and sometimes more invasive than conventional tests.' [2]. However, a number of studies emphasize the usefulness of cardiopulmonary exercise testing for determination of impairment and disability specifically from occupational exposure [30, 42, 43, 46, 48, 50–53]. An appropriate perspective, it can be argued from these studies, is that exercise testing complements clinical evaluation, improves the accuracy of resting pulmonary function, and supplements roentgenographic studies. Exercise testing adds to diagnostic accuracy, both quantitatively (measurement of work capacity, peak $\dot{V}O_2$, and sustained work capacity) and qualitatively (identification of the cause of exercise limitation).

Exercise Testing and Decision Making on Impairment

We [46] had the opportunity to perform exercise studies and obtain clinical information on 348 current or former shipyard workers, all men, who complained of exercise limitation but whose FEV_1 was at least 40% predicted and FEV_1/VC more than 40%, and had no obvious cardiac dysfunction. In this retrospective analysis, we compared the consultant's conclusion about impairment and cause of impairment based on chest radiographs, pulmonary function tests, resting electrocardiogram, and clinical information with the conclusion reached with the aid of the cardiopulmonary exercise test data. Normal work capacity (no impairment) was defined as being within the 95% confidence limit for normal peak $\dot{V}O_2$ [10, 54]. Interpretation of exercise tests was standardized for cardiovascular limitation, ventilatory limitation, and noncirculatory, nonrespiratory disorders, including poor effort and musculoskeletal problems [46].

Non-exercise evaluations led to the conclusion that 148 subjects would have normal work capacity, but 46 of these (31%) had a peak $\dot{V}O_2$ below the 95% confidence limit. On the other hand, 66 men were predicted to have low work capacity, but of these, only 43 (67%) were correctly categorized. Among those whose exercise capacity could not be estimated, 60% had normal peak $\dot{V}O_2$ and 37% were abnormally low. Thus, the sensitivity of non-exercise data was 31% for impairment, with a specificity of 49%. The non-exercise test information had a positive predictive value for impairment of 65% for this population; the corresponding negative predictive value was 69%. It should be noted that impairment in this study was defined as an abnormal peak $\dot{V}O_2$, the usual clinical definition, rather than in terms of functional capacity or exercise reserve. Resting pulmonary function tests had low sensitivity for predicting abnormal exercise arterial blood gases. For example, single-breath diffusion capacity for carbon monoxide (abnormal <80% predicted), had a sensitivity of 45% and specificity of 91% for abnormal exercise alveolar-arterial PO_2 difference (>35 mm Hg). For predicting abnormal dead space/tidal volume ratio (>0.30 at maximum exercise), diffusing capacity for carbon monoxide had 18% sensitivity and 94% specificity.

The cause of exercise limitation should have a major effect on the ability to predict impairment because only pulmonary function (and clinical features suggesting severe limitation) should be particularly helpful. Furthermore, as in other studies [37, 39], nonventilatory causes of limitation are likely to be common in this patient population. Only 25 of 138 with impairment were limited by obstructive or restrictive lung disease, while 69% (95/138) had a cardiovascular cause of exercise limitation. These data are similar to those of Agostoni et al. [48] who found that 37% of 120 former asbestos workers had cardiac limitation rather than ventilatory limitation.

In a further retrospective analysis of these data, we matched smoking and never-smoking shipyard workers by age and duration of asbestos exposure [52]. Smokers had significantly lower VC, FEV_1, FEV_1/VC, and DLCO than nonsmokers, and smokers more frequently had lower peak $\dot{V}O_2$ and O_2 pulse and more often had an abnormally increased maximum exercise $P(A-a)O_2$. Specifically, 45% (33/73) of smokers had a peak $\dot{V}O_2$ less than 80% of predicted compared to only 20.5% (15/73) of nonsmokers. Smokers were more likely to have impairment caused by heart disease (49%), poor effort (21%) or musculoskeletal causes (12%) than by airway obstruction (6%).

Exercise Testing and Quantitation of Impairment

The 1986 ATS Statement [3] concluded that degree of impairment could be classified from resting lung function as normal, mildly impaired, moderately impaired, or severely impaired (table 2) in those with lung disease. If exercise testing were added, then useful stratification could be achieved on the basis of peak $\dot{V}O_2$, expressed as ml/kg/min. It was estimated that office work required about 5–7 ml/kg/min, moderate labor about 15 ml/kg/min, and strenuous labor 20–30 ml/kg/min. For manual labor at a comfortable working place, a work rate at approximately 40% of peak $\dot{V}O_2$ was chosen. Interestingly, this is similar to the sustainable work rate level in normal subjects as estimated by the lactic acidosis threshold.

A report of a working group of the European Society for Clinical Respiratory Physiology [55] decided that equating the degree of respiratory impairment from pulmonary function tests with the degree of reduced exercise capacity was not ideal. They noted also that the World Health Organization definition of respiratory disability required assessment of both losses of lung function from pulmonary function tests and information about exercise performance [6]. Except for those with severe respiratory impairment (resting pulmonary function), the working group recommended assessing exercise capacity from symptom-limited exercise testing, with measurement or estimation of peak $\dot{V}O_2$. They proposed a scale of percentage 'respiratory disability' with a score ranging from 0 to 100%, referring to the estimated loss of function as determined from exercise testing. The peak $\dot{V}O_2$ at the lower limit of the 95% CI was chosen as the point of 0% disability (using 1.64 SD below the mean predicted value). For 100% disability, the group chose a peak $\dot{V}O_2$ of 0.5 liters/min or about twice the resting $\dot{V}O_2$ for normal subjects (a very severely limited exercise capacity corresponding to only a few walking steps at a time). They presented data from 157 men with respiratory impairment (using ATS pulmonary function criteria) and found that 28% had no impairment from exercise testing by their calculation; 38% had 1–19% respiratory disability; 11% had severe disability (60–79% respiratory disability); and 1% had 100% respiratory disability.

Cotes et al. [56] subsequently compared this method with an established empirical rating for total cardiorespiratory disability derived from clinical information, chest radiograph, and FEV_1 and FVC. Sixty-two former coal miners, asbestos workers, or others with potential occupational lung disorders were studied. Disability scores (%) were calculated using measured peak $\dot{V}O_2$ and peak $\dot{V}O_2$ estimated from age, $\dot{V}O_2$ at 1 liter/min, and FEV_1 [55]. The two scores correlated well with each other ($r = 0.72$), and both correlated reasonably with the empirical rating ($r = 0.51$). However, addition of radiographic evidence of progressive massive fibrosis, FEV_1, and clinical grade of breathlessness further reduced variance ($r^2 = 0.49$) between the new rating system and the empirical disability score. Furthermore, in subjects with a discrepancy between the estimated and measured peak $\dot{V}O_2$, information from the exercise test helped explained the difference.

Recently, Neder et al. [57] proposed expressing disability using what they termed loss of aerobic capacity ($\dot{V}O_2$, % predicted) rather than remaining capacity (peak $\dot{V}O_2$ ml/kg/min), in contrast with some of the ATS recommen-

Table 4. Relative value of resting and exercise testing for impairment evaluation

	Resting studies	Cardiopulmonary exercise
Is ventilatory capacity during exercise reduced?	++	+++
Is maximum work capacity reduced?	++ (if ventilatory-limited)	++++
What is the physiological basis for reduced work capacity?	+	+++
Are there subtle pulmonary gas exchange abnormalities present?	+	++++
Does cardiac function limit exercise?	++ (if severely reduced)	+++

Table 5. Suggested strategy for using cardiopulmonary exercise testing in impairment evaluation

Subject or patient	Cardiopulmonary exercise test suggested
Asymptomatic, no exertional dyspnea or exercise intolerance	disproportionate complaints about work-related exercise intolerance concern about subtle pulmonary gas exchange abnormalities that may relate to an occupational exposure
Mild respiratory impairment	
Mild-to-moderate respiratory impairment	above reasons symptoms inconsistent with degree of impairment defined by resting pulmonary function testing
Moderate respiratory impairment	above reasons resting tests may have underestimated the degree of impairment because of pulmonary vascular involvement, unsuspected coexisting disease, or inability to estimate ventilatory requirement for exercise
Severe respiratory impairment	usually none, but may be useful in some subjects in whom impairment is overestimated
Any	accurate determination of exercise capacity is desired need for apportioning cause of impairment

dations. They reasoned that considerable loss of capacity could be sustained in a young, non-obese individual with a high predicted normal peak $\dot{V}O_2$, but even then that individual may have only mild or no impairment by peak $\dot{V}O_2$, ml/kg/min. On the other hand, an older, obese subject may have only a small decrease in peak $\dot{V}O_2$, % predicted, but have severe impairment by peak $\dot{V}O_2$, ml/kg/min (e.g. <15 ml/kg/min). The authors reviewed data from 75 subjects with silica exposure. Only 19 (25.3%) had a peak $\dot{V}O_2$ >25 ml/kg/min (normal by ATS criteria) but 53.3% of the same 75 subjects had a peak $\dot{V}O_2$ >70% of predicted (defined as normal). Out of 56 subjects with impairment defined by the ATS exercise criteria (peak $\dot{V}O_2$ <25 ml/kg/min), 21 had no impairment using the peak $\dot{V}O_2$, % predicted. As hypothesized, older subjects and those who were overweight were more likely to be discordant. The authors concluded that in evaluation of impairment, comparison to predicted peak $\dot{V}O_2$ was more useful than using the recommendation of peak $\dot{V}O_2$, ml/kg/min.

Recommendations for Exercise Testing in Impairment and Disability Evaluation

Although there are no absolute indications for the addition of exercise testing to medical history, physical examination, resting pulmonary function tests, and chest roentgenogram for assessment of respiratory impairment, certain guidelines appear to be justifiable. These are summarized in tables 4 and 5. Exercise testing is not indicated in those who lack complaints of exercise dyspnea, fatigue, or intolerance. Those with clearly severe respiratory impairment, such as those who meet the ATS criteria for impairment by FEV_1 or DLCO, also do not require exercise testing.

Cardiopulmonary exercise testing is indicated when accurate measurement of work capacity is desired or when symptoms or exercise intolerance are inconsistent with clinical findings and resting tests. There is strong evidence that evaluation and quantitation of impairment is enhanced by use of exercise testing, notably because of the lack of success of resting pulmonary function tests to predict exercise capacity, and we and others have found that both over- and underestimation of work capacity is found in subjects being assessed for impairment. In addition, exercise arterial blood gases, especially with calculation of alveolar-arterial PO_2 difference and dead space/tidal volume ratio, are very sensitive tests of subtle lung disease. In some patients, exercise testing is useful for diagnosis as well as measurement of impairment. This is especially true in those with co-existing disorders or unsuspected cardiovascular or pulmonary vascular disorders. In summary, cardiopulmonary exercise testing provides objective determination of exercise capacity, increased sensitivity for pulmonary gas exchange abnormalities, and the ability to identify unsuspected or unanticipated non-pulmonary causes of impairment.

References

1 Sood A, Beckett WS: Determination of disability for patients with advanced lung diseases. Clin Chest Med 1997;18:471–482.
2 American Medical Association; in Cocchiarella L, Andersson GBJ (eds): Guides to the Evaluation of Permanent Impairment, ed 5. Chicago, AMA Press, 2001.
3 American Thoracic Society: Evaluation of impairment/disability secondary to respiratory disorders. Am Rev Respir Dis 1986;133:1205–1209.
4 Cotes JE, Reed JW, Elliott C: Breathing and exercise requirements of the work place; in Whipp BJ, Wasserman K (eds): Exercise: Pulmonary Physiology and Pathophysiology. New York, Marcel Dekker, 1991, p 495.
5 Hansen JE, Wasserman K: Disability evaluation; in Murray JF, Nadel JA (eds): Textbook of Respiratory Medicine, ed 1. Philadelphia, Saunders, 1988, p 699.
6 World Health Organization: International Classification of Impairments, Disabilities, and Handicaps. Geneva, World Health Organization, 1980.
7 Harber P, Fedoruk MJ: Work placement and worker fitness: Implications of the Americans with disabilities act for pulmonary medicine. Chest 1994;105:1564–1571.
8 Sue DY, Wasserman K: Impact of integrative cardiopulmonary exercise testing on clinical decision making. Chest 1991;99:981–992.
9 Wasserman K, Whipp BJ: Exercise physiology in health and disease. Am Rev Respir Dis 112: 219–249.
10 Wasserman K, Hansen JE, Sue DY, Casaburi R, Whipp BJ: Principles of Exercise Testing and Interpretation, ed 3. Baltimore, Lippincott Williams & Wilkins, 1999.
11 Weber KT, Janicki JS (eds): Cardiopulmonary Exercise Testing: Physiologic Principles and Clinical Applications. Philadelphia, Saunders, 1986.
12 Hansen JE, Sue DY, Oren A, Wasserman K: Relation of oxygen uptake to work rate in normal men and men with circulatory disorders. Am J Cardiol 1987;59:669–674.
13 Hansen JE, Casaburi R, Cooper DM, Wasserman K: Oxygen uptake as related to work rate increment during cycle ergometer exercise. Eur J Appl Physiol 1988;57:140–145.
14 Koike A, Hiroe M, Adachi H, Yajima T, Itoh H, Takamoto T, Taniguchi K, Marumo F: Cardiac output-O_2 uptake relation during incremental exercise in patients with previous myocardial infarction. Circulation 1992;85:1713–1719.
15 Beaver WL, Wasserman K: Muscle RQ and lactate accumulation from analysis of the $\dot{V}CO_2$-$\dot{V}O_2$ relationship during exercise. Clin J Sports Med 1991;1:27.
16 Koike A, Weiler-Ravell D, McKenzie DK, Zanconato S, Wasserman K: Evidence that the metabolic acidosis threshold is the anaerobic threshold. J Appl Physiol 1990;68:2521–2526.
17 Wasserman K: The anaerobic threshold to evaluate exercise performance. Am Rev Respir Dis 1984;129(suppl):S35–S40.
18 Wasserman K, Beaver WL, Whipp BJ: Gas exchange theory and the lactic acidosis (anaerobic) threshold. Circulation 1990;81(suppl II): 14–30.
19 Wasserman K, Koike A: Is the anaerobic threshold truly anaerobic? Chest 1992;101 (suppl):211S–218S.
20 Beaver WL, Wasserman K, Whipp BJ: A new method for detecting the anaerobic threshold by gas exchange. J Appl Physiol 1986;60:2020–2027.
21 Dickstein K, Barvik S, Aarsland T, Snapinn S, Karlsson J: A comparison of methodologies in detection of the anaerobic threshold. Circulation 1990;81(suppl II):38–46.
22 Sue DY, Wasserman K, Moricca RB, Casaburi R: Metabolic acidosis during exercise in chronic obstructive pulmonary disease. Chest 1988;94:931–938.
23 Marciniuk DD, Sridhar G, Clemens RE, Zintel TA, Gallagher CG: Lung volumes and expiratory flow limitation during exercise in interstitial lung disease. J Appl Physiol 1994;77:963–973.
24 Gallagher CG: Exercise limitation and clinical exercise testing in chronic obstructive pulmonary disease. Clin Chest Med 1994;15:305–326.
25 Sue DY, Oren A, Hansen JE, Wasserman K: Single-breath diffusing capacity for carbon monoxide as a predictor of exercise gas exchange. New Engl J Med 1987;316:1301–1306.
26 Wagner PD: Ventilation-perfusion matching during exercise. Chest 101;(suppl):192S–198S.
27 Campbell SC: A comparison of the maximum voluntary ventilation with forced expiratory volume in one second: An assessment of subject cooperation. J Occup Med 1982;24:531–533.
28 Gandevia B, Hugh-Jones P: Terminology for measurements of ventilatory capacity. Thorax 1957;1:290–293.
29 Marciniuk DD, Gallagher CG: Clinical exercise testing in interstitial lung disease. Clin Chest Med 1994;15:287–304.
30 Cotes JE, Zejda J, King B: Lung function impairment as a guide to exercise limitation in work-related lung disorders. Am Rev Respir Dis 1988;137:1089–1093.
31 Ortega F, Montemayor T, Sanchez A, Cabello F, Castillo J: Role of cardiopulmonary exercise testing and the criteria used to determine disability in patients with severe chronic obstructive pulmonary disease. Am J Respir Crit Care Med 1994;150:747–751.
32 Vyas MN, Banister EW, Morton JW, Grzybowski S: Response to exercise in patients with chronic airway obstruction. II. Effects of breathing 40% oxygen. Am Rev Respir Dis. 1971;103:401–412.
33 Pineda H, Haas F, Axe K, Haas A: Accuracy of pulmonary function tests in predicting exercise tolerance in chronic obstructive pulmonary disease. Chest 1984;86:564–567.
34 Jones NL, Jones G, Edwards RHT: Exercise tolerance in chronic airway obstruction. Am Rev Respir Dis 1971;103:477–491.
35 Foglio K, Carone M, Pagani M, Bianchi L, Jones PW, Ambrosino N: Physiological and symptom determinants of exercise performance in patients with chronic airway obstruction. Respir Med 2000;94:256–263.
36 Carlson DJ, Ries AL, Kaplan RM: Prediction of maximum exercise tolerance in patients with COPD. Chest 1991;100:307–311.
37 Rampulla C, Baiocchi S, Dacosto E, Ambrosino N: Dyspnea on exercise. Pathophysiologic mechanisms. Chest 1992;101(suppl):248S–252S.
38 Spiro SG, Dowdeswell IRG, Clark TJH: An analysis of submaximal exercise responses in patients with sarcoidosis and fibrosing alveolitis. Br J Dis Chest 1981;75:169–180.
39 Hansen JE, Wasserman K: Pathophysiology of activity limitation in patients with interstitial lung disease. Chest 1996;109:1566–1576.

40 Harris-Eze AO, Sridhar G, Clemson RE, Zintel TA, Gallagher CG, Marciniuk DD: Role of hypoxemia and pulmonary mechanics in exercise limitation in interstitial lung disease. Am J Respir Crit Care Med 1996;154:994–1001.
41 Keogh BA, Lakatos E, Price D, Crystal RG: Importance of the lower respiratory tract in oxygen transfer: Exercise testing in patients with interstitial and destructive lung disease. Am Rev Respir Dis 1984;129(2 Pt 2):S76–80.
42 Agusti AGN, Roca J, Rodriguez-Roisin R, Xaubet A, Agusti-Vidal A: Different patterns of gas exchange response to exercise in asbestos and idiopathic pulmonary fibrosis. Eur Respir J 1988;1:510–516.
43 Markos J, Musk AW, Finucane KE: Functional similarities of asbestosis and cryptogenic fibrosing alveolitis. Thorax 1988;43:708–714.
44 Wang XR, Araki S, Yano E, Wang MZ, Wang ZM: Dyspnea and exercise testing in workers exposed to silica. Indust Health 1995;33:163–171.
45 Shih JF, Wilson JS, Broderick A, Watt JL, Galvin JR, Merchant JA, Schwartz DA: Asbestos-induced pleural fibrosis and impaired exercise physiology. Chest 1994;105:1370–1376.
46 Oren A, Sue DY, Hansen JE, Torrance DJ, Wasserman K: The role of exercise testing in impairment evaluation. Am Rev Respir Dis 1987;135:230–235.
47 Neder JA, Nery LE, Castelo A, Andreoni S, Lerario MC, Sachs A, Silva AC, Whipp BJ: Prediction of metabolic and cardiopulmonary responses to maximum cycle ergometry: A randomised study. Eur Respir J 1999;14:1304–1313.
48 Agostoni P, Smith DD, Schoene RB, Robertson HT, Butler J: Evaluation of breathlessness in asbestos workers. Results of exercise testing. Am Rev Respir Dis 1987;135:812–816.
49 Howard J, Mohsenifar Z, Brown HV, Koerner SK: Role of exercise testing in assessing functional respiratory impairment due to asbestos exposure. J Occup Med 1982;24:685–689.
50 Pearle J: Exercise performance and functional impairment in asbestos-exposed workers. Chest 1981;80:701–705.
51 Risk C, Epler GR, Gaensler EA: Exercise alveolar-arterial oxygen pressure difference in interstitial lung disease. Chest 1984;85:69–74.
52 Sue DY, Oren A, Hansen JE, Wasserman K: Lung function and exercise performance in smoking and nonsmoking asbestos-exposed workers. Am Rev Respir Dis 1985;132:612–618.
53 Wiedemann HP, Gee JBL, Balmes JR, Loke J: Exercise testing in occupational lung disease. Clin Chest Med 1984;5:157–171.
54 Hansen JE, Sue DY, Wasserman K: Predicted values for clinical exercise testing. Am Rev Respir Dis 1984;129:S49–S55.
55 Cotes JE: Rating respiratory disability: A report on behalf of a working group of the European society for clinical respiratory physiology. Eur Respir J 1990;3:1074–1077.
56 Cotes JE, Chinn DJ, Reed JW, Hutchinson JE: Experience of a standardised method for assessing respiratory disability. Eur Respir J 1994;7:1074–1076.
57 Neder JA, Nery LE, Bagatin E, Lucas SR, Ancao MS, Sue DY: Differences between remaining ability and loss of capacity in maximum aerobic impairment. Brazil J Med Biol Research 1998;31:639–646.

Darryl Y. Sue, MD
Department of Medicine
Harbor-UCLA Medical Center
Box 400, 1000 W. Carson St.
Torrance, CA 90509-2910 (USA)
Tel. +1 310 222 2401, Fax +1 310 320 9688
E-Mail sue@humc.edu

Weisman IM, Zeballos RJ (eds): Clinical Exercise Testing.
Prog Respir Res. Basel, Karger, 2002, vol 32, pp 231–241

Role of Cardiopulmonary Exercise Testing in the Preoperative Evaluation for Lung Resection

A.H. Diacon C.T. Bolliger

Lung Unit, Department of Internal Medicine, University of Stellenbosch, Tygerberg, Cape Town, South Africa

Summary

To date, the majority of lung resection candidates in industrialized nations suffer from lung cancer. Most of them are former or current smokers and therefore at risk for chronic obstructive lung disease (COPD) and coronary artery disease (CAD), conditions associated with increased surgical mortality and morbidity. On the other hand, lung cancer mortality approaches 100% when not treated surgically, and postoperative complications can, therefore, almost always be accepted unless they are fatal. Although the assessment before lung resection has been studied over many years, no single or combined parameter has been shown to sufficiently predict the surgical outcome. In recent years, cardiopulmonary exercise testing (CPET) is increasingly used to assess the surgical risk. Moreover, CPET in combination with split function studies is used to predict postoperative exercise capacity. Many candidates for lung resection, however, can be operated without complex testing like CPET and split function studies, which are not universally available and costly. Patients with normal or only slightly impaired pulmonary function and no cardiovascular risk factors tolerate pulmonary resections up to a pneumonectomy without any problems, and exercise testing is not indicated in these cases. Candidates for lung resection with abnormal cardiopulmonary function should be further evaluated with CPET and split function studies according to a predefined protocol, and the individual risk assessed in respect to the planned extent of resection. Typically, exercise capacity after lobectomy is only slightly reduced, or not at all. Pneumonectomy leads to a loss of approximately 20% in exercise capacity. In this chapter, we outline the principles and current recommendations in the assessment of the lung resection candidate, with special emphasis on the role of CPET.

Introduction

Some decades ago, the majority of patients undergoing lung surgery were suffering from the sequelae of tuberculosis. With the advent of effective antituberculous drugs and the dramatic increase in the incidence of lung cancer worldwide, the majority of today's lung resection candidates suffer from lung cancer, for whom surgery is the only curative form of treatment. Fortunately, advances in surgical techniques and postoperative care have made lung resections accessible for older patients and those with limited cardiopulmonary reserves. Though a limited surgical mortality may be acceptable in a disease with close to 100% mortality in itself, appropriate patient selection and risk management have consequently become a core issue in lung cancer surgery.

The ideal parameter for the evaluation of the surgical risk in lung resection would be technically simple, inex-

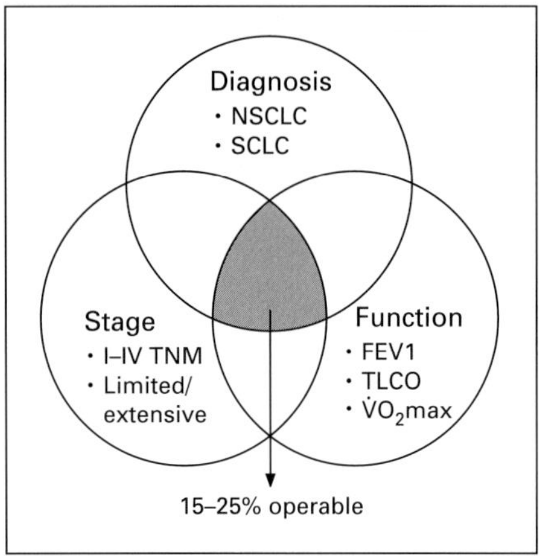

Fig. 1. Management of lung cancer. The circles represent the three entities that determine the management of a patient with lung cancer NSCLC = Non-small cell lung cancer; SCSL = small cell lung cancer; FEV_1 = forced expiratory volume in the 1st second; TLCO = transfer factor for lung carbon monoxide; VO_2max = maximal oxygen consumption. With permission from Bolliger [72].

pensive, highly reproducible and universally available. Many a parameter has been considered for the selection of patients for lung surgery. The use of vital capacity for the prediction of the surgical risk was reported as early as in 1955 [1]. Subsequently, various factors derived from history and symptoms, lung function, pulmonary hemodynamics and radiological imaging have been proposed. While invasive hemodynamic parameters are currently considered obsolete for classical lung resection surgery, none of the other single parameters has shown a satisfactory predictive value for the outcome after lung resection.

Cardiopulmonary exercise testing (CPET), in contrast, comprehends many specific physiologic factors in one test. CPET evaluates directly the cardiopulmonary reserves and imitates the stress of undergoing surgery to a certain extent. In recent years, CPET was extensively studied and generally accepted for the prediction of perioperative risk and the long term postoperative outcome after lung resection. However, most lung resection candidates with normal or only slightly impaired lung function and good general condition can be resected safely without CPET, which is not universally available and costly. Therefore, a stepwise approach to the functional assessment of the lung resection candidate is practical and various combinations of CPET with other parameters are recommended. Beginning with simple clinical parameters, basic pulmonary function testing (PFT), including measurement of transfer factor of the lung for carbon monoxide (TLCO), patients at risk for complications can be identified and further investigated with CPET and, if necessary, split function studies for the estimation of predicted postoperative (ppo) values. This evaluation process can be incorporated into a comprehensive algorithm in order to facilitate decision making and avoid unnecessary testing.

In this chapter, we discuss the single steps of the functional evaluation of the lung resection candidate with emphasis on the role of CPET. In addition, we present a validated practical algorithm for the functional assessment of the lung resection candidate.

Evaluation of Lung Resection Candidates

General Approach to the Lung Resection Candidate

Most lung resection candidates today are lung cancer patients. In this condition, the initial three steps are assessment of tumor type, tumor stage and operability (fig. 1). Some definitions of the terms used in this chapter are briefly summarised below:

Tumor type refers mainly to the discrimination of small-cell lung cancer (SCLC) versus non-small-cell lung cancer (NSCLC). Only the latter is usually treated with lung resection. In SCLC, the mainstay of therapy is chemo- and radiotherapy.

Tumor staging of NSCLC according to the TNM system takes the extent of the tumor into account. In lung cancer patients, resectability is compulsory for curative surgery. *Resectability* means the possibility to surgically remove the tumor completely. Preoperative surgical planning is normally based on radiological (chest X-ray, chest CT, positron emission tomography) and endoscopic (transbronchial needle aspiration, mediastinoscopy) staging, whereby local tumor extent and mediastinal lymph node involvement are assessed. The extent of planned resection, usually lobectomy or pneumonectomy, substantially contributes to the final decision, whether to proceed to surgical resection or to evaluate alternative treatment methods. In candidates with severely impaired lung function, the possibility of tissue sparing procedures such as atypical sublobar or sleeve resection must be weighed against the increased risk of local tumor recurrence.

This article focuses on the functional reserves for which the term *operability* is used. Certain authors make a further distinction between 'operability' and 'functional resectability'. The first addresses the ability of the patient to tolerate the stress of the operation and the early postoperative phase (30 days). The latter looks at the permanent loss of cardiopulmonary function. However, the term 'functional resectability' has not been used widely and tends to lead to confusion. In practise, it is simpler and more generally accepted to use the term 'operability' for both these aspects and to reserve the term 'resectability' for the surgical aspect concerned with the question whether the tumor can be totally removed based on anatomical information.

Although the bulk of the literature describes predominantly malignant disease, the principles outlined below are generally also applicable to non cancer cases. The extent of resection, however, is often less in benign disease, because radical excision respecting the rules of cancer surgery is not necessary.

Most lung resection candidates are former or current smokers and at increased risk for ischemic heart disease and chronic obstructive lung disease. In general, it is of utmost importance, that the patient is investigated and treated in the best possible condition. Patients with chronic obstructive lung disease should receive optimized antiobstructive therapy before undergoing surgery [2]. Smokers should be advised to quit and be offered counseling for this, preferably at least 8 weeks before surgery [3]. Repeat assessment of functional measurements may be necessary after improving medical therapy (i.e. in a pulmonary rehabilitation program). Due to the often rapid progress of disease in lung cancer patients the period or 'window for functional improvement' is usually limited to 6–8 weeks. Insufficient treatment both reduces the patient's chances to be eligible for lung resection and increases the risk of perioperative complications.

Operative Morbidity and Mortality

The perioperative risk refers to the immediate or short term risk leading to perioperative morbidity and mortality. Overall perioperative mortality rates for pneumonectomies ranges from 5% up to 17% and for lobectomies from <1% to 5% [4, 5]. An overall mortality rate of <5% is considered to be good and <2% excellent. Because lung cancer is a disease with a mortality approaching 100% if not treated surgically, a certain degree of non-fatal postoperative complications can almost always be accepted. Major complication categories in lung resection are cardiac and pulmonary.

Cardiac Complications

An abnormal electrocardiogram (ECG) has been associated with postoperative myocardial infarction, arrhythmias and heart failure since the early 1960s [6, 7]. However, the cardiac risk of lung resection candidates has not received much attention in recent years, despite major advances in treatment options with coronary catheter interventions (PTCA) or coronary artery bypass grafting (CABG). Recent American guidelines for the assessment of the cardiovascular risk in non-cardiac surgery combine various clinical risk predictors with the presumed risk of the planned surgical procedure. Intrathoracic surgery has, according to these guidelines, an inherent moderate risk of 1–5% for fatal or nonfatal cardiac complications [8]. Therefore, every lung resection candidate should be evaluated for potential cardiac disease and treated accordingly before surgery is performed.

Table 1. Generally accepted risk factors for postoperative complications

Higher planned extent of resection
Poor exercise performance
Poor predicted postoperative FEV_1
Poor predicted postoperative TLCO
Age >70 years
pCO_2 >45 mm Hg

Pulmonary Complications

Postoperative pulmonary complications generally include atelectasis, pneumonia, pulmonary embolism, prolonged mechanical ventilation, CO_2 retention, and death [4, 9, 10]. Pulmonary complications can frequently occur after major nonpulmonary surgery and contribute to mortality and length of hospital stay [11]. Poor exercise capacity is a recognised predictor for pulmonary complications in elective general surgery [12, 13]. Exercise testing, however, is not routinely used to assess the pulmonary risk in non lung resection surgery.

The risk of pulmonary complications is inherently higher in lung resection, because some functional lung tissue is almost always resected. Contrary to non-pulmonary surgery, many risk factors have been studied for lung parenchymal resection. Generally accepted risk factors are listed in table 1. Impaired lung mechanics, gas exchange and exercise capacity are clearly associated with poor surgical outcome, and the risk of pulmonary complications is higher with greater extent of resection [14–17]. Older patients and patients with CO_2 retention or impaired TLCO, however, can undergo parenchymal resection with acceptable risk when assessed with exercise testing and should therefore not be excluded from surgery based on these factors alone [18–20].

Assessment of Operability

Pulmonary Function Testing

Since the first report about the usefulness of vital capacity for predicting surgical outcome in 1955, many static and dynamic lung function variables have been proposed over time [1, 21]. However, only FEV_1 has stood the test of time as the best single predictor of postoperative pulmonary complications [5, 22–25]. Very few perioperative complications occurred in a large series of patients selected based on FEV_1 >2 l for pneumonectomy, FEV_1 >1 l for lobectomy and FEV_1 >0.6 l for segmentectomy [5]. Regrettably, most reports on FEV_1 focus on absolute values rather that % of predicted (% pred). The latter approach has the advantage of taking age, sex and height into consideration, a notion that will probably gain importance with the current massive increase in female lung cancer patients.

TLCO was suggested early as a risk predictor, and proposed values were from <50% pred to <60% pred as prohibitive for pneumonectomy or major pulmonary resections [26, 27]. In a recent study, the correlation of lower TLCO% pred with a higher rate of pulmonary complications after lung resection was confirmed [28]. TLCO as an isolated parameter, however, did not gain much importance until the emergence of split function studies (see below) [4].

Prediction of Postoperative Function with Split Function Studies

Lung resection candidates with normal lung function tolerate resections up to an entire lung quite well and can, with certain restrictions, lead a normal postoperative life in their private as well as in their professional environment. However, the majority of lung resection candidates are patients with cancer caused by smoking, which also leads to COPD. Such patients have impaired functional reserves and are therefore at risk for permanent disability after extensive resection of lung tissue. It has been shown, that resections of not more than one lobe usually lead to a mild early postoperative functional impairment with little permanent deficit in PFT (≤10%) and preserved exercise capacity [29–31]. Pneumonectomies lead to a permanent loss of lung function of roughly one third and a moderate drop in exercise capacity (±20%) [31–33].

Based on the extent of planned resection and the preoperative functional reserves, a forecast of the remaining postoperative proportion of functional parameters can be undertaken. One might be tempted, for example for a lobectomy, to simply deduct a fifth of the preoperative function to calculate the predicted postoperative (ppo) value. However, prediction of postoperative functional parameters is not a simple arithmetic matter. It must be taken into account that the disease process is normally unevenly distributed and that the contribution of the lung tissue to be resected to overall lung function is variable. Furthermore, considerable compensation for lost lung parenchyma can occur over time.

Several methods to calculate ppo function have been proposed. To date, technetium-99 macroaggragate perfusion scans (split function studies) are widely in use for this purpose. This technique allows quantification of the individual contribution of the parenchyma to be resected to overall function, is easy to perform and generally available. The formula to calculate a ppo value based on perfusion studies is, as proposed by Olsen: value ppo = preoperative value × (1 – contribution of the parenchyma to be resected) [34].

Many authors have confirmed the accuracy of the estimated functional loss in FEV_1 and other lung function parameters after resection [35]. With the advent of the ppo concept, FEV_1 ppo has received increasing interest. Though not a consistent finding, various studies had better results for prediction of perioperative complications with FEV_1 ppo than with baseline FEV_1 [25, 36–38]. However, there is no consensus about 'how much' FEV_1 ppo is required as a minimum for safe resection, and values of 700–1,000 ml or 30% pred have been proposed [25, 36, 37].

With the same formula as described by Olsen, TLCO ppo can be calculated. A minimal value of TLCO ppo of 40% pred has been suggested. One report showed that both FEV_1 ppo and TLCO ppo in % pred alone and in combination were good indicators for postoperative complications [4]. In another study, the product of FEV_1 ppo × TLCO ppo in % pred was highly predictive of complications [39]. In contrast, baseline lung function was not predictive in both reports.

Based on the literature of several decades, it is fair to conclude that no single parameter has been established as the superior predictor of the perioperative risk. Presently, the most convincing concept is to use a combination of functional tests. In general, the approach to use percentage of predicted rather than absolute values is probably superior to arbitrary absolute values, because differences in gender, age and body mass are taken into account.

Cardiopulmonary Exercise Testing

Cardiopulmonary exercise testing assesses both the cardiovascular and pulmonary reserves and, additionally, simulates the stress of a thoracic operation to a certain

Table 2. Studies with minimal achievement

Author	Type of exercise	Patients	Conclusions
Van Nostrand, 1968 [73]	stair climbing	213	≤1 flight: high mortality
Berggren, 1984 [74]	cycle ergometry	82 ≥70 years old	>83 W during 6 min: low risk
Bagg, 1984 [75]	12 min walking	22	no prediction of respiratory complications
Olsen, 1991 [76]	stair climbing	54	<3 flights: high complication rate
Bolton, 1992 [77]	stair climbing	70	≥3 flights: accept. risk for lobectomy ≥5 flights: accept. risk for pneumonectomy
Holden, 1992 [48]	6 min walking stair climbing	16 high risk 16 high risk	>1,000 feet: acceptable risk >44 steps: acceptable risk
Pollock, 1993 [41]	stair climbing (standardised)	31 men with COPD	>4.6 flights correspond to VO_2max >20 ml/kg/min: low risk
Pate, 1996 [37]	stair climbing	12 high risk	≥3 flights: acceptable risk

extent. CPET has gained increasing importance since a report in 1982, when maximum exercise capacity was found to be superior to resting lung mechanics (FEV_1, FVC) in predicting operative mortality in a small number of patients [40]. Various exercise protocols have been proposed, which can roughly be divided into three distinct groups by the type of exercise intensity demanded from the patient: minimal achievement, submaximal, and maximal or symptom-limited tests.

Minimal Achievement Tests. The principle of a minimal achievement test is to declare a subject fit for a certain extent of resection, if a predefined minimal achievement is accomplished. Tests such as stair climbing or walking over 6 or 12 min have the advantage to be simple and cheap. Different protocols have been proposed (table 2). Most of these tests are poorly standardised, however, and allow identification of low risk patients rather than exact risk stratification in compromised patients. The lack of adequate cardiac monitoring is an additional disadvantage, and the exact type of limitation can not be reliably detected. However, it was shown in patients with COPD, that a standardised symptom-limited maximal stair climb test helps estimation of VO_2max [41]. In the absence of sophisticated equipment, such a test is certainly acceptable to select patients fit for resection. In borderline patients, however, more elaborate studying is necessary.

Submaximal Tests. To avoid the physical stress of a test to exhaustion, submaximal tests have been proposed. In a submaximal test, the subject is exercised up to a predefined level, and the observed values are used to calculate the operative risk based on previous experience. However, most of these tests involve invasive instrumentation, which is probably the reason why they have not become very popular [42–45]. An algorithm for preoperative functional evaluation based on a submaximal test has been proposed by a Japanese group [46].

Maximal Tests. The bulk of the literature has been about incremental maximal or symptom-limited tests using a ramp protocol. In such a test setting, the patient is motivated to exercise until exhaustion or until an exercise induced symptom such as dyspnea or leg fatigue make it impossible to continue. The highest oxygen consumption achieved is called VO_2max or peakVO_2. Maximal protocols are easy to standardise, non-invasive, and VO_2max is reproducible [47]. Although VO_2max has been shown to predict postoperative outcome in many reports, different cut-off values for safe resections make general recommendations somewhat difficult (table 3). Furthermore, comparison of reports is complicated by incongruent definitions of end points, differences in testing protocols, small size or special selection of samples and inconsistent reporting in absolute values or percent of predicted [23, 28, 48, 49]. Nevertheless, a preoperative VO_2max of >20 ml/kg/min is generally accepted to date as safe for any resection up to pneumonectomy, and a value of <10 ml/kg/min as predictive for a very high complication rate, irrespective of the extent of resection. In analogy to pulmonary function tests, VO_2max values should be expressed in % predicted, which also takes age and sex into consideration.

The postoperative loss of exercise capacity is usually overestimated when looking at PFT values alone. After lobectomy, there is no long term loss in VO_2max, whereas after pneumonectomy a loss of 20–23% is observed [31, 32, 50]. In recent years, the predicted postoperative

Table 3. Studies with preoperative exercise testing

Author, year	Patients	Mortality	Findings/remarks	Recommendations
Eugene, 1982 [40]	19	16%	VO_2max <1,000 ml: 75% mortality	VO_2max <1,000 ml: high risk
Smith, 1984 [9]	22	0	VO_2max <15 ml/kg/min: 100% complication rate	VO_2max >20 ml/kg/min: low risk VO_2max <15 ml/kg/min: high risk
Bechard, 1987 [10]	50	4%	VO_2max <10 ml/kg/min: 29% mortality	VO_2max <10 ml/kg/min: high risk
Morice, 1992 [18]	37 (high risk)	0/8 pts	offered surgery to patients with VO_2max >15 ml/kg/min	VO_2max >15 ml/kg/min: acceptable risk
Dales, 1993 [49]	117	<1%	risk higher if: VO_2max <1,250 ml FEV_1 <60% pred ventilatory reserve <25 l	use VO_2max >1,250 ml and ventilatory reserve >25 l
Epstein, 1993 [65]	42	2%	VO_2max <500 ml/m²/min: higher complication rate	use risk index
Bolliger, 1995 [51]	25 (high risk)	12%	calculates ppo VO_2max	ppoVO_2max <10 ml/kg/min: high risk
Bolliger, 1995 [53]	80	4%	VO_2max <60% pred: higher complicaton rate	VO_2max <60% pred: high risk VO_2max <60% pred: prohibitive >1 lobe VO_2max <43% pred: prohibitive any resection
Pate, 1996 [37]	12 (high risk)	8.3%	low complication rate despite high risk	VO_2max >10 ml/kg/min: acceptable risk
Richter Larsen, 1997 [78]	97	9.3%	complications higher in patients with VO_2max <50% predicted	VO_2max <12 ml/kg/min: high risk
Ribas, 1998 [79]	65 (high risk)	6.2%	complications higher if paO_2 decreases during exercise	use FEV_1ppo, TLCO ppo, O_2 desaturation VO_2max not predictive
Wyser, 1999 [52]	137	1.5%	prospective evaluation VO_2max in 68 high-risk patients	VO_2max >75% pred: low risk VO_2max ppo >35% pred: low risk
Brutsche, 2000 [17]	125	1.6%	VO_2max <60% pred: higher complication rate	VO_2max <60% pred: high risk VO_2max >90% pred: low risk
Wang, 2000 [80]	57	4%	VO_2max <15 ml/kg/min: higher complication rate	use exercise-induced increase in TLCO, FEV_1% pred, TLCO % pred, VO_2max/kg

VO_2max = Maximal oxygen uptake; ppo = predicted postoperative. Adapted from Reilly [81].

VO_2max (VO_2max ppo) has been proposed to assess the surgical risk. Interestingly, the same simple formula used to predict FEV_1 ppo and TLCO ppo was found useful for this prediction [51]. However, VO_2max ppo and its proposed value of 10 ml/kg/min as prohibitive for any resection still warrant confirmation in a large number of patients [52]. An additional advantage of calculating VO_2max ppo is the estimation of a patient's postoperative professional working capacity.

In conclusion, symptom-limited maximal exercise testing has the advantage of good standardisation and reproducibility. The equipment is affordable and testing is not invasive, and the value of VO_2max in predicting perioperative complications is clearly established.

Clinical Application

Despite the availability of modern tests like split function studies and CPET, most patients without cardiac disease can undergo resections up to pneumonectomy based on simple PFT. To avoid unnecessary cost, it is important to take a stepwise approach to the evaluation of the lung resection candidate. An ideal tool for this purpose is an algorithm, including all necessary preoperative variables (PFT, ppo function, and CPET). The algorithm should result in a clear-cut recommendation, whether lung resection is possible and if yes, to what extent.

CPET is now recognised widely as the test of choice for patients with abnormal basic lung function values. It is

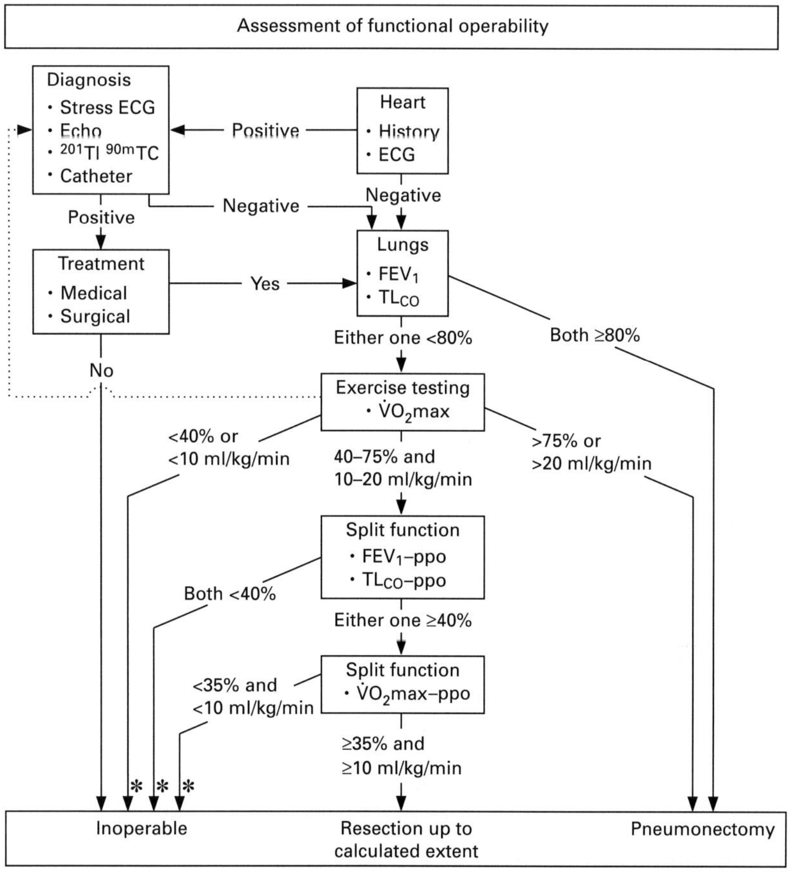

Fig. 2. Proposed algorithm for the assessment of operability of lung resection candidates. Patients undergo successive steps from top to bottom, until they qualify for varying extents of resection or are deemed inoperable. The 'safety loop' for patients with cardiac problems is indicated in the upper left-hand corner. The dashed line leading from exercise testing back to the cardiac workup is for patients with a negative cardiac history and a normal ECG, who show symptoms or signs of ischemia during exercise. * Consider eligibility for combined tumor resection and lung volume reduction surgery in carefully selected patients. TI = Thallium; TC = technetium; VO_2max = maximal oxygen consumption during exercise; ppo = predicted postoperative; FEV_1 = forced expiratory volume in the 1st second; TLCO = transfer factor for lung carbon monoxide. With permission from Bolliger and Perruchoud [35].

not clear, however, what extent of lung function impairment can still be tolerated for lung resection without additional CPET.

The algorithm presented in this chapter was proposed by Bolliger et al. [53] after evaluation of a consecutive series of 80 lung resection candidates with multiple regression analysis. The best predictor for postoperative complications was VO_2max % pred, which was slightly better than VO_2max absolute. Of 9 patients with VO_2max of <60% pred, 8 had complications, including all 3 who died. In a high risk subgroup of 25 patients who underwent split function studies, VO_2max % pred and VO_2max ppo were predictive, while FEV_1 ppo and TLCO ppo were not significantly different in patients with or without complications [51]. The initially suggested algorithm was slightly amended after prospective evaluation in a follow-up series of 137 consecutive patients [52]. Adherence to this algorithm resulted in a reduction of mortality and complication rates from 4 to 1.5% and from 20 to 11%, respectively, while the proportion of patients deemed inoperable remained unchanged (fig. 2).

Patients who have a negative cardiac history and a normal ECG can undergo lung resection without further assessment of the cardiac risk. Any patient with active or suspected cardiac disease should first undergo a thorough cardiac work-up and, if necessary, even coronary bypass surgery in case of ischemic heart disease [54]. Only patients whose cardiac condition is amenable to treatment can undergo further investigation for pulmonary resection.

Since resection of the diseased lung up to pneumonectomy seldom results in a functional loss of >50% [55], and postoperative values of >40% for FEV_1 and TLCO are safe [4, 39], the algorithm allows resections up to a pneumonectomy without any further tests, if FEV_1 and TLCO are both >80% predicted. If either FEV_1 or TLCO is

<80% pred, exercise testing with the measurement of VO_2max is performed. Rarely, exercise testing will pick up ischemic heart disease in patients with a negative cardiac history and a normal ECG. This will also lead to a cardiac work-up (interrupted line in the algorithm). If VO_2max is >75% pred or >20 ml/kg/min, patients qualify for resection up to a pneumonectomy; if it is <40% pred or 10 ml/kg/min they are inoperable.

All patients with VO_2max values in between undergo split-function studies with the aid of a pulmonary perfusion scan to determine their predicted postoperative function (ppo-function). Firstly, FEV_1 ppo and TLCO ppo are analyzed; if the values for both parameters are <40% pred, patients are deemed inoperable. If either one is >40% pred, then VO_2max ppo becomes the decisive factor. With a VO_2max ppo of either <35% pred or <10 ml/kg/min patients are also deemed inoperable; whereas patients with a VO_2max ppo >35% pred and >10 ml/kg/min are operable up to the extent which was used for the prediction of postoperative function.

Another algorithm focused on high risk patients with FEV_1 or TLCO of <60% pred has most recently been proposed by Weisman, aiming to reduce cost for additional testing without jeopardizing the overall outcome [56]. Naturally, different approaches to the use of CPET are possible, and local availability of testing facilities or cost factors may influence the choice of a specific method.

In many institutions, an interdisciplinary discussion of patients proposed for lung resection, involving pulmonologist, radiologist, thoracic surgeon and (radio)-oncologist, has proven very useful. Based on cancer staging, resectability and operability estimates, a comprehensive management plan should be established. The operating surgeon must be informed about the extent of resection functionally possible, and in selected cases atypical resection techniques must be considered to optimise risk management.

Establishment of functional operability is a dynamic process and investigations must sometimes be repeated to keep up with the current state of each patient. Especially with preoperative (neoadjuvant) treatment protocols for NSCLC, several weeks can go by between initial assessment and surgery. The data on surgical outcome after neoadjuvant treatment are conflicting, and a negative impact on the operative risk seems possible, particularly after combined chemo-radiotherapy with irradiation doses of >45 Gy [57–61]. Based on our experience, preoperative chemotherapy can lead to functional deterioration and inoperability, but the converse can also be true, for example if a previously obstructed bronchus becomes patent again after treatment. To our knowledge, no published data on the issue of operability after neoadjuvant treatment are available to date, so that each case should be reassessed for operability as well as for resectability before surgery.

Controversial Issues

Patients Unable to Exercise

A limitation of exercise testing is that not all patients can exercise with standardised equipment such as cycle ergometers and treadmills. This group is very heterogeneous. Some patients are able to perform an exercise test with alternative equipment, i.e. a rowing ergometer. Other patients will have to be evaluated with PFT and split function studies alone. However, patients unable to exercise because of orthopedic problems, vascular disease or chronic neurologic disorders generally have a clearly decreased level of fitness and eligibility for major surgery must be determined with caution. In one report, inability to perform cycle ergometry was found to be a independent predictor of bad outcome after lung resection [62].

Quantitative CT Scanning

A new approach to the prediction of postoperative function is quantitative computed tomography. One group found excellent correlation for FEV_1 and FVC in a group of 34 patients [63]. In a most recent study, the usefulness of quantitative CT scanning comparing various techniques for estimating ppo function was confirmed, although perfusion studies remained the most accurate [64]. Because lung cancer patients regularly undergo CT scanning for preoperative staging, this technique has the potential to replace perfusion scans in the evaluation of the majority of patients relegating additional perfusion scans for patients with moderate-severe impairment of cardiopulmonary reserves only.

Cardiopulmonary Risk Index

Epstein et al. [65] proposed a cardiopulmonary risk index (CPRI) for the preoperative risk-assessment of lung resection candidates. The CPRI assigns points for various cardiac and pulmonary risk factors. The CPRI has been compared to VO_2max and both have shown to be predictive for perioperative complications. Other authors, however, could not confirm the predictive value of the CPRI [66]. Furthermore, some parameters used are rather subjective. Although some prediction of risk seems possible, the value of the CPRI for the selection of pulmonary resection candidates is not clearly defined.

New Horizons with Lung Volume Reduction Surgery?

Lung volume reduction surgery (LVRS) is performed in selected extremely symptomatic emphysematous patients in order to improve lung function, quality of life and exercise capacity [67]. During LVRS, the most dysfunctional parts of one or both lungs are removed mainly by means of wedge resection. Because emphysema and lung cancer share cigarette smoking as a common risk factor, coincidence can occur. Therefore, the combination of cancer surgery with LVRS, which improves overall lung function postoperatively, might become a promising new treatment option in selected lung cancer patients previously deemed inoperable. However, most tumors resected to date in combination with LVRS have been detected incidentally during work-up for LVRS. Therefore, these tumors are in a very early stage and prognosis after surgical resection is favorable. Early reports are promising, but data for long term survival are not available to date [68, 69]. In lung cancer surgery, it is well known that resections of less than a lobe are associated with a smaller chance of curative resection even in T1, N0, stage I NSCLC [70, 71]. Whether the risk of less radical surgery outweighs the benefit from LVRS is currently not known. This problem warrants investigation in prospective studies including lung cancer patients with anatomically resectable tumors previously deemed inoperable due to limited cardiopulmonary reserves.

Conclusion

CPET has gained an important role in the preoperative assessment of lung resection candidates. While PFTs and cardiac studies adequately assess specific risk components, CPET allows simultaneous measurement of pulmonary and cardiovascular parameters in a single test. With additional pulmonary perfusion scans, accurate predicted postoperative values for FEV_1, TLCO and, most recently, VO_2max can be calculated. In combination with the planned extent of resection, the individual risk of the pulmonary resection candidate can be assessed.

The current trend seems to favor split-function studies and exercise testing with the measurement of VO_2max. The majority of reports found VO_2max a good independent risk predictor. Maximal exercise tests are fairly easy to standardise, and, in our opinion, VO_2max represents the single best parameter to evaluate both the pulmonary as well as the cardiovascular reserves. Excessive testing can be avoided by adherence to an integrated algorithm, providing rational decision-making based on established risk factors.

References

1 Gaensler EA, Cugell DW, Lindgren I: The role of pulmonary insufficiency in mortality and invalidism following surgery for pulmonary tuberculosis. J Thorac Surg 1955;29:163.

2 Smetana GW: Preoperative pulmonary evaluation. N Engl J Med 1999;340:937–944.

3 Warner MA, Offord KP, Warner ME, Lennon RL, Conover MA, Jansson-Schumacher U: Role of preoperative cessation of smoking and other factors in postoperative pulmonary complications: A blinded prospective study of coronary artery bypass patients. Mayo Clin Proc 1989;64:609–616.

4 Markos J, Mullan BP, Hillman DR, Musk AW, Antico VF, Lovegrove FT, Carter MJ, Finucane KE: Preoperative assessment as a predictor of mortality and morbidity after lung resection. Am Rev Respir Dis 1989;139:902–910.

5 Miller JI Jr: Physiologic evaluation of pulmonary function in the candidate for lung resection. J Thorac Cardiovasc Surg 1993;105:347–351; discussion 351–342.

6 Didolkar MS, Moore RH, Takita H: Evaluation of the risk in pulmonary resection for bronchogenic carcinoma. Am J Surg 1974;127: 700–703.

7 Mittman C: Assessment of operative risk in thoracic surgery. Am Rev Respir Dis 1961;84: 197–207.

8 Eagle KA, Brundage BH, Chaitman BR, Ewy GA, Fleisher LA, Hertzer NR, Leppo JA, Ryan T, Schlant RC, Spencer WH 3rd, Spittell JA Jr, Twiss RD, Ritchie JL, Cheitlin MD, Gardner TJ, Garson A Jr, Lewis RP, Gibbons RJ, O'Rourke RA, Ryan TJ: Guidelines for perioperative cardiovascular evaluation for noncardiac surgery: Report of the American College of Cardiology/American Heart Association Task Force on Practice Guidelines. Committee on Perioperative Cardiovascular Evaluation for Noncardiac Surgery. Circulation 1996;93: 1278–1317.

9 Smith TP, Kinasewitz GT, Tucker WY, Spillers WP, George RB: Exercise capacity as a predictor of post-thoracotomy morbidity. Am Rev Respir Dis 1984;129:730–734.

10 Bechard D, Wetstein L: Assessment of exercise oxygen consumption as preoperative criterion for lung resection. Ann Thorac Surg 1987;44: 344–349.

11 Lawrence VA, Dhanda R, Hilsenbeck SG, Page CP: Risk of pulmonary complications after elective abdominal surgery. Chest 1996;110: 744–750.

12 Williams-Russo P, Charlson ME, MacKenzie CR, Gold JP, Shires GT: Predicting postoperative pulmonary complications. Is it a real problem? Arch Intern Med 1992;152:1209–1213.

13 Older P, Hall A, Hader R: Cardiopulmonary exercise testing as a screening test for perioperative management of major surgery in the elderly. Chest 1999;116:355–362.

14 Lockwood P: Lung function test results and the risk of post-thoracotomy complications. Respiration 1973;30:529–542.

15 Moghissi K, Connolly CK: Resection rates in lung cancer patients. Eur Respir J 1996;9:5–6.

16 Damhuis RA, Schutte PR: Resection rates and postoperative mortality in 7,899 patients with lung cancer. Eur Respir J 1996;9:7–10.

17 Brutsche MH, Spiliopoulos A, Bolliger CT, Licker M, Frey JG, Tschopp JM: Exercise capacity and extent of resection as predictors of surgical risk in lung cancer. Eur Respir J 2000; 15:828–832.

18 Morice RC, Peters EJ, Ryan MB, Putnam JB, Ali MK, Roth JA: Exercise testing in the evaluation of patients at high risk for complications from lung resection. Chest 1992;101:356–361.
19 Gerson MC, Hurst JM, Hertzberg VS, Doogan PA, Cochran MB, Lim SP, McCall N, Adolph RJ: Cardiac prognosis in noncardiac geriatric surgery. Ann Intern Med 1985;103:832–837.
20 Bolliger CT, Soler M, Stulz P, Gradel E, Muller-Brand J, Elsasser S, Gonon M, Wyser C, Perruchoud AP: Evaluation of high-risk lung resection candidates: Pulmonary haemodynamics versus exercise testing. A series of five patients. Respiration 1994;61:181–186.
21 American College of Physicians: Preoperative pulmonary function testing. Ann Intern Med 1990;112:793–794.
22 Boushy SF, Billig DM, North LB, Helgason AH: Clinical course related to preoperative and postoperative pulmonary function in patients with bronchogenic carcinoma. Chest 1971;59: 383–391.
23 Colman NC, Schraufnagel DE, Rivington RN, Pardy RL: Exercise testing in evaluation of patients for lung resection. Am Rev Respir Dis 1982;125:604–606.
24 Keagy BA, Lores ME, Starek PJ, Murray GF, Lucas CL, Wilcox BR: Elective pulmonary lobectomy: Factors associated with morbidity and operative mortality. Ann Thorac Surg 1985;40:349–352.
25 Wernly JA, DeMeester TR, Kirchner PT, Myerowitz PD, Oxford DE, Golomb HM: Clinical value of quantitative ventilation-perfusion lung scans in the surgical management of bronchogenic carcinoma. J Thorac Cardiovasc Surg 1980;80:535–543.
26 Nagasaki F, Flehinger BJ, Martini N: Complications of surgery in the treatment of carcinoma of the lung. Chest 1982;82:25–29.
27 Ferguson MK, Little L, Rizzo L, Popovich KJ, Glonek GF, Leff A, Manjoney D, Little AG: Diffusing capacity predicts morbidity and mortality after pulmonary resection. J Thorac Cardiovasc Surg 1988;96:894–900.
28 Wang J, Olak J, Ultmann RE, Ferguson MK: Assessment of pulmonary complications after lung resection. Ann Thorac Surg 1999;67: 1444–1447.
29 Ali MK, Mountain CF, Ewer MS, Johnston D, Haynie TP: Predicting loss of pulmonary function after pulmonary resection for bronchogenic carcinoma. Chest 1980;77:337–342.
30 Loddenkemper R, Gabler A, Gobel D: Criteria of functional operability in patients with bronchial carcinoma: Preoperative assessment of risk and prediction of postoperative function. Thorac Cardiovasc Surg 1983;31:334–337.
31 Bolliger CT, Jordan P, Soler M, Stulz P, Tamm M, Wyser C, Gonon M, Perruchoud AP: Pulmonary function and exercise capacity after lung resection. Eur Respir J 1996;9:415–421.
32 Van Mieghem W, Demedts M: Cardiopulmonary function after lobectomy or pneumonectomy for pulmonary neoplasm. Respir Med 1989;83:199–206.
33 Pelletier C, Lapointe L, LeBlanc P: Effects of lung resection on pulmonary function and exercise capacity. Thorax 1990;45:497–502.
34 Olsen GN, Block AJ, Tobias JA: Prediction of postpneumonectomy pulmonary function using quantitative macroaggregate lung scanning. Chest 1974;66:13–16.
35 Bolliger CT, Perruchoud AP: Functional evaluation of the lung resection candidate. Eur Respir J 1998;11:198–212.
36 Olsen GN, Block AJ, Swenson EW, Castle JR, Wynne JW: Pulmonary function evaluation of the lung resection candidate: A prospective study. Am Rev Respir Dis 1975;111:379–387.
37 Pate P, Tenholder MF, Griffin JP, Eastridge CE, Weiman DS: Preoperative assessment of the high-risk patient for lung resection. Ann Thorac Surg 1996;61:1494–1500.
38 Kristersson S, Lindell SE, Svanberg L: Prediction of pulmonary function loss due to pneumonectomy using ^{133}Xe-radiospirometry. Chest 1972;62:694–698.
39 Pierce RJ, Copland JM, Sharpe K, Barter CE: Preoperative risk evaluation for lung cancer resection: Predicted postoperative product as a predictor of surgical mortality. Am J Respir Crit Care Med 1994;150:947–955.
40 Eugene J, Brown SE, Light RW, Milne NE, Stemmer EA: Maximum oxygen consumption: A physiologic guide to pulmonary resection. Surg Forum 1982;33:260–262.
41 Pollock M, Roa J, Benditt J, Celli B: Estimation of ventilatory reserve by stair climbing. A study in patients with chronic airflow obstruction. Chest 1993;104:1378–1383.
42 Pierce RJ, Pretto JJ, Rochford PD, McDonald CF, Hanan JA, Barter CE: Lobar occlusion in the preoperative assessment of patients with lung cancer. Br J Dis Chest 1986;80:27–36.
43 Nakagawa K, Nakahara K, Miyoshi S, Kawashima Y: Oxygen transport during incremental exercise load as a predictor of operative risk in lung cancer patients. Chest 1992;101:1369–1375.
44 Miyoshi S, Nakahara K, Ohno K, Monden Y, Kawashima Y: Exercise tolerance test in lung cancer patients: The relationship between exercise capacity and postthoracotomy hospital mortality. Ann Thorac Surg 1987;44:487–490.
45 Olsen GN, Weiman DS, Bolton JW, Gass GD, McLain WC, Schoonover GA, Hornung CA: Submaximal invasive exercise testing and quantitative lung scanning in the evaluation for tolerance of lung resection. Chest 1989;95: 267–273.
46 Nakahara K, Monden Y, Ohno K, Miyoshi S, Maeda H, Kawashima Y: 1985:A method for predicting postoperative lung function and its relation to postoperative complications in patients with lung cancer. 1992 update. Ann Thorac Surg 1992;54:1016–1017.
47 Janicki JS, Gupta S, Ferris ST, McElroy PA: Long-term reproducibility of respiratory gas exchange measurements during exercise in patients with stable cardiac failure. Chest 1990; 97:12–17.
48 Holden DA, Rice TW, Stelmach K, Meeker DP: Exercise testing, 6-min walk, and stair climb in the evaluation of patients at high risk for pulmonary resection. Chest 1992;102: 1774–1779.
49 Dales RE, Dionne G, Leech JA, Lunau M, Schweitzer I: Preoperative prediction of pulmonary complications following thoracic surgery. Chest 1993;104:155–159.
50 Corris PA, Ellis DA, Hawkins T, Gibson GJ: Use of radionuclide scanning in the preoperative estimation of pulmonary function after pneumonectomy. Thorax 1987;42:285–291.
51 Bolliger CT, Wyser C, Roser H, Soler M, Perruchoud AP: Lung scanning and exercise testing for the prediction of postoperative performance in lung resection candidates at increased risk for complications. Chest 1995;108:341–348.
52 Wyser C, Stulz P, Soler M, Tamm M, Muller-Brand J, Habicht J, Perruchoud AP, Bolliger CT: Prospective evaluation of an algorithm for the functional assessment of lung resection candidates. Am J Respir Crit Care Med 1999;159: 1450–1456.
53 Bolliger CT, Jordan P, Soler M, Stulz P, Gradel E, Skarvan K, Elsasser S, Gonon M, Wyser C, Tamm M, et al: Exercise capacity as a predictor of postoperative complications in lung resection candidates. Am J Respir Crit Care Med 1995;151:1472–1480.
54 Foster ED, Davis KB, Carpenter JA, Abele S, Fray D: Risk of noncardiac operation in patients with defined coronary disease: The Coronary Artery Surgery Study (CASS) registry experience. Ann Thorac Surg 1986;41:42–50.
55 Hall DR: Regional lung function after pneumonectomy. Thorax 1974;29:425–431.
56 Weisman IM: Cardiopulmonary exercise testing in the preoperative assessment for lung resection surgery. Semin Thorac Cardiovasc Surg 2001;13:116–125.
57 Bunn PA Jr, Mault J, Kelly K: Adjuvant and neoadjuvant chemotherapy for non-small cell lung cancer: A time for reassessment? Chest 2000;117:119S–122S.
58 Siegenthaler MP, Pisters KM, Merriman KW, Roth JA, Swisher SG, Walsh GL, Vaporciyan AA, Smythe WR, Putnam JB Jr: Preoperative chemotherapy for lung cancer does not increase surgical morbidity. Ann Thorac Surg 2001;71: 1105–1111.
59 Schilder RJ, Goldberg M, Millenson MM, Movsas B, Rogatko A, Rogers B, Langer CJ: Phase II trial of induction high-dose chemotherapy followed by surgical resection and radiation therapy for patients with marginally resectable non-small cell carcinoma of the lung. Lung Cancer 2000;27:37–45.
60 Sonett JR, Krasna MJ, Suntharalingam M, Schuetz J, Doyle LA, Lilenbaum R, Gamliel Z: Safe pulmonary resection after chemotherapy and high-dose thoracic radiation. Ann Thorac Surg 1999;68:316–320.
61 Rusch VW, Benfield JR: Neoadjuvant therapy for lung cancer: A note of caution. Ann Thorac Surg 1993;55:820–821.
62 Epstein SK, Faling LJ, Daly BD, Celli BR: Inability to perform bicycle ergometry predicts increased morbidity and mortality after lung resection. Chest 1995;107:311–316.

63 Wu MT, Chang JM, Chiang AA, Lu JY, Hsu HK, Hsu WH, Yang CF: Use of quantitative CT to predict postoperative lung function in patients with lung cancer. Radiology 1994;191: 257–262.
64 Bolliger CT, Guckel C, Engel H, Stoehr S, Wyser C, Habicht J, Jordan P, Tamm M, Soler M, Perruchoud AP: Predicted postoperative function after lung resection: Comparison of quantitative CT, scintigraphy, and anatomical calculations. AJRCCM 2000;161:A269.
65 Epstein SK, Faling LJ, Daly BD, Celli BR: Predicting complications after pulmonary resection: Preoperative exercise testing vs a multifactorial cardiopulmonary risk index. Chest 1993;104:694–700.
66 Melendez JA, Carlon VA: Cardiopulmonary risk index does not predict complications after thoracic surgery. Chest 1998;114:69–75.
67 Cooper JD, Trulock EP, Triantafillou AN, Patterson GA, Pohl MS, Deloney PA, Sundaresan RS, Roper CL: Bilateral pneumectomy (volume reduction) for chronic obstructive pulmonary disease. J Thorac Cardiovasc Surg 1995; 109:106–116.
68 McKenna RJ Jr, Fischel RJ, Brenner M, Gelb AF: Combined operations for lung volume reduction surgery and lung cancer. Chest 1996; 110:885–888.
69 DeRose JJ Jr, Argenziano M, El-Amir N, Jellen PA, Gorenstein LA, Steinglass KM, Thomashow B, Ginsburg ME: Lung reduction operation and resection of pulmonary nodules in patients with severe emphysema. Ann Thorac Surg 1998;65:314–318.
70 Landreneau RJ, Sugarbaker DJ, Mack MJ, Hazelrigg SR, Luketich JD, Fetterman L, Liptay MJ, Bartley S, Boley TM, Keenan RJ, Ferson PF, Weyant RJ, Naunheim KS: Wedge resection versus lobectomy for stage I (T1 N0 M0) non-small-cell lung cancer. J Thorac Cardiovasc Surg 1997;113:691–698; discussion 698–700.
71 Ginsberg RJ, Rubinstein LV: Randomized trial of lobectomy versus limited resection for T1 N0 non-small cell lung cancer. Lung Cancer Study Group. Ann Thorac Surg 1995;60:615–622.
72 Bolliger CT: Pre-operative assessment of the lung cancer patient. SAMJ 2001;91:120–123.
73 Van Nostrand D, Kjelsberg MO, Humphrey EW: Preresectional evaluation of risk from pneumonectomy. Surg Gynecol Obstet 1968; 127:306–312.
74 Berggren H, Ekroth R, Malmberg R, Naucler J, William-Olsson G: Hospital mortality and long-term survival in relation to preoperative function in elderly patients with bronchogenic carcinoma. Ann Thorac Surg 1984;38:633–636.
75 Bagg LR: The 12-min walking distance; its use in the pre-operative assessment of patients with bronchial carcinoma before lung resection. Respiration 1984;46:342–345.
76 Olsen GN, Bolton JW, Weiman DS, Hornung CA: Stair climbing as an exercise test to predict the postoperative complications of lung resection. Two years' experience. Chest 1991;99: 587–590.
77 Bolton JW, Weiman DS, Haynes JL, Hornung CA, Olsen GN, Almond CH: Stair climbing as an indicator of pulmonary function. Chest 1987;92:783–788.
78 Richter Larsen K, Svendsen UG, Milman N, Brenoe J, Petersen BN: Exercise testing in the preoperative evaluation of patients with bronchogenic carcinoma. Eur Respir J 1997;10: 1559–1565.
79 Ribas J, Diaz O, Barbera JA, Mateu M, Canalis E, Jover L, Roca J, Rodriguez-Roisin R: Invasive exercise testing in the evaluation of patients at high-risk for lung resection. Eur Respir J 1998;12:1429–1435.
80 Wang JS, Abboud RT, Evans KG, Finley RJ, Graham BL: Role of CO diffusing capacity during exercise in the preoperative evaluation for lung resection. Am J Respir Crit Care Med 2000;162:1435–1444.
81 Reilly JJ Jr: Evidence-based preoperative evaluation of candidates for thoracotomy. Chest 1999;116:474S-476S.

Andreas H. Diacon, MD
Department of Internal Medicine
Tygerberg Hospital, University of Stellenbosch
PO Box 19063, 7505 Tygerberg (RSA)
Tel. +27 21 938 9556, Fax +27 21 931 7442
E-Mail diacon@mac.com

Weisman IM, Zeballos RJ (eds): Clinical Exercise Testing.
Prog Respir Res. Basel, Karger, 2002, vol 32, pp 242–253

The Role of Cardiopulmonary Exercise Testing for Patients with Suspected Metabolic Myopathies and Other Neuromuscular Disorders

Kevin R. Flaherty[a] Idelle M. Weisman[b] R. Jorge Zeballos[c]
Fernando J. Martinez[a]

[a]University of Michigan Health System, Department of Internal Medicine, Division of Pulmonary and Critical Care Medicine, Ann Arbor, Mich.; [b]Human Performance Laboratory, Department of Clinical Investigation, Pulmonary-Critical Care Service, William Beaumont Army Medical Center, El Paso, Tex., and Department of Medicine, Pulmonary-Critical Care Division, University of Texas Health Science Center at San Antonio, San Antonio, Tex.; [c]Human Performance Laboratory, Department of Clinical Investigation, William Beaumont Army Medical Center, and Department of Anesthesiology, Texas Tech University Health Sciences Center, El Paso, Tex., USA

Summary

Neuromuscular diseases (NMDs) can be associated with significant exercise limitation. As cardiopulmonary exercise testing (CPET) examines the integrated response to exercise, it has been investigated in multiple NMDs, proving itself particularly valuable in the evaluation of metabolic disorders, which exhibit typical patterns of exercise response. Disorders of carbohydrate metabolism usually demonstrate limitations of aerobic capacity and abnormalities of glycogen utilization. Lipid disorders seem to be associated with lesser aerobic limitation, while disorders of mitochondrial function seem to be associated with the greatest limitation in aerobic capacity. Furthermore, a hyperventilatory and hypercirculatory pattern seems to typify exercise response in these latter patients. As such, CPET can be used in the initial evaluation of patients with suspected carbohydrate or lipid metabolism as well as those with defects of mitochondrial function.

The opinions or assertions contained herein are the private views of the authors and are not to be construed as official or as reflecting the views of the Department of the Army or the Department of Defense.

Neuromuscular diseases can be associated with an abnormal muscle response to exercise. As such, these disorders may present with weakness, myalgia, abnormal fatigue, or exertional breathlessness [1, 2]. These disorders can be classified as those that are associated with impaired muscle energy metabolism, those associated with impaired muscle bulk, and those associated with impaired control of muscle contraction [2]. A general enumeration of these disorders is presented in table 1. As reviewed elsewhere in this book, exercise requires a close integration between skeletal muscle function, cardiovascular function with associated oxygen delivery, and ventilatory function with oxygenation of blood. As such, it is not surprising that myopathic disorders can significantly impact exercise capacity. This chapter reviews the pathophysiologic implications of myopathic disorders on exercise capacity and reviews clinical indications of exercise testing in the diagnosis and management of these disorders.

Disorders of Muscle Energy Metabolism

Metabolic myopathies are disorders of muscle energy metabolism. These disorders have been grouped into three broad categories: (1) defective carbohydrate utilization, (2) abnormal lipid utilization, and (3) mitochondrial

Table 1. General classification of muscle disorders

Disorders of muscle energy metabolism
Disorders of carbohydrate metabolism
Myophosphorylase deficiency
Phosphorylase kinase deficiency
Phosphofructokinase deficiency
Disorders of lipid metabolism
Fatty acid oxidation defects
Carnitine palmitoyltransferase deficiency
Disorders of mitochondrial function
Disorders of muscle bulk
Muscular dystrophies
Chronic motor neuropathies and neuropathies
Inflammatory disorders
Disorders of muscle activation
Focal or multifocal brain lesions
Neurodegenaritive disorders
Psychiatric disorders

myopathies [3]. As such, abnormalities of muscle metabolism can affect the breakdown and utilization of carbohydrates, lipid utilization, or mitochondrial oxidation [3]. A basic understanding of substrate utilization at the level of the skeletal muscle provides a useful framework to understand the varying exercise response noted in metabolic myopathies.

The force-generating elements of the muscle cell are the myofibrils. Contraction occurs with the cyclical association between the myosin thick filament and the actin thin filament; each reversible cycle of association is associated with hydrolysis of a molecule of ATP [2]. As such, the hydrolysis of ATP to ADP and inorganic phosphate (P_i) provides the source of energy for contraction. Phosphocreatine (P_{Cr}) buffers the ATP concentration during a rapid increase in energy use by muscle; only after P_{Cr} is depleted does a significant portion of the energy for contraction come from the hydrolysis of ATP. Unfortunately, the concentration of ATP in muscle is sufficient to provide only a few seconds of maximal exercise [2]. Metabolic pathways within the cell that guarantee the supply of ATP include glycolysis and fatty acid oxidation [4]. These are illustrated in figure 1.

Glycolysis is the principal pathway utilized in the nutritionally replete state. Glycogen stores are limited, however, and are depleted rapidly. Oxidative metabolism of glycogen requires an adequate blood flow and oxygen supply but produces a much higher yield of ATP than anaerobic glycolysis [2]. Anaerobic glycogenolysis, which can be used during periods of oxygen deficiency, is associated with the accumulation of metabolic end products [5]. Figure 1 demonstrates the typical sequence of events during the conversion of glucose to pyruvate in the cytoplasm. Pyruvate is subsequently transferred into the mitochondria where further conversion takes place to acetyl coenzyme A (CoA) by the action of pyruvate dehydrogenase (PD) [4]. Acetyl CoA enters the tricarboxylic acid cycle (TCA) and the reduced form of nicotinamide adenine dinucleotide (NADH) is generated. The enzymatic activity of PD is a key regulatory step; inhibition of PD results in accumulation of pyruvate, which is metabolized to lactate. Factors inhibiting PD activity include NADH, acetyl CoA, ATP and an anaerobic environment [4, 6, 7].

Free fatty acids (FFA) become an important source of oxidative metabolism with prolonged exercise (>30 min) as well as during fasting. In this form of oxidation, FFA, particularly long chain FFA (LCFAs), are conjugated to carnitine-producing acylcarnitine which is transferred into the mitochondria by carnitine palmitoyltransferase (CPT) [8]. As such, carnitine has two important functions, facilitating transport of LCFAs into mitochondria and modulating the intramitochondrial coenzyme A (CoA)/acyl-CoA ratio [9]. In the mitochondria, further conversion occurs to acetyl CoA and flavin adenine dinucleotide ($FADH_2$) by acyl dehydrogenases. In the nutritionally replete state, acetyl CoA enters the TCA cycle while in the fasting state it is metabolized to β-hydroxybutyrate.

Oxidative phosphorylation of ADP to ATP takes place within the inner mitochondrial membrane by five protein complexes that utilize NADH from the TCA cycle and $FADH_2$ from FFA oxidation. These five enzyme complexes contain approximately 100 different protein subunits [10] and include: complex I (NADH dehydrogenase), complex II (succinate dehydrogenase), complex III (cytochrome *c* reductase), Complex IV (cytochrome *c* oxidase) and complex V (ATP synthase). This respiratory chain produces ATP by creating a proton gradient across the inner mitochondrial membrane [10].

It is apparent from this brief review that abnormalities in any of these pathways can affect ATP generation and subsequent skeletal muscle function. For example, abnormalities of PD function alter glucose metabolism leading to excess metabolism of lactate from pyruvate. Similarly, abnormalities in β-fatty acid oxidation compromise the use of FFA for ATP production. This will produce particular functional abnormalities in the fasting state or after a meal high in fat content [4]. Most importantly, diseases that affect oxidative phosphorylation can markedly impair ATP generation and skeletal muscle function during exercise.

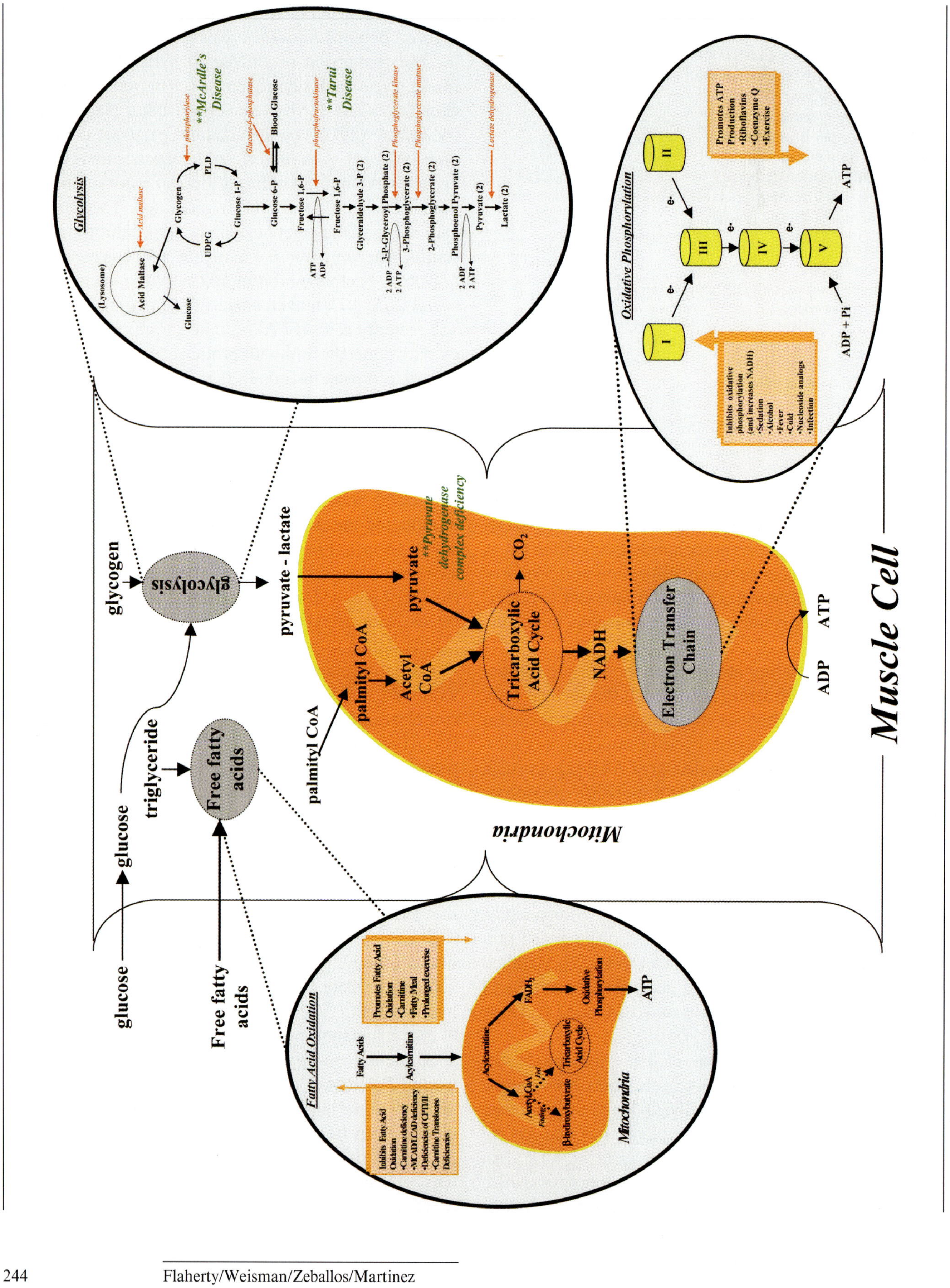

Muscle Cell
glucose
glucose
Free fatty acids
triglyceride
Free fatty acids
glycogen
glycolysis
pyruvate - lactate
palmityl CoA
palmityl CoA
Acetyl CoA
pyruvate
**Pyruvate dehydrogenase complex deficiency
Tricarboxylic Acid Cycle
CO_2
NADH
Electron Transfer Chain
ADP
ATP
Mitochondria
Glycolysis
(Lysosome)
Acid Maltase
Glucose
Acid maltase
Glycogen
UDPG
PLD
phosphorylase
**McArdle's Disease
Glucose 1-P
Glucose 6-P
Glucose-6-phosphatase
Blood Glucose
Fructose 1,6-P
phosphofructokinase
**Tarui Disease
ATP
ADP
Fructose 1,6-P
Glyceraldehyde 3-P (2)
2 ADP
2 ATP
3-P-Glyceroyl Phosphate (2)
Phosphoglycerate kinase
3-Phosphoglycerate (2)
Phosphoglycerate mutase
2-Phosphoglycerate (2)
Phosphoenol Pyruvate (2)
Pyruvate (2)
Lactate dehydrogenase
Lactate (2)
Oxidative Phosphorylation
I
II
III
IV
V
e-
ADP + Pi
ATP
Inhibits oxidative phosphorylation (and increases NADH)
•Sedation
•Alcohol
•Fever
•Cold
•Nucleoside analogs
•Infection
Promotes ATP Production
•Riboflavins
•Coenzyme Q
•Exercise
Fatty Acid Oxidation
Fatty Acids
Acylcarnitine
Acylcarnitine
Acylcarnitine
Acetyl CoA
Fasting
Fed
β-hydroxybutyrate
Tricarboxylic Acid Cycle
$FADH_2$
Oxidative Phosphorylation
ATP
Mitochondria
Inhibits Fatty Acid Oxidation
•Carnitine deficiency
•MCAD/LCAD deficiency
•Deficiencies of CPT I/II
•Carnitine Translocase Deficiencies
Promotes Fatty Acid Oxidation
•Carnitine
•Fatty Meal
•Prolonged exercise

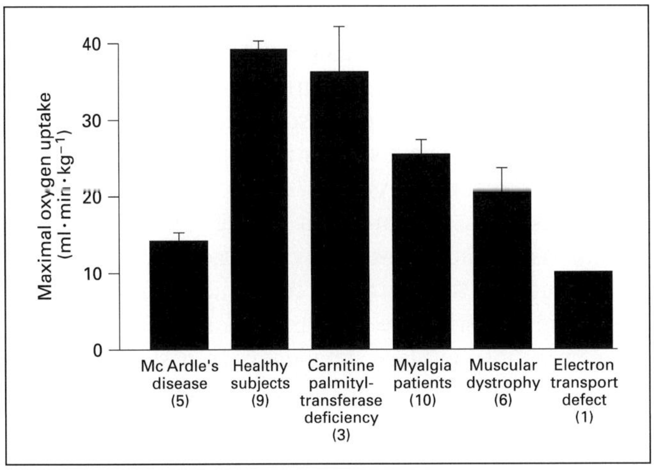

Fig. 2. Maximal oxygen uptake in McArdle patients compared with healthy subjects, patients with carnitine palmityltransferase deficiency, patients with myalgias, patients with muscular dystrophy and patients with electron transport defects [from 28, with permission].

Disorders of Carbohydrate Metabolism

The glycogenoses are disorders of glycogen or glucose metabolism, and usually present with exertional muscle fatigue, myalgia, contractures, or myoglobunuria [11]. Numerous disorders are recognized as recently reviewed by Amato [12]. As noted in figure 1, there are several potential sites for abnormalities of carbohydrate metabolism.

Muscle Phosphorylase Deficiency

The prototypical disorder of muscle glycogenolysis is McArdle's disease (type V glycogen storage disorder or muscle phosphorylase deficiency) which is attributed to mutations in the muscle glycogen phosphorylase gene [13]. The onset of symptoms typically occurs between ages 10 and 30 years [11]. Although patients appear normal at rest, intense or isometric exercise provokes muscle cramps, painful contractures with myoglobinuria, and occasionally renal failure [14]. Interestingly, many patients describe a 'second-wind' phenomenon where initial submaximal exercise provokes fatigue and myalgia which is followed by decreased limitation during subsequent exercise [11, 15]. Initial laboratory examination may demonstrate elevated creatinine kinase levels at rest which can rise dramatically with attacks of myoglobinuria [3, 11].

Fig. 1. Schematic illustration of the metabolic pathways (glycolysis, fatty acid oxidation, and oxidative phosphorylation) and selected associated disorders within a muscle cell.

The hallmark defect in muscle glycogenolysis is a failure of lactate to rise during ischemic exercise. This rather straightforward test involves inflating a blood pressure cuff 10 mm Hg above systolic pressure while the patient squeezes a hand ergometer. Serial blood levels of ammonia and lactate are measured; in normal subjects the ammonia and lactate levels increase by at least 3- to 4-fold- and return to normal levels within 10–15 min of completing exercise [16]. In patients with glycogen storage myopathy, lactate levels do not rise and, in fact, lactate levels may fall although ammonia levels do rise [5, 16]. The measurement of changes in ammonia levels serves as a control to evaluate the adequacy of patient effort [11]. In addition, changes in pH parallel lactate production, so a lack of normal decline in pH is seen [5]. Given these physiologic abnormalities, it is expected that maximal exercise testing may provide important insights and add valuable diagnostic information.

The published literature suggests that patients with muscle myophosphorylase deficiency exhibit a decreased maximal VO_2 to approximately one-third to one-half of the value achieved by sedentary control subjects [3, 5, 17–22]. This is illustrated in figure 2. The limitation in VO_2 seems to reflect substrate limitation and impaired oxidative phosphorylation [5, 23]. The latter is felt to reflect impaired substrate delivery to mitochondria [23]. The biochemical defect in this disorder highlights the important role of glycogen as the fuel utilized to rapidly establish an oxidative steady state [5]. Its absence leads to marked fluctuation in exercise capacity according to the availability of alternative fuels. For example, infusions of glucose during exercise in patients with McArdle's disease improves maximal VO_2, the maximal a-v O_2 difference and abolishes the excessive ATP degradation in working muscles [5, 24]. As a correlate, infusion of FFA, thereby increasing their availability during exercise, also leads to similar improvements during exercise [5]. The physiologic correlate of these changes is the 'second-wind' phenomenon. This refers to the characteristic increase in exercise capacity that is seen spontaneously in patients with McArdle's disease during prolonged exercise [25]. Two distinct phases of exercise have been described during prolonged, submaximal exercise [15]. The first phase ('adaptation phase') is seen during the initial 15 min of exercise at a workload 30% of VO_2max; the second phase ('second wind') followed during which patients were able to continue exercise without difficulty. The 'second wind' phase was characterized by an increase in cardiac output

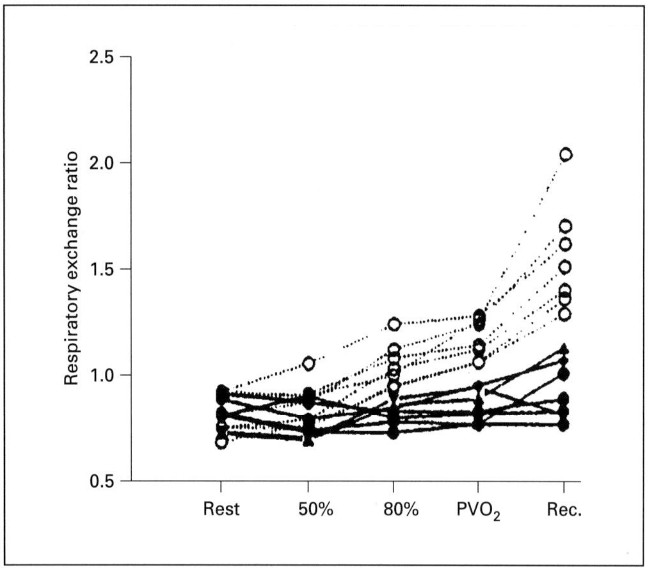

Fig. 3. Values of respiratory exchange ratio (RER) for 7 subjects with McArdle's (solid symbols) and 7 control subjects (open symbols) at rest, 50% peak VO_2, 80% peak VO_2, and after 3 min of recovery [from 17, with permission].

and metabolic changes causing increases in blood-borne glucose and FFA delivery to peripheral muscle.

A unique manifestation of the biochemical defect in myophosphorylase function and the inability to utilize glycogen during exercise is a failure of the respiratory exchange ratio (RER) to rise above one despite maximal exercise [17, 22]. This is reflected in figure 3 where the response to exercise in patients with McArdle's disease is contrasted with normal controls [17]. This may serve as a diagnostic finding in patients examined for typical symptoms. In addition, the biochemical defect impairs the ability of skeletal muscle to generate lactic acid during exercise [22]. In fact, muscle lactate can decrease during exercise in McArdle's disease patients [26]. Despite the inability to generate lactic acid, a ventilatory threshold has been described by some [3, 19, 27], although not by others [17]. As such, the hyperventilation noted during exercise may be related to other factors including discomfort and alternate metabolic signals [17]. In addition to hyperventilation, McArdle's disease patients demonstrate a hyperdynamic response during exercise. As such, an exaggerated heart rate response and cardiac output response have been described [15, 28].

Phosphofructokinase Deficiency

Deficiency of phosphofructokinase, Tarui disease, presents in a similar fashion to McArdle's disease with exercise-induced pain and contracture [11], although it is a rarer disorder [29]. In contrast to McArdle's disease, exercise intolerance occurs earlier and is more severe; a compensated hemolysis can also be seen [14]. Many of the responses to testing are similar to patients with myophosphorylase deficiency. As such, lactate does not rise (and often falls) with ischemic arm testing [5]. Similarly, the normal rise in the lactate/pyruvate ratio is not seen.

As expected, the functional consequences during maximal exercise testing are similar to those seen in patients with myophosphorylase deficiency. In a study of 7 patients with phosphofructokinase deficiency (PFKD), 5 with selective deficiency of CPT (CPTD) and 6 healthy controls, maximal VO_2 and arteriovenous oxygen deficiency were markedly lower in those with PFKD (fig. 4) [30]. Similarly, the rise in RER is attenuated [5]. Interestingly, peak exercise cardiac output and heart rate were similar among the three groups (fig. 4) [30]. These data suggest that the subnormal maximal VO_2 is primarily due to subnormal capacity for muscle O_2 extraction [30]. The main difference between PFKD and myophosphorylase deficiency is the inability of muscle deficient in PFK to utilize glucose. As a result of this inability to utilize glucose, muscle function during exercise should be closely tied to the ability to utilize FFA. This was confirmed by Haller and Lewis [31] who studied 4 PFK-deficient patients during intravenous glucose infusion, overnight fasting, and intravenous infusion of triglycerides and heparin. These interventions led to marked fluctuations in plasma FFA; lower FFA levels resulted in a lower maximal arteriovenous difference and lower maximal VO_2 [31]. This phenomenon has been termed the 'out-of-wind' phenomenon to describe deterioration in exercise capacity after high carbohydrate ingestion in PFKD patients.

Disorders of Lipid Metabolism

Fatty acids present an important fuel for muscle function, particularly with prolonged exertion and in the fasting state. The β-oxidation of fatty acids takes place in the mitochondria; the translocation of these FFA requires carnitine and CPT [8]. As such, two defects can be associated with impaired function of lipid metabolism during exercise, carnitine deficiency syndromes, and defects of CPT.

Carnitine Deficiency

Carnitine deficiency occurs when there is an insufficient amount of intracellular carnitine to accomplish the

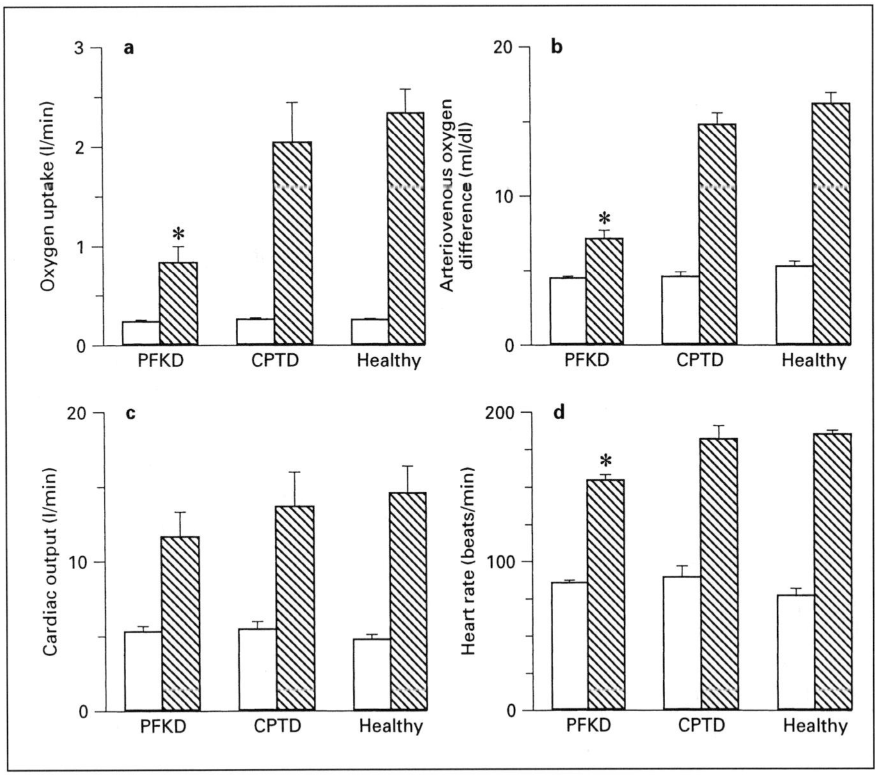

Fig. 4. Mean O_2 uptake (**a**), arteriovenous O_2 difference (**b**), cardiac output (**c**), and heart rate (**d**) at rest (□) and during peak exercise (▨) in patients with muscle phosphofructokinase deficiency (PFKD) and carnitine palmitoyltransferase deficiency (CPTD). * Significantly ($p < 0.001$) lower peak exercise values for PKFD patients than for CPTD patients or healthy subjects [from 30, with permission].

primary functions of carnitine [9]. Carnitine deficiency may occur as a primary deficiency although more frequently it is seen as a secondary deficiency [9, 32]. There are numerous causes of secondary systemic carnitine deficiency including Acyl-CoA dehydrogenase deficiency, organic acidemias, mitochondrial respiratory disorders and numerous systemic disorders [9, 32]. In 22 of 77 patients with mitochondrial myopathies, abnormal carnitine distribution was noted in muscle; this was equally seen in individuals with lipid storage myopathy (31.5%) and those with ragged red fibers (see below; 25.6%) [33]. Interestingly, this same group has reported improvement in these patients with *L*-carnitine supplementation [34].

Carnitine Palmitoyltransferase Deficiency (CPTD)

CPT exists as two genetically and catalytically distinct enzymes (CPT I and CPT II) [35]. Inherited defects in the CTP II gene cause a spectrum of disorders with symptoms including attacks of myalgia, cramps, and muscle stiffness or tenderness [8]. As expected from the biologic defect, symptoms are most commonly precipitated by prolonged exertion. In addition, symptoms can be precipitated with fasting, cold exposure or a high fat intake [8]. In contrast to the glycogenoses, ischemic exercise testing results in a normal lactate response. Maximal exercise testing has suggested that maximal VO_2 is generally not impaired (see fig. 2 and 4). Similarly, peak cardiac output and heart rate are similar to matched control subjects (see fig. 4) [30], as are other responses linked to oxidative phosphorylation [3, 5, 30, 36, 37]. Interestingly, the RER has been reported to be higher than normal, corresponding to the dependence on carbohydrate metabolism [5, 37, 38].

Disorders of Mitochondrial Function

The term mitochondrial myopathy refers to various syndromes with diverse pathologic, histochemical, and biochemical characteristics. These syndromes are often multisystemic with varying signs and symptoms affecting any organ system [39, 40]. The final pathogenesis of the different syndromes is a decline in mitochondrial adenosine triphosphate (ATP)-generating capacity leading to a deficit in energy production [41]. Exercise intolerance is one manifestation described in some patients [3, 41]. As muscle requires oxidative phosphorylation for ATP production, mitochondrial dysfunction can also produce muscular symptoms such as myalgia or weakness. Although these disorders were previously thought to be rare [39], a recent study estimated the prevalence of patients with mitochondrial myopathy and unexplained exertional limitation to be 8.5% [1].

The diagnosis of a metabolic or mitochondrial myopathy is complicated by the wide array of presenting signs and symptoms that can affect any organ system and vary in severity between patients [39]. The exact criteria required to make a diagnosis are also somewhat variable. A recent review recommended the following major diagnostic criteria: (1) abnormal histology (more than 2% ragged-red fibers in a muscle biopsy; (2) abnormal enzymatic activity (more than 20% reduction compared to age-matched controls), and (3) identification of genetic mutations with undisputed pathogenicity [42]. A detailed discussion of the histologic features, enzymatic assays, and genetic mutations is beyond the scope of this chapter but can be found in several recent excellent reviews [16, 43–46]. Physiologic testing can potentially be utilized as a screening tool for patients with suspected mitochondrial myopathy prior to performing a muscle biopsy.

Pulmonary Function Testing

Dandurand et al. [41] evaluated pulmonary function and blood lactate levels in 13 patients with mitochondrial myopathies, 7 patients with nonmetabolic myopathies, and 12 healthy control subjects. In general, pulmonary function tests were normal and similar between disease groups although the mean functional residual capacity was greater (119% predicted vs. 90% predicted; $p = 0.006$) for patients with mitochondrial myopathies compared to nonmetabolic myopathy patients. Flaherty et al. [1] recently evaluated 28 patients with unexplained dyspnea that were found to have mitochondrial myopathies and compared physiologic parameters to 11 healthy controls. No differences were noted in spirometry, lung volumes, or gas transfer. However, the maximal voluntary ventilation was lower in patients as compared to controls (111 vs. 186 l/min; $p < 0.0001$). These data suggest that mitochondrial myopathies may be present in patients with unexplained dyspnea and normal resting pulmonary function.

Respiratory Muscle Function

Several case reports have suggested that patients with mitochondrial myopathy may manifest respiratory muscle weakness [47, 48]. These reports describe 3 patients (ages 27–70) that presented with acute respiratory failure requiring prolonged weaning from ventilatory support. Interestingly, Dandurand et al. [41] did not report a significant prevalence of respiratory muscle weakness in their patients with either mitochondrial myopathy or nonmitochondrial myopathy. They described a maximal inspiratory pressure (MIP) below the normal range in 0/14 patients with mitochondrial myopathy and 2/6 patients with nonmitochondrial myopathy. Similarly, a maximum expiratory pressure (MEP) was below the normal range in only 4/14 of the patients with mitochondrial myopathy and 2/6 patients with nonmitochondrial myopathy.

In the 28 patients described by Flaherty et al. [1], a lower MIP (77 vs. 115% predicted; $p = 0.01$) and maximal transdiaphragmatic pressure ($P_{di}max$) (80 vs. 144 cm H_2O; $p = 0.0004$) was seen in patients with mitochondrial myopathies compared to normal controls. No difference in transdiaphragmatic sniff pressure (P_{di} sniff) was noted. Furthermore, patients were divided into a group that stopped exercise primarily due to dyspnea ($n = 16$) and a group that stopped exercise primarily due to fatigue ($n = 11$). There was a trend for patients that stopped due to dyspnea to have lower respiratory muscle pressures as measured by MIP (64 vs. 95% predicted; $p = 0.06$), maximal expiratory force (45 vs. 57% predicted; $p = 0.22$), P_{di} sniff (70 vs. 100 cm H_2O; $p = 0.01$), and $P_{di}max$ (61 vs. 115 cm H_2O; $p = 0.01$). Patients that stopped exercise primarily due to dyspnea also had a lower MVV (93 vs. 128 l/min; $p = 0.01$) compared to patients that stopped exercise due to fatigue.

These studies suggest that respiratory muscle weakness may be present in patients with a mitochondrial myopathy. Furthermore, respiratory muscle weakness may be more prevalent in patients that manifest respiratory symptoms compared to patients that complain primarily of fatigue.

Exercise Testing

Dandurand et al. [41] evaluated exercise performance and blood lactate levels in 13 patients with mitochondrial myopathies, 7 patients with nonmetabolic myopathies, and 12 health control subjects. Exercise results did not differ between disease groups. Patients with mitochondrial myopathy demonstrated a shorter duration of exercise (6.9 vs. 11.6 min, $p < 0.001$), lower percent predicted maximal work capacity (47 vs. 127, $p < 0.001$), lower percent predicted VO_2max (61 vs. 115, $p < 0.001$), lower VO_2/kg at maximal workload (17 vs. 39, $p < 0.001$), lower percent predicted VO_2 at anaerobic threshold (AT) (35 vs. 71, $p < 0.001$), lower percent predicted peak heart rate (85 vs. 101, $p < 0.001$), and lower percent predicted minute ventilation (52 vs. 76, $p < 0.01$) [41]. Interestingly, 12/13 patients with mitochondrial myopa-

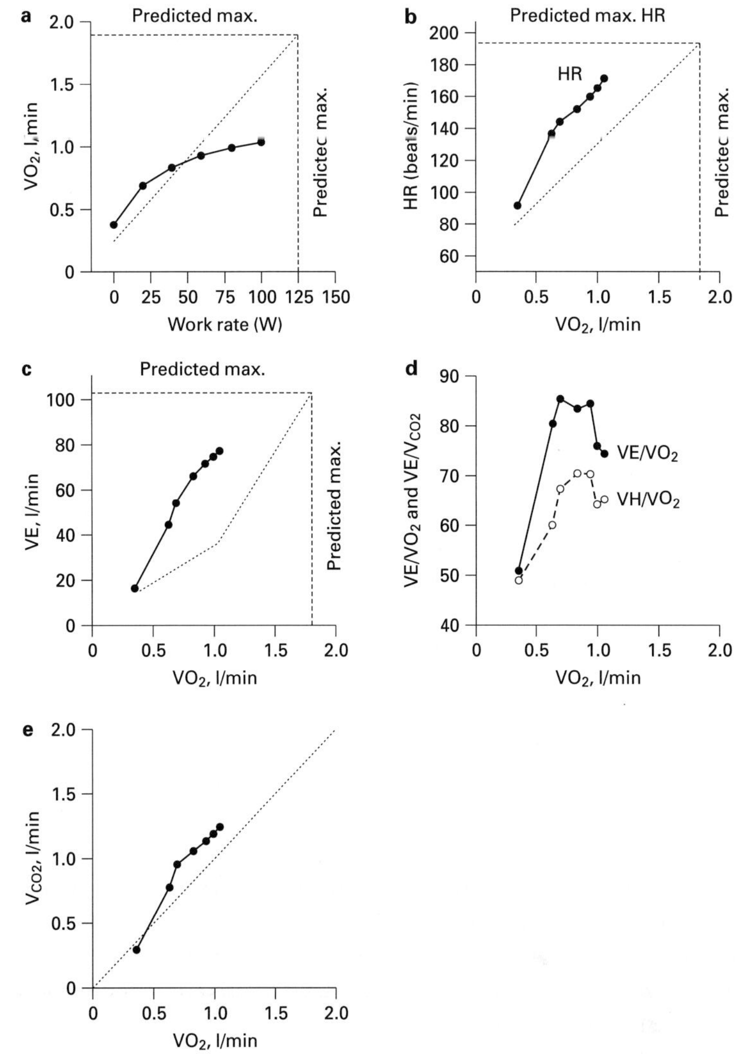

Fig. 5. Illustrative case of a 36-year-old female with a 1-year history of progressive exertional dyspnea, previously a 100-mile/week cyclist, with biopsy-proven mitochondrial myopathy. A markedly reduced aerobic capacity (**a**), hypercirculatory response (**b**), hyperventilatory response (**c, d**) and an indeterminate anaerobic threshold (**e**) are evident [from 1, with permission].

thies exhibited abnormal heart rate responses compared to 3/12 healthy controls and 3/7 nonmetabolic myopathy patients ($p = 0.02$). Heart rate abnormalities included fixed elevations and an abnormally elevated heart rate for a given work rate; a single patient had a heart rate below predicted [41].

In the series of Flaherty et al. [1] mitochondrial myopathy patients achieved a lower maximum VO_2 (67 vs. 104% predicted; $p < 0.0001$), lower AT (46 vs. 65% predicted VO_2max; $p = 0.03$), elevated heart rate response (defined as change in heart rate/change in VO_2, 91 vs. 41; $p = 0.01$), lower maximal minute ventilation (71 vs. 104 l/min; $p < 0.001$), and elevated VE/VO_2 (59 vs. 41; $p = 0.02$) and VE/VCO_2 (55 vs. 42; $p = 0.002$) at peak exercise. Importantly, individual responses were variable with 5 patients achieving a VO_2max greater than 90% of predicted. The response of a typical patient is illustrated in figure 5.

Hooper et al. [49] also described the exercise response for 3 patients with mitochondrial myopathy that presented with unexplained dyspnea. The exercise response was variable with VO_2max ranging from 22 to 84% predicted. In response to steady-state exercise, all patients demonstrated an early and rapid elevation of heart rate to greater

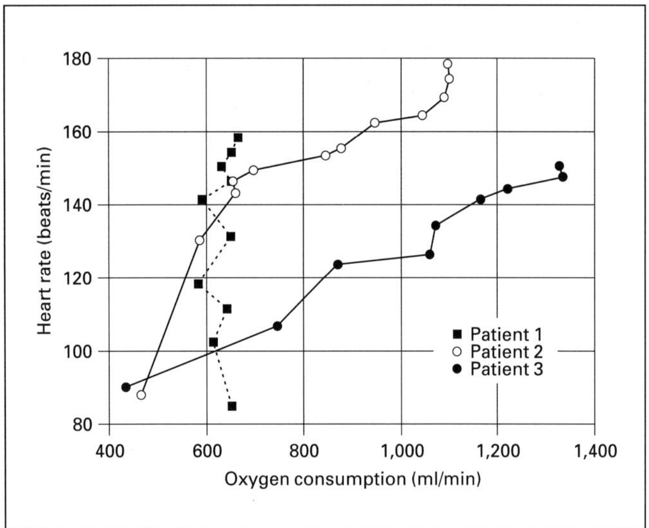

Fig. 6. Relationship between heart rate and VO_2 during progressive incremental exercise testing in 3 patients with mitochondrial enzyme deficiency presenting as exercise limitation in normal-appearing adults [from 49, with permission].

than 80% of predicted maximum (fig. 6). No evidence of cardiac dysfunction was present despite detailed testing which included right heart catheterization during exercise [49]. A single case report has confirmed an increased O_2 delivery but abnormal O_2 extraction (markedly reduced $C(a\text{-}v)O_2$) supporting abnormal skeletal muscle oxidative metabolism [50]. An additional study, using noninvasive estimates of cardiac output during maximal and submaximal exercise, confirmed exercise intolerance related to impaired peripheral oxygen extraction [51]. It is evident that a hyperdynamic circulatory response appears to be one of the more consistent findings in patients with metabolic myopathies [3, 50]. This may relate to the regulatory role that abnormalities in muscle oxidative metabolism may play on the cardiovascular response as a reflection of the normal coupling between O_2 utilization and delivery [51, 52]. Unfortunately, this hypercirculatory response is not specific for mitochondrial myopathies; some investigators have described impaired muscle oxidative metabolism in patients with exercise intolerance of unexplained origin [53].

Deficiency of oxidative metabolism results in more glycolytic anaerobic activity leading to increased lactate production within the tissue [54]. Several investigators have evaluated the ability of lactate levels, both at rest and with exercise, to identify patients with mitochondrial myopathies. It has also been suggested that the lactate to pyruvate level (normally <20) [54], and the subanaerobic threshold exercise test (SATET) [55], may be useful in screening patients for potential mitochondrial myopathies. The sensitivity and specificity of the SATET test was evaluated by Nashef and Lane [55] in 29 normal volunteers and 6 patients with mitochondrial myopathy. The AT and predicted work rate were calculated [56] and subjects exercised at 60 rpm for up to 15 min at 90% of their predicted work rate for AT. Venous lactate levels were collected pre-, post- and 30 min post-exercise. Only 2/29 controls had a peak lactate of >5 m*M*; all patients had a peak lactate level >5 m*M*. Using 5 m*M* as a cut-point, the sensitivity of this test was 100% and the specificity was 93% for identifying patients with mitochondrial myopathies [55].

Finsterer et al. [57] also evaluated the test characteristics for a lactate stress test for the diagnosis of mitochondrial myopathy. In this study, 31 healthy controls, 10 patients with nonmitochondrial myopathy, and 26 patients with mitochondrial myopathy were evaluated. Subjects exercised on a cycle ergometer for 15 min at a constant work rate of 30 W. Venous lactate was assayed at baseline; 5, 10, and 15 min after starting exercise; and 15 min after the completion of exercise. No control subjects and only 1 of the 10 nonmitochondrial myopathy patients experienced an increase in lactate level. This contrasted to 18 of the 31 patients with mitochondrial myopathy that had an abnormal lactate stress test. This corresponded to a sensitivity of 69% and a specificity of 90% for the diagnosis of a mitochondrial myopathy. These studies demonstrate that an elevated lactate level at a low workload can be seen in patients with mitochondrial myopathies. Although the sensitivity is not 100%, this finding may be useful to help screen patients for the presence of a mitochondrial myopathy prior to proceeding with a muscle biopsy and could help distinguish patients with a mitochondrial myopathy from patients with disorders of muscle glycogenolysis.

A hyperventilatory response has frequently been noted in mitochondrial disorders (see fig. 5) [1]. The etiology is unknown, but has been postulated to occur in response to the excess of CO_2 produced by the buffering of lactate [49]. An alternate hypothesis suggests that hyperventilation relates to an increase in respiratory drive originating in metabolically sensitive chemoreceptors localized in peripheral skeletal muscles, similar to the mechanism described to explain the hypercirculatory response [52].

It is evident from these data that patients with a mitochondrial myopathy, on average, present with a reduced peak VO_2, a hyperdynamic cardiac response, a normal to low AT, and a higher minute ventilation per level of VO_2. It is likely that deconditioning plays some part in this abnormal response [41, 58, 59]. After 8 weeks of training, a 30% increase in aerobic capacity, reduction in blood lactic acid and improvement in ADP recovery has been reported in patients with mitochondrial myopathy [59]. This improvement is greater (30%) than seen in patients with nonmetabolic myopathy (16%) and normal controls (10%) after 8 weeks of exercise training [58]. Importantly, the aerobic capacity of these patients after training was still reduced as compared to the sedentary normal control group before training.

Recent data have shed further light on the pathophysiologic basis of symptomatic limitation in patients with mitochondrial myopathies. Mitochondrial myopathy patients terminating exercise because of fatigue demonstrate less impairment of respiratory muscle function than those stopping exercise because of breathlessness [1]. In addition, increased breathlessness in these patients appears to relate to abnormal respiratory muscle recruitment during exercise.

Disorders of Muscle Bulk

Given the requirement of preserved muscle function to maintain a normal exercise capacity, several groups have examined the role of CPET in disorders of muscle bulk or strength. Carroll et al. [60] examined exercise capacity in 15 controls and 29 patients with a variety of neuromuscular diseases (10 metabolic myopathies, 8 muscular dystrophies and 11 miscellaneous disorders). Patients with neuromuscular disease exhibited a decreased VO_2max. Those with nonmetabolic myopathies achieved a maximal VO_2 of 19.2 ml/kg compared with 36.6 ml/kg in the control subjects. Similarly, Dandurand et al. [41] studied 7 patients with miscellaneous, nonmetabolic myopathies (inflammatory myopathies) noting a mean VO_2max % predicted of 62.1% which was similar to that achieved by 15 patients with mitochondrial disease but significantly lower than the 115.7% achieved by 12 healthy normals. Although the maximal achieved heart rate was similar in mitochondrial and nonmetabolic myopathy patients, the latter group experienced less frequent abnormalities (3/7 patients) than the former group (12/13 patients). Similarly, observed VE was similar between both groups of myopathic patients and a rapid, shallow breathing pattern was frequently seen in both patient groups (11/13 mitochondrial myopathy patients and 7/7 nonmetabolic myopathy patients). Lastly, peak lactate and the AT occurred at similar levels in both myopathic patient groups. The authors suggested that the pattern was most consistent with deconditioning in both groups. A similar level of aerobic limitation has been documented in a separate study of 11 patients with polymyositis [61]. Although 8 of 11 patients had normal pulmonary function, 9 of the patients exhibited a decreased maximal VO_2. The authors suggested that occult pulmonary hypertension could account for some of the observed limitation (7/11 exhibited echocardiographic evidence of pulmonary vascular abnormality). The importance of deconditioning is supported by the improvement in aerobic capacity documented with short-term training in patients with mitochondrial myopathies and patients with nonmetabolic myopathies (predominantly muscular dystrophies) [58]. After an 8-week rehabilitation program, patients with nonmetabolic myopathies improved submaximal workload achieved (4.90–5.64 METs), heart rate during exercise (148–134 beats/min), and lactate post-exercise (3.0–2.25 mmol/l) [58].

Several groups have reported similar data in patients with late sequelae of poliomyelitis. Stanghelle et al. [62] examined 68 consecutive patients with post-polio syndrome (31 exercised with arm ergometry and 37 with bicycle ergometry). Although mean FVC was normal for the patient group, a pronounced reduction in maximal VO_2 was seen (32 with $VO_2max < 60\%$ predicted and 16 $< 50\%$ predicted); this was particularly evident in females. Fifteen patients were felt to have 'pulmonary limitation' based on a maximal VE/MVV ratio above 70%. The authors suggested a strong component of deconditioning. Willen et al. [63] extended these findings by studying 32 patients with post-polio syndrome. Decrements in maximal VO_2 were seen among males (69% predicted) and females (79% predicted). Interestingly, AT was lower in males (34% maximal VO_2) than females (47% maximal VO_2). Strong correlations were noted between leg muscle strength and peak VO_2 and workload. As in other nonmetabolic myopathies, patients with post-polio symptoms have demonstrated improvement in aerobic capacity with exercise training suggesting some component of poor conditioning [64]. Additional data have been reported in a group of 5 patients with significant respiratory muscle involvement (mean VC 38% predicted) as a sequelae of polio [65]. All patients exhibited decreased exercise tolerance with a respiratory limitation in all but 1 of the patients. Importantly, all patients demonstrated impaired diaphragmatic function at rest and a decrease in peak gastric pressure during inspiration at peak exercise. Although a definitive conclusion cannot be reached, this pattern of breathing supports increased accessory muscle recruitment during exercise. As such, nonmetabolic disorders are generally associated with impaired aerobic capacity, strongly suggestive of poor conditioning. With more severe disease, respiratory limitation is more likely to be seen, particularly in the presence of respiratory muscle involvement.

Conclusion

Given the importance of skeletal muscle to normal exercise response, CPET is frequently abnormal in patients with myopathies. Metabolic and nonmetabolic myopathies demonstrate stereotypical responses although the contribution of deconditioning confounds the interpretation of testing in both groups of disorders.

References

1 Flaherty KR, Wald J, Weisman IM, Zeballos RJ, Schork MA, Blaivas M, Rubenfire M, Martinez FJ: Unexplained exertional limitation. Characterization of patients with a mitochondrial myopathy. Am J Respir Crit Care Med 2001;164:425–432.
2 Taivassalo T, Reddy H, Matthews PM: Muscle responses to exercise in health and disease. Neurol Clin 2000;18:15–34.
3 Elliot DL, Neil RM, Buist M, Goldberg L, Kennaway NG, Phil D, Powell BR, Kuehl KS: Metabolic myopathies: Evaluation by graded exercise testing. Medicine 1989;68:163–172.
4 Clay AS, Behnia M, Brown KK: Mitochondrial disease. A pulmonary and critical-care medicine perspective. Chest 2001;120:634–648.
5 Haller RG, Bertocci LA: Exercise evaluation of metabolic myopathies; in Engel A, Franzini-Armstrong C (eds): Myology. Basic and Clinical, ed 2. New York, McGraw-Hill, 1994.
6 Taivassalo T, Matthews PM, DeStefano N, Sripathi N, Genge A, Karpati G, Arnold DL: Combined aerobic training and dichloroacetate improve exercise capacity and indices of aerobic metabolism in muscle cytochrome oxidase deficiency. Neurology 1996;47:529–534.
7 DeStefano N, Matthews PM, Ford B, Genge A, Karpati G, Arnold DL: Short-term dichloroacetate treatment improves indices of aerobic metabolism in patients with mitochondrial disorders. Neurology 1995;45:1193–1198.
8 Zierz S: Carnitine palmitoyltransferase deficiency; in Engel A, Franzini-Armstrong C (eds): Myology. Basic and Clinical, ed 2. New York, McGraw-Hill, 1994, pp 1577–1585.
9 Breningstall GN: Carnitine deficiency syndromes. Ped Neurol 1990;6:75–81.
10 Larsson NG, Oldfors A: Mitochondrial myopathies. Acta Physiol Scand 2001;171:385–393.
11 Martin A, Haller RG, Barohn R: Metabolic myopathies. Curr Opin Rheumatol 1994;6: 552–558.
12 Amato AA: Acid maltase deficiency and related disorders. Neurol Clin 2000;18:151–163
13 Kubisch C, Wicklein EM, Jentsch TJ: Molecular diagnosis of McArdle disease: revised genomic structure of the myophosphorylase gene and identification of a novel mutation. Hum Mut 1998;12:27–32.
14 DiMauro S, Tsujino S: Nonlysosomal glycogenoses; in Engel A, Franzini-Armstrong C (eds): Myology. New York, McGraw-Hill, 1994, pp 1554–1576.
15 Braakhekke JP, De Bruin MI, Stegeman DF, Wevers RA, Binkhorst RA, Joostein EMG: The second wind phenomenon in McArdle's disease. Brain 1986;109:1087–1101.
16 Pourmand R: Metabolic myopathies: a diagnostic evaluation. Neurol Clin 2000;18:1–13.
17 Riley M, Nicholls DP, Nugent AM, Steele IC, Bell N, Davies PM, Stanford CF, Patterson VH: Respiratory gas exchange and metabolic responses during exercise in McArdle's disease. J Appl Physiol 1993;75:745–754.
18 Haller RG, Lewis SF, Cook JD, Blomqvist CG: Myophosphorylase deficiency impairs muscle oxidative metabolism. Ann Neurol 1985;17: 196–199.
19 Hagberg JM, Coyle EF, Carroll JE, Miller JM, Martin WH, Brooke MH: Exercise hyperventilation in patients with McArdle's disease. J Appl Physiol: Environ Exercise Physiol 1982; 52:991–994.
20 Kissel JT, Beam W, Bresolin N, et al: Physiologic assessment of phosphorylate mutase deficiency. Neurology 1985;35:828–833.
21 Andersen KI, Lund-Johansen P, Clausen G: Metabolic and circulatory responses to muscular exercise in a subject with glycogen storage disease (McArdle's disease). Scand J Clin Lab Invest 1969;24:105–113.
22 Chaussain M, Camus F, Defoligny C, Eymard B, Fardeau M: Exercise intolerance in patients with McArdle's disease or mitochondrial myopathies. Eur J Med 1992;1:457–463.
23 DeStefano N, Argov Z, Matthews PM, Karpati G, Arnold DL: Impairment of muscle mitochondrial oxidative metabolism in McArdle's disease. Muscle Nerve 1996;19:764–769.
24 Mineo I, Kono N, Yamada Y, Hara N, Kiyokawa H, Hamaguchi T, Kawachi M, Yamasaki T, Nakajima H, Kuwajima M, et al: Glucose infusion abolishes the excessive ATP degradation in working muscles of a patient with McArdle's disease. Muscle Nerve 1990;13:618–620.
25 Pearson C, Rimer D, Mommaerts WFHM: A metabolic myopathy due to absence of muscle phosphorylase. Am J Med 1961;30:502–517.
26 Lofberg M, Lindholm H, Naveri H, Majander A, Suomalainen A, Paetau A, Sovijarvi A, Harkonen M, Somer H: ATP, phosphocreatine and lactate in exercising muscle in mitochondrial disease and McArdle's disease. Neuromusc Disord 2001;11:370–375.
27 Hagberg JM, King DS, Rogers MA, Montain SJ, Jilka SM, Kohrt WM, Heller SL: Exercise and recovery ventilatory and VO_2 responses of patients with McArdle's disease. J Appl Physiol 1990;68:1393–1398.
28 Lewis SF, Hall RG: The pathophysiology of McArdle's disease: clues to regulation in exercise and fatigue. J Appl Physiol 1986;61:391–401.
29 Vora S, Durham S, deMartinville B, George DL, Francke U: Assignment of the human gene for muscle-type phosphofructokinase (PFKM) to chromosome 1 (Region CEN-Q32) using somatic cell hybrids and monoclonal anti-M antibody. Somat Cell Genet 1982;8:95–104.
30 Lewis SF, Vora S, Haller RG: Abnormal oxidative metabolism and O_2 transport in muscle phosphofructokinase deficiency. J Appl Physiol 1991;70:391–398.
31 Haller RG, Lewis SF: Glucose-induced exertional fatigue in muscle phosphofructokinase deficiency. N Engl J Med 1991;324:364–367.
32 Infante JP, Huszagh VA: Secondary carnitine deficiency and impaired docosahexaenoic (22:6n-3) acid synthesis: a common denominator in the pathophysiology of diseases of oxidative phosphorylation and β-oxidation. FEBS Letters 2000;468:1–5.
33 Campos Y, Huertas R, Bautista J, Gutierrez G, Segura D, Villanueva M, Cabello A, Alesso L, Arenas J: Muscle carnitine deficiency and lipid storage myopathy in patients with mitochondrial myopathy. Muscle Nerve 1993;16:778–781.
34 Campos Y, Huertas R, Lorenzo G, Bautista J, Gutierrez G, Aparicio M, Alesso L, Arenas J: Plasma carnitine insufficiency and effectiveness of L-carnitine therapy in patients with mitochondrial myopathy. Muscle Nerve 1993; 16:150–153.
35 Vladutiu GD: Biochemical and molecular correlations in carnitine palmitoyltransferase II deficiency. Muscle Nerve 1999;22:949–951.

36 Haller RG, Lewis SF, Cook JD, Blomqvist CG: Hyperkinetic circulation during exercise in neuromuscular disease. Neurology 1983;33: 1283–1287.
37 Carroll JE, Brooke MH, DeVivo DC, Kaiser KK, Hagberg JM: Biochemical and physiologic consequences of carnitine palmityltransferase deficiency. Muscle Nerve 1978;1:103–110.
38 Layzer RB, Havel RJ, McIlroy MB: Partial deficiency of carnitine palmityltransferase: Physiologic and biochemical consequences. Neurology 1980;30:627–633.
39 Chinnery PF, Turnbull DM: Mitochondrial medicine. QJM 1997;90:657–667.
40 Andreu AL, Hanna MG, Reichmann H, Bruno C, Penn AS, Tanji K, Pallotti F, Iwata S, Bonilla E, Lach B, et al: Exercise intolerance due to mutations in the cytochrome b gene of mitochondrial DNA. N Engl J Med 1999;341:1037–1044.
41 Dandurand RJ, Matthews PM, Arnold DL, Eidelman DH: Mitochondrial disease: Pulmonary function, exercise performance, and blood lactate levels. Chest 1995;108:182–189.
42 Walker UA, Collins S, Byrne E: Respiratory chain encephalomyopathies: A diagnostic classification. Eur Neurol 1996;36:260–267.
43 Shoffner JM: Metabolic myopathies: Mitochondrial myopathy diagnosis. Neurol Clin 2000;18:105–123.
44 Vladutiu GD: Metabolic myopathies: The molecular diagnosis of metabolic myopathies. Neurol Clin 2000;18:53–104.
45 Zeviani M, Tiranti V, Piantadosi C: Reviews in molecular medicine: Reviews in mitochondrial disorders. Medicine 1998;77:59–72.
46 Simon DK, Johns DR: Mitochondrial disorders: Clinical and genetic features. Annu Rev Med 1999;50:111–127.
47 Cros D, Palliyath S, DiMauro S, Ramirez C, Shamsnia M, Wizer B: Respiratory failure revealing mitochondrial myopathy in adults. Chest 1992;101:824–828.
48 O'Brien A, Blaivas M, Albers J, Wald J, Watts C: A case of respiratory muscle weakness due to cytochrome *c* oxidase enzyme deficiency. Eur Respir J 1998;12:742–744.
49 Hooper RG, Thomas AR, Kearl RA: Mitochondrial enzyme deficiency causing exercise limitation in normal-appearing adults. Chest 1995;107:317–322.
50 Haller RG, Henriksson KG, Jorfeldt L, Hultman E, Wibom R, Sahlin K, Areskog N, Gunder M, Ayyad K, Blomqvist CG, et al: Deficiency of skeletal muscle succinate dehydrogenase and aconitase. J Clin Invest 1991;88: 1197–1206.
51 Vissing J, Galbo H, Haller RG: Exercise fuel mobilization in mitochondrial myopathy: A metabolic dilemma. Ann Neurol 1996;40:655–662.
52 Haller RG, Lewis SF, Estabrook RW, DiMauro S, Servidei S, Foster DW: Exercise intolerance, lactic acidosis, and abnormal cardiopulmonary regulation in exercise associated with adult skeletal muscle cytochrome *c* oxidase deficiency. J Clin Invest 1989;84:155–161.
53 Argov Z, DeStefano N, Taivassalo T, Chen J, Karpati G, Arnold DL: Abnormal oxidative metabolism in exercise intolerance of undetermined origin. Neuromusc Disord 1997;7:99–104.
54 Argov Z: Functional evaluation techniques in mitochondrial disorders. Eur Neurol 1998;39: 65–71.
55 Nashef L, Lane RJM: Screening for mitochondrial cytopathies: The sub-anaerobic threshold exercise test (SATET). J Neurol Neurosurg Psychiatry 1989;52:1090–1094.
56 Reinhard U, Muller PH, Schmulling RM: Determination of anaerobic threshold by the ventilation equivalent in normal individuals. Respiration 1979;38:36–42.
57 Finsterer J, Shorny S, Capek J, Cerny-Zacharias C, Pelzl B, Messner R, Bittner RE, Mamoli B: Lactate stress test in the diagnosis of mitochondrial myopathy. J Neurol Sci 1998;159: 176–180.
58 Taivassalo T, DeStefano N, Chen J, Karpati G, Arnold DL, Argov Z: Short-term aerobic training response in chronic myopathies. Muscle Nerve 1999;22:1239–1243.
59 Taivassalo T, DeStefano N, Argov Z, Matthews PM, Chen J, Genge A, Karpati G, Arnold DL: Effects of aerobic training in patients with mitochondrial myopathies. Neurology 1998;50:1055–1060.
60 Carroll JE, Hagberg JM, Brooke MH, Shumate JB: Bicycle ergometry and gas exchange measurements in neuromuscular diseases. Arch Neurol 1979;36:457–461.
61 Hebert CA, Byrnes TJ, Baethge BA, Wolf RE, Kinasewitz GT: Exercise limitation in patients with polymyositis. Chest 1990;98:352–357.
62 Stanghelle JK, Festvag L, Aksnes AK: Pulmonary function and symptom-limited exercise testing in subjects with late sequelae of poliomyelitis. Scand J Rehab Med 1993;25:125–129.
63 Willen C, Cider A, Sunnerhagen KS: Physical performance in individuals with late effects of polio. Scand J Rehab Med 1999;31:244–249.
64 Halstead LS, Rossi CD: Post-polio syndrome: results of a survey of 539 survivors. Orthopedics 1985;8:845–850.
65 Weinberg J, Borg J, Bevegard S, Sinderby C: Respiratory response to exercise in postpolio patients with severe inspiratory muscle dysfunction. Arch Phys Med Rehabil 1999;80: 1095–1100.

Fernando J. Martinez, MD
1500 E. Medical Center Drive
3916 Taubman Center
Ann Arbor, MI 48109 (USA)
Tel. +1 734 763 2540, Fax +1 734 936 5048
E-Mail fmartine@umich.edu

Weisman IM, Zeballos RJ (eds): Clinical Exercise Testing.
Prog Respir Res. Basel, Karger, 2002, vol 32, pp 254–263

Role of Cardiopulmonary Exercise Testing in Lung and Heart-Lung Transplantation

Trevor J. Williams William R. Slater

Lung Transplant Service Medical, Department of Respiratory Medicine, Alfred Hospital, Monash University, Prahran (Melbourne), Australia

Summary

Lung transplantation has evolved over the last 2 decades as an important treatment option for severe pulmonary and pulmonary vascular disease. Initially, survival and duration of survival were the only outcome measures measured. Function outcomes including cardiopulmonary exercise testing have only more recently been reported. Exercise capacity seems to correlate very poorly with measured lung function, but early onset lactic acidosis and premature exercise termination at a substantially reduced VO_2 peak are seen almost universally. Cardiac and ventilatory limitation are only sporadically seen. It appears that peripheral muscle dysfunction due to pre- and posttransplant factors is the most frequent cause of exercise limitation. Although clear criteria for exercise testing of lung transplant recipients have yet to be developed, cardiopulmonary exercise testing (CPET) will help clarify the degree and mechanism of exercise limitation, aiding decision making as to the timing of transplantation. Furthermore, posttransplantation the assessment of vocational and exercise capacity as well as detection of allograft dysfunction can be greatly aided by CPET.

Introduction

Solid organ transplantation has been one of the great medical miracles of the 20th century. The notion of replacing diseased organs dates back many centuries. The first attempt at lung replacement is attributed to the surgeon/physiologist Vladimir Demikhov who, having returned from WWII, performed a remarkable series of experiments in the second half of the 1940s. After initially performing heterotopic heart transplantation he moved on to perform heart-lung transplantation (HLTx) in over 50 dogs [1], although the lungs demonstrated the capacity for gas exchange, within 1 week all dogs died because of progressive ventilatory failure. These experiments were both instructive and remarkable. The recognition that complete denervation of both lungs seems to result in progressive respiratory failure led Demikhov to single lung transplantation with the first dog autotransplant surviving 1 month.

In 1963, Hardy et al. [2] described the first attempt at human single lung transplantation (SLTx). Although the man died 18 days later of renal failure, the ability for the transplanted lung to contribute to gas exchange in the recipient was clearly demonstrated. Through the 1960s and 1970s, approximately 40 attempts at lung transplantation were made worldwide, the longest reported survival in this era was a SLTx recipient with silicosis who survived 10 months [3] spending all but a few weeks in hospital during this time. The 1980s saw the first long-term quality survival in lung transplant recipients. In 1982, the Stanford University Group led by Reitz et al. [4] reported two long-term survivors, one having eventually survived for 5 years, having received HLTx for pulmonary vascular disease. The following year, the Toronto Lung Transplant Group successfully performed SLTx resulting in almost a decade of quality survival in that recipient [5].

Double lung transplantation was first performed successfully in 1985 as an 'en bloc' procedure [6] although the incidence of anastomotic complications was alarmingly high. The procedure was subsequently modified in 1989 to the bilateral (sequential) lung transplant (BLTx) procedure utilizing a clam shell incision and usually obviating the requirement for cardiopulmonary bypass [7]. Live donor lung transplantation was first performed in the early 1990s using the procedure developed by Starnes and co-workers at the University of Southern California. It has generally been performed utilizing a single lobe from each of two living donors which is transplanted ipsilaterally and orthotopically into a smaller single recipient [8, 9].

Measurement of Outcomes in Lung Transplantation

Survival

In the first two decades of human lung transplantation from 1963, the length of survival from the point of engraftment was the principle and often only outcome variable measured. Patient survival immediately postoperatively, followed by reports of increasing lengths of time out of hospital became the key reported outcome variables. Earlier on, however, reference was made to physiological effects including the ability of the transplanted lung to support gas exchange, and interestingly an understanding of potential complications of two different lungs with quite different mechanical properties as occurs in single lung transplantation for emphysema [10].

By the end of the 1980s there had been a dramatic increase in the number of lung transplant procedures occurring worldwide to the point that meaningful actuarial assessments of survival could be made in large patients populations. Two major registries have been reporting outcomes: the International Society of Heart and Lung Transplant Registry and the St Louis International Lung Transplant Registry. Although there were differences in terms of completeness of data in each of the registries, by 1995 the Registries were reporting 1- and 5-year survivals of 62–78% and 40–50% in lung transplantation and HLTx [11, 12]. It became evident that two important trends in survival analysis were occurring. There had been a progressive improvement in survival virtually completely attributable to improved 90-day survival, without evidence of improvement in survival in long-term survivors who had already survived the initial posttransplant period. The second important feature was that survival did seem to vary considerably depending on pretransplant diagnosis with patients with emphysema and cystic fibrosis having better survival posttransplant than those with pulmonary fibrosis or pulmonary hypertension.

Lung Function

Towards the end of the 1980s and early 1990s transplant groups around the world had sufficient long-term survivors that outcomes from lung transplantation including lung function could be reported. These generally showed a dramatic effect on lung function by lung transplantation with HLTx and BLTx resulting in only mildly restricted spirometry with only a slight reduction in diffusing capacity and a normal PA-a O_2 gradient. Improvement in spirometry occurs during the first 2 years following bilateral lung transplantation unless complications supervened [13, 14].

Spirometry following SLTx is almost always abnormal, generally reflecting the underlying pretransplant pathology. Patients receiving SLTx for obstructive lung disease generally have an FEV_1 around 50–65% of predicted but with quite a broad range. Generally, for SLTx recipients diffusing capacity is significantly reduced and PA-a O_2 gradient significantly widened. Spirometry improves little in SLTx recipients beyond 3 months posttransplantation [13, 14]. Live donor lobar transplantation is typically associated with a mild restrictive ventilatory defect and diffusing capacity at the lower end of the normal range [8, 9]. The spirometry and diffusing capacity reported generally reflect stable patients without significant complication after lung transplantation. Many factors, however, will impact on lung function including the presence of pleural complications, diaphragmatic injury or injury to the lung allograft caused by rejection or allograft infection. The most feared complication in the long-term recipient is the development of chronic rejection in the form of bronchiolitis obliterans syndrome (BOS) manifesting as a progressive obstructive ventilatory defect.

Functional Class

Those directly involved in lung transplant programs have little doubt of the substantial improvement in functional class of successfully transplanted individuals. Nevertheless, data reporting New York Heart Association (NYHA) functional class show all patients are NYHA Class III or IV pretransplantation with 70% of patients improved to NYHA class 1 and 21% to NYHA class II assessed 2–4 years posttransplant, i.e. 91% were at least one NYHA class better [15].

More recently, formal measures of quality of life have been reported with Gross et al. [16] showing a substantial

Table 1. Exercise responses for single (SLTx), bilateral (BLTx) and heart-lung (HLTx) transplant recipient expressed as mean reported in each study [as referenced]

	SLTx	BLTx	HLTx
Six-minute walk test			
6 MWT, m	480–670 [51, 52]	600–700 [51, 52]	NR
Incremental CPETx			
Peak work rate, % predicted	30–45 [24, 53–55]	30–46 [24, 53, 54]	30 [54]
Peak VO_2, % predicted	41–58 [19, 20, 24, 54, 55]	40–59 [19, 20, 24, 54]	38–52 [19, 22, 54]
Symptoms (Borg scale)	legs > breathing [14]	legs > breathing [14]	legs > breathing [14]
Peak HR, % predicted	69–81 [19, 20, 24, 54, 55]	67–90 [19, 20, 24, 54]	59–83 [19, 22, 54]
Peak O_2 pulse, % predicted	60–65 [20, 54]	59–70 [20, 54]	63–64 [22, 54]
VE_{max}/MVV, %	47–63 [19, 20, 24, 55, 56]	33–53 [19, 20, 24, 56]	39 [19]
SaO_2% rest/peak exercise	94–97/90–94 [19, 20, 24]	95–97/94–97 [19, 20, 24]	NR/97 [19]
$PAO_2 - PaO_2$ (max ex), mm Hg	25–41 [54, 55]	31 [54]	18–33 [22, 54]
V_D/V_T	increased [54, 55]	increased [54]	increased [22, 54]
AT as % of predicted VO_2max	31–41 [19, 24]	42–43 [19, 24]	34 [19]

NR = Not reported.

positive impact of lung transplantation on the dimensions of physical functions, health perception, social function and role function using the MOS20 health profile. These benefits appear to be maintained until BOS supervenes. Generally, however, return to work results have been disappointing with Craven et al. [17] reporting only 38% of recipients returning to paid employment following lung transplantation.

Six-Minute Walk Test

The results of the six-minute walk test have been quite extensively reported as an outcome measure following lung transplantation. Generally, patients range from 200 to 400 m in 6 min pretransplant, improving to 500–700 m posttransplant, maintaining this benefit unless serious complications supervene [14]. Due to its simplicity, this test has developed wide currency in reporting outcome from lung transplantation.

Incremental Cardiopulmonary Exercise Testing (Table 1)

Treadmill exercise studies of utilizing the Bruce Protocol have been reported occasionally. Williams et al. [13] reported that no patient prior to transplantation completed Bruce Stage I despite the use of supplemental oxygen. Overall, almost 75% of all recipients achieved Bruce Stage II or better posttransplant. The outcome in double-lung transplant recipients appeared slightly better than single-lung transplant recipients (stage 2.7 ± 0.3 vs. 2.0 ± 0.25; mean ± SEM).

Progressive incremental cardiopulmonary exercise testing (CPET) with measurement of ventilation, VO_2 and VCO_2 have been rarely reported in those awaiting lung transplantation. Theodore et al. [93] reported results of 10 patients with severe pulmonary vascular disease having a group mean VO_2 peak of 9.4 ml/kg/min (24% of predicted) using a treadmill exercise protocol. This substantial degree of exercise limitation has also been confirmed by two other reports [13, 18] using incremental bicycle ergometer protocols. Nevertheless, these were generally patients well enough to participate in CPET protocols without requiring supplemental oxygen and if anything may overestimate the maximum exercise capacity of the group.

A number of authors have now reported a significant reduction in VO_2 peak using CPET protocols measured approximately 3 months posttransplant (usually following formal rehabilitation) [18–24]. The mean VO_2 peak reported ranged from 14 to 18 ml/kg/min in these studies (a range of 45–52% predicted). Similar results have also been reported in pediatric lung transplant recipients [25]. A similar degree of exercise limitation seems to occur (despite differences in the magnitude of lung function improvement) in HLTx, BLTx and SLTx recipients [23, 24]. There does not appear to be any systematic impact of pretransplant diagnosis on posttransplant exercise capacity [21]. Stiebellehner et al. [26] have demonstrated that lung transplant recipients are capable of demonstrating significant (albeit small) responses to supervised training programs. Nevertheless, beyond 3 months, lung function generally improves slightly, but exercise capacity seems to improve very little, with no authors reporting a patient group returning to normal exercise capacity.

Exercise Responses and Exercise Limitation after Lung Transplantation

Although there are significant differences in terms of exercise responses comparing HLTx, BLTx, and SLTx recipients, a number of common features are to be found on incremental exercise testing. Resting heart rate is generally high, the anaerobic threshold occurs very early in exercise and patients generally report leg tiredness as the predominant symptom at exercise termination [23, 24]. Although many factors may impact on oxygen delivery to exercising muscle (e.g. cardiac response, oxygenation of mixed venous blood by the lung, haemoglobin concentration), the unifying factor appears to be an abnormality of oxygen uptake or utilization by peripheral muscles.

Cardiac Response

In HLTx recipients, cardiac denervation is present and, there is at least a theoretical concern of the possibility that abnormal cardiac responses result in exercise limitation. The denervated heart response to exercise is abnormal with a high resting heart rate, and initial increases in cardiac output being entirely due to contractility [27]. A combination of a low cardiac output at peak exercise and high lactate initially lead to speculation as to the possibility to cardiac limitation in patients with a transplanted heart [28]. Kavanagh et al. [29] noted that these cardiac outputs were not measured at the same absolute workload when compared to controls, and that arterio-venous oxygen difference was normal suggesting cardiac output and oxygen delivery was normal at matched work rate. Subsequently, Jensen et al. [30] using acetylene-breathing methods confirmed a normal relationship between cardiac output and oxygen consumption in cardiac transplant recipients. The cardiac allograft is susceptible to early ischemic injury, rejection or transplant coronary disease which need to be considered in HLTx as cardiac causes of premature exercise termination.

Right-ventricular impairment may contribute to exercise limitation particularly in those with high pulmonary vascular resistance receiving SLTx [31–33]. Nevertheless, it appears that cardiac limitation is a rare and sporadic event among lung transplant recipients and does not generally explain the almost universal reduction in exercise capacity.

Exercise-Induced Hypoxemia

Generally, desaturation is seen only in SLTx at peak exercise [23, 24]. HLTx or BLTx recipients who are free of complications do not desaturate at peak exercise. Any desaturation in HLTx or BLTx recipients at peak exercise indicates graft dysfunction. In single lung transplant recipients, mild desaturation does not indicate allograft dysfunction.

Ventilation

HLTx and BLTx recipients (unless with significant allograft dysfunction) do not approach ventilatory limitation at the point of exercise termination. Martinez et al. [34] studied 7 single lung transplant recipients for obstructive lung disease and showed expiratory flow limitation utilizing exercise flow-volume studies. Generally, single lung transplant recipients approach or reach ventilatory limitation at the point of exercise cessation.

Exercising Skeletal Muscle Dysfunction

There is now mounting evidence that exercise limitation following lung transplantation is due primarily to abnormalities of the exercising skeletal muscles. A number of abnormalities have now been reported and a combination of pre- and posttransplant factors seems likely. The reduced skeletal muscle oxidative capacity is probably due to a combination of a number of factors.

The quadriceps femoris muscle mass is substantially reduced in severe COPD [35], and this seems to persist posttransplant. A number of factors may be responsible including nutrition [36], the effects of drugs particularly corticosteroids [37], disuse/deconditioning, and endocrine effects of severe respiratory disease (e.g. low testosterone levels in males with severe COPD) [38].

Using ^{31}P magnetic resonance spectroscopy, Evans et al. [39] demonstrated a lower resting skeletal muscle pH with an earlier and more rapid fall of pH on exercise, suggesting early anaerobic metabolism comparing lung transplantation recipients and matched controls. A subsequent study using near infrared spectroscopy [40] showed that myoglobin oxygen saturation is normal despite very early onset of anaerobic metabolism strongly, suggesting that oxygen utilisation rather than delivery was limiting.

A recently reported study of quadriceps femoris biopsies in stable lung transplant recipients [41] has shown a number of abnormalities including a marked reduction in type 1 fiber proportion as has previously been reported in patients with severe emphysema [42, 43]. The reduction in type 1 fiber proportion is very significant (25 vs. 56%) comparing lung transplant recipients to normal sedentary controls. Marked reduction in the mitochondrial enzymes glutamate dehydrogenase, citrate synthase and oxyglutertate dehydrogenase, as well as 3-hydroxacyl CoA hydrogenase (HADH) was also demonstrated. Furthermore, marked reduction in mitochondrial ATP production to an array of substrates was seen. At rest, muscle fibers had higher lactate concentrations and IMP content consistent with a high reliance on anaerobic metabolism. Whether these changes represent a primary muscle defect or simply the effects of prolonged reduction in activity is unclear. It seems likely that the calcineurin antagonist cyclosporin A is responsible in part for the marked reduction in mitochondrial oxidative capacity as has been demonstrated both in vivo and in vitro in rats [44, 45]. Nevertheless, they probably do explain the very early rise in plasma lactate concentration and premature exercise termination in this group of patients.

Other abnormalities in the skeletal muscle of lung transplant have been suggested. Although potassium homeostasis is abnormal [46], no abnormality of Na/K pump density or activity or Na/K ATPase enzyme activity is seen [47]. Sarcoplasmic reticulum function (Ca release, uptake on Ca ATPase activity) seems reduced when account is taken of the decreased type I fiber proportion [48].

In summary, the common factor limiting exercise in stable fully rehabilitated patients following lung transplantation is leg fatigue. SLTx recipients approach or reach ventilatory limitation (with mild desaturation) at the point of exercise termination. Stable HLTx and BLTx recipients do not have evidence of ventilatory limitation nor desaturation and generally appear limited by their exercising muscles. Nevertheless, the unifying factor across all lung transplant recipients appears to be a peripheral defect of oxygen utilization is the quadriceps femoris muscles.

Conduct of Cardiopulmonary Exercise Tests in Lung Transplant Recipients

CPET presents significant challenges in patients with severe lung disease both before and after lung transplantation. The exercise responses are almost always abnormal and the focus is generally on assessing the contribution of ventilatory, cardiac and peripheral factors to exercise limitation.

Pretransplant CPET is infrequently performed because exercise is inevitably severely limited due to the underlying disease. Exercise is usually terminated before the anaerobic threshold can be determined. Frequently, severe exercise-induced hypoxemia leads to premature termination of the CPET. Attempting to supplement oxygen during the CPET adds significantly to the complexity of testing and is often quite impractical for some laboratories. A second important technical point is to make sure increments are appropriate – typically 5–10 W/min is suitable – as the rate of incremental increase in workload may impact on final measured W_{peak} and VO_2peak [49]. Generally, CPET is performed to confirm that the degree of exercise limitation reported by the patient is matched by objective measurement. In the illustrative case 1, lung transplantation when initially referred was likely to have been quite premature, despite the patient's complaints of severe exercise-induced breathlessness. Indeed at that time lung transplantation would likely worsen exercise capacity. Poor exercise capacity relative to measured lung function [50] may define a group at increased risk of dying on the waiting list, as reported in cystic fibrosis patients.

After lung transplantation, a CPET after full rehabilitation is very useful in allowing the physician to advise as to exercise capacity and capacity to perform certain vocations. The lung function test correlates very poorly with exercise capacity. Again, an appropriately low work rate increment (10–15 W/min) is required to give optimal test duration. This early posttransplant exercise test also provides a useful baseline – subsequent slight changes with respect to exercise-induced desaturation or reduced ventilatory reserve may reflect early dysfunction of the pulmonary allograft.

To help in the understanding of the indications, conduct, features and interpretation of CPET in the lung transplant recipient, 4 illustrative cases are presented.

Illustrative Cases

Case 1: Right SLTx for Idiopathic Pulmonary Fibrosis

A 49-year-old male presenting with exercise-induced dyspnea. A high resolution CT scan shows basal fibrosis with minimal ground glass opacity. Video-assisted thoracoscopic lung biopsy confirms a usual interstitial pneumonitis pathological picture. He was commenced on prednisolone 25 mg daily p.o. and azathioprine 25 mg daily p.o. but his condition slowly deteriorated. In view of symptoms, unfavorable pathology and failure to improve on therapy he was referred for lung transplant assessment.

CPET 1: Two Years Prior to Lung Transplantation. An incremental CPET was performed because the degree of

Table 2. Case 1: right SLTx for idiopathic pulmonary fibrosis

	CPET 1 2 years pre-SLTx	CPET 2 2 months pre-SLTx	CPET 3 3 months post-SLTx	CPET 4 12 months post-SLTx	Predicted values
$FEV_{1.0}$, liters	3.75	2.40	3.32	2.60 (BOS1)	3.58
VC, liters	4.70	2.78	4.23	3.78	4.85
FER, %	80	86	78	69	>75
D_LCO, ml/min/mm Hg	16.9	10.2	20.2	15.5	28.3
W_{max}, watts	180	115	132	132	158
HR, /min					
Rest	66	74	96	79	
Peak	180	123	155	141	178
VO_2/HR, ml/beat					
Rest	4.2	6.6	4.9	5.3	
Peak	15.9	10.8	8.7	11.0	
V_E peak, liters/min	129	71	96	103	
(% of predicted MVV)	(91)	(84)	(116)		
VO_2 at AT, ml/kg/min	28.6	12.5	10.4	14.5	
(% of predicted VO_2 max at AT)	(90)	(41)	(34)	(48)	
VO_2peak, ml/kg/min	37.1	17.5	16.4	20.2	33.1
V_E/VO_2 pre-AT	33	46	48	47	<34
SaO_2, %					
Rest	96	97	100	99	
Peak	86	78	97	93	
Borg					
Breathlessness	9	7	8	8	
Legs	5	5	5	3	

A 49-year-old male who received a right SLTx for idiopathic pulmonary fibrosis. CPET was performed both pre- and posttransplantation.

exercise limitation seemed out of keeping with the patient's measured lung function, which showed normal spirometry with a moderately reduced diffusion capacity. An incremental bicycle ergometer exercise test with 20-W/min increments was performed to volitional exertion. Breathlessness was the predominant symptom at exercise termination. Above normal work-rate and VO_2 was achieved. Heart rate was limiting and ventilation approached limiting levels. Mild desaturation was seen progressively through the exercise test. The exercise response was abnormal but immediate listing for transplantation was deferred because this was likely to result in substantial worsening of exercise capacity.

CPET 2: Two Months Prior to SLTx. A steady deterioration had occurred over the ensuing 18 months and he was actively listed for SLTx 3 months prior to this exercise test. Spirometry now showed a moderately restrictive ventilatory defect with marked reduction in diffusion capacity. A repeat incremental exercise test with 16.5-W/min increments was performed, demonstrating a low peak work and VO_2. Breathlessness was the predominant symptom at exercise termination. Heart rate was not limiting, but minute ventilation approached limiting levels, with marked desaturation occurring progressively throughout the exercise test. Ventilation was clearly excessive below an early anaerobic threshold. The conclusion drawn was that progression of disease was clearly evident and transplantation was indicated on prognostic grounds, without concern that lung transplantation would negatively impact on exercise capacity.

CPET 3: Three Months after SLTx. At 3 months after right SLTx, spirometry shows a mild restrictive ventilation defect with a mildly impaired diffusion capacity. A repeat incremental bicycle ergometer exercise test was performed. Work rate was mildly reduced, but VO_2 substantially reduced (53% predicted) at peak exercise. Heart rate was not limiting but ventilation exceeded predicted maximum. Very mild desaturation was noted. Excessive ventilation was seen below a very early anaerobic threshold. Anaerobic threshold was even earlier than 2 months prior to transplantation. Although successfully transplanted, only a slight impact had been made on maximum exercise capacity.

CPET 4: Twelve Months after SLTx. Exercise capacity was reassessed 12 months after right single lung transplantation. He had developed significant chronic rejection (BOS class 1 – BOS 1). Spirometry shows mild mixed obstructive and restrictive ventilatory defect with moderately reduced diffusion capacity. A repeat incremental exercise test showed mildly reduced work and moderately reduced VO_2 (61% predicted) at peak exercise. Heart rate was not limiting although ventilation approached limiting levels, with modest desaturation noted. Excessive ventilation was seen prior to a slightly early anaerobic threshold. The development of BOS 1 had not impacted on his exercise capacity and a significant improvement in anaerobic threshold and VO_2 peak was seen from 3 to 12 months posttransplant. Interestingly, the VO_2 peak at 12 months was only 54% of the VO_2 peak 2 years prior to transplantation, with a substantially earlier anaerobic threshold.

Comment. Transplantation was indicated on prognostic grounds and did slightly improve exercise capacity from that measured 2 months pretransplant. Most striking was the low VO_2 peak and early anaerobic threshold when compared to those measured 2 years prior to transplantation (table 2).

Table 3. Case 2: SLTx for obstructive lung disease

	Measured	Predicted
$FEV_{1.0}$, liters	1.76	2.43
VC, liters	2.22	3.17
FER, %	79	>75
D_LCO, ml/min/mm Hg	21.1	22.6
W_{max}, Watts	82.5	112
HR, /min		
Rest	82	
Peak	148	176
VO_2/HR		
Rest		
Peak	5.3	7.6
VE_{Peak}, /min	62	
(% MVV)	(100)	
VO_2 at AT, ml/kg/min	9.3	
(% of predicted VO_2 max)	(40)	
VO_2peak, ml/kg/min	16.0	29.0
VE/VO_2 pre-AT	35	<34
SaO_2, %		
Rest	99	
Peak	98	
Borg		
Breathlessness	6	
Legs	5	

A 51-year-old female 3 months after left SLTx for severe obstructive lung disease.

Illustrative Case 2 SLTx for Obstructive Lung Disease

History. A 51-year-old lady who presents with a long history of chronic asthma, and who developed severe fixed airflow obstruction despite appropriate therapy. She received a left SLTx and made an uneventful postoperative recovery, completing 2 months of supervised rehabilitation.

CPET at Three Months Posttransplant. Spirometry shows a mild-moderate restrictive ventilatory defect, with evidence of minimal airflow obstruction on tests of small airway function. Diffusion capacity is normal. An incremental bicycle ergometer exercise test was performed (16.5-W/min increments) to volitional exhaustion. A mildly reduced work rate and moderately reduced VO_2 peak were seen. Exercise termination was predominantly due to leg tiredness. Heart rate was not limiting but ventilation reached 100% predicted at exercise termination, although no significant desaturation occurred. Excessive ventilation was seen below a very early anaerobic threshold.

Comment. The spirometry is somewhat atypical as the predominant abnormality is a restrictive ventilatory defect despite the substantial airflow obstruction in the native lung. The main findings on exercise are typical of SLTx, that is an early anaerobic threshold and exercise termination at or near MVV (table 3).

Illustrative Case 3 BLTx for Cystic Fibrosis

History. A 23-year-old lady presenting with a steady deterioration in lung function and recurrent admissions due to exacerbations of cystic fibrosis. She received BLTx and had an uneventful postoperative course. She commenced supervised rehabilitation 3 days per week at 2 weeks posttransplantation, continuing to 3 months posttransplantation.

CPET at Three Months after BLTx. Spirometry and diffusion capacity are normal. An incremental bicycle exercise test using 10-W/min increments to volitional exhaustion. Leg tiredness was the predominant symptom at exercise termination. A low peak work and peak VO_2 (54% predicted) were achieved. Neither cardiac nor respiratory function appeared limiting. Anaerobic threshold was reached very early in exercise, although below this ventilation appeared normal in relation to VO_2.

Table 4. Case 3: BLTx for cystic fibrosis

	Measured	Predicted
$FEV_{1.0}$, liters	3.36	3.31
VC, liters	3.45	3.78
FER, %	97	>75
D_LCO, ml/min/mm Hg	22.3	26.5
W_{max}, Watts	100	158
HR, /min		
Rest	77	
Peak	162	195
VO_2/HR, ml/beat		
Rest	5.2	
Peak	6.8	
VE_{Peak}, liters/min	50	118
VO_2 at AT, ml/kg/min	14.7	
(% of predicted VO_2 max)	(37)	
VO_2peak, ml/kg/min	21.0	39.0
VE/VO_2 pre-AT	30	<34
SaO_2, %		
Rest	96	
Peak	97	
Borg		
Breathlessness	5	
Legs	7	

A 23-year-old female, 3 months after BLTx for cystic fibrosis.

Table 5. Case 4: HLTx for VSD/pulmonary hypertension

	Measured	Predicted
$FEV_{1.0}$, liters	4.28	4.53
VC, liters	5.17	5.39
FER, %	83	>75
D_LCO, ml/min/mm Hg	23.7	33.4
W_{max}, Watts	116	247
HR, /min		
Rest	100	
Peak	130	196
VO_2/HR, ml/beat		
Rest	5.9	
Peak	11.2	
VE_{Peak}, liters/min	66	150
VO_2 at AT, ml/kg/min	16.4	
(% of predicted VO_2 max)	(30)	
VO_2peak, ml/kg/min	25.0	49.0
VE/VO_2 pre-AT	32	<34
SaO_2, %		
Rest	97	
Peak	97	
Borg		
Breathlessness	3	
Legs	7	

A 21-year-old man, fully recovered from a HLTx for ventricular septal defect and pulmonary hypertension tested 18 months posttransplant.

Comment. This is a typical response to incremental exercise in a BLTx recipient. Exercise terminated well short of cardiac or ventilatory limitation due to leg tiredness. The anaerobic threshold occurred very early in exercise (table 4).

Illustrative Case 4 HLTx for VSD/Pulmonary Hypertension

History. A 21-year-old male with severe pulmonary hypertension secondary to a ventricular septal defect who was listed for transplantation due to progressive right ventricular failure. He received a HLTx and recovered rapidly and uneventfully. A CPET was performed 18 months posttransplant having returned to full time employment as a professional fisherman 12 months previously.

CPET at 18 Months after HLTx. Spirometry is normal and diffusion capacity mildly reduced. An incremental bicycle ergometer exercise test was performed with 16.5-W/min increments. Leg tiredness was the predominant symptom at exercise termination. A high resting heart rate with blunted chronotropic response to exercise is seen, but no evidence of cardiac limitation was evident. Neither ventilatory limitation nor desaturation were evident at peak exercise. Ventilation was not excessive in relation to VO_2 below a very early anaerobic threshold.

Comment. Despite a functionally excellent result from HLTx, substantially reduced maximum exercise capacity, presumed due to impaired oxygen uptake or utilization, is evident. A high heart rate at rest and blunted response to exercise is seen due to cardiac denervation (table 5).

Conclusion

Lung transplantation has evolved to the point where survival is expected and we are now focusing on the quality of outcome. Substantial exercise limitation is present on CPET both before and after lung transplantation. The mechanism of exercise limitation changes from ventilatory limitation pretransplantation to peripheral limitation posttransplantation. CPET will help clarify the degree and mechanism of exercise limitation where a discrepancy between lung function and exercise capacity is suspected or expected.

References

1 Shumacker HBJ: A surgeon to remember: Notes about Vladimir Demikhov. Ann Thorac Surg 1994;58:1196–1198.

2 Hardy JD, Webb WR, Dalton ML, Walker GR: Lung homotransplantation in man. JAMA 1963;186:1065–1074.

3 Derom F, Barbier F, Ringoir S, Versieck J, Rolly G, Berzsenyi G, et al: Ten-month survival after lung homotransplantation in man. J Thorac Cardiovasc Surg 1971;61:835–846.

4 Reitz BA, Wallwork JL, Hunt SA, Pennock JL, Billingham ME, Oyer PE, et al: Heart-lung transplantation: Successful therapy for patients with pulmonary vascular disease. N Engl J Med 1982;306:557–564.

5 Unilateral lung transplantation for pulmonary fibrosis. Toronto Lung Transplant Group. N Engl J Med 1986;314:1140–1145.

6 Patterson GA, Cooper JD, Goldman B, Weisel RD, Pearson FG, Waters PF, et al: Technique of successful clinical double-lung transplantation. Ann Thorac Surg 1988;45:626–633.

7 Pasque MK, Cooper JD, Kaiser LR, Haydock DA, Triantafillou A, Trulock EP: Improved technique for bilateral lung transplantation: Rationale and initial clinical experience. Ann Thorac Surg 1990;49:785–791.

8 Barr ML, Schenkel FA, Cohen RG, Chan KM, Barbers RG, Marboe CC, et al: Living-related lobar transplantation: Recipient outcome and early rejection patterns. Transplant Proc 1995; 27:1995–1996.

9 Starnes VA, Barr ML, Cohen RG, Hagen JA, Wells WJ, Horn MV, et al: Living-donor lobar lung transplantation experience: Intermediate results. J Thorac Cardiovasc Surg 1996;112: 1284–1290.

10 Stevens PM, Johnson PC, Bell RL, Beall AC Jr, Jenkins DE: Regional ventilation and perfusion after lung transplantation in patients with emphysema. N Engl J Med 1970;282:245–249.

11 St.Louis International Lung Transplant Registry Report: St. Louis, Washington University School of Medicine, 1996.

12 Hosenpud JD, Novick RJ, Breen TJ, Keck B, Daily P: The Registry of the International Society for Heart and Lung Transplantation: Twelfth official report – 1995. J Heart Lung Transplant 1995;14:805–815.

13 Williams TJ, Grossman RF, Maurer JR: Long-term functional follow-up of lung transplant recipients. Clin Chest Med 1990;11:347–358.

14 Williams TJ, Snell GI: Early and long-term functional outcomes in unilateral, bilateral, and living-related transplant recipients. Clin Chest Med 1997;18:245–257.

15 Pasque MK, Trulock EP, Cooper JD, Triantafillou AN, Huddleston CB, Rosenbloom M, et al: Single lung transplantation for pulmonary hypertension: Single institution experience in 34 patients. Circulation 1995;92:2252–2258.

16 Gross CR, Savik K, Bolman RM III, Hertz MI: Long-term health status and quality of life outcomes of lung transplant recipients. Chest 1995;108:1587–1593.

17 Craven JL, Bright J, Dear CL: Psychiatric, psychosocial, and rehabilitative aspects of lung transplantation. Clin Chest Med 1990;11:247–257.

18 Ross DJ, Waters PF, Mohsenifar Z, Belman MJ, Kass RM, Koerner SK: Hemodynamic responses to exercise after lung transplantation. Chest 1993;103:46–53.

19 Levy RD, Ernst P, Levine SM, Shennib H, Anzueto A, Bryan CL, et al: Exercise performance after lung transplantation. J Heart Lung Transplant 1993;12:27–33.

20 Miyoshi S, Trulock EP, Schaefers HJ, Hsieh CM, Patterson GA, Cooper JD: Cardiopulmonary exercise testing after single and double lung transplantation. Chest 1990;97:1130–1136.

21 Orens JB, Becker FS, Lynch JP, III, Christensen PJ, Deeb GM, Martinez FJ: Cardiopulmonary exercise testing following allogeneic lung transplantation for different underlying disease states. Chest 1995;107:144–149.

22 Theodore J, Morris AJ, Burke CM, Glanville AR, VanKessel A, Baldwin JC, et al: Cardiopulmonary function at maximum tolerable constant work rate exercise following human heart-lung transplantation. Chest 1987;92: 433–439.

23 Williams TJ, Howard M, Roget J, Esmore DS: Exercise capacity after combined heart-lung transplantation. Transplant Proc 1992;24: 2018.

24 Williams TJ, Patterson GA, McClean PA, Zamel N, Maurer JR: Maximal exercise testing in single and double lung transplant recipients. Am Rev Respir Dis 1992;145:101–105.

25 Nixon PA, Fricker FJ, Noyes BE, Webber SA, Orenstein DM, Armitage JM: Exercise testing in pediatric heart, heart-lung, and lung transplant recipients. Chest 1995;107:1328–1335.

26 Stiebellehner L, Quittan M, End A, Wieselthaler G, Klepetko W, Haber P, et al: Aerobic endurance training program improves exercise performance in lung transplant recipients. Chest 1998;113:906–912.

27 Pope SE, Stinson EB, Daughters GT, Schroeder JS, Ingels NB Jr, Alderman EL: Exercise response of the denervated heart in long-term cardiac transplant recipients. Am J Cardiol 1980;46:213–218.

28 Savin WM, Haskell WL, Schroeder JS, Stinson EB: Cardiorespiratory responses of cardiac transplant patients to graded, symptom-limited exercise. Circulation 1980;62:55–60.

29 Kavanagh T, Yacoub MH, Mertens DJ, Kennedy J, Campbell RB, Sawyer P: Cardiorespiratory responses to exercise training after orthotopic cardiac transplantation. Circulation 1988;77:162–171.

30 Jensen RL, Yanowitz FG, Crapo RO: Exercise hemodynamics and oxygen delivery measurements using rebreathing techniques in heart transplant patients. Am J Cardiol 1991;68: 129–133.

31 Carere R, Patterson GA, Liu P, Williams T, Maurer J, Grossman R: Right and left ventricular performance after single and double lung transplantation. The Toronto Lung Transplant Group. J Thorac Cardiovasc Surg 1991;102: 115–122.

32 Globits S, Burghuber OC, Koller J, Schenk P, Frank H, Grimm M, et al: Effect of lung transplantation on right and left ventricular volumes and function measured by magnetic resonance imaging. Am J Respir Crit Care Med 1994;149: 1000–1004.

33 Katz WE, Gasior TA, Quinlan JJ, Lazar JM, Firestone L, Griffith BP, et al: Immediate effects of lung transplantation on right ventricular morphology and function in patients with variable degrees of pulmonary hypertension. J Am Coll Cardiol 1996;27:384–391.

34 Martinez FJ, Orens JB, Whyte RI, Graf L, Becker FS, Lynch JP III: Lung mechanics and dyspnea after lung transplantation for chronic airflow obstruction. Am J Respir Crit Care Med 1996;153:1536–1543.

35 Bernard S, Whittom F, Leblanc P, Jobin J, Belleau R, Berube C, et al: Aerobic and strength training in patients with chronic obstructive pulmonary disease. Am J Respir Crit Care Med 1999;159:896–901.

36 Kelsen SG, Ference M, Kapoor S: Effects of prolonged undernutrition on structure and function of the diaphragm. J Appl Physiol 1985;58:1354–1359.

37 Decramer M, Lacquet LM, Fagard R, Rogiers P: Corticosteroids contribute to muscle weakness in chronic airflow obstruction. Am J Respir Crit Care Med 1994;150:11–16.

38 Kamischke A, Kemper DE, Castel MA, Luthke M, Rolf C, Behre HM, et al: Testosterone levels in men with chronic obstructive pulmonary disease with or without glucocorticoid therapy. Eur Respir J 1998;11:41–45.

39 Evans AB, Al Himyary AJ, Hrovat MI, Pappagianopoulos P, Wain JC, Ginns LC, et al: Abnormal skeletal muscle oxidative capacity after lung transplantation by 31P-MRS. Am J Respir Crit Care Med 1997;155:615–621.

40 Tirdel GB, Girgis R, Fishman RS, Theodore J: Metabolic myopathy as a cause of the exercise limitation in lung transplant recipients. J Heart Lung Transplant 1998;17:1231–1237.

41 Wang XN, Williams TJ, McKenna MJ, Li JL, Fraser SF, Side EA, et al: Skeletal muscle oxidative capacity, fiber type, and metabolites after lung transplantation. Am J Respir Crit Care Med 1999;160:57–63.

42 Jakobsson P, Jorfeldt L, Brundin A: Skeletal muscle metabolites and fibre types in patients with advanced chronic obstructive pulmonary disease (COPD), with and without chronic respiratory failure. Eur Respir J 1990;3:192–196.

43 Jobin J, Maltais F, Doyon JF, Leblanc P, Simard PM, Simard AA, et al: Chronic obstructive pulmonary disease: Capillarity and fiber-type characteristics of skeletal muscle. J Cardiopulm Rehabil 1998;18:432–437.

44 Hokanson JF, Mercier JG, Brooks GA: Cyclosporine A decreases rat skeletal muscle mitochondrial respiration in vitro. Am J Respir Crit Care Med 1995;151:1848–1851.
45 Mercier JG, Hokanson JF, Brooks GA: Effects of cyclosporine A on skeletal muscle mitochondrial respiration and endurance time in rats. Am J Respir Crit Care Med 1995;151:1532 1536.
46 Hall MJ, Snell GI, Side EA, Esmore DS, Walters EH, Williams TJ: Exercise, potassium, and muscle deconditioning post-thoracic organ transplantation. J Appl Physiol 1994;77:2784–2790.
47 Williams TJ, Fraser SF, McKenna MJ, Li JL, Wang XN, Carey MF, et al: Skeletal muscle sodium-potassium pump activity is normal post lung transplant. Am J Respir Crit Care Med 1996;153:A828.
48 Li JL, McKenna MJ, Wang XN, Fraser SF, Carey MF, Side EA, et al: Low skeletal muscle sarcoplasmic reticulum calcium release post lung transplantation. Am J Respir Crit Care Med 1996;153:A828.
49 Debigare R, Maltais F, Mallet M, Casaburi R, Leblanc P: Influence of work rate incremental rate on the exercise responses in patients with COPD. Med Sci Sports Exerc 2000;32:1365–1368.
50 Nixon PA, Orenstein DM, Kelsey SF, Doershuk CF: The prognostic value of exercise testing in patients with cystic fibrosis. N Engl J Med 1992;327:1785–1788.
51 Cooper JD, Patterson GA, Trulock EP: Results of single and bilateral lung transplantation in 131 consecutive recipients. Washington University Lung Transplant Group. J Thorac Cardiovasc Surg 1994;107:460–470.
52 Grossman RF, Frost A, Zamel N, Patterson GA, Cooper JD, Myron PR, et al: Results of single-lung transplantation for bilateral pulmonary fibrosis. The Toronto Lung Transplant Group. N Engl J Med 1990;322:727–733.
53 Lands LC, Smountas AA, Mesiano G, Brosseau L, Shennib H, Charbonneau M, et al: Maximal exercise capacity and peripheral skeletal muscle function following lung transplantation. J Heart Lung Transplant 1999;18:113–120.
54 Schwaiblmair M, Reichenspurner H, Muller C, Briegel J, Furst H, Groh J, et al: Cardiopulmonary exercise testing before and after lung and heart-lung transplantation. Am J Respir Crit Care Med 1999;159:1277–1283.
55 Systrom DM, Pappagianopoulos P, Fishman RS, Wain JC, Ginns LC: Determinants of abnormal maximum oxygen uptake after lung transplantation for chronic obstructive pulmonary disease. J Heart Lung Transplant 1998;17:1220–1230.
56 Lands LC, Smountas AA, Mesiano G, Brosseau L, Shennib H, Charbonneau M, et al: Maximal exercise capacity and peripheral skeletal muscle function following lung transplantation. J Heart Lung Transplant 1999;18:113–120.

Dr. Trevor J. Williams
Department of Respiratory Medicine
Alfred Hospital
Prahran (Melbourne) 3181 (Australia)
Tel. +61 3 9276 2489, Fax +61 3 9276 3434
E-Mail trevor.williams@med.monash.edu.au

Weisman IM, Zeballos RJ (eds): Clinical Exercise Testing.
Prog Respir Res. Basel, Karger, 2002, vol 32, pp 264–272

Exercise Responses in Systemic Conditions

Obesity, Diabetes, Thyroid Disorders, and Chronic Fatigue Syndrome

Kathy E. Sietsema

UCLA School of Medicine, Harbor-UCLA Medical Center, Torrance, Calif., USA

Summary

A wide variety of systemic conditions affect exercise capacity and may present with exercise intolerance. Obesity reduces exercise tolerance principally through the increased metabolic demands of ambulation, but may also be associated with alterations of ventilatory function, and with circulatory impairment which is often linked to associated hypertension. Diabetes alters the function of multiple organ systems by virtue of vascular, neuropathic and metabolic mechanisms. Thyroid hormone affects function of virtually every organ system and either excess or deficiency may result in impairment of circulatory responses and alteration of skeletal muscle structure and function. The physiologic processes involved in chronic fatigue syndrome are less well understood, but exercise intolerance is universal in this condition and significant reductions in exercise capacity may be present. Understanding the effects of these diverse conditions on metabolic and organ system function is essential for recognizing their expression in parameters derived from cardiopulmonary exercise testing.

Introduction

Several distinct systemic conditions are addressed in the following discussion. Exercise testing is not performed for primary diagnosis of any of these conditions, nor are there established recommendations or guidelines for use of exercise data in clinical decision making for affected patients. Each, however, is associated with exercise intolerance, and may be represented among patients evaluated for exertional dyspnea or fatigue. In addition, some are common co-existing conditions that may complicate the clinical evaluation of a patient with other diagnoses, or the interpretation of his or her exercise test. It is therefore useful to consider what is known regarding how these conditions may themselves modify exercise responses. A comprehensive review of the effects of these conditions on exercise function is beyond the scope of this chapter, which will focus primarily on those findings that are most likely to be reflected in gas exchange and other measurements made during clinical cardiopulmonary exercise testing. Where possible, recently published reviews are identified for more detailed reference.

Obesity

Obesity is an increasingly prevalent problem with profound health effects. Aside from the well-recognized associations with diabetes, atherosclerotic disease and hypertension, obesity may have direct effects on organ system functions that affect responses to exercise testing. In general, these are increasingly evident with increasing severity of obesity, so not all processes identified in this discussion apply to all obese patients. Obesity refers to an excess of fat, and therefore is most meaningfully defined and quantified by measures of the mass and distribution of adipose tissue. Measures of body composition are not universally and readily available in all clinical settings, however, and therefore obesity is often inferred from the relationship of weight to height, such as by the body mass index (BMI, weight in kg/height in m^2), or percent of ideal weight derived from nomograms. While these approaches do not actually distinguish fat from lean mass, they are generally useful for describing different magnitudes of obesity. Obesity also raises important issues about the expression and interpretation of exercise data for addressing clinical questions.

Physiologic Effects of Obesity Relevant to Cardiopulmonary Exercise Testing

It is well-recognized that obesity can affect pulmonary function [1]. Respiratory system compliance is reduced by the increased mass of the chest wall and resistance to descent of the diaphragm represented by increased abdominal mass [1]. Work of breathing is therefore increased [2]. Lung volumes may be reduced as a consequence, and increase towards normal following weight loss [3]. Some investigators have found, at least among young adult subjects, that reduction in vital capacity or total lung capacity is uncommon unless obesity is severe, i.e. a weight (kg) to height (cm) ratio of 1.0 or greater, corresponding roughly to weights at least double the ideal value. Functional residual capacity is reduced with much lesser degrees of obesity [4], however, and correlates negatively with the extent of overweight. Residual volume is preserved, so expiratory reserve volume is reduced, also in proportion to the degree of obesity. Hypoxemia, or increased $P(A\text{-}a)O_2$ difference is a recognized consequence of obesity [5], even in the absence of obesity hypoventilation or sleep disordered breathing, and is attributed to ventilation perfusion mismatching due to relative underventilation of the lung bases. Hypoxemia is greater in the supine position, and may normalize with upright posture [6].

An association between heart failure and obesity has been noted for many years, and strong epidemiologic relationships exist between obesity, hypertension, and hypertensive heart disease. Alterations in cardiac structure and function, including increased left-ventricular mass and reductions in parameters of systolic and diastolic function have also been reported in obese subjects who are normotensive, however [7]. An intrinsic cardiomyopathy of obesity has thus been proposed, the characteristics of which have recently been reviewed [8]. Obese subjects have an expanded blood volume, even in the absence of heart failure, and resting cardiac output is increased [9, 10]. Left-ventricular mass is increased and correlates with severity of obesity [11]. In contrast to the concentric hypertrophy of hypertension, uncomplicated obesity is characterized by eccentric hypertrophy [8]. Left-ventricular filling pressures are reported to be high–normal at rest in severely obese patients, and increase further with exercise, implying associated pulmonary congestion and/or edema [9]. Exercise blood pressure is higher in obese compared to lean subjects, even among those who are normotensive at rest [12]. Changes in right-ventricular structure and function occur when alveolar hypoventilation or sleep apnea syndromes complicate obesity, but are beyond the scope of this discussion. Many of the cardiovascular changes described in obesity appear to be reversible with weight loss [9, 12].

Metabolic effects of obesity include an increase in resting metabolic rate due to the added metabolic activity of the fat mass [13]. The metabolic cost of ambulation is increased to an even greater degree due to the work required to support the added body mass. From well-established principles of exercise training, this situation might be expected to result in increased exercise capacity for obese subjects due to the chronic training effects of the metabolic requirements of doing ambulatory activities. Indeed, modeling of data from healthy populations of varying body composition suggests that an increase in fat mass is associated with compensatory changes in muscle mass to support the added weight, such that peak VO_2 values normalized to lean mass are similar to those of lean subjects [14]. Measured fat-free mass is thus a better predictor of maximal VO_2 than is total mass, although the relationship between mass and exercise capacity is likely more complex than the linear relationships often employed in clinical practice [15, 16]. Other metabolic factors relevant to obesity include insulin resistance, which not only affects carbohydrate metabolism, but is also associated with impairment in peripheral vascular reactivity.

Findings on Cardiopulmonary Exercise Testing Related to Obesity

Resting VO_2 is increased because of increased metabolically active tissue mass [13]. In the initial transition from rest to exercise there is also an exaggerated increase in VO_2 compared to lean subjects, due to the greater work involved in supporting and propelling the weight (on a treadmill) or simply lifting large legs against gravity (on a cycle ergometer) [17]. Once these initial high metabolic demands are taken into account, however, the oxygen cost of further increases in work rate follows the same slope in obese as in lean subjects [18]. That is to say, the slope of the relationship between VO_2 and work rate is normal, as long as data from the initial rest to exercise transition are excluded. Any apparent reductions in mechanical efficiency, reflected in a greater than normal slope, are likely due to ergonomic factors related to work expended in postural control [19], or excessive work of breathing associated with high levels of ventilation near peak exercise [17], as mechanical efficiency of skeletal muscle in obese subjects is similar to that of lean subjects [20].

As noted above, peak VO_2 in obese subjects has a similar relationship to lean body mass as in normal subjects, although the lean mass may in fact be increased to some degree in response to the chronic training effect of carrying excess weight. Among the practical issues of exercise testing of obese individuals, then, are how to predict what maximal VO_2 should be, and how to express the measured values. Commonly used predicting equations are based on regression analyses of normal subjects who were, for the most part, nonobese. Weight is a positive factor in these equations and using the obese patient's actual weight for this may result in inappropriately high predicted values. Substituting 'ideal' weight, calculated from height, in these calculations results in lower predicted values, but these may be inappropriately low as they do not take into account the expected normal training response that the ambulatory obese subject should derive from being overweight. Because of this a hybrid approach has been recommended in which ideal weight is incorporated into established formulae, but the calculated value is then increased by 6 ml/min for each kg of excess weight [21]. This value was derived from analysis of the excess VO_2 required for unloaded cycling for obese subjects [22] rather than direct observations of peak VO_2 values. It was consistent, however, with the small increase in peak VO_2 above that predicted from ideal weight among subjects included in an analysis by the same investigators of 77 apparently healthy men [23]. None of the men in that analysis were severely obese, and the validity of this approach has not been assessed in larger populations, nor specifically in more severely obese individuals, or in women.

From the above it follows that absolute values of both peak VO_2 and the VO_2 at the lactate threshold should be at least as high, arguably higher, in an obese subject compared to an otherwise identical lean individual. However, both the weight indexed VO_2 values for these parameters, and the work rates associated with them, will likely be lower in obese subjects. Obese children, for example, have a greater absolute peak VO_2, but lower peak VO_2/kg, than their lean contemporaries [14]. This raises the issue of how exercise values should be reported for obese persons. The widely used convention of indexing peak VO_2 to body weight results in values that are low, even for disease-free obese subjects. Distinction thus need be made between the use of peak VO_2 as an expression of cardiovascular capacity and its use to describe work capacity. The former can most meaningfully expressed as peak VO_2 per lean mass, or as a percent of a reasonably calculated predicted value, while the latter might be expressed as peak VO_2 indexed to actual body weight, as this reflects capacity for ambulatory activity. The choice of expression therefore depends on whether the clinical question relates to physiologic capacity of the organism as a whole, or the capacity for doing external work above and beyond the work involved in supporting the organism.

Ventilatory patterns may be altered by obesity. The lower end-expiratory lung volume at rest leaves less room for reducing end expiratory volumes during exercise, and, indeed, moderately obese subjects are found to not decrease end-expiratory volumes during exercise, in contrast to nonobese subjects [24]. This being the case, increases in tidal volume can only be accomplished by increasing inspiratory volumes, and this response appears attenuated, perhaps due to the work of breathing associated with increasing tidal volume in the face of decreased thoracic compliance. Not surprisingly, such limitation in tidal volume are more evident in patients with truncal as compared to peripheral obesity [25]. Although reduced tidal volumes could lead to a higher VD/VT in obese subjects, ventilatory equivalents at rest and exercise at least for moderately obese subjects are reported to be similar to those of lean subjects during upright exercise [17, 20]. In contrast to most patients with intrinsic lung disease, obese patients exhibit a decrease in abnormalities of oxygenation during exercise compared to rest [6]. This has been attributed to improved ventilation-perfusion matching due to increased tidal volumes and reversal of basal atelectasis which is more prominent at rest or in the supine position.

Systemic blood pressure is higher during exercise in obese compared to lean subjects, even for subjects who are normotensive at rest [12]. There do not appear to be systematic effects of obesity on the heart rate response to exercise, although heart rate may well be high relative to work rate, commensurate with the increased metabolic rate. In the presence of heart failure, whether attributable to longstanding hypertension, to hypoxema-induced right-sided heart failure resulting from hypoventilation or sleep apnea syndromes, or to cardiovascular effects intrinsic to obesity itself, all of the findings characteristic of heart failure on exercise testing may be expected.

Diabetes

Diabetes is an important risk factor for a number of diseases which independently limit exercise function, including coronary artery disease, peripheral arterial disease, and chronic renal insufficiency. Each of these impairs exercise function, and are addressed in other sections of this book. Even in the absence of overt secondary disease processes, however, diabetics may have altered organ system function that could affect exercise responses. Autonomic control is impaired by diabetic neuropathy. Altered insulin sensitivity affects peripheral vascular resistance and metabolic responses. Microvascular changes associated with diabetes can have adverse effects on myocardial function, and pulmonary or peripheral gas exchange. Though some of these processes may differ systematically between type I and type II diabetics, there are more similarities than differences between these groups with respect to acute responses to short term exercise, and the following discussion is based on observations from both.

Physiologic Effects of Diabetes Relevant to Cardiopulmonary Exercise Testing

Cardiac dysfunction is recognized in diabetics without evidence of obstructive coronary artery disease [26, 27]. Diabetic cardiomyopathy is characterized by impaired left-ventricular diastolic relaxation, which may be identified in a high proportion of diabetics [28, 29], and occurs early in the course of the disease [30]. Diastolic impairment is identified even in the absence of hypertension or systolic dysfunction [28, 30], but the extent of dysfunction is increased with co-existing systemic hypertension [31]. Among diabetics, the presence and degree of diastolic dysfunction has been correlated with reduced exercise capacity [29]. Although resting systolic function is generally normal in asymptomatic diabetics without clinical evidence of coronary disease, impaired systolic responses to exercise are also reported [32]. This may be attributable to myocardial adrenergic denervation [32] or to microvascular disease. There are some data to indicate that cardiac function in uncomplicated diabetics correlates with the adequacy of glycemic control [26, 33].

Reductions in spirometric volumes are reported with diabetes, and correlate with the duration of diabetes when other factors are controlled for [34, 35]. Alterations in insulin sensitivity and carbohydrate metabolism due to diabetes are clearly important to sustained exercise during which substrate availability is at issue, but of lesser importance in the context of the short protocols used in clinical cardiopulmonary exercise testing.

Findings on Cardiopulmonary Exercise Testing Related to Diabetes

Some investigators have reported that physically active diabetics without secondary complications may have normal peak work capacity [36] or peak VO_2 [37] compared to healthy subjects with similar activity patterns. In many series, however, especially when not matched for high levels of physical activity, diabetics have reduced peak exercise VO_2 compared to age and gender matched healthy controls [38–42]. Greater reductions in peak VO_2 are reported for diabetics with evidence of autonomic neuropathy than for those without [37, 43]. Patients with neuropathy have lower peak heart rates and lower exercise blood pressure, and do not increase cardiac output normally at peak exercise [43]. Correlation has been identified between reduction of peak VO_2 and the presence and severity of diabetic retinopathy and urinary albumin excretion, implying a relationship to microvascular disease [44]. Thus, both autonomic control of circulation and microvascular disease are implicated in exercise impairment in diabetes. In addition to a reduction in peak VO_2, diabetics are reported to have slower adaptation to submaximal exercise [45], more shallow increase in VO_2 relative to work rate during graded testing [38, 40] and prolonged time course of recovery of heart rate following maximal exercise [36]. Despite reported decreases in spirometric volumes and diffusing capacity [34, 35, 42], adverse effects of diabetes on the efficiency of pulmonary gas exchange or arterial blood gases during exercise have not been reported [42, 46].

On cardiopulmonary exercise testing therefore diabetics may demonstrate low values for peak VO_2, peak work rate, and peak heart rate compared with predicted. A reduction in peak heart rate may be low due to cardiovascular autonomic dysfunction and thus cannot be taken to indicate submaximal effort on testing. For the same reason, heart rate responses may not be appropriate benchmarks for exercise prescription in this population. Other indices sensitive to cardiovascular response, including the peak O_2 pulse and the anaerobic threshold may be reduced to the extent that cardiac output is impaired. A lower than average slope of VO_2 relative to work rate may be observed, and may reflect prolonged dynamic responses. Reductions of the slope to values below the normal range likely reflect impairment in cardiovascular responses. The ventilatory response to exercise, the ventilatory equivalents, and arterial blood gas values should be similar to normal unless there is additional co-existing pulmonary disease.

Thyroid Disorders

Both hyperthyroidism and hypothyroidism are identified as causes of exertional dyspnea. In neither case are the underlying mechanisms entirely clear. Thyroid hormone has diverse actions, affecting virtually every organ system, however, including effects on cardiac and skeletal muscle, vascular tone, and nervous system responses, each of which are relevant to exercise function.

Physiologic Effects of Thyroid Disorders Relevant to Cardiopulmonary Exercise Testing

Hyperthyroidism is associated with elevations in metabolic rate, with attendant increases in resting values of pulmonary gas exchange, ventilation, and cardiac output. Conversely, these variables are decreased in hypothyroidism, although the changes may be more difficult to detect, at least at rest. Cardiovascular effects of thyroid disorders have recently been reviewed [47].

In hyperthyroidism, cardiac output is increased disproportionately to the increased metabolic rate due to the added effects of reduced vascular resistance, increased blood volume, increased heart rate and enhancement of both contractility and diastolic relaxation of the heart [47]. There is some controversy regarding whether hyperthyroidism per se leads to cardiac dysfunction. Although left-ventricular systolic function at rest is increased in hyperthyroidism, a decrease in left-ventricular ejection fraction during exercise compared to rest has been reported in some hyperthyroid patients [48, 49]. Clinical heart failure is nevertheless uncommon in this condition, and, when it occurs, may be related to sustained tachycardia rather than contractile dysfunction [47]. Changes in skeletal muscle are described in experimental hyperthyroidism, including a shift of fiber type distribution towards fast twitch type [50], reduction of muscle mass due to negative protein balance [50], and more rapid depletion of glycogen during exercise [51]. Given the preservation of cardiac output and muscle blood flow during exercise [52], these changes in skeletal muscle are proposed as the principle bases of reduced exercise endurance in hyperthyroidism [50, 51].

Hypothyroidism is associated with more readily demonstrated impairments in cardiac function than hyperthyroidism, though the clinical findings of altered cardiovascular activity at rest are generally less apparent. Both systolic [53] and diastolic [54] function of the heart are depressed in hypothyroidism due to loss of inotropic and lusitropic actions of thyroid hormone on myocardium [47]. Despite this, common echocardiographic measures of global ventricular function may remain normal until hypothyroidism is severe [55, 56]. Additional impairment in cardiac function in hypothyroidism may be attributable to altered cardiac loading conditions [55] due to increased systemic vascular resistance and decreased blood volume [47]. Skeletal muscle oxidative enzyme capacity is reduced markedly in hypothyroidism [57] and contractile properties of the muscle are impaired. Exercise of small muscle masses is associated with higher blood lactate levels [58] and altered phosphocreatine responses [59] for patients with hypothyroidism compared to euthyroid controls. Overt skeletal muscle myopathy, manifest as proximal muscle weakness, pain and cramping [60] is a well-recognized manifestation of hypothyroidism. Respiratory as well as locomotor muscles [61] may be affected in hypothyroidism. In addition to reduced respiratory muscle strength, abnormalities of respiratory control are also recognized in thyroid deficiency [62], and either may result in reduced ventilatory volumes and hypercapnia.

Consistent with the preceding observations, hypothyroidism appears to impair exercise performance more substantially than hyperthyroidism. Baldwin et al. [57] report a 32% reduction in maximal VO_2 in thyroid-deficient rats compared with control animals. In contrast, short-term experimental hyperthyroidism in humans resulted a reduction of peak VO_2 of approximately 5% among otherwise healthy young volunteers [50]. In the latter experiments, heart rate and cardiac output were elevated at rest and throughout exercise, and VO_2 at any given work rate was higher in the hyperthyroid state. For both hypothyroid and acutely hyperthyroid rats, lactate threshold occurred at a lower work rate of exercise than for euthyroid animals [63].

Findings on Cardiopulmonary Exercise Testing Related to Thyroid Disorders

Studies of exercise function in patients with untreated hyperthyroidism reveal similar findings to the experimental models described above. Specifically, heart rate and VO_2 are high at rest, and remains high relative to any given work rate [64–66]. Kahaly et al. [67] studied 42 hyperthyroid patients with echocardiography and found that cardiac output, ejection fraction and stroke volume are all high at rest, and systemic vascular resistance low. With exercise, the increase in cardiac output was less than in the euthyroid condition, though peak values were marginally higher. Stroke volume declined from rest to exercise in untreated hyperthyroidism; treatment with popranolol decreased resting but not maximal values, restoring the pattern of increase from rest to exercise. Consistent with this, the same authors reported [65] that O_2 pulse was normal at rest, but low during exercise and only partially corrected by treatment with β-adrenergic blockade. The rate of increase of VO_2 relative to the increase in work rate has been variously reported to be elevated in hyperthyroid compared to euthyroid subjects [66] or within the normal range [64, 65]. Some investigators report a decrease in the slope when the same patients are restudied under euthyroid conditions [64, 66], but others do not [65]. In contrast to the study of short-term experimental hyperthyroidism [50], patients with clinical disease have been reported to have similar VO_2 values at the anaerobic threshold and peak exercise when euthyroid compared to when they had been hyperthyroid [65, 66]. Because VO_2 is elevated at rest and relative to work rate in hyperthyroidism, the increase in VO_2 from rest to peak exercise, and the work rates associated with anaerobic threshold and peak exercise are higher under euthyroid conditions compared to hyperthyroid. Ventilation is high at rest in the hyperthyroid states, but not significantly different at peak exercise under the two conditions [65].

There are relatively few reports of exercise responses in hypothyroid humans. Short-term hypothyroidism appears to have minor effects on cardiac contractile properties [55]. Exercise cardiac output is reduced compared to control conditions [55] but it is not clear whether this reduction is disproportionate to the reduction in metabolic rate. In subclinical hypothyroidism, subtle abnormalities of left-ventricular function are reported during exercise [68, 69], but it is doubted that these are of clinical significance. Even in symptomatic patients first presenting with thyroid deficiency, abnormalities of left-ventricular diastolic function may be difficult to detect except in the more severely affected patients [56]. Despite this, reports of impaired skeletal muscle function [58] in subjects with subclinical hypothyroidism suggests that maximal exercise capacity is likely to be reduced.

From the above it can be expected that marked abnormalities may be recognized on cardiopulmonary exercise tests in patients with hyperthyroidism. Resting levels of VO_2, VCO_2, heart rate and ventilation will all be elevated, and will remain high relative to normal values for a given level of submaximal work. The increase in VO_2 relative to work rate may be higher than average, but does not necessarily exceed the upper limits of normal. Peak VO_2 is reduced little, if at all, by uncomplicated hyperthyroidism; however, peak work rate will likely be reduced due to the shift of VO_2 relative to work rate. Despite the hyperdynamic circulation, O_2 pulse may be reduced because of a disproportionate increase in heart rate and cardiac output relative to VO_2. In hypothyroidism, in contrast, heart rate is low at rest and the response to exercise is attenuated. Peak VO_2 and lactate threshold are both likely to be significantly reduced in symptomatic hypothyroidism, though there are few data related to this in human subjects. Additional data regarding exercise responses in subclinical hypothyroidism would be of particular interest as the need for therapy for these patients is not fully defined.

Chronic Fatigue Syndrome

Although the etiology of chronic fatigue syndrome (CFS) remains unclear, there is an extensive literature characterizing its clinical features, and outlining standard criteria for case definitions for clinical research purposes [70, 71]. Common to the several working case definitions are fatigue of at least 6 months' duration which persists despite rest and reduction in activities, and a negative evaluation for other conditions that would account for the symptoms. Patients commonly report orthostatic and exercise intolerance and complain that even short periods of exertion result in exaggerated symptoms of fatigue for days thereafter. Exercise intolerance is thus a central feature of CFS, but despite considerable interest, the basis for it has not been identified.

Physiologic Effects of Chronic Fatigue Syndrome Relevant to Cardiopulmonary Exercise Testing

Although a great many contradictory reports have been generated regarding one or another abnormality of organ system function among selected patients, the overall consensus is that there is no specific abnormality of neuromuscular, cardiovascular or respiratory function underlying the condition.

Clinical studies have been complicated by the apparent heterogeneity of the patient population, with many reported findings affecting only a portion of a study group. Some of the more consistent findings that are reported include certain laboratory studies such as mild reductions in 24-hour cortisol excretion [72], decreased activity of natural killer cells [73, 74], and other alterations in immune effector cells or their products [74, 75]. These findings have been taken as support for the concept that patients with CFS have chronic activation of the immune system, but the basis for this and the relationship of these abnormalities to specific symptoms remain to be defined.

Findings on Cardiopulmonary Exercise Testing Related to CFS

A number of series of patients with CFS undergoing cardiopulmonary exercise testing have been reported. Several relatively small series of patients found average peak VO_2 values [76, 77] or peak work capacity [78] to be only mildly reduced compared to age- and gender-matched control subjects, or compared to published normal values [79, 80]. A larger series [81] of 427 patients and 204 age- and gender-matched sedentary control subjects reports a more significant reduction in peak VO_2, with the mean value of 20.5 ml/min/kg corresponding to only 64% of the value for control subjects. These investigators and others [77] have identified that a higher proportion of patients than control fail to demonstrate findings confirming that maximal effort had been attained during testing. However, analysis of the subset of patients with reasonably high peak heart rate and RER values still showed peak VO_2 to be significantly lower than in the control subjects [81]. The discrepancy in peak VO_2 values reported by various investigators may reflect recruitment bias towards higher functioning patients for inclusion in some series. There is, however, clearly a spectrum of exercise performance even among patients meeting the same case definition criteria. The relatively well-preserved exercise function of some symptomatic patients argues against the acute cardiorespiratory responses demonstrated on exercise testing to be the fundamental basis of clinical symptoms in CFS.

Some series, but not all [77], report higher heart rates for patients compared to controls at a given submaximal level of upright exercise. One [82] found lower heart rate responses during supine exercise. Peak heart rates are sometimes [80, 81], but not always [77–79], less than predicted. When subnormal peak heart rates have been noted, this has been variously interpreted to reflect premature limitation of exercise at a submaximal level due to central (i.e. nonmuscular) fatigue [79], or to reflect an intrinsic defect in chronotropic response [81], perhaps due to altered autonomic control. The question of autonomic dysfunction is also raised by another report of a high prevalence of abnormal results on tilt testing [83]. These findings have subsequently been contradicted by others [84], however, and additional studies of cardiovascular autonomic responses in CFS patients at rest have not shown consistent abnormalities [85, 86].

Whether the low peak heart rates and peak VO_2 values represent intrinsic effects of CFS or are the secondary results of poor maximal performance remains unclear. The lactate threshold has been reported to be normal in a series in which peak VO_2 was only mildly reduced [77], but both the work rate and heart rate corresponding to lactate threshold were low in the series finding lower peak VO_2 values [81]. The rate of increase of VO_2 relative to work rate is only reported in a few studies, and has been normal [77, 80]. No abnormality in ventilatory responses to exercise are reported from these studies.

Some investigators conclude that patients with CFS resemble severely deconditioned normal subjects. Deconditioning would not be surprising, as meeting the case definitions almost requires that patients be inactive, and patients represented in the studies had often been symptomatic for many years. Cause and effect with respect to exercise capacity and exercise behavior in this stetting remains to be established, however.

To summarize, exercise testing in patients with CFS often reveals mild-to-moderate reductions in peak VO_2, high submaximal heart rates, but low peak heart rate. As there are no pathognomonic findings of CFS on cardiopulmonary exercise testing, the role of testing is largely for evaluating alternative diagnoses, or for prescribing exercise training. With respect to the latter, it may be noted that despite the history of symptom exacerbation by exercise, incremental testing has been done without clinically important aggravation of the patients' conditions. There are findings to support a decline in cognitive function following a bout of maximal exercise [87, 88], as well as a decrease in spontaneous activity over subsequent days as reflected in accelerometer readings [89]. Both of these observations are consistent with symptomatic reports of prolonged post-exercise aesthenia in this condition. Nevertheless, Mullis et al. [80] concluded that of 130 patients undergoing maximal testing, none had lasting deterioration in their condition following testing, and only 3% reported exacerbation of symptoms. This is of practical importance as exercise training has been reported to improve sense of well-being and level of fitness of patients with CFS [90].

References

1 Luce JM: Respiratory complications of obesity. Chest 1980;78:626–631.

2 Sharp JT, Henry JP, Sweany SK: The total work of breathing in normal and obese men. J Clin Invest 1964;43:728–734.

3 Thomas PS, Cowen ER, Hulands G, Milledge JS: Respiratory function in the morbidly obese before and after weight loss. Thorax 1989;44: 382–386.

4 Ray CS, Sue DY, Bray G, Hansen JE, Wasserman K: Effects of obesity on respiratory function. Am Rev Respir Dis 1983;128:501–506.

5 Holley HS, Milic-Emili J, Becklake MR, Bates DV: Regional distribution of pulmonary ventilation and perfusion in obesity. J Clin Invest 1967;46:475–481.

6 Hakala K, Mustajoki P, Aittomaki J, Sovijarvi A: Improved gas exchange during exercise after weight loss in morbid obesity. Clin Physiol 1996;16:229–238.

7 Alpert MA, Lambert CR, Terry BE, Cohen MV, Mukerji V, Massey CV, Hashimi MW, Panayiotou H: Interrelationship of left ventricular mass, systolic function and diastolic filling in normotensive morbidly obese patients. Int J Obes Relat Metab Disord 1995;19:550–557.

8 Alpert MA: Obesity cardiomyopathy: Pathophysiology and evolution of the clinical syndrome. Am J Med Sci 2001;321:225–236.

9 Kaltman AJ, Goldring RM: Role of circulatory congestion in the cardiorespiratory failure of obesity. Am J Med 1976;60:645–653.

10 Alexander JK, Dennis DW, Smith WG, Amad KH, Ducan WC, Austin RD: Blood volume, cardiac output and distribution of systemic blood flow in extreme obesity. Cardiovasc Res Center Bull 1962;1:39–43.

11 Lauer MS, Anderson KM, Kannel WB, Levy D: The impact of obesity on left ventricular mass and geometry. The Framingham Heart Study. JAMA 1991;266:231–236.

12 Ben-Dov I, Grossman E, Stein A, Shachor D, Gaides M: Marked weight reduction lowers resting and exercise blood pressure in morbidly obese subjects. Am J Hypertens 2000;13:251–255.

13 Nielsen S, Hensrud DD, Romanski S, Levine JA, Burguera B, Jensen MD: Body composition and resting energy expenditure in humans: Role of fat, fat-free mass and extracellular fluid. Int J Obes Relat Metab Disord 2000;24: 1153–1157.

14 Goran M, Fields DA, Hunter GR, Herd SL, Weinsier RL: Total body fat does not influence maximal aerobic capacity. Int J Obes Relat Metab Disord 2000;24:841–848.

15 Nevill AM, Holder RL: Scaling, normalizing, and per ratio standards: An allometric modeling approach. J Appl Physiol 1995;79:1027–1031.

16 Batterham AM, Vanderburgh PM, Mahar MT, Jackson AS: Modeling the influence of body size on $V(O_2)$ peak: Effects of model choice and body composition. J Appl Physiol 1999;87: 1317–1325.

17 Whipp BJ, Davis JA: The ventilatory stress of exercise in obesity. Am Rev Respir Dis 1984; 129:S90–92.

18 Freyschuss U, Melcher A: Exercise energy expenditure in extreme obesity: Influence of ergometry type and weight loss. Scand J Clin Lab Invest 1978;38:753–759.

19 Dempsey JA, Reddan W, Balke B, Rankin J: Work capacity determinants and physiologic cost of weight-supported work in obesity. J Appl Physiol 1966;21:1815–1820.

20 Anton-Kuchly B, Roger P, Varene P: Determinants of increased energy cost of submaximal exercise in obese subjects. J Appl Physiol 1984; 56:18–23.

21 Wasserman K, Hansen JE, Sue DY, Casaburi R, Whipp BJ: Normal values; in Principles of Exercise Testing and Interpretation, ed 3. Philadelphia, Lippincott Williams & Wilkins, 1999, pp 143–164.

22 Wasserman K, Whipp BJ: Excercise physiology in health and disease. Am Rev Respir Dis 1975;112:219–249.

23 Hansen JE, Sue DY, Wasserman K: Predicted values for clinical exercise testing. Am Rev Respir Dis 1984;129:S49–55.

24 Babb TG, Buskirk ER, Hodgson JL: Exercise end-expiratory lung volumes in lean and moderately obese women. Int J Obes 1989;13:11–19.

25 Li J, Li S, Feuers RJ, Buffington CK, Cowan GS: Influence of body fat distribution on oxygen uptake and pulmonary performance in morbidly obese females during exercise. Respirology 2001;6:9–13.

26 Uusitupa MI, Mustonen JN, Airaksinen KE: Diabetic heart muscle disease. Ann Med 1990; 22:377–386.

27 Fein FS, Sonnenblick EH: Diabetic cardiomyopathy. Cardiovasc Drugs Ther 1994;8:65–73.

28 Zabalgoitia M, Ismaeil MF, Anderson L, Maklady FA: Prevalence of diastolic dysfunction in normotensive, asymptomatic patients with well-controlled type 2 diabetes mellitus. Am J Cardiol 2001;87:320–323.

29 Poirier P, Garneau C, Bogaty P, Nadeau A, Marois L, Brochu C, Gingras C, Fortin C, Jobin J, Dumesnil JG: Impact of left ventricular diastolic dysfunction on maximal treadmill performance in normotensive subjects with well-controlled type 2 diabetes mellitus. Am J Cardiol 2000;85:473–477.

30 Di Bonito P, Cuomo S, Moio N, Sibilio G, Sabatini D, Quattrin S, Capaldo B: Diastolic dysfunction in patients with non-insulin-dependent diabetes mellitus of short duration. Diabet Med 1996;13:321–324.

31 Nicolino A, Longobardi G, Furgi G, Rossi M, Zoccolillo N, Ferrara N, Rengo F: Left ventricular diastolic filling in diabetes mellitus with and without hypertension. Am J Hypertens 1995;8:382–389.

32 Scognamiglio R, Avogaro A, Casara D, Crepaldi C, Marin M, Palisi M, Mingardi R, Erle G, Fasoli G, Dalla Volta S: Myocardial dysfunction and adrenergic cardiac innervation in patients with insulin-dependent diabetes mellitus. J Am Coll Cardiol 1998;31:404–412.

33 Astorri E, Fiorina P, Contini GA, Albertini D, Magnati G, Astorri A, Lanfredini M: Isolated and preclinical impairment of left ventricular filling in insulin-dependent and non-insulin-dependent diabetic patients. Clin Cardiol 1997;20:536–540.

34 Davis TM, Knuiman M, Kendall P, Vu H, Davis WA: Reduced pulmonary function and its associations in type 2 diabetes: The Fremantle Diabetes Study. Diabetes Res Clin Pract 2000;50:153–159.

35 Barrett-Connor E, Frette C: NIDDM, impaired glucose tolerance, and pulmonary function in older adults: The Rancho Bernardo Study. Diabetes Care 1996;19:1441–1444.

36 Radice M, Rocca A, Bedon E, Musacchio N, Morabito A, Segalini G: Abnormal response to exercise in middle-aged NIDDM patients with and without autonomic neuropathy. Diabet Med 1996;13:259–265.

37 Veves A, Saouaf R, Donaghue VM, Mullooly CA, Kistler JA, Giurini JM, Horton ES, Fielding RA: Aerobic exercise capacity remains normal despite impaired endothelial function in the micro- and macrocirculation of physically active IDDM patients. Diabetes 1997;46:1846–1852.

38 Regensteiner JG, Sippel J, McFarling ET, Wolfel EE, Hiatt WR: Effects of non-insulin-dependent diabetes on oxygen consumption during treadmill exercise. Med Sci Sports Exerc 1995; 27:875–881.

39 Baraldi E, Monciotti C, Filippone M, Santuz P, Magagnin G, Zanconato S, Zacchello F: Gas exchange during exercise in diabetic children. Pediatr Pulmonol 1992;13:155–160.

40 Bottini P, Tantucci C, Scionti L, Dottorini ML, Puxeddu E, Reboldi G, Bolli GB, Casucci G, Santeusanio F, Sorbini CA: Cardiovascular response to exercise in diabetic patients: Influence of autonomic neuropathy of different severity. Diabetologia 1995;38:244–250.

41 Katoh J, Hara Y, Kurusu M, Miyaji J, Narutaki K: Cardiorespiratory function as assessed by exercise testing in patients with non-insulin-dependent diabetes mellitus. J Int Med Res 1996;24:209–213.

42 Wanke T, Formanek D, Auinger M, Zwick H, Irsigler K: Pulmonary gas exchange and oxygen uptake during exercise in patients with type 1 diabetes mellitus. Diabet Med 1992;9:252–257.

43 Roy TM, Peterson HR, Snider HL, Cyrus J, Broadstone VL, Fell RD, Rothchild AH, Samols E, Pfeifer MA: Autonomic influence on cardiovascular performance in diabetic subjects. Am J Med 1989;87:382–388.

44 Estacio RO, Regensteiner JG, Wolfel EE, Jeffers B, Dickenson M, Schrier RW: The association between diabetic complications and exercise capacity in NIDDM patients. Diabetes Care 1998;21:291–295.

45 Regensteiner JG, Bauer TA, Reusch JE, Brandenburg SL, Sippel JM, Vogelsong AM, Smith S, Wolfel EE, Eckel RH, Hiatt WR: Abnormal oxygen uptake kinetic responses in women with type II diabetes mellitus. J Appl Physiol 1998;85:310–317.

46 Minette P, Buysschaert M, Rahier J, Veriter C, Frans A: Pulmonary gas exchange in life-long nonsmoking patients with diabetes mellitus. Respiration 1999;66:20–24.

47 Klein I, Ojamaa K: Thyroid hormone and the cardiovascular system. N Engl J Med 2001; 344:501–509.
48 Forfar JC, Muir AL, Sawers SA, Toft AD: Abnormal left ventricular function in hyperthyroidism: Evidence for a possible reversible cardiomyopathy. N Engl J Med 1982;307: 1165–1170.
49 Iskandrian AS, Rose L, Hakki AH, Segal BL, Kane SA: Cardiac performance in thyrotoxicosis: Analysis of 10 untreated patients. Am J Cardiol 1983;51:349–352.
50 Martin WH, Spina RJ, Korte E, Yarasheski KE, Angelopoulos TJ, Nemeth PM, Saffitz JE: Mechanisms of impaired exercise capacity in short duration experimental hyperthyroidism. J Clin Invest 1991;88:2047–2053.
51 McAllister RM, Delp MD, Laughlin MH: Thyroid status and exercise tolerance: Cardiovascular and metabolic considerations. Sports Med 1995;20:189–198.
52 McAllister RM, Sansone JC, Laughlin MH: Effects of hyperthyroidism on muscle blood flow during exercise in rats. Am J Physiol 1995; 268:H330–335.
53 Bough EW, Crowley WF, Ridgway C, Walker H, Maloof F, Myers GS, Daniels GH: Myocardial function in hypothyroidism: Relation to disease severity and response to treatment. Arch Intern Med 1978;138:1476–1480.
54 Wieshammer S, Keck FS, Waitzinger J, Henze E, Loos U, Hombach V, Pfeiffer EF: Acute hypothyroidism slows the rate of left ventricular diastolic relaxation. Can J Physiol Pharmacol 1989;67:1007–1010.
55 Wieshammer S, Keck FS, Waitzinger J, Kohler J, Adam W, Stauch M, Pfeiffer EF: Left ventricular function at rest and during exercise in acute hypothyroidism. Br Heart J 1988;60: 204–211.
56 Tielens ET, Pillay M, Storm C, Berghout A: Changes in cardiac function at rest before and after treatment in primary hypothyroidism. Am J Cardiol 2000;85:376–380.
57 Baldwin KM, Ernst SB, Herrick RE, Hooker AM, Mullin WJ: Exercise capacity and cardiac function in trained and untrained thyroid-deficient rats. J Appl Physiol 1980;49:1022–1026.
58 Monzani F, Caraccio N, Siciliano G, Manca L, Murri L, Ferrannini E: Clinical and biochemical features of muscle dysfunction in subclinical hypothyroidism. J Clin Endocrinol Metab 1997;82:3315–3318.
59 Argov Z, Renshaw PF, Boden B, Winokur A, Bank WJ: Effects of thyroid hormones on skeletal muscle bioenergetics: In vivo phosphorus-31 magnetic resonance spectroscopy study of humans and rats. J Clin Invest 1988;81:1695–1701.
60 Khaleeli AA, Griffith DG, Edwards RH: The clinical presentation of hypothyroid myopathy and its relationship to abnormalities in structure and function of skeletal muscle. Clin Endocrinol (Oxf) 1983;19:365–376.
61 Martinez FJ, Bermudez-Gomez M, Celli BR: Hypothyroidism. A reversible cause of diaphragmatic dysfunction. Chest 1989;96:1059–1063.
62 Zwillich CW, Pierson DJ, Hofeldt FD, Lufkin EG, Weil JV: Ventilatory control in myxedema and hypothyroidism. N Engl J Med 1975;292: 662–665.
63 Zarzeczny R, Pilis W, Langfort J, Kaciuba-Uscilko H, Nazar K: Influence of thyroid hormones on exercise tolerance and lactate threshold in rats. J Physiol Pharmacol 1996;47:503–513.
64 Ben-Dov I, Sietsema KE, Wasserman K: O_2 uptake in hyperthyroidism during constant work rate and incremental exercise. Eur J Appl Physiol Occup Physiol 1991;62:261–267.
65 Kahaly GJ, Nieswandt J, Wagner S, Schlegel J, Mohr-Kahaly S, Hommel G: Ineffective cardiorespiratory function in hyperthyroidism. J Clin Endocrinol Metab 1998;83:4075–4078.
66 Kimura H, Kawagoe Y, Kaneko N, Fessler HE, Hosoda S: Low efficiency of oxygen utilization during exercise in hyperthyroidism. Chest 1996;110:1264–1270.
67 Kahaly GJ, Wagner S, Nieswandt J, Mohr-Kahaly S, Ryan TJ: Stress echocardiography in hyperthyroidism. J Clin Endocrinol Metab 1999;84:2308–2313.
68 Arem R, Rokey R, Kiefe C, Escalante DA, Rodriguez A: Cardiac systolic and diastolic function at rest and exercise in subclinical hypothyroidism: Effect of thyroid hormone therapy. Thyroid 1996;6:397–402.
69 Forfar JC, Wathen CG, Todd WT, Bell GM, Hannan WJ, Muir AL, Toft AD: Left ventricular performance in subclinical hypothyroidism. Q J Med 1985;57:857–865.
70 Bates DW, Buchwald D, Lee J, Kith P, Doolittle TH, Umali P, Komaroff AL: A comparison of case definitions of chronic fatigue syndrome. Clin Infect Dis 1994;18(suppl 1):S11–15.
71 Fukuda K, Straus SE, Hickie I, Sharpe MC, Dobbins JG, Komaroff A: The chronic fatigue syndrome: A comprehensive approach to its definition and study. International Chronic Fatigue Syndrome Study Group. Ann Intern Med 1994;121:953–959.
72 Demitrack MA, Dale JK, Straus SE, Laue L, Listwak SJ, Kruesi MJ, Chrousos GP, Gold PW: Evidence for impaired activation of the hypothalamic-pituitary-adrenal axis in patients with chronic fatigue syndrome. J Clin Endocrinol Metab 1991;73:1224–1234.
73 Whiteside TL, Friberg D: Natural killer cells and natural killer cell activity in chronic fatigue syndrome. Am J Med 1998;105:27S–34S.
74 Barker E, Fujimura SF, Fadem MB, Landay AL, Levy JA: Immunologic abnormalities associated with chronic fatigue syndrome. Clin Infect Dis 1994;18(suppl 1):S136–141.
75 Buchwald D, Komaroff AL: Review of laboratory findings for patients with chronic fatigue syndrome. Rev Infect Dis 1991;13(suppl 1): S12–18.
76 Riley MS, O'Brien CJ, McCluskey DR, Bell NP, Nicholls DP: Aerobic work capacity in patients with chronic fatigue syndrome. BMJ 1990;301:953–956.
77 Sisto SA, LaManca J, Cordero DL, Bergen MT, Ellis SP, Drastal S, Boda WL, Tapp WN, Natelson BH: Metabolic and cardiovascular effects of a progressive exercise test in patients with chronic fatigue syndrome. Am J Med 1996; 100:634–640.
78 Gibson H, Carroll N, Clague JE, Edwards RH: Exercise performance and fatiguability in patients with chronic fatigue syndrome. J Neurol Neurosurg Psychiatry 1993;56:993–998.
79 Kent-Braun JA, Sharma KR, Weiner MW, Massie B, Miller RG: Central basis of muscle fatigue in chronic fatigue syndrome. Neurology 1993;43:125–131.
80 Mullis R, Campbell IT, Wearden AJ, Morriss RK, Pearson DJ: Prediction of peak oxygen uptake in chronic fatigue syndrome. Br J Sports Med 1999;33:352–356.
81 De Becker P, Roeykens J, Reynders M, McGregor N, De Meirleir K: Exercise capacity in chronic fatigue syndrome. Arch Intern Med 2000;160:3270–3277.
82 Montague TJ, Marrie TJ, Klassen GA, Bewick DJ, Horacek BM: Cardiac function at rest and with exercise in the chronic fatigue syndrome. Chest 1989;95:779–784.
83 Bou-Holaigah I, Rowe PC, Kan J, Calkins H: The relationship between neurally mediated hypotension and the chronic fatigue syndrome. JAMA 1995;274:961–967.
84 Poole J, Herrell R, Ashton S, Goldberg J, Buchwald D: Results of isoproterenol tilt table testing in monozygotic twins discordant for chronic fatigue syndrome. Arch Intern Med 2000;160:3461–3468.
85 Soetekouw PM, Lenders JW, Bleijenberg G, Thien T, van der Meer JW: Autonomic function in patients with chronic fatigue syndrome. Clin Auton Res 1999;9:334–340.
86 De Becker P, Dendale P, De Meirleir K, Campine I, Vandenborne K, Hagers Y: Autonomic testing in patients with chronic fatigue syndrome. Am J Med 1998;105:22S–26S.
87 LaManca JJ, Sisto SA, DeLuca J, Johnson SK, Lange G, Pareja J, Cook S, Natelson BH: Influence of exhaustive treadmill exercise on cognitive functioning in chronic fatigue syndrome. Am J Med 1998;105:59S–65S.
88 Blackwood SK, MacHale SM, Power MJ, Goodwin GM, Lawrie SM: Effects of exercise on cognitive and motor function in chronic fatigue syndrome and depression. J Neurol Neurosurg Psychiatry 1998;65:541–546.
89 Sisto SA, Tapp WN, LaManca JJ, Ling W, Korn LR, Nelson AJ, Natelson BH: Physical activity before and after exercise in women with chronic fatigue syndrome. QJM 1998;91: 465–473.
90 Fulcher KY, White PD: Randomised controlled trial of graded exercise in patients with the chronic fatigue syndrome. BMJ 1997;314: 1647–1652.

Kathy E. Sietsema, MD
Division of Respiratory and Critical Care Physiology and Medicine
Harbor-UCLA Medical Center
1000 West Carson Street
Torrance, CA 90509 (USA)
Tel. +1 310 222 3803, Fax +1 310 328 9849
E-Mail ksietsema@rei.edu

Weisman IM, Zeballos RJ (eds): Clinical Exercise Testing.
Prog Respir Res. Basel, Karger, 2002, vol 32, pp 273–281

Clinical Exercise Testing during Pregnancy and the Postpartum Period

Mary L. O'Toole Raul Artal

Women's Exercise Research Laboratory, Department of Obstetrics, Gynecology and Women's Health, Saint Louis University, St. Louis, Mo., USA

Summary

Cardiopulmonary exercise testing of pregnant women may be done for either diagnostic or nondiagnostic reasons. The most common reason to exercise test healthy young women, pregnant or not, is to acquire information with which to develop individualized exercise prescriptions. Pregnant women can be tested either during weight-bearing activity (e.g., treadmill walking) or during an activity that is independent of body weight (e.g., cycle ergometry). Semi-recumbent cycle ergometry appears to be the most comfortable modality. Short incremental protocols (8–12 min) to maximal subjective effort provide good information and appear to be safe during all stages of pregnancy for both mother and fetus. Single-stage submaximal protocols are also safe and may provide useful information, particularly when substrate or hormonal responses are of interest. For proper interpretation of results, individuals involved in conducting exercise testing of pregnant women should be aware of the anatomical and physiological changes that may alter cardiopulmonary responses to exercise during pregnancy.

Introduction

Many young women consider physical activity to be an integral part of their lives and wish to continue regular activity throughout their pregnancies. Many other young women are sedentary, but see pregnancy as a time to develop healthy lifestyle habits including participation in regular physical activity. Other young women have or develop medical conditions during their pregnancies for which regular physical activity would be beneficial. Individuals from each of these groups may benefit from cardiopulmonary exercise testing to assist in the planning of physical activity during pregnancy.

As with other populations, cardiopulmonary exercise testing of pregnant women may be done for either diagnostic or nondiagnostic reasons. Diagnostic tests are done to establish the safety of participation while nondiagnostic tests may be used to assess fitness, provide a basis for exercise prescription or monitor progress in an exercise program. Pregnant women, however, present unique concerns regarding exercise testing and participation. Unlike usual diagnostic tests for disease conditions, the well-being of the fetus and the exercising mother must be established. Thus, all tests, while not strictly diagnostic, are used to establish safety of exercise participation during pregnancy. Pregnancy is associated with profound anatomical and physiological changes that alter cardiopulmonary responses both at rest and during exercise. Individuals involved in conducting cardiopulmonary exercise testing of pregnant women must be aware of these changes in order to choose appropriate testing modalities and protocols as well as to be able to correctly interpret exercise test results.

Anatomic/Physiologic Changes Associated with Pregnancy

The most obvious changes with the potential to affect exercise test responses during pregnancy are the increase in body weight and fat. Average weight gain during pregnancy is approximately 12.5 kg, approximately a 20% increase in body weight for most women [1]. Weight gain increases with increasing gestation such that expected weight gain during the first trimester is only 1–3 kg, while 6–8 kg increases occur during the second trimester and 3.5–4 kg increases are usual during the third trimester. Of this, 2.5 kg is estimated to be increased maternal fat [2, 3]. Although the time course for changes in maternal body fat are difficult to precisely quantify, most evidence suggests that percent body fat increases during the first and second trimesters, then plateaus or decreases slightly during the third trimester [1, 4].

The gains in weight and body fat result in changes in posture, balance, and locomotor patterns. Protrusion of the abdomen with accompanying increased lumbar lordosis and anterior pelvic rotation results in altered spinal mechanics and displacement forward of the woman's line of gravity. These changes result in low back pain for approximately 50% of pregnant women and may alter their ability to perform an adequate exercise test during walking on a treadmill [5]. An upward displacement of the diaphragm alters pulmonary mechanics so that residual volume, expiratory reserve volume and functional residual capacity are all reduced at rest. However, inspiratory capacity is increased so that vital capacity is not changed and resting pulmonary function is well preserved [6–8]. Increase diaphragmatic work and greater use of accessory muscle of breathing do result in an increased work of breathing that is partially compensated for by decreased bronchial smooth muscle tone and reduced pulmonary resistance [9].

In addition to the anatomic changes, pregnancy affects the pulmonary system by increasing ventilatory sensitivity. The respiratory center has a decreased threshold to respond to PCO_2 and an increased sensitivity to any rise in PCO_2 [6, 7, 11–13]. These changes are thought to be secondary to increased circulating progesterone levels and result in larger tidal volumes and minute ventilations. Resting arterial PO_2 levels rise to approximately 100 mm Hg and arterial PCO_2 levels decrease to 30–32 mm Hg. Respiratory alkalosis results and is only partially compensated for by urinary excretion of bicarbonate.

Pregnancy also causes changes in the cardiovascular system that have an impact on responses during exercise testing. Such changes include an increase in blood volume, heart rate, and stroke volume as well as resultant cardiac output, and a decrease in systemic vascular resistance [11, 14, 15]. Blood volume expands to 40–50% above resting levels, reaching a peak towards the end of the second trimester [16]. Increases in both plasma volume (approximately 50%) and red cell volume (20%) contribute to the increase in blood volume [17–19]. Associated increases in end-diastolic volumes in conjunction with slightly increased contractility result in larger stroke volumes than during the nonpregnant state [20]. Resting heart rates start to rise as early as 8 weeks of gestation (approximately 8 bpm) and reach a peak by 32 weeks of gestation that is about 20 bpm higher than in the nonpregnant state [21, 22]. Most studies show that maternal stroke volume increases by 10% by the end of the first trimester and is followed by a 20% increase in heart rate during the second and third trimesters [23]. The increased cardiac output results in a chronic volume overload of the heart. As in other situations with chronic volume overload, the left-ventricular chamber increases in size with little or no change in wall thickness [24–26]. Despite this increase in cardiac output, mean arterial pressure decreases by 5–10 mm Hg by the middle of the second trimester and then gradually increases back to prepregnancy levels [13]. The decreased blood pressures are mediated by venous relaxation, greater venous capacitance and reduced peripheral resistance [27, 28]. In particular, there is an increase in the vasculature of the uterine circulation and decreases in vascular resistance in the skin, kidney and uteroplacental circulations [23]. These hemodynamic changes appear to establish a circulatory reserve necessary to provide nutrients and oxygen to both mother and fetus at rest and during moderate exercise.

Clinical Screening Prior to Exercise Testing during Pregnancy

Pretest screening should be designed to determine whether sufficient physiologic reserve exists to accommodate maternal and fetal needs plus additional demands of exercise testing. A thorough pretest medical history should include both past and present information. Suggested components for this exam include any medical diagnoses, findings from previous physical exams, a thorough history of any symptoms, recent illnesses, orthopedic problems, medication use, other habits such as use of caffeine, alcohol or tobacco, exercise history, work history with emphasis on physical demands, and family history of

Table 1. Contraindications to exercise testing*

Absolute
Recent significant change in resting ECG suggestive of ischemia, myocardial infarction or other acute cardiac event
Unstable angina
Uncontrolled arrhythmias causing symptoms or hemodynamic compromise
Severe symptomatic aortic stenosis
Uncontrolled congestive heart failure
Acute pulmonary embolus or pulmonary infarction
Acute myocarditis or pericarditis
Suspected or known dissecting aneurysm
Acute infection
Relative
Left main coronary stenosis
Stenotic valvular heart disease of moderate severity
Significant electrolyte abnormalities
Severe arterial hypertension at rest (systolic BP >200 mm Hg; diastolic BP >110 mm Hg)
Tachy- or bradyarrhythmias
Hypertrophic cardiomyopathy or other forms of outflow tract obstruction
Disorders (neuromuscular, musculoskeletal or rheumatoid) that are exacerbated by exercise
High-degree atrioventricular block
Ventricular aneurysm
Uncontrolled metabolic disease (e.g. diabetes, thrytoxicosis or myxedema)
Chronic infectious disease (e.g. mononucleosis, hepatitis, AIDS)

* Adapted from ref. [29].

Table 2. Contraindications to exercise testing or participation during pregnancy

Absolute
Hemodynamically significant heart disease
Constrictive lung disease
History of three or more spontaneous abortions
Incompetent cervix/cerlage
Multiple gestation
Persistent second-or-third-trimester bleeding
Placenta previa
Premature labor during the prior or current pregnancy
Ruptured membranes
Pregnancy-induced hypertension
Relative
Anemia Breech presentation in last trimester
Cardiac arrhythmia or palpitations
Chronic bronchitis
Uncontrolled diabetes
Morbid obesity
Extreme underweight
History of bleeding during current pregnancy
History of extremely sedentary lifestyle
History of intrauterine growth restriction
History of precipitous labor
Hypertension
Orthopedic limitations
Seizure disorder
Thyroid disease
Heavy smoker

cardiopulmonary or metabolic disease [29]. Contraindications to exercise testing because of medical conditions in the nonpregnant state are equally applicable during pregnancy (table 1). In addition, certain obstetrical conditions may develop in a pregnant woman regardless of her previous activity or fitness level that disqualify her from safely participating in an exercise test. Use of the PARmed-X for Pregnancy may be an aid in identifying these obstetrical conditions [30]. Table 2 is suggested as a guide to determining the appropriateness of exercise testing or participation during pregnancy for individual patients [see also ref. 31].

Exercise Test Considerations

Reasons to Exercise Test Pregnant Women

The most common reason to exercise test healthy women is to acquire information with which to develop individualized exercise prescriptions. This is true for pregnant as well as nonpregnant women. The 'gold standard' tests for this purpose are tests to assess cardiopulmonary fitness by measuring maximal aerobic capacity (VO_2max). These tests are typically incremental tests with work rates starting at low intensity and progressing up to maximal effort. In nonpregnant individuals, incremental submaximal tests to a preset endpoint (such as 85% age-predicted maximal heart rate) are sometimes used to predict maximal exercise capacity and develop individualized exercise plans. Because of progressive changes in hemodynamics, pulmonary function, and energy cost of exercise during the course of gestation, submaximal tests are less useful during pregnancy and may be quite misleading when used for this purpose (see below). Exercise tests may also be used and to monitor progress in response to an exercise training program and to adjust the exercise prescription appropriately over time. In nonpregnant women, either maximal or submaximal tests may be reliably used. In pregnant women, submaximal tests may be used in most cases. However, if precise quantification of fitness changes during pregnancy is important (such as in research studies), maximal exercise tests are necessary.

In addition to using exercise testing to guide healthy pregnant women in an exercise program, exercise testing may be used to guide exercise training for women with gestational diabetes. Testing procedures are similar to those used with healthy women with the addition of blood glucose monitoring before and after exercise. Exercise tests that monitor substrate utilization and/or hormonal, cardiovascular or pulmonary responses over a prolonged period of time to a single submaximal intensity (see below) may also be useful in guiding exercise of women with gestational diabetes. Additional uses of exercise tests during pregnancy are to evaluate suspected deficits in cardiopulmonary or metabolic function and to monitor disease-related decreases in physical function.

Selection of Testing Mode

Pregnant women can be tested either during weight-bearing activity, such as treadmill walking or during an activity that is independent of body weight, such as cycle ergometry.

Weight-Bearing Exercise. Treadmill walking is a commonly used weight-bearing exercise testing mode. The main advantage of treadmill testing is that it provides a familiar type of exercise stress (i.e. walking). Treadmill tests can be used for women with marked differences in fitness level because of the wide range of speeds and grades available. The treadmill test should be chosen when the individualized exercise prescription is to be a walking program. Several disadvantages are associated with treadmill testing. Good balance and locomotor skills are necessary for safe and accurate testing. Although most treadmills have a front and at least one side rail for individuals to steady themselves, accurate cardiopulmonary and metabolic measurements will only result when the test is done without holding the handrails. Other disadvantages of treadmill testing include the expense of a treadmill, inability to move it easily and difficulty in making some measurements, such as taking blood pressure. For these reasons, treadmill testing may not be appropriate for pregnant women late in gestation when balance is difficult, when pregnancy-induced hypertension may be present or for sequential measurements through the course of pregnancy.

Weight-Supported Exercise. Cycle ergometers provide an option for non-weight-bearing testing and may be more useful during pregnancy. Cycle ergometers may be traditional upright leg cycles, semi-recumbent cycles or arm cycles. Regardless of specific type, resistance can usually be adjusted in small amounts. Older mechanically braked ergometers (e.g. Monark) require proper pedal speed to be maintained to obtain the desired resistance. This may be difficult for some women, particularly late in pregnancy when the protruding abdomen may interfere will leg cycling movements. Most newer models, however, are electromagnetically braked so that appropriate resistance will result across a wide range of pedal rates. Cycle ergometers are relatively inexpensive, require little space and are easily transportable. Upright cycling has frequently been used to test pregnant women. We have also used the semi-recumbent cycle for sedentary, overweight pregnant women because of its more comfortable seat and body position. Physiologic monitoring is considerably easier during cycling compared with treadmill testing. Arm ergometers have been used with pregnant women and have been shown to be safe (no uterine contractions during or immediately postexercise) [32]. However, we do not recommend routine use of arm ergometry to test pregnant women because of the small muscle mass used and resultant local arm and shoulder fatigue.

Maximal Exercise Tests

Protocol Selection. The basic pattern of maximal test protocols for pregnant women is not different from that for nonpregnant women. Selection of a specific protocol should be in accord with the purpose of the test, the outcome measure(s) of interest and the individual being tested. For example, if the purpose is to individualize a walking program, a treadmill protocol would be appropriate. If, on the other hand, sedentary obese patients are to be tested, a semirecumbent cycle ergometer protocol may be more appropriate. Treadmill protocols that call for constant speed with increases in grade have been used with pregnant women [33] as have those using a constant treadmill incline with increases in speed [34]. The treadmill protocol that we prefer to use with pregnant women is the ACT (Activity Counseling Trial) protocol [35]. Briefly, in the ACT protocol, participants are taught to walk on the treadmill at a low speed until they can walk without holding on to the handrails. This is particularly important for pregnant women whose balance may be altered by her pregnancy. Treadmill speed is then increased slowly until a speed that elicits a heart rate equivalent to 60–70% of age-predicted maximal heart rate is identified. After a brief rest, the test begins at the identified speed and zero percent grade. The test proceeds with 2% grade increments every 2 min (approximately 1 MET/stage increments) until maximal effort is reached. This protocol is a particularly good option for women who have been active

Table 3. General indications for stopping an exercise test in low-risk adults*

Onset of angina or angina-like symptoms
Significant drop (20 mm Hg) in systolic blood pressure or failure of systolic blood pressure to rise with an increase in exercise intensity
Excessive rise in blood pressure (SBP > 260 mm Hg; DBP > 115 mm Hg)
Signs of poor perfusion: light-headedness, confusion, ataxia, pallor, cyanosis, nausea, or cold and clammy skin
Failure of heart rate to increase with increase in intensity
Noticeable change in heart rhythm
Subject requests to stop
Physical or verbal manifestations of severe fatigue
Failure of the testing equipment

* Adapted from ref. [29].

Table 4. Warning signs to stop exercising while pregnant*

Shortness of breath
Dizziness
Headache (may be early sign of pre-eclampsia or pregnancy-induced hypertension)
Chest pain
Muscle weakness
Calf pain or swelling (need to rule out thrombophelbitis)
Regular good-quality contractions that change the cervix
Decreased fetal movement
Amniotic fluid leakage
Generalized swelling (early sign of pre-eclampsia)
Pain of hips, back, or symphysis pubis

* Adapted from Artal and Sherman [10] and Kulpa [55].

walkers or joggers prior to pregnancy. It is also appropriate for more sedentary women who wish to participate in a walking program during pregnancy. When administered correctly, this protocol results in maximal effort being reached in 8–12 min regardless of initial fitness level.

Most commonly, maximal exercise tests during pregnancy use upright leg cycle ergometer protocols. Protocols that have been reported are remarkably similar. After a 2- to 4-min warm-up during which the patient pedals against little or no resistance, resistance is increased by 20–30 W/min to volitional fatigue [34, 36–40]. Upright leg cycle ergometry protocols have been used successfully from 16 to 35 weeks of gestation to 12 weeks postpartum. In addition to upright cycling protocols, we have found the leg cycling test on a semi-recumbent cycle ergometer to be more comfortable for obese, pregnant women, particularly during the third trimester. The semi-recumbent cycle protocol utilized in our laboratory employs 10-Watt increments (approximately 0.5 MET increments) each minute. We have found this protocol to be useful in evaluating women with gestational diabetes who tend to be overweight or obese and sedentary. Spinnewijn et al. [40] have used a tethered swimming protocol to evaluate exercise performance in a weightless environment. In this protocol, the swimmer swims breast stroke attached to a pulley system with adjustable weights. Initial resistance is 0.5 kg with 0.5 kg being added each minute until the swimmer can no longer sustain the pull. Regardless of the protocol chosen, it is advisable to have an experienced obstetrical nurse use a cardiotocometer to monitor the fetus for 15–20 min before and after the exercise test. Measurements of fetal baseline heart rate, frequency of accelerations and decelerations, and fetal heart rate variability can then be used, according to the guidelines developed by the National Institute of Child Health and Human Development, to document lack of harm to the fetus from the exercise test [41].

Safety of Maximal Exercise Testing Protocols. Maximal testing using short protocols (8–12 min) appears to be safe during all stages of pregnancy for both mother and fetus [36, 42]. Usual monitoring during maximal testing of pregnant women should include a 12-lead ECG, heart rate (HR), blood pressure (BP), and rating of perceived exertion (RPE). When energy expenditure, substrate utilization or pulmonary function are of interest, gas exchange measurements should be added. The same precautions and indications for stopping an exercise test that are used with nonpregnant individuals should be observed (table 3).

Additionally, reasons to stop an exercise test of a pregnant woman include the warning signs listed in table 4.

However, in the absence of signs or symptoms of exercise intolerance, a pregnant woman should be able to safely continue a cardiopulmonary exercise test until she reaches subjective maximal effort (volitional fatigue). Fetal heart rate responses to a short, maximal exercise test have been reported to be minimal and transient. The most common response is a mild tachycardia immediately after exercise that returns to baseline levels within 20–30 min [43–48]. Caution is advised, however, that these data are derived from normal pregnancies in healthy women. Screening, including estimates of fetal weight, should be made before clearing an apparently healthy, pregnant woman for a maximal exercise test.

Expected Responses to Maximal Exercise Tests during Pregnancy. Studies have compared physiologic responses to maximal cardiopulmonary exercise testing of pregnant women with responses of nonpregnant women. Both cross-sectional and longitudinal study designs have been used to study maximal responses at various times throughout gestation and postpartum. Some data [34] support the use of postpartum values as control values (i.e. not different from pre-pregnancy values), while others [49] suggest that true control values (not recently pregnant) and postpartum values may result in different outcomes in ventilatory and metabolic comparisons. These authors also reported on a sub-sample of women (n = 4) who were studied 3 months before gestation to 6 months postpartum. The average 7-week postpartum values at maximal exercise were not different from prepregnancy or 6-month postpartum values, suggesting that comparison of pregnancy values with either pre- or postpregnancy values provides an appropriate control. Upright cycling has been the most common testing mode, but data are also available for treadmill testing and tethered swimming.

There is consensus that cycling VO_2peak is unaffected by pregnancy [34, 36, 40, 50–52]. Peak power (Watts) may be slightly less (4%) at 35 (but not at 15 or 25) weeks of gestation in comparison with 7 weeks postpartum [34]. Maximal heart rate may be unchanged [36] or slightly lower [34, 40] during pregnancy. Efficiency of leg cycling at maximal effort appears to be unchanged during pregnancy [34, 36]. Cross-sectional analyses suggest that maximal CO_2 production (VCO_2max) is slightly lower and may be sufficiently low to decrease maximal respiratory exchange ratio (RER max) [36]. Longitudinal analysis demonstrated that VCO_2max progressively decreased (6, 9 and 11% at 15, 25 and 35 weeks of gestation) during pregnancy [34]. RER max appears to be approximately 5–7% lower late in pregnancy in comparison with nonpregnant conditions [34, 36]. Maximal minute ventilation can be expected to be approximately 5–7% greater during pregnancy, mainly as a result of a higher maximal tidal volume and no change in breathing frequency. Thus, the ventilatory equivalent of oxygen (V_E/VO_2) should increase and the ventilatory equivalent of carbon dioxide (V_E/VCO_2) should decrease. This was documented in a longitudinal study [34], but was not evident in data from a recent, cross-sectional study [36]. In the cross-sectional study, none of the respiratory gas exchange variables that were measured (V_E, $P_{ET}O_2$, $P_{ET}CO_2$) were different between pregnant and nonpregnant women at maximal exercise [36]. Peak lactates have been reported to be decreased in pregnant women [36, 39, 50, 53]. The lower peak lactate in combination with lower respiratory exchange ratios suggest that carbohydrate utilization is reduced, perhaps as a protective mechanism to spare glucose for the fetus. A lesser O_2 debt (excess postexercise oxygen consumption) has been reported and suggests that smaller changes in temperature, catecholamines, calcium ions, fatty acids, or restoration of glycogen, ATP and creatine phosphate stores have occurred [36]. These responses may aid in maintenance of fetal well being during strenuous exercise.

Treadmill testing has been used less frequently to assess physiologic function at maximal exertion in pregnant women. Artal et al. [33] studied responses to maximal weight-bearing exercise (treadmill walking) in pregnant women late in the 2nd trimester or early 3rd trimester in comparison with non-pregnant women. At maximal exercise, they found lower tidal volume, VO_2max, VCO_2max and RER max in the pregnant women than the controls. In contrast, Lotgering et al. [34] reported that maximal power and maximal oxygen uptake were unchanged by pregnancy. It seems likely that these differences may be the result of inherent differences between cross-sectional [33] and longitudinal [34] study designs. Lotgering et al. [34] reported that findings for weight-bearing exercise (treadmill) were similar to those for non-weight-bearing exercise (cycle ergometry). One observed difference was that VCO_2max appeared to be more blunted during treadmill exercise causing RER_{max} to be lower during treadmill exercise than cycle ergometry. Artal et al. [33] noted that the ventilatory equivalent for oxygen was statistically unchanged, but that there was a consistent trend for it to be slightly increased (fig. 1). Thus, data from both studies suggest that maximal weight-bearing exercise results in greater augmented respiratory sensitivity in comparison to non-weight-bearing exercise. As would be expected from nonpregnant responses, values for all other physiologic variables studied were higher during treadmill exercise than during cycle ergometry [34].

Two studies have investigated the physiologic responses to swimming during pregnancy in comparison to postpartum responses [40, 50]. Spinnewijn et al. [40] reported no difference in VO_2peak or HR peak between pregnancy and postpartum. As with other modes of exercise, VCO_2peak was lower (~ 10%) during pregnancy and resulted in a lower RER peak. Both V_E peak (~ 4%) and V_t peak (~ 8%) were slightly increased, but statistically unchanged. Also similar to results with other exercise modes, peak lactates were lower during pregnancy. McMurray et al. [50] had previously reported marked differences in responses (17% lower VO_2 peak to swimming

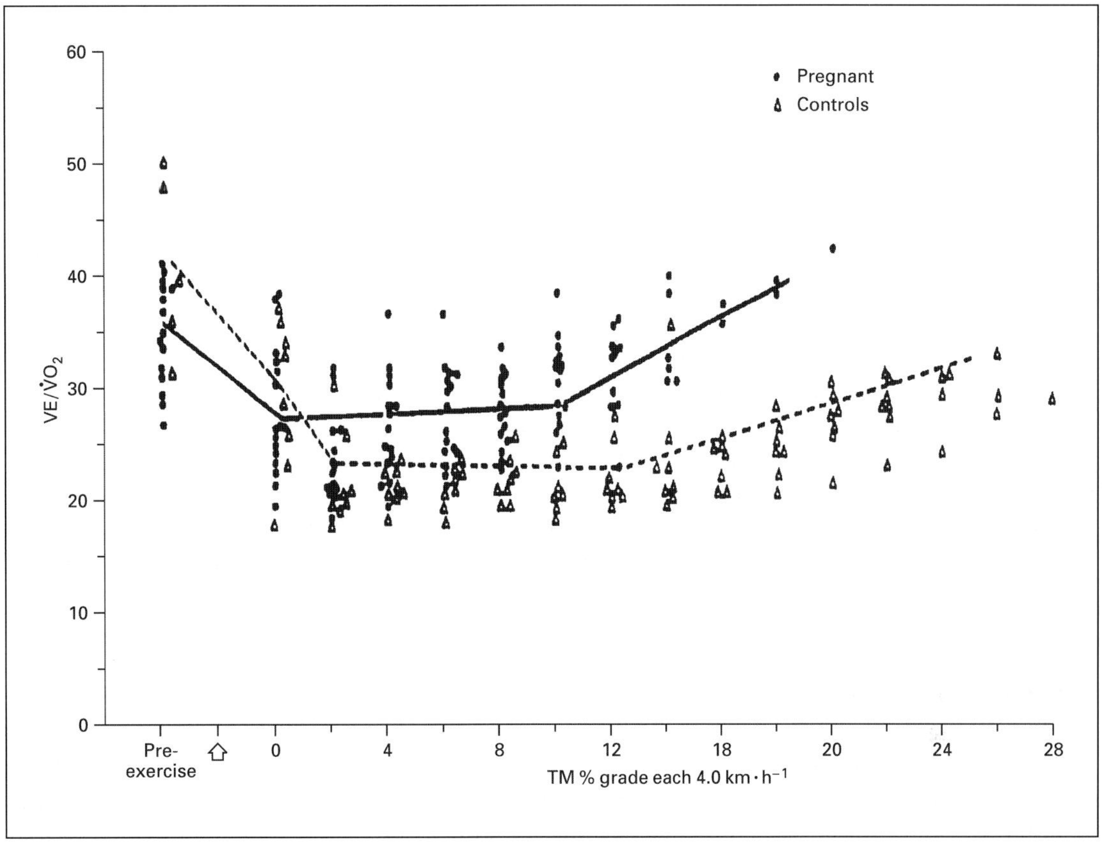

Fig. 1. Ventilatory equivalent of oxygen (V_E/VO_2) before and during symptom-limited treadmill walking to maximal effort in pregnant vs. nonpregnant controls. From Artal et al. [33].

during pregnancy, but methodical differences in testing protocols likely caused these apparent differences. Spinnewijn et al. [40] reported that during pregnancy, swimming VO_2peak was 11% lower and VCO_2peak was 25% lower in comparison with cycling values. In accord with these lower values, RER peak, V_E peak, V_t peak and peak lactate were also lower in swimming than cycling. These responses are similar to those expected in nonpregnant individuals.

Submaximal Exercise Tests

Protocol Selection. Not all cardiopulmonary exercise testing of pregnant women needs to be maximal exercise testing. Submaximal tests are appropriate when information about safety or the impact of a therapeutic intervention at a particular exercise intensity is required. Steady-state responses reflect homeostatic adjustment to a submaximal exercise level and can be used to assess appropriateness of cardiovascular, pulmonary or metabolic responses. Several submaximal stages can be used or a single stage can be used. During a single-stage test, the participant exercises on an ergometer (treadmill, leg cycle ergometer, etc.) for a prolonged period of time at a single, submaximal exercise intensity. Measures of cardiovascular variables such as heart rate and blood pressure are the mainstays of single-stage tests and are assessed over time. Other uses include tracking substrates (e.g. glucose, lactate, fatty acids), electrolytes (e.g. sodium, potassium) and/or hormones (e.g. insulin, epinephrine) for a prolonged period of time. Single-stage tests may also be used to measure energy expenditure (caloric cost) of a specific exercise intensity. They may also be used to assess the relative contribution of carbohydrate and fat as substrate during that exercise intensity and may be particularly useful in quantifying caloric expenditure of an activity.

Expected Responses to Submaximal Exercise Tests during Pregnancy. Comparisons of physiologic responses to submaximal exercise during pregnancy with responses by nonpregnant controls suggest that few differences can be expected during non-weight-bearing exercise when individuals are carefully matched. In active women (all regularly exercised 3–6 times per week), ventilatory threshold during cycle ergometry was not different between pregnant and nonpregnant groups, nor was the respiratory compensation threshold or work efficiency [36, 39]. Other physiologic responses at single submaximal exercise intensity, defined as an oxygen uptake of 100 ml less than the ventilatory threshold, were compared in these subjects. There was no significant effect of pregnancy on cardiovascular (HR), metabolic (VO_2) or respiratory responses except for significantly increased ventilatory equivalents for oxygen and carbon dioxide and significantly decreased end tidal and arterial carbon dioxide levels in the pregnant women [36]. These data support the well-documented increase in respiratory drive during pregnancy and demonstrate that the increased drive continues to be operative during submaximal exercise.

Exercise Testing and Prescription during the Postpartum Period

Many of the physiologic and morphologic changes of pregnancy persist 4–6 weeks postpartum. Thus, pre-pregnancy exercise routines should be resumed gradually based on a woman's physical capability. The competitive athlete with an uncomplicated pregnancy may resume training as early a 2 weeks postpartum. No known maternal complications are associated with resumption of training [54]. There are, however, anecdotal reports of failure of infants to gain weight as rapidly as expected in strenuously training mothers. Failure to gain weight is associated with decreased milk production that may be secondary to inadequate fluid or nutritional intake to balance training-induced outputs. Nursing women should feed the infant before exercising in order to avoid the discomfort of engorged breasts [55]. Additionally, nursing before exercise will avoid the potential problems associated with increased acidity of milk secondary to any build-up of lactic acid. A recent study of the short-term effects of dieting plus aerobic exercise on lactation performance concluded that this was a safe practice that resulted in optimal weight loss without affecting lactation performance [56]. Finally, a return to physical activity following pregnancy has been associated with decreased postpartum depression, but only if the exercise is stress relieving and not stress provoking [57].

Conclusions

Pregnancy is associated with profound anatomical and physiological changes that alter cardiopulmonary responses to clinical exercise testing. Nevertheless, exercise tests can be used during pregnancy for the same reasons they are used in a nonpregnant population (e.g. diagnostic reasons, development of individualized exercise prescriptions, and monitoring progress in a training program) as long as appropriate testing modalities and protocols are used. Semirecumbent cycle ergometry appears to be the most comfortable modality, but treadmill walking or upright cycle ergometry may also be used. Short protocols (8–12 min) to maximal subjective effort appear to be safe during all stages of pregnancy for both mother and fetus. Single-stage submaximal protocols also provide useful information particularly when therapeutic interventions, substrate utilization (especially for diabetics), or hormonal responses are of interest. Individuals responsible for the conduct and interpretation of exercise testing in pregnant women should be aware of expected responses to submaximal and maximal exercise during pregnancy.

References

1 Girandola RN, Khodiguian N, Artal R, Wiswell RA: Body composition in pregnancy; in Artal R, Wiswell RA, Drinkwater BL (eds): Exercise and Pregnancy. Baltimore, Williams & Wilkins, 1991, pp 99–108.
2 Brown JE: Nutrition for Your Pregnancy. Minneapolis, University of Minnesota Press, 1983.
3 Palin D, Rankine D: Nutrition in pregnancy – national guidelines: A summary. J Can Diet Assoc 1987;47:209.
4 Wolfe L: Pregnancy; in Skinner JS (ed): Exercise Testing and Exercise Prescription for Special Cases, ed 2. Philadelphia, Lea & Febiger, 1993, pp 363–385.
5 Artal R, Friedman MJ, McNitt-Gregg JL: Orthopedic problems in pregnancy. Physician Sportsmed 1990;18:93–105.
6 Alaily AB, Carroll KB: Pulmonary ventilation in pregnancy. Br J Obstet Gynaecol 1978;85: 518–524.
7 Knuttgen HG, Emerson K Jr: Physiological response to pregnancy at rest and during exercise. J Appl Physiol 1974;36:549–553.
8 Ratigan TR: Anatomic and physiologic changes of pregnancy: Anesthetic considerations. J Am Assoc Nurse 1983;51:38–42.
9 Gee JB, Packer BS, Millen JE, Robin ED: Pulmonary mechanics during pregnancy. J Clin Invest 1967;46:945–952.
10 Artal R, with Sherman C: Exercise during pregnancy: Safe and beneficial for most. Physician Sportsmed 1999;27(8):51–75.

11 Artal R, Wiswell RA, Drinkwater BL (eds): Exercise in Pregnancy, ed 2. Baltimore, Williams & Wilkins, 1991.
12 Pernoll ML, Metcalfe J, Kovach PA, Wachtel R, Dunham MJ: Ventilation during rest and exercise in pregnancy and postpartum. Resp Physiol 1975;25:295–310.
13 Romem Y, Masaki DI, Artal R: Physiological and endocrine adjustments to pregnancy; in Artal R, Wiswell RA, Drinkwater BL (eds): Exercise and Pregnancy. Baltimore, Williams & Wilkins, 1991, pp 9–29.
14 Clark SL, Cotton DB, Lee W, Bishop C, Hill T, Southwick J, Pivarnik J, Spillman T, DeVore GR, Phelan J: Central hemodynamic assessment of normal term pregnancy. Am J Obstet Gynecol 1989;161:1439–1442.
15 Wolfe LA, Ohtake PJ, Mottola MF, McGrath MJ: Physiological interactions between pregnancy and aerobic exercise. Exerc Sport Sci Rev 1989;17:295–351.
16 Morton MJ: Maternal hemodynamics in pregnancy; in Artal R, Wiswell RA, Drinkwater BL (eds): Exercise and Pregnancy. Baltimore, Williams & Wilkins, 1991.
17 Pirani BB, Campbell DM, MacGillivray I: Plasma volume in normal first pregnancy. J Obstet Gynaecol Br Commonw 1973;80:884–887.
18 Lund CJ, Donovan JC: Blood volume during pregnancy. Am J Obstet Gynecol 1967;98:394–403.
19 Scott DE: Anemia in pregnancy. Obstet Gynecol Annu 1972;1:219–244.
20 Longo LD: Maternal blood volume and cardiac output during pregnancy: A hypothesis of endocrinologic control. Am J Physiol 1983;245:R720–R729.
21 Bader RA, Bader ME, Rose PJ, Braunwald E: Haemodynamics at rest and during exercise in normal pregnancy as studied by cardiac catheterization. J Clin Invest 1955;34:1524.
22 Wilson M, Morganti AG, Zervoudakis I, Letcher RL, Romney BM, Von Oeyon P, Papera S, Sealey JE, Laragh JH: Blood pressure, the unine-aldosterone system and sex steroids throughout normal pregnancy. Am J Med 1980;68:97.
23 Pivaranik JM: Cardiovascular responses to aerobic exercise during pregnancy and postpartum. Semin Perinatol 1996;20:242–249.
24 Katz R, Karliner JS, Resnik R: Effects of a natural volume overload state (pregnancy) in left ventricular performance in normal human subjects. Circulation 1978;48:434.
25 Mashini IS, Albazzaz SJ, Fadel HE, Abdulla AM, Hadi HA, Harp R, Devoe LD: Serial noninvasive evaluation of cardiovascular hemodynamics during pregnancy. Am J Obstet Gynecol 1987;156:1208–1213.
26 Rubler S, Damani PM, Pinto ER: Cardiac size and performance during pregnancy estimated with echocardiography. Am J Cardiol 1977;40:534–540.
27 Goodrich SM, Wood JE: Peripheral venous distensibility and velocity of venous blood flow during pregnancy or during oral contraceptive therapy. Am J Obstet Gynecol 1964;90:740.
28 Goodrich SM, Wood JE: The effect of estradiol-17beta on peripheral venous distensibility and velocity of venous blood flow. Am J Obstet Gynecol 1966;96:407–412.
29 American College of Sports Medicine: ACSM's Guidelines for Exercise Testing and Prescription, ed 6. Philadelphia, Lippincott Williams & Wilkins, 2000, pp 36, 50, 80.
30 Canadian Society for Exercise Physiology: Physical Activity Readiness Medical Examination for Pregnancy. Ottawa, Canadian Society for Exercise Physiology, 1996.
31 American College of Obstetricians and Gynecologists: Exercise during Pregnancy and the Postpartum Period, Tech Bull #189. Washington, American College of Obstetricians and Gynecologists, 1994.
32 Jovanovic-Peterson L, Durak EP, Peterson CM: Randomized trial of diet versus diet plus cardiovascular conditioning on glucose levels in gestational diabetes. Am J Obstet Gynecol 1989;161:415–419.
33 Artal R, Wiswell R, Romem Y, Dorey F: Pulmonary responses to exercise in pregnancy. Am J Obstet Gynecol 1986:154:378–383.
34 Lotgering FK, Van Doorn MB, Struijk PC, Pool J, Wallenburg HCS: Maximal aerobic exercise in pregnant women: Heart rate, O_2 consumption, CO_2 production, and ventilation. J Appl Physiol 1991;70:1016–1023.
35 Blair SN, Applegate WB, Dunn AL, Ettinger WH, Haskell WL, King AC, Morgan TM, Shih JA, Simons-Morton DG: Activity Counseling Trial (ACT): Rationale, design, and methods. Med Sci Sports Exerc 1998;30:1097–1106.
36 Heenan AP, Wolfe LA, Davies GAL: Maximal exercise testing in late gestation: Maternal responses. Obstet Gynecol 2001;97:127–134.
37 South-Paul JE, Rajjagopal KR, Tenholder MF: The effect of participation in a regular exercise program upon aerobic capacity during pregnancy. Obstet Gynecol 1988;71:175–179.
38 Lotgering FK, Struijk PC, Van Doorn MB, Spinnewijn WEM, Wallenburg HCS: Anaerobic threshold and respiratory compensation in pregnant women. J Appl Physiol 1995;78:1772–1777.
39 Wolfe LA, Walker RMC, Bonen A, McGrath MJ: Effects of pregnancy and chronic exercise on respiratory responses to graded exercise. J Appl Physiol 1994;76:1928–1936.
40 Spinnewijn WEM, Wallenburg HCS, Struijk PC, Lotgering FK: Peak ventilatory responses during cycling and swimming in pregnant and nonpregnant women. J Appl Physiol 1996;81:738–742.
41 Electronic fetal heart rate monitoring: Research guidelines for interpretation. National Institute of Child Health and Human Development Research Planning Workshop. Am J Obstet Gynecol 1997;177:1385–1390.
42 Macphail A, Davies GAL, Victory R, Wolfe LA: Maximal exercise testing in late gestation: Fetal responses. Obstet Gynecol 2000;96:565–570.
43 Wolfe LA, Brenner IKM, Mottola MF: Maternal exercise, fetal well-being, and pregnancy outcome. Exerc Sport Sci Rev 1994;22:145–194.
44 Artal R, Rutherford S, Romem Y, Kammula RK, Dorey FJ, Wiswell RA: Fetal heart rate responses to maternal exercise. Am J Obstet Gynecol 1986;155:729–733.
45 Watson WJ, Katz VL, Hackney AC, Gall MM, McMurray RG: Fetal responses to maximal swimming and cycling exercise during pregnancy. Obstet Gynecol 1991;77:382–386.
46 Webb KA, Wolfe LA, McGrath MJ: Effects of acute and chronic maternal exercise on fetal heart rate. J Appl Physiol 1994;77:2207–2213.
47 O'Neill ME: Maternal rectal temperature and fetal heart rate responses to upright cycling in late pregnancy. Br J Sports Med 1996;30:32–35.
48 Manders MAM, Sonder GJB, Mulder EJH, Visser GHA: The effects of maternal exercise on fetal heart rate and movement patterns. Early Hum Dev 1997;48:237–247.
49 Jaque-Fortunato SV, Wiswell RA, Khodiguian N, Artal R: A comparison of the ventilatory responses to exercise in pregnant, postpartum and nonpregnant women. Seminar Perinatol 1996;20:263–276.
50 McMurray RG, Hackney AC, Katz VL, Gall M, Watson WJ: Pregnancy-induced changes in the maximal physiological responses during swimming. J Appl Physiol 1991;71:1454–1459.
51 Sady SP, Carpenter MW, Thompson PD, Sady MA, Haydon B, Coustan DR: Cardiovascular response to cycle exercise during and after pregnancy. J Appl Physiol 1989;66:336–341.
52 Sady MA, Haydon BB, Sady SP, Carpenter MW, Thompson PD, Coustan DR: Cardiovascular response to maximal cycle exercise during pregnancy and at two and seven months postpartum. Am J Obstet Gynecol 1990;162:1181–1185.
53 Clapp JF III, Wesley M, Sleamaker RH: Thermoregulatory and metabolic responses to jogging prior to and during pregnancy. Med Sci Sports Exerc 1987;19:124–130.
54 Hale RW, Milne L: The elite athlete and exercise in pregnancy. Semin Perinat 1996;20:277–284.
55 Kulpa P: Exercise during pregnancy and post partum; in Agostini R (ed): Medical and Orthopedic Issues of Active and Athletic Women. Philadelphia, Hanley & Belfus, 1994, pp 191–199.
56 McCrory MA, Nommsen-Rivers LA, Mole PA, Lonnerdal B, Dewey KG: Randomized trial of short-term effects of dieting compared with dieting plua aerobic exercise on lactation performance. Am J Clin Nutr 1999;69:959–967.
57 Koltyn KF, Schultes SS: Psychological effects of an aerobic exercise session and a rest session following pregnancy. J Sports Med Phys Fitness 1997;37:287–291.

Mary L. O'Toole, PhD
Department of Obstetrics, Gynecology and Women's Health
6420 Clayton Road, Suite 290
St. Louis, MO 63117 (USA)
Tel. +1 314 781 2543, Fax +1 314 645 6173
E-Mail otoolem@slucare1.sluh.edu

Weisman IM, Zeballos RJ (eds): Clinical Exercise Testing.
Prog Respir Res. Basel, Karger, 2002, vol 32, pp 282–299

Clinical Exercise Testing in Children

John Fahey[a] Dan Nemet[b] Dan M. Cooper[b]

[a]Department of Pediatrics, Section of Cardiology, Yale University School of Medicine, New Haven, Conn., and [b]Center for the Study of Health Effects of Exercise in Children, University of California, Irvine, College of Medicine, Orange, Calif., USA

Summary

In children, exercise is not merely play but a fundamental biologic regulator of growth and development. Recognizing this, the pediatric exercise laboratory will need to focus not only on traditional cardiorespiratory responses to exercise, but also on testing strategies that gauge the dynamic relationship between exercise and growth. The pediatric exercise laboratory performs critical diagnostic procedures relevant to childhood lung (e.g. cystic fibrosis or asthma), cardiac (e.g. congenital heart disease), and metabolic diseases (e.g. diabetes). In addition, exercise testing in children will increasingly be relied upon to develop exercise therapies for children with conditions ranging from obesity to mitochondrial disease. The clinician referring a child for pediatric exercise consultation must gain insight not only into the child's functional capability at the moment, but also, whether or not the level of physical activity of his or her patient optimizes the many long-term benefits of exercise for the overall process of growth and development.

Introduction

Children are, arguably, the most naturally physically active human beings. However, surprisingly little is yet understood about the role of exercise in: (1) the growth and development of healthy children; (2) gaining diagnostic insight into pediatric pathophysiology, and (3) providing novel therapies for children with chronic disease and disability. We now believe that exercise in children is not merely play, but rather, is essential for healthy growth and development. There is mounting research identifying physiological, molecular, and structural mechanisms that link exercise with processes of growth and development in health and disease. Moreover, there appear to be significant long-term health consequences for the child who is unable to optimally engage in physical activity because of environmental, social and psychological, or physiological barriers. In this chapter, we review essential knowledge that links physical activity with growth and that provides the basis for innovative uses of exercise in children from both a diagnostic and a therapeutic perspective.

Exercise and Physical Activity in Healthy Children

It is now known that exercise in healthy younger children is characterized by many brief pulses (about 85 per hour, mean of 20 s duration) that vary greatly in intensity [1]. The majority of these exercise bouts are relatively low intensity, but in about 20%, the exercise intensity is likely to be above the anaerobic or lactate threshold [2–4] (fig. 1). During these high-intensity exercise bouts, perturbations in circulating levels of growth hormone (GH) [5], insulin-like growth factor-I (IGF-I) [6], and inflammatory mediators (e.g. interleukin-6) might occur [7]. Current research suggests that physical activity may influence growth and development by activating these anabolic and catabolic mediators.

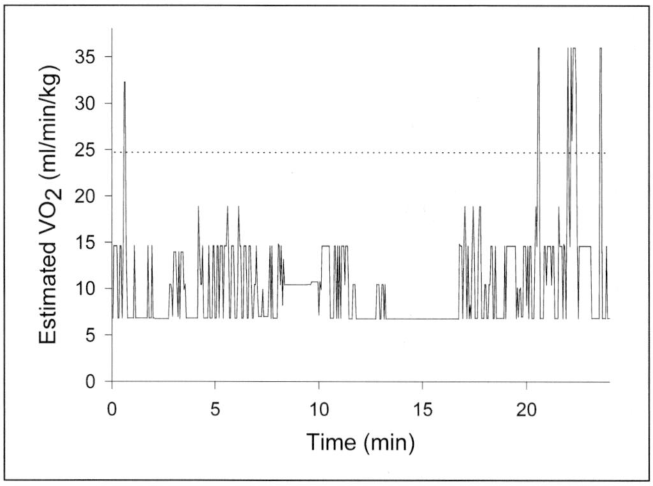

Fig. 1. Representative example of activity patterns derived from direct observation in a 7-year-old boy over a 24-min period. Bouts of physical activity are randomly spaced. Most bouts were in the low-intensity range (below the LT – the dashed line, estimated for children this age); however, a substantial portion of the energy expenditure due to physical activity results from the less frequent, high-intensity bouts. Reprinted with permission from Berman et al. [1].

With very few exceptions, all children, whether or not they have a chronic illness, should be encouraged to be active and fit. But what has been difficult to do is to arrive at physiologically sound definitions for 'fitness' in both the healthy child and in the child with chronic disease. In this context, laboratory tests of exercise capability in children have become increasingly relevant. Exercise testing can reproducibly measure respiratory, cardiac, and metabolic function under stress, and the values derived from a given child can then be compared with normal data. This information can be used to better define the exercise 'prescription' because the initial response characteristics serve as baseline values to gauge the later effects of training or other therapies. Other fundamental questions that can be answered by exercise testing are: (1) at what level of intensity does exercise become dangerous; (2) what are the mechanisms that limit physical activity in a particular child, and (3) to what extent can these limitations be ameliorated by exercise itself?

Approaches to Exercise Testing in Children

Although children are naturally active, exercise testing in children and adolescents was initially an outgrowth of the larger experience in adults. The history of modern physiologically based exercise testing was derived from efforts to understand maximal exercise response for several reasons. First, in the early part of the 20th Century, biomedical scientists were occupied with discovering how to make better soldiers and physical laborers – activities that required substantial energy expenditure. Secondly, observations from the same time period showed that humans achieved a true maximal oxygen uptake (VO_2) (i.e. a point at which the individual could increase external work with no accompanying increase in oxygen uptake). This was very intriguing to investigators who felt that the VO_2max must indicate critically important features of the physiological response to exercise.

As a consequence, equipment and testing protocols designed for adults are still frequently used to test children in many laboratories. There are, however, several important considerations that require different testing approaches in evaluating children. The laboratory must be able to accommodate large discrepancies in subject age, size, strength, coordination, fitness level and attention span. The personnel must be comfortable in working with younger children and adolescents. The 6-year-old boy may be eager to perform, but intimidated and scared by the equipment and monitors; the 16-year-old girl may want to do her best, but worried about how much sweat the exercise testing bout may produce. Pediatric exercise laboratories must have a variety of innovative protocols and equipment that can be readily modified. Cycle ergometers must have adjustable seats, handle bars, and pedals. The treadmills must have additional or adjustable side rails. Finally, it must be recognized that the VO_2max test which focused on peak function may not be suitable to determine limitations in function. Ironically, determining impaired metabolic and physiologic responses to exercise is a major goal of exercise testing in the child with chronic disease or disability.

In addition, the physiologic responses of children during exercise are different than in adults, and, indeed, mature. 'Normal' values must be found that adequately account for growth related changes in body mass, intrinsic muscle function, and neuromotor maturation. An overview of some valid normal values for exercise testing in children can be found in a variety of sources [8, 9]. Ultimately, each pediatric exercise laboratory must ensure that any reference value for normal values is validated and appropriate for the ethnic and socioeconomic mix of children tested in a particular geographical area. Ideally, the pediatric exercise laboratory should be a separate facility, with dedicated personnel and equipment, presenting a 'child friendly' environment.

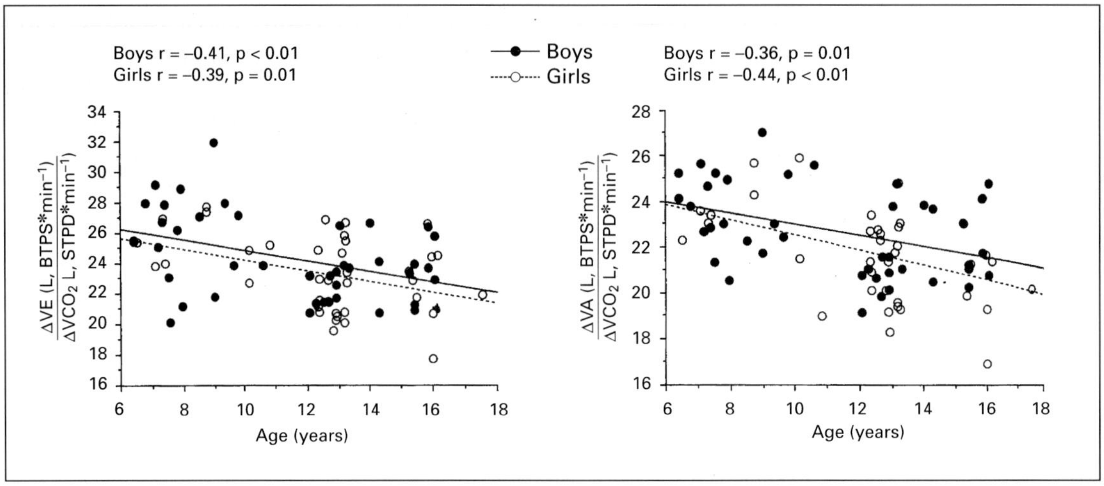

Fig. 2. Relationship between V_E-VCO_2 slope during exercise and age in children and adolescents. These data confirm earlier observations from Cooper et al. [3]. Ventilation per VCO_2 production is greater in younger children. Reprinted with permission from Nagano et al. [20].

Maturation of the Physiologic Responses of Children to Exercise

Research over the past 50–70 years has demonstrated key areas in which the cardiorespiratory responses to exercise differ between prepubertal children and adults. These include:

(1) Reduced mechanical efficiency and increased oxygen cost of work [10, 11].

(2) Generally faster oxygen uptake, heart rate, and ventilatory kinetics at the onset of and in recovery from a bout of exercise [11].

(3) Inability to achieve as high a level of lactate and hydrogen ion concentration (or to increase intramuscular Pi/PCr ratios by magnetic resonance spectroscopy) [12].

(4) Increased ventilatory cost of carbon dioxide production [13].

As for adults, in order for children to perform progressively increasing workload protocols, there must be progressive, proportional increases in both cardiac output and ventilation in order to deliver oxygen to the exercising muscles and eliminate carbon dioxide from the venous blood. Similar to adult responses, children can achieve 5-fold increases in cardiac output [14–16], and 12-fold increases in minute ventilation [13, 17] over resting values. However, the changes that produce these increases are quite different. Stroke volume, when indexed to body surface area, seems to be the same in children and adults both at rest and during exercise [18]. In spite of this, children typically have higher heart rates during exercise when compared to adults. Young children have higher resting heart rates than adults, with resultant elevation of the exercise heart rates. Further, children have significantly higher maximal heart rates, in the range of 200–215 beats/min, persisting until late adolescence (thereafter, maximal heart rates tend to decrease with age). For all of these reasons, heart rates tend to be significantly higher during pediatric exercise tests and should not be interpreted as a sign of distress or dysfunction. As in adults, the systolic blood pressure rises progressively during progressive exercise, while the diastolic blood pressure either stays the same or only slightly increases. In general, the systolic blood pressure rarely exceeds 200 mm Hg in a healthy pediatric population [14].

The ventilatory response to exercise is also different in children. Ventilatory responses are appropriately normalized to CO_2 production since it is the latter that is physiologically driving ventilation during exercise. Numerous studies of exercise in children (including our own) have clearly demonstrated that the slope of the relationship between ventilation and CO_2 production (fig. 2) is greater in children compared with adults. The mechanism for this is likely related to a lower CO_2 set point, relatively less CO_2 storage in the body fat and muscle, and altered sensitivity of respiratory control centers [10, 13, 19, 20].

Like adults, children will achieve a lactate or anaerobic threshold [3], but because of their relatively inability to produce large concentrations of lactate [21] and to lower pH, relatively greater respiratory 'noise', and their increased V_E relative to VCO_2, it is more technically difficult in children to precisely determine the threshold using noninvasive gas exchange measurements (i.e. the slope changes in R, $PetO_2$, or V_E/VO_2 are simply not as great as in adults). Similarly, while in adults, oxygen uptake continues to increase even for constant work rate, above-AT exercise, the slope of the oxygen uptake response for above-AT constant work rate exercise (phase 3) in children is quite low and often difficult to observe [10]. Although the precise mechanisms for these maturational differences in lactate kinetics are not known, some workers have suggested that immature anaerobic glycolytic pathways may well lead to the relative inability of children to produce lactate at levels equivalent to those found in adults.

Exercise Measurements

At least three leads of the standard surface electrocardiogram should be routinely and continuously monitored, and the examiner should have the ability to view various combinations of the twelve available leads. Lead placement is the same in children as in adults, as is the skin preparation. Smaller leads are available for children to avoid overlap or misplacement. The heart rate is measured from the electrocardiogram. Blood pressure is measured at each level of exercise using an appropriately sized blood pressure cuff. The recommendation is that the bladder of the cuff completely encircles the arm, and the cuff should cover two-thirds of the distance from the antecubital fossa to the axilla. Too small a cuff will produce falsely elevated measurements, whereas too large a cuff will minimally depress the blood pressure measurement [22]. Obviously, a large assortment in cuff sizes must be available, and the examiner should err on the side of too large a cuff if there is a question.

The use of respiratory gas analyzers has become routine in pediatric exercise laboratories. Variables such as VO_2, VCO_2, ventilation, tidal volume, and respiratory rate can be monitored continuously during the tests, on a breath-by-breath basis. Mouthpieces are available in a variety of sizes, allowing metabolic measurements in children as young as 6–7 years of age. Tightly fitting masks are also available for small children who do not tolerate the mouthpiece or nose clip, but the tendency for leaks is greater. Equipment to perform resting and postexercise spirometry, and inspiratory and expiratory flow volume loops can usually be easily obtained.

Noninvasive cardiac output and stroke volume measurements during exercise are possible in pediatric patients, although used more for research than clinical studies. The techniques are the same as used for adults. Both CO_2 rebreathing and acetylene-helium rebreathing techniques have been employed successfully in children [23, 24]. These require the absence of significant ventilation-perfusion mismatching, as well as no intracardiac or intrapulmonary shunting; both of which significantly limit the usefulness of this type of measurement in the pediatric laboratory. In addition, these techniques also require a high degree of patient cooperation. Other techniques may have more use for the pediatric patient. Doppler and two-dimensional echocardiographic measurements are frequently easier in children since they tend to have better acoustic windows [25]. Electrical bioimpedance measurements have recently been significantly improved, require no patient cooperation, and may be used in children as small as 15 kg, but are awaiting correlation with more accepted techniques.

Oxygen saturation measurements have become almost a routine part of exercise testing, especially in pediatric pulmonary and cardiac patients, since the introduction of pulse oximetry. Both finger and ear oximeters have been used, but both have the disadvantage of being inaccurate at higher work rates due to motion artifact or tight gripping of the handlebars during cycle ergometry. These problems can be largely overcome using a reflectance oxygen probe, which is placed over the temporal artery on the forehead and held in place with a headband [26].

Protocols for Exercise Testing

There is no single, standardized exercise protocol routinely used or recommended for exercise testing in the pediatric population, and with good reason. The protocol must be selected, and sometimes modified, based on the information required, as well as the age, health and fitness level of the subject. There are two general types of exercise testing: (1) progressively increasing workloads to maximum, with no rest period between changes in work increments, and (2) a brief constant work rate [8].

Progressively increasing workloads to maximum are the most common in use in pediatric laboratories, and may use either a treadmill or cycle ergometer. There are many benefits to these protocols and they can answer a variety of clinical questions. They can measure the level of aerobic fitness (VO_2max). Maximal stress yields confidence about the safety of strenuous exercise for patients, parents, and caretakers. They maximally stress the respiratory system, and can precipitate both exercise-induced stridor and/or bronchospasm. They also maximally stress the heart by maximizing myocardial oxygen demands (i.e. maximal rate-pressure product).

There are, however, drawbacks, limitations, and criticisms of this form of maximal exercise testing. It is felt to be an 'unnatural' form of exercise, and not representative of patterns of physical activity of normal children [27]. Neither children, adults, nor virtually any mammal normally exercise to maximum, and VO_2max may only occur in the exercise laboratory. The study requires cooperation on the part of the patient, substantial coaxing on the part of the laboratory technician, and a true maximal study is very difficult to obtain in the young child, either on the treadmill or the cycle. In fact, only about 20–30% of children actually achieve a true plateau of oxygen uptake, diagnostic of VO_2max. Finally, in children with chronic heart or lung disease, it is the rare laboratory technician who will cajole and coax the subjects to the same extent as he or she would a healthy child, particularly in the higher exercise intensities where pH is lower and the child is likely to experience uncomfortable levels of dyspnea and fatigue.

Although the clinical utility of maximal values can be questioned, much useful information is available from progressive exercise protocols. Gas exchange and HR responses continuously change during progressive tests, and often the relationships between these changing variables (referred to as dynamic relationships) can be quantified using straightforward analytic techniques. As noted above, the LAT in children and young adults can be determined noninvasively from the dynamic responses of gas exchange during progressive exercise [3, 28]. Simple linear regression analysis of HR and VO_2 can provide noninvasive indicators of cardiac function [29–31]. The slope of the regression changes systematically with maturation and with diseases (e.g. congenital heart disease [32]). Similarly, linear regression analysis of V_E and VCO_2 can be used to assess respiratory efficiency and control during exercise [33]. The real clinical value of progressive exercise testing for children may prove to be in the rich cardiorespiratory data obtained during the submaximal phases rather than from the final, single, data point at peak or maximal power.

There is to date less experience with brief, constant work rate tests [32]. Nonetheless, there are practical benefits to these protocols, and there is a growing body of research demonstrating the efficacy of these protocols in identifying impaired cardiorespiratory responses to exercise in children with a variety of diseases and disabilities (see below). It has been argued, for example, that onset and offset gas exchange and heart rate kinetics (i.e. the time required for physiological systems to respond to and recover from exercise) are as important as maximal values in assessing impairment. Brief exercise protocols more closely mimic exercise patterns of children and are more likely to be tolerated than either maximal exercise tests or long bouts of sustained, heavy exercise. This approach has been used successfully in children with chronic disease (fig. 3, 4).

Recovery kinetics may determine the child's ability to do repetitive bouts of exercise, and therefore be more predictive of functional ability. This form of testing is not as stressful to the children and they are easier for the children to perform [27]. It may be that combinations of several types of exercise testing will be needed for the long-term management of children with significant cardiac or pulmonary disease (fig. 5–7).

Pediatric stress tests can be performed using either the cycle or the treadmill. Cycle ergometers are more commonly used for pediatric stress tests than for adult tests. Many laboratories have both available since each has advantages and disadvantages. Cycle ergometers have several significant advantages for clinical exercise testing. Due to the stability of the trunk and arms, there tends to be less artifact in the measurement of the ECG and blood pressure. It is easier to do metabolic measurements as the mouthpiece can be supported by a mechanical arm and the children do not bear the weight or have to wear a cumbersome halo device. There is easier access to the patient, making cardiac output and echocardiographic measurements more convenient. The cycle is also easier and quieter with essentially no risk of injury to the patient and is preferred if laboratory space is limited. The seat height and handle bar height are adjustable. However, it is frequently inconvenient to change the length of the pedal arm. Many children less than 6 years of age cannot sustain pedaling at even the lowest work rates, and a treadmill must be used. A final but critical point is that with the cycle ergometer, the external work performed is known precisely while on the treadmill, the actual work done can at best only be estimated.

Treadmills have the advantage that children can easily walk and then run at a slow pace. Meaningful tests can be performed on children as young as three years of age. As more muscle groups are used in running as opposed to cycling, VO_2max values tend to be about 10% higher on the treadmill when compared to the cycle ergometer. There are several disadvantages to the treadmill. Safety

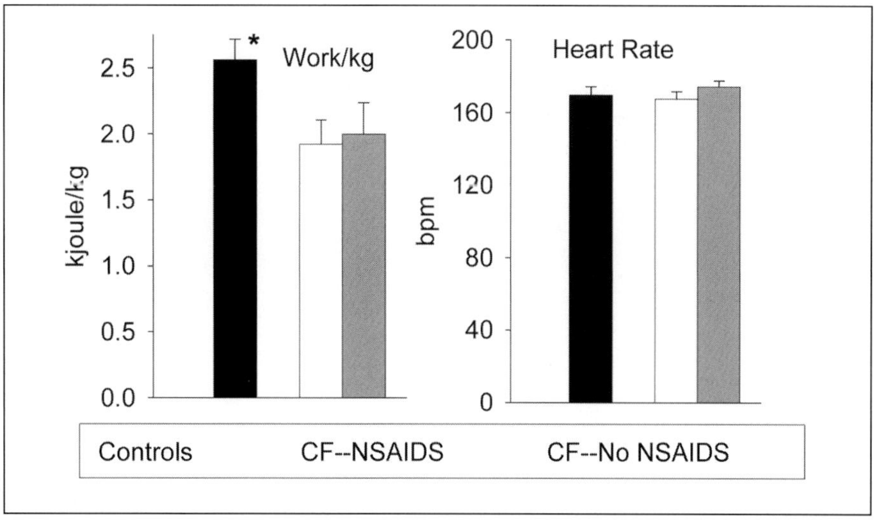

Fig. 3. Comparison among total work performed, total work per body weight, and heart rate by end-exercise in controls and CF subjects using multiple, constant work rate protocols scaled to each child's LT. Total work performed was significantly higher in controls (* $p < 0.001$). However, both CF (i.e. with and without nonsteroidal anti-inflammatory agents – NSAIDS) and control groups reached the same heart rate by end-exercise. No effect of ibuprofen use was observed in the CF subjects. Data reprinted with permission from Tirakitsoontorn [2001].

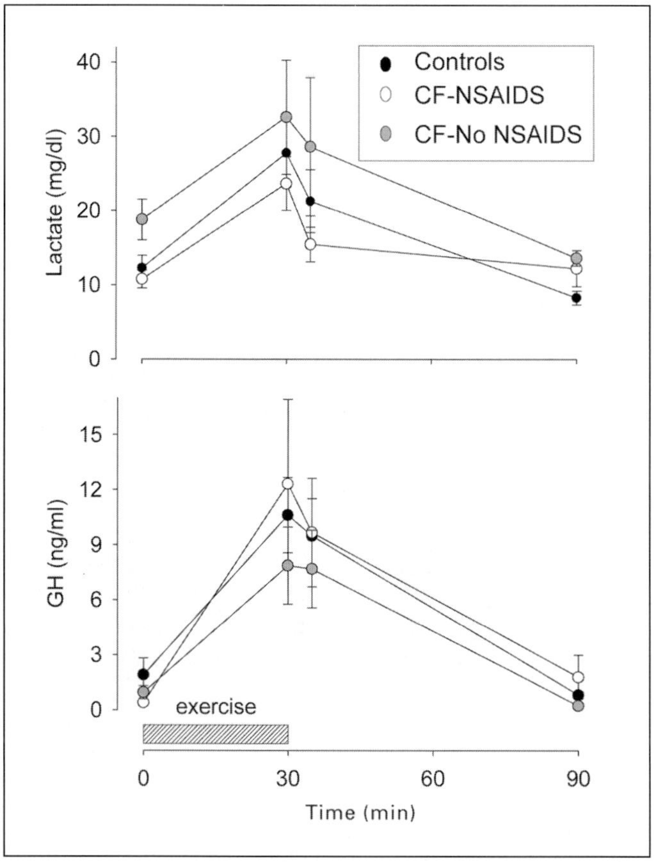

Fig. 4. Effect of exercise on plasma lactate and serum GH in both controls and CF subjects. GH and lactate levels increased significantly during exercise and were the same in both control and CF groups. No effect of ibuprofen was observed in the CF subjects. This approach demonstrates the potential utility of brief, scaled, constant work rate protocols in gauging metabolic responses to exercise in children. Data reprinted with permission from Tirakitsoontorn [2001].

concerns are greater on the treadmill due to the risks of falling on the moving belt. An observer must be positioned behind young children to support them if they fall or stumble. Increased body movement leads to a great deal of artifact on the ECG. The blood pressure is harder to measure when the patient is running. Treadmills are frequently loud and threatening to young children. Treadmills are more expensive and require more space in the lab.

There are a variety of standardized protocols that have been used for cycle ergometry in children. As noted, most pediatric exercise laboratories use progressive protocols (incremental or ramp-type) in which the child exercises to the limit of his or her tolerance. One should gauge the rate of work rate increase so that the total time on the cycle ergometer should be about 10–14 min, allowing sufficient data density for accurate analysis. In healthy children, the rate of increase might range from 5–10 W/min in 6-year-olds to 15–25 W/min in 18-year-olds. As clinicians gain experience, their ability to select the 'right' work rate increment improves.

The Bruce protocol is the most commonly used treadmill protocol in the pediatric exercise laboratory [34]. Developed for adults, this protocol consists of 3-min stages with an increase at each stage in both the speed and grade of the treadmill. There is no modification in the protocol for age or size. Most pediatric laboratories have modified the Bruce protocol for small children by including two stages at the beginning of the protocol with low belt speed and lower grades. Another treadmill protocol used for children is the James protocol [35]. As for the James protocol, the 3-min stages make metabolic measurements difficult. Children also find the 3-min stages at

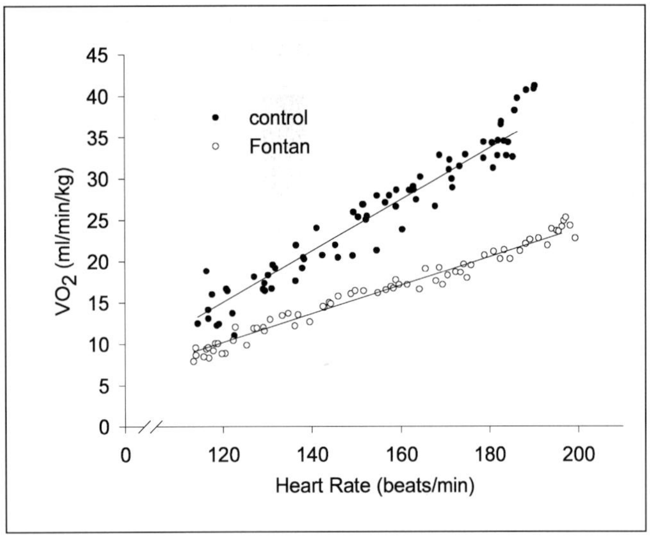

Fig. 5. Relationship between VO_2 and HR during progressive exercise in individual 12-year-old control and Fontan subjects. In both cases, there was a characteristic largely linear relationship between the two variables (solid lines indicate best-fit lines by linear regression). As demonstrated in these two subjects, the slope of the relationship (VO_2/HR) was lower in the Fontan patients. Data reprinted with permission from Troutman et al. [32].

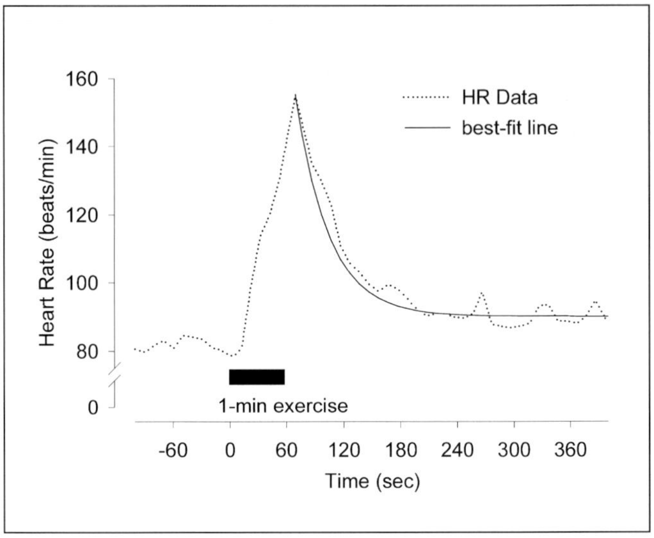

Fig. 6. HR response before, during, and in the recovery from 1 min of exercise in a 14-year-old Fontan subject. The recovery kinetics were quantified using a single exponential as shown. Data reprinted with permission from Troutman et al. [32].

the lower work levels boring and become distracted. The studies are excessively long in highly fit individuals due to the nonstressful early stages.

The Balke protocol uses a constant treadmill speed with increases in treadmill grade every minute [36]. The treadmill speed is chosen based on patient age. This protocol is well suited for unfit, obese, or chronically ill children where most of the test is spent walking. This is a disadvantage for the highly fit subjects. Modified 'running' Balke protocols can be developed starting at a higher initial grade, and choosing a faster treadmill velocity. Metabolic measurements are also easier with the Balke protocol and its modifications [37].

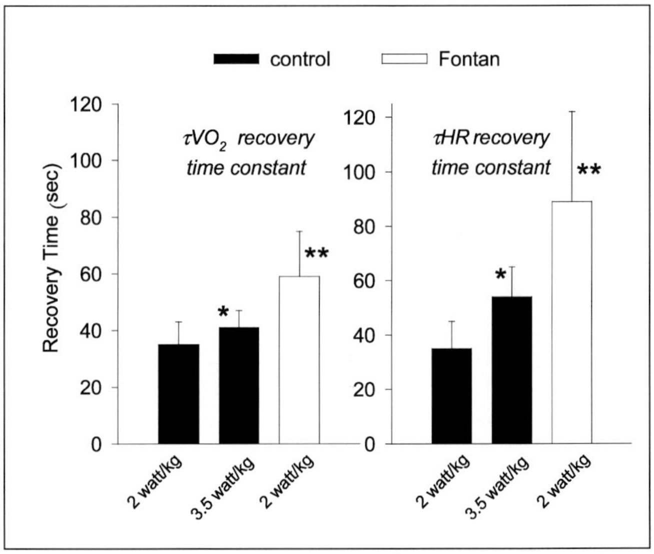

Fig. 7. HR and O_2 recovery times for control and Fontan subjects. In controls, recovery times were longer following the higher work rate protocols (* $p < 0.05$). In Fontan subjects, recovery times were prolonged compared with both the same absolute (2 W/kg) and relative (3.5 W/kg) protocols in control subjects (** $p < 0.001$). Data reprinted with permission from Troutman et al. [32].

Indications for Pediatric Exercise Tests

Indications for exercise testing in pediatric patients are varied and often much different than in the adult population. Exercise testing may be needed for diagnostic purposes or to institute a therapeutic exercise program. Interesting examples are included in table 1.

A useful approach toward the indications for exercise testing in children is to group them based on the special interests of the physicians or other health care profession-

Table 1. Examples of current clinical uses of exercise in children and adolescents

Diagnostic	
Elucidation of bronchial reactivity	
Growth hormone deficiency	
Preparticipation sports physical in children	
Establishing reduced physical activity as an etiology for obesity	
Evaluating fitness and the efficacy of therapy in patients with a variety of congenital heart diseases	
Evaluating long-term outcomes of surgical repair of single-ventricle congenital heart lesions	
Determination of optimal hematocrit in patients with congenital anemia	
Quantifying the functional disability caused by chronic diseases of childhood and developing an exercise prescription	
Predicting outcomes in cystic fibrosis	
Establishing the diagnosis of the long QT syndrome	
Therapeutic and rehabilitation	
Training respiratory muscles in patients with chronic lung disease	
An adjunct to chest physiotherapy in patients with cystic fibrosis	
Stabilization of glycemia in insulin-dependent diabetes	
An adjunct to diet in the treatment of childhood obesity	
Nonpharmacologic treatment of juvenile hypertension	
Increasing school and social participation in children with osteogenesis imperfecta	
Amelioration of exercise induced asthma	
Pediatric cardiac rehabilitation	
Improving functional performance in children with cerebral palsy	

als who are making the referrals. For example, the questions to be answered by the test may be much different if the child is referred by a pediatric pulmonologist as opposed to a pediatric cardiologist. However, it is not uncommon to find multiplicity of mechanisms – the child referred by the general pediatrician for 'feeling faint' during exercise may prove to have exercise-induced bronchospasm. Using this approach, the patient referrals could be broken down into four categories: (1) pediatric pulmonary; (2) pediatric cardiology; (3) other pediatric subspecialties, and (4) general pediatrics. Each will be dealt with in a separate section. There will obviously be overlap between the categories; for example, shortness of breath with exercise may be a question asked in all categories, and this grouping will only serve as a framework.

Pediatric Pulmonary Referrals

Pediatric pulmonologists deal with a variety of chronic lung and airway diseases. The most important chronic pediatric lung diseases are asthma, cystic fibrosis, and chronic lung disease associated with prematurity [e.g. bronchopulmonary dysplasia (BPD) and gastroesophageal reflux (GER)]. In addition, upper airway obstruction is probably more common in the pediatric age range, and may be classified as congenital, acquired, or functional. Symptoms associated with exercise may occur with all of these diseases.

Asthma and Exercise

Currently, the most common use of diagnostic exercise testing is in the evaluation of exercise-induced asthma (EIA). EIA, a common feature of asthma especially in children, is characterized by a short and sometimes severe asthmatic attack following exercise. As EIA occurs in about 60–80% of asthmatic children it can be used as one of the diagnostic tests to establish the disease; moreover, an exercise challenge is a more specific indicator of asthma than either histamine or methacholine challenges [38].

During exercise, lung function changes little or may even improve. Toward the end of exercise or few minutes after, lung function begins to fall. The maximum fall in lung function occurs 5–10 min after the end of exercise after which recovery in lung function will take place in about 30–45 min. In a small proportion of asthmatic subjects a late phase reaction may develop [39–41].

The upper limit of post-exercise fall in FEV_1 (mean + 2 SD) in normal children was found to be 6–8% [42]. In asthmatic children the severity of EIA may be influenced by the severity of asthma [43] and by pre-exposure to allergens [44]. Moreover, the severity, duration and type of exercise may influence the severity of EIA. Running, as compared to swimming under the same inspired air conditions and work intensity, will result in much more EIA [45]. It is also important to note that the recovery from EIA differs in younger compared with older children. For example, Hofstra et al. [46] recently demonstrated that 7- to 10-year-olds with EIA improved FEV_1 by a mean of 1.60%/min following the challenge, but improvement in 11- to 12-year-olds was significantly prolonged (0.54%/min). Practical guidelines for the performance of exercise challenge testing for the diagnosis of asthma are reviewed elsewhere [8].

Cystic Fibrosis and Exercise

The clinician attempting to prescribe a program of exercise training for children and adolescents with cystic fibrosis (CF) faces a dilemma. Exercise may promote health in CF in part by stimulating growth factors and tissue anabolism (enhanced bone mineralization, increased muscle hypertrophy, mitochondrial density and

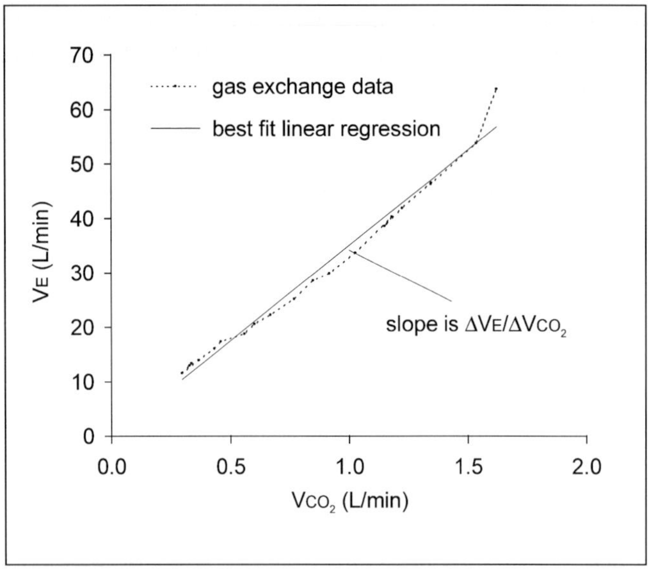

Fig. 8. The relationship between V_E-VCO_2 during a progressive exercise test in a 9-year-old girl with CF. Since V_E is driven by VCO_2, these data tend to have a high signal-to-noise ratio. The slope of the V_E-VCO_2 relationship is easily calculated using standard linear regression techniques. Reprinted with permission from Moser et al. [53].

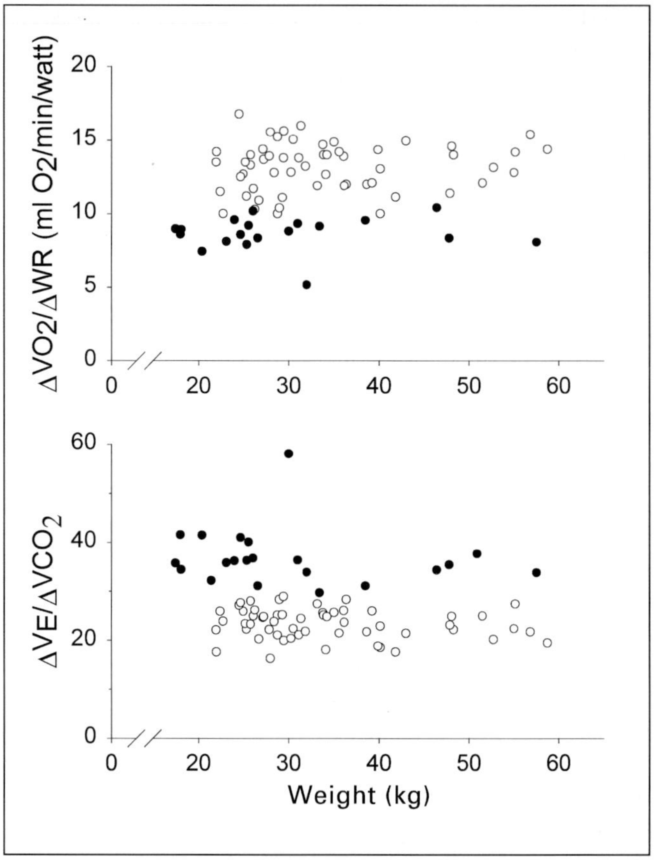

Fig. 9. Dynamic variables of progressive exercise tests in CF subjects (closed circles) and controls (open circles) as a function of body weight. $\Delta VO_2/\Delta WR$ data are shown in the upper panel, and $\Delta V_E/\Delta VCO_2$ in the lower panel. Both variables were significantly abnormal in CF subjects. Reprinted with permission from Moser et al. [53].

capillarization, and increased insulin sensitivity). However, even in healthy children, it is now known that the very same process of exercise, if sufficiently intense, can stimulate inflammatory cytokines and lead to a catabolic state [7, 47–49]. Finding the optimal level of physical activity in children and adolescents with CF is difficult because the underlying disease is associated with increased basal energy expenditure [50–53], hypoxemia, malnutrition, and inflammation, all of which promote tissue catabolism even at rest.

Cystic fibrosis is a multisystem disease, with the lung, gut, and pancreas being most severely affected. There is an increased viscosity of secretions that block the airways. Additionally, inflammatory processes in the lung (secondary to chronic bacterial and viral infections) lead to further viscosity increases and worse obstruction. Pulmonary disease progresses through bronchitis/bronchiolitis, bronchiectasis, emphysema, and restrictive changes, and accounts for 95% of the deaths of patients with cystic fibrosis. It is a progressive disease that eventually results in hypoxemia and pulmonary hypertension. Individuals with cystic fibrosis experience an average 2% per year decline in their FEV_1. Many patients with mild lung dysfunction have normal exercise tolerance. As the disease progresses and lung function deteriorates, exercise tolerance diminishes.

Children and adolescents with cystic fibrosis are known to have reduced exercise tolerance, but despite this there appear to be therapeutic benefits of exercise in these subjects. Indeed, fitter CF patients may have an improved outcome [54]. The precise mechanism of the exercise impairment remains largely unknown, but clearly, nutritional and cardiorespiratory factors play a role [55].

Although VO_2peak or max is usually reduced in CF patients, more recent studies have begun to identify those factors which may contribute to the exercise limitation in these children. Using progressive exercise protocols on the cycle ergometer and breath-to-breath measurements of gas exchange, $\Delta VO_2/\Delta HR$ was found to be low in CF subjects and $\Delta V_E/\Delta VCO_2$ high (fig. 8, 9). The slope of the

VO_2-HR relationship is determined by the stroke volume and the arteriovenous oxygen content difference. This slope is typically reduced when the stroke volume response to exercise is impaired, such as in children with single-ventricle lesions corrected surgically by the Fontan procedure [32]. Although left-ventricular dysfunction is not typically found in mild-to-moderate CF, stroke volume during exercise has been shown to be reduced in CF adults with severe lung disease (FEV_1 <55% predicted) [56]. $\Delta\dot{V}O_2/\Delta HR$ may be useful in identifying early abnormalities in cardiac function in CF subjects.

A much more substantial abnormality was the large increase in the slope of $\Delta\dot{V}_E/\Delta\dot{V}CO_2$. The elevated slope suggests excessive ventilation in CF subjects compared with controls as shown by the modified alveolar gas equation:

$$\dot{V}_E = [863 \times PaCO_2^{-1} \times (1 - V_D/V_T)^{-1}] \times \dot{V}CO_2$$

where $\dot{V}_E$ is minute ventilation; $\dot{V}CO_2$ is CO_2 production, $PaCO_2$ is arterial CO_2 tension, and V_D/V_T is dead space to tidal volume ratio. The two most likely explanations for excessive ventilation are increased V_D/V_T and changes in chemoreceptor set point for $PaCO_2$. In CF patients, previous investigators using other approaches have found exercise abnormalities both in chemoreceptor set point [57] and increased ventilatory dead space [58, 59]. The measurement of $\Delta\dot{V}_E/\Delta\dot{V}CO_2$ during exercise may prove to be a noninvasive, relatively effort independent, and useful means to gauge dynamic respiratory function in these patients.

A novel finding of recent studies was that the reduction in peak $\dot{V}O_2$ in CF was observed even when normalized to muscle size (measured by MRI determined cross-sectional area). Thus, reduced muscle mass alone (resulting, perhaps, from nutritional or ongoing inflammatory processes) could not account for all of the impairment of peak $\dot{V}O_2$ observed in CF. These observations indicate that the impaired exercise response in CF is related to altered oxygen delivery or intrinsic abnormality of muscle function in CF subjects.

Bronchopulmonary Dysplasia and Exercise

Premature infants who survive severe neonatal respiratory distress syndrome may develop a more chronic form of lung disease, termed bronchopulmonary dysplasia (BPD) [60]. The condition is characterized by persistence of respiratory distress, pulmonary radiographic abnormalities, and the need for supplemental oxygen for at least 4 weeks after birth. The etiology of BPD is multifactorial. The principal risk factors appear to be the degree of prematurity with its related structural and functional pulmonary immaturity, the presence and severity of respiratory distress syndrome, the duration and intensity of oxygen therapy, and positive pressure mechanical ventilation. The vast majority of infants with BPD do not require oxygen therapy by 2 years of age. However, a variety of chronic impairments in lung function have been reported [61, 62]. Many will have hyperinflation as evidenced by a large residual volume and a high ratio of residual volume to total lung capacity. Evidence for airway obstruction and airway hyperreactivity is commonly found. Exercise-induced asthma may be present in as many as 50% of BPD survivors. Many of these chronic respiratory symptoms may persist into adulthood [63]. As more premature infants are surviving, this is an ever-increasing group of patients who will need chronic pulmonary follow-up.

Exercise testing is an important part of the follow-up and response to therapy. These children tend to lower values of VO_2max and lactate threshold compared to controls. Values of minute ventilation and tidal volume tended to be lower during exercise, and these children may have a limited ability to increase ventilation with exercise. Arterial oxygen desaturation with exercise was not uncommon, occurring in as many as one-third of the patients. As mentioned, exercise-induced asthma was common. As for cystic fibrosis, these exercise abnormalities are not predicted by resting pulmonary function tests. The effects of exercise training for these patients have not been evaluated.

Upper Airway Obstruction and Exercise

Upper airway obstruction may also limit exercise performance in children. This is frequently overlooked as a cause of exercise-related dyspnea. The obstruction may occur above, at, or below the vocal cords. The airway may be congenitally deformed, as in micrognathia associated with the Pierre-Robin syndrome, or dysfunctional, as in laryngomalacia and tracheomalacia [64–66]. The airway may be secondarily obstructed. Granuloma formation either on or just below the vocal cords may be the result of prolonged intubation and lead to exercise related stridor. Children who have had a tracheostomy frequently have residual subglottic narrowing following decannulation. Vocal cord paralysis may follow chest surgery in children, usually following tumor resection or repair of congenital cardiac malformations. Stridor may be functional as well, with no signs at rest, and only manifest during stress or exercise [67–69]. This is seen in vocal cord dysfunction were the vocal cords move paradoxically during stress [70, 71]. Abnormal movement of the arytenoid region during extreme exertion may result in 'exercise-induced laryngomalacia', a syndrome associated with severe dyspnea and stridor during intense exercise. This syndrome may only be diagnosed in the exercise laboratory and may require laryngoscopy during exercise to make the diagnosis.

The exercise laboratory is probably underutilized for work-up and/or follow-up of children with the above or similar conditions. Any question of exercise-related symptoms in this group should certainly be tested.

Pediatric Cardiology Referrals

Children with congenital heart disease account for about 80–90% of pediatric cardiology patients. Currently, there are successful surgical or transcatheter options for repair or palliation of all forms of congenital heart disease, and the mortality rate for infants with congenital heart disease is less than 10%. Current estimates would predict that soon there will be more adults with congenital heart disease than children with congenital heart disease. In addition, there are only a very few circumstances that would require these patients, adults or children, to be restricted from athletics. Exercise testing is routinely recommended in these patients prior to sports participation. It is beyond the scope of this chapter to review all forms of congenital heart disease and their unique problems, and only general functional problems will be discussed.

Acquired heart diseases are an important minority of patients in pediatrics, and include patients with Kawasaki disease, cardiomyopathy and myocarditis, and rheumatic heart disease. With the exception of hypertrophic cardiomyopathy, these patients are also encouraged to be active, with few or no restrictions, and exercise testing is an important part of their work-up as well.

Specific recommendations for exercise testing prior to sports participation have been published for both children and adults with congenital heart disease or acquired heart disease. The 'Bethesda Conference' recommendations are excellent guidelines, and deal with each form of heart disease individually [72, 73].

Heart Rate Response to Exercise

Blunting of the heart rate response during maximal and submaximal exercise has been reported following surgical repair of all forms of congenital heart disease, from the simple (atrial and ventricular septal defects) to the complex (tetralogy of Fallot, Fontan operations for single ventricle [74]). The mechanism of such chronotropic incompetence is unknown and probably multifactorial. Damage to the SA nodal artery during cannulation for heart-lung bypass, direct damage to the SA node or its artery during the surgical repair, and part of the natural history of the disease have all been implicated. Maximal heart rates in the range of 140–160 beats/min are seen and can obviously contribute to or be responsible for exercise limitation [75–77]. As noted above, it is also possible to utilize submaximal and novel approaches to exercise testing in order to gain useful information regarding underlying pathophysiology in children with congenital heart disease [32].

Blunted heart rate responses may also occur in some forms of congenital heart disease even without surgery, most notably congenitally corrected transposition (L-transposition) of the great arteries. In addition, anti-arrhythmic medications, especially beta-blockers, can also blunt the heart rate response to exercise. Exercise testing is routinely performed to assess both the control of the arrhythmia during exercise and to ensure that the heart rate is not excessively inhibited. Children with complete heart block, either congenital or surgically induced, obviously have depressed heart rate responses both at rest and during exercise. Determination of the heart rate response can help decide if a pacemaker would be indicated.

All children with pacemakers have exercise testing in order to adjust the pacemaker parameters to produce an adequate heart rate response during exercise [78, 79]. Current pacemakers have maximal rates in the range of 180 beats/min. Dual chamber pacemakers (sensing and pacing in both the atria and the ventricles) may develop the equivalent of 2:1 heart block as the sinus node rate goes above 180 beats/min, and can produce severe symptoms with exercise. Careful adjustment of the upper rate limit behavior of dual chamber pacemakers during exercise testing is required to prevent this problem.

Blood Pressure Response to Exercise

In the postoperative cardiac patient, it is important to determine if previous surgery may have involved either of the subclavian arteries. For coarctation of the aorta, the left subclavian artery may have been used as part of the repair (subclavian patch aortoplasty), the left arm arterial supply is via collaterals, and the blood pressure is not accurate in the left arm. Similarly, if the patient has tetralogy of Fallot, either subclavian artery may have been used for a Blalock-Taussig shunt, and the blood pressure will not be accurate in that arm. If there is any doubt, the blood pressure should be taken in both arms prior to the exercise test.

The blood pressure response to exercise is exceedingly important for the follow-up and management of patients after repair of aortic coarctation. Although upper extremity blood pressure usually returns to normal after repair, in as many as 30–65% of postcoarctectomy patients there is an exaggerated systolic blood pressure response during graded exercise [80, 81]. This is usually not associated with symptoms or ECG changes. However, patients with this response tend not to regress their left-ventricular hypertrophy following repair, and this may be an indication to institute anti-hypertensive therapy [82].

It is never normal for the systolic blood pressure to decrease during a progressive exercise test and usually indicates an inability to increase cardiac output. This is an indication to stop an exercise test. Classically, this was seen in severe aortic stenosis and pulmonary stenosis. However, patients are no longer left with severe aortic or pulmonary stenosis and this should now be exceedingly rare. However, such a response may be seen in hypertrophic cardiomyopathy if there is subaortic obstruction due to asymmetric septal hypertrophy. Also, patients with dilated cardiomyopathy may exhibit the same response. For both groups, this is an ominous sign and may be a risk factor for sudden death.

Evaluation for Myocardial Ischemia

Obviously, this is the most common indication for exercise testing in adult cardiology due to the prevalence of atherosclerotic coronary artery disease in the adult population. Significant atherosclerosis is rare in the pediatric age range. However, the coronary arteries may be abnormal in a variety of pediatric patients. Monitoring for ECG changes of myocardial ischemia is the same in children as in adults.

The coronary arteries may be congenitally abnormal, as in patients with anomalous left coronary artery from the pulmonary artery. There may be a single coronary artery system, with either the left coming off the right or the right coming off the left and coursing aberrantly. Alternatively, the coronary arteries may be manipulated as part of surgical repair of a congenital heart defect. During the arterial switch operation for simple transposition of the great arteries, both coronary arteries are removed, mobilized and reimplanted in the new aortic root, and are therefore at risk for stenosis. Similarly, the coronary arteries may be reimplanted during the Ross operation for repair of aortic valve disease. It is now routine to reimplant the left coronary in infants if it arises from the pulmonary artery [83]. These children will require periodic exercise testing to assess for coronary insufficiency throughout their lives.

Children who have had Kawasaki disease comprise another major group of children at risk for coronary disease. Kawasaki disease is an inflammatory disease of unknown etiology affecting only children, and may lead to coronary artery aneurysm formation. If untreated, 15–20% of children with Kawaski disease will develop coronary artery aneursym; if treated early with gammaglobulin, the incidence is reduced to 3–5%. Coronary aneurysms put the children at risk for coronary thrombosis, coronary stenosis, and myocardial infarction [84, 85]. Exercise testing, both with and without nuclear testing, will be necessary throughout the children's lives [86].

Evaluation for Arrhythmias

Open-heart surgery to repair congenital cardiac defects leaves a surgical scar on either the right atrium or right ventricle, and may be a potential source of arrhythmias for these patients [76, 77, 87, 88]. The arrhythmia potential is increased if there is any residual hemodynamic burden on the myocardium. There may be a volume load on the hearts due to valvar insufficiency or residual atrial or ventricular septal defects. There may be pressure loads if there are residual stenoses at the valvar or supravalvar level. Some arrhythmias are precipitated by the increased myocardial oxygen demands associated with aerobic exercise. It is very common to perform maximal exercise tests on postoperative cardiac patients, either to work-up symptoms (palpitations, lightheadedness, syncope), to monitor the effectiveness of anti-arrhythmic therapy, or for clearance prior to athletic participation [72].

Patients with extensive atrial surgery are at high risk for atrial arrhythmias (atrial fibrillation, atrial flutter). This includes patients with atrial switch operations (Mustard, Senning operations) for simple transposition of the great arteries [87, 89]. Moreover, patients with Fontan operation for single ventricle very commonly have atrial arrhythmias. Patients with ventricular incisions are at risk for ventricular tachycardia. There is almost no current operation for congenital heart disease that involves an incision in the left ventricle. Patients with tetralogy of Fallot commonly have an incision along the right ventricular outflow tract in order to relieve sub-pulmonic obstruction. Ventricular tachycardia is common in this group of patients, and there is a significant risk of sudden death in the group as a whole [90–92]. It is more common if the right ventricle is dilated, as is seen in the group with significant pulmonary insufficiency. Most patients in this group have exercise tests every 2–3 years even if asymptomatic [73].

Pediatric patients may also have arrhythmias without congenital heart disease. Supraventricular tachycardia, with and without associated Wolf-Parkinson-White syndrome is common. Patients are evaluated pre- and post-therapy with exercise testing. Patients with cardiomyopathy, both hypertrophic and dilated, may have life-threatening ventricular arrhythmias. Hypertrophic cardiomyopathy is a very high-risk group with a high risk (1–2% per year) of sudden death. Although hypertrophic cardiomyopathy used to be a contraindication to exercise stress testing, most patients today will have an exercise test for risk assessment and/or response to therapy.

Evaluation for Exercise Limitation, Sports Participation

The preparticipation physical has been a part of most pediatric sports activities for many years, but substantial controversy remains regarding its efficacy and cost effectiveness [93–97]. Few, if any, prospective studies have been done to determine standards for preparticipation physicals. Finally, the use of stress exercise testing in the preparticipation physical has not been adequately addressed.

Nonspecific complaints of exercise limitation, easy fatigability, or shortness of breath with exercise are common in children with congenital or acquired heart disease. Obviously, the concern is for abnormalities due to the underlying heart disease. Pulmonary function testing and metabolic measurements during the exercise test should be performed whenever possible. Abnormalities in the heart rate or blood pressure response as noted above may occur, and arrhythmias are a risk. Many of these children will have had multiple surgeries and/or prolonged periods of intubation. It is not uncommon to find a restrictive pattern on the baseline pulmonary function test due to previous thoracotomies and sternotomies, or pleural sclerosing procedures to treat chronic pleural effusions. Inspiratory stridor may occur due to vocal cord granuloma of subglottic stenosis due to the previous intubations. Vocal cord paralysis or paresis may have occurred during one of the surgeries. Exercise-induced asthma may also occur. The exercise limitation may be ventilatory and not cardiac in origin.

Commonly, however, the exercise test may be normal, with the exception of a low VO_2max. Deconditioning in this group of children is multifactorial. The children may be afraid to exercise. They may be encouraged not to exercise by anxious parents or medical caregivers. A normal exercise test may be useful in showing the children and their parents that it is not dangerous to exercise. A careful exercise program can then be outlined.

Other Subspecialty Referrals

The Endocrinology and Metabolic Services may be a significant source of referrals. The recent increase in the incidence of type 2 diabetes in children and adolescents is an alarming manifestation of the broader problem of physical inactivity, poor diet, and obesity afflicting young people throughout the world [98]. The development of frank diabetes in children and adolescents will be associated with intensive and costly medical therapy, and long-term chronic disease is almost certain. Determining the level of fitness in obese children and an accompanying realistic exercise and nutrition program is a major task of the modern pediatric exercise physiology laboratory.

Children with type 1 diabetes mellitus are encouraged to be active and fit [99, 100]. Exercise-related symptoms are usually attributed to abnormal metabolism of exogenous insulin, but, increasingly, new studies are leading to a more broad-based understanding of the effect of exercise on the hormonal response to stress [101, 102]. Similar to children with other chronic conditions, children with type 1 diabetes are likely to benefit from exercise testing with metabolic measurements to determine the optimal role of exercise and physical activity for a particular child and his or her level of fitness.

The Renal Service follows most patients with hypertension. Essential hypertension is uncommon in the pediatric age range, accounting for less than 30% of children with hypertension. The majority of children with hypertension have renal disease [103, 104]. As for aortic coarctation of the aorta, the blood pressure response to children with hypertension may be exaggerated. Optimal blood pressure control should include both resting and exercise blood pressure.

Finally, there is growing understanding of the use of exercise testing in evaluating mitochondrial myopathies [105]. In many of these disorders, a lifelong, nonspecific history of poor fitness or inability to 'keep up with other children' during exercise is often encountered. Using the exercise laboratory to identify excessive acidosis with exercise (which can be done with simultaneous blood sampling or by careful analysis of gas exchange) will increasingly play an important role in this relatively new area of clinical awareness.

General Pediatric Referrals

There are three general pediatric problems that may be very difficult to sort out, and do not fall under any particular subspecialty: (1) shortness of breath with exercise; (2) chest pain, and (3) syncope. They may eventually be referred to the exercise laboratory from a variety of sources.

Exercise-related dyspnea is common. Frequently, the children will already have had a trial of an inhaled beta-agonist with the assumption that the breathlessness is related to exercise-induced asthma. A maximal exercise test with metabolic measurements and measurement of VO_2max can usually sort out the problem and direct therapy. The test must be strenuous enough to reproduce the breathlessness. Exercise-induced asthma should be easily documented or ruled out. More rare problems like arrhythmia or exercise-induced stridor will be detected. Deconditioning, documented by a low VO_2max, can also be diagnosed, and is probably more common than exercise-induced asthma. Recommendations for aerobic conditioning can be made at the same time.

Chest pain is a very common complaint in both children and adolescents. It may occur at rest or with exercise. The media have been successful in associating chest pain and 'heart attacks' in the adult population. Both parents and children make the same association for the pediatric age group. However, cardiac-related chest pain accounts for less than 4% of all chest pain in children.

Musculoskeletal chest wall pain is the most common. This pain may be worse with exercise due to the increased ventilation with exercise, and the association of the pain with exercise does not make it more likely to be cardiac in origin. Exercise-induced asthma may present with chest pain, due to the deep inspiratory 'tightness' that occurs with bronchospasm. Obviously, the pain is usually postexercise. Gastric reflux may present with low sternal or left precordial chest pain. This may be aggravated by exercise, meals, or lying down. Cardiac pain usually occurs with two circumstances. Pericardial pain due to inflammation (pericarditis) usually causes acute severe, substernal chest pain. The pain is described as squeezing or tightening, and is worse with movement and breathing. It is highly unlikely that these children would be referred for an exercise study. Anginal chest pain is uncommon in pediatrics, and as for adults, represents a mismatch between myocardial supply and demand. The coronary arteries may be congenitally abnormal (abnormal takeoff) or have acquired defects (Kawasaki disease) and these have been discussed previously. Marked ventricular hypertrophy may lead to underperfusion of the subendocardial layers of the heart and lead to myocardial ischemia and exertional angina. Severe valvar stenosis is now a rare problem out of the newborn period, and hypertrophic cardiomyopathy is now the leading cause of ventricular hypertrophy.

Referral of children with chest pain for exercise testing is common, especially if no clear etiology of the pain can be established by history or physical exam. Occasionally, the exercise test is diagnostic, i.e. if exercise-induced asthma is found, chest wall pain is reproduced following exercise, or ECG changes develop. More commonly, the test is normal but reassuring [106–109].

Syncope is also common in the pediatric age group. The vast majority is vasovagal in origin and unrelated to exercise. Syncope during exercise or in the immediate postexercise period is more worrisome and deserves a complete work-up [110]. Syncope while exercising may be due to a tachyarrhythmia, either atrial or ventricular. Syncope while exercising may also signal an inability to increase cardiac output adequately to meet the increased metabolic demands of exercise. Inability to increase stroke volume with exercise can be associated with valve stenosis (aortic, pulmonary, mitral), hypertrophic cardiomyopathy, dilated cardiomyopathy, primary pulmonary hypertension, or excessive diuretic therapy. Inadequate increases in heart rate may be associated with exercise-induced heart block. Blunting of the heart rate response with exercise has been discussed previously, and may be associated with prior heart surgery and anti-arrhythmic therapy. Exercise syncope was a common presentation for exercise-induced laryngomalacia. Sustaining exercise above the anaerobic threshold can lead to lightheadedness and syncope either during or immediately postexercise, and can be seen in athletes during training or competition. Therefore, a maximal exercise test with careful monitoring of heart rate, ECG, blood pressure, ventilation and oxygen consumption should be performed as part of the work-up for exercise related syncope. Occasionally a relatively low VO_2max in a competitive athlete is the only abnormality found.

Contraindications and Reasons to Terminate an Exercise Test

There are both absolute and relative reasons to defer or cancel an exercise test. As for any test, the risks must be weighed against the importance of the information to be gained [14]. Absolute contraindications usually involve an acute and evolving process, frequently inflammatory,

Table 2. Absolute contraindications to exercise testing

1	Acute myocarditis, pericarditis, or endocarditis
2	Acute rheumatic fever
3	Acute phase of Kawasaki disease
4	Acute myocardial infarction
5	Severe systemic hypertension
6	Active pneumonia
7	Exacerbation of asthma
8	Active hepatitis

Table 3. Relative contraindications to exercise testing

1	Severe left-ventricular outflow tract obstruction, including hypertrophic cardiomyopathy
2	Severe right-ventricular outflow tract obstruction
3	Congestive heart failure
4	Ischemic coronary artery disease
5	Advanced ventricular arrhythmias
6	Pacemakers with defibrillation capabilities
7	Pulmonary vascular obstructive disease
8	End-stage cystic fibrosis patients

and exercise itself may potentially be harmful. Some of these absolute contraindications are listed in table 2.

Relative contraindications imply that the exercise test poses potential risks to the child. The physician in charge of the exercise laboratory should be in contact with the referring physician regarding the relative risks and benefits for the particular patient, the exact question to be answered, potential alternatives to or modifications of exercise to answer the question at lower risk, and specific indications to end the test early. Examples or relative contraindications are included in table 3. Any such list should be amended for each individual laboratory based on the capabilities of the technical personnel and the characteristics of the referral population.

There are four general reasons to terminate an exercise test:

(1) The patient requests to end the test.

(2) Diagnostic findings have been established or a predetermined end point has been reached.

(3) Failure of monitoring equipment which could compromise patient safety.

(4) Signs or symptoms occur that pose a significant risk for the patient if exercise continues.

Worrisome symptoms would include dizziness, stridor or any excessive dyspnea, and headache. Signs which should lead the examiner to terminate the test include: ST segment depression of greater than 3 mm indicating myocardial ischemia, a progressive decrease in systolic blood pressure, or a rise in systolic blood pressure above 250 mm Hg. The development of an arrhythmia, either supraventricular or ventricular tachycardia, or the onset of heart block should require exercise termination. An increase in ventricular ectopy with exercise is worrisome but should be decided on an individual basis whether the exercise should continue.

Safety Issues

Exercise testing can be performed in children at low risk, even in patients with significant cardiac or pulmonary disease [111]. Complications are rare but do occur, and proper safety precautions are important to any pediatric exercise laboratory. A pediatric 'crash' cart should be available in the laboratory. A defibrillator with both pediatric and adult paddles is mandatory. Oxygen and suction should be available, as should equipment for bag-valve-mask ventilation. A nebulizer and asthma medications should be available.

All staff members should be certified in cardiopulmonary resuscitation. It is optimal to have two staff members conduct each test. One should take blood pressure and observe the ECG, while the other monitors the ergometer and observes the child. A staff member should stand behind the child during treadmill testing due to the risk of falling. If a test is deemed to be low risk for complications, a physician does not need to be present for the test but should be immediately available. The American Heart Association has issued guidelines for groups of patients who are felt to be at low risk for exercise complications. The medical director of the laboratory should review all referrals to the exercise laboratory prior to scheduling, determine which studies have significant risk, and ensure that a qualified physician will be present for the test. Finally, all children and their parents or legal guardians should sign an informed consent prior to the exercise testing procedures.

References

1 Berman N, Bailey RC, Barstow TJ, Cooper DM: Spectral and bout detection analysis of physical activity patterns in healthy, prepubertal boys and girls. Am J Hum Biol 1998;10:289–297.

2 Wasserman K, Whipp BJ, Koyal SN, Beaver WL: Anaerobic threshold and respiratory gas exchange during exercise. J Appl Physiol 1973;35:236–243.

3 Cooper DM, Weiler-Ravell D, Whipp BJ, Wasserman K: Oxygen uptake and heart rate during exercise as a function of growth in children. Pediatr Res 1984;18:845–851.

4 Cooper DM, Weiler-Ravell D, Whipp BJ, Wasserman K: Aerobic parameters of exercise as a function of body size during growth in children. J Appl Physiol 1984;56:628–634.

5 Seip RL, Weltman A, Goodman D, Rogol AD: Clinical utility of cycle exercise for the physiologic assessment of growth hormone release in children. Am J Dis Child 1990;144:998–1000.

6 Cappon J, Brasel JA, Mohan S, Cooper DM: Effect of brief exercise on circulating insulin-like growth factor-I. J Appl Physiol 1994;76:1418–1422.

7 Scheett TP, Milles PJ, Ziegler MG, Stoppani J, Cooper DM: Effect of exercise on cytokines and growth mediators in prepubertal children. Pediatr Res 1999;46:429–434.

8 Cooper DM, Springer C: Pulmonary function assessment in the laboratory during exercise; in Chernick V, Boat TF (eds): Kendig's Disorders of the Respiratory Tract in Children, ed 6. Philadelphia, Saunders, 1988, pp 214–237.

9 Armstrong N: Paediatric Exercise Science and Medicine. Oxford, Oxford University Press, 2000, pp 1–472.

10 Armon Y, Cooper DM, Flores R, Zanconato S, Barstow TJ: Oxygen uptake dynamics during high-intensity exercise in children and adults. J Appl Physiol 1991;70:841–848.

11 Zanconato S, Cooper DM, Armon Y: Oxygen cost and oxygen uptake dynamics and recovery with one minute of exercise in children and adults. J Appl Physiol 1991;71:993–998.

12 Zanconato S, Buchthal S, Barstow TJ, Cooper DM: ^{31}P-magnetic resonance spectroscopy of leg muscle metabolism during exercise in children and adults. J Appl Physiol 1993;74:2214–2218.

13 Cooper DM, Kaplan M, Baumgarten L, Weiler-Ravell D, Whipp BJ, Wasserman K: Coupling of ventilation and CO_2 production during exercise in children. Pediatr Res 1987;21:568–572.

14 Washington RL, Bricker JT, Alpert BS, Daniels SR, Deckelbaum RJ, Fisher EA, Gidding SS, Isabel-Jones J, Kavey RE, Marx GR, et al: Guidelines for exercise testing in the pediatric age group. From the Committee on Atherosclerosis and Hypertension in Children, Council on Cardiovascular Disease in the Young, the American Heart Association. Circulation 1994;90:2166–2179.

15 Eriksson BO, Grimby G, Saltin B: Cardiac output and arterial blood gases during exercise in pubertal boys. J Appl Physiol 1971;31:348–352.

16 Rowland T, Popowski B, Ferrone L: Cardiac responses to maximal upright cycle exercise in healthy boys and men. Med Sci Sports Exerc 1997;29:1146–1151.

17 Godfrey S, Davies CT, Wozniak E, Barnes CA: Cardio-respiratory response to exercise in normal children. Clin Sci 1971;40:419–431.

18 Rowland T, Whatley BJ: Cardiac dynamics during upright cycle exercise in boys. Am J Hum Biol 2000;12:749–757.

19 Springer C, Barstow TJ, Cooper DM: Effect of hypoxia on ventilatory control during exercise in children and adults. Pediatr Res 1989;25:285–290.

20 Nagano Y, Baba R, Kuraishi K, Yasuda T, Ikoma M, Nishibata K, Yokota M, Nagashima M: Ventilatory control during exercise in normal children. Pediatr Res 1998;43:704–707.

21 Beneke R, Heck H, Schwarz V, Leithauser R: Maximal lactate steady state during the second decade of age. Med Sci Sports Exerc 1996;28:1474–1478.

22 Gomez-Marin O, Prineas RJ, Rastam L: Cuff bladder width and blood pressure measurement in children and adolescents. J Hypertens 1992;10:1235–1241.

23 Paterson DH, Cunningham DA, Plyley MJ, Blimkie CJ, Donner AP: The consistency of cardiac output measurement (CO_2 rebreathe) in children during exercise. Eur J Appl Physiol Occup Physiol 1982;49:37–44.

24 Pianosi P, Garros D: Comparison of impedance cardiography with indirect Fick (CO_2) method of measuring cardiac output in healthy children during exercise. Am J Cardiol 1996;77:745–749.

25 Marx GR, Hicks RW, Allen HD: Measurement of cardiac output and exercise factor by pulsed Doppler echocardiography during supine bicycle ergometry in normal young adolescent boys. J Am Coll Cardiol 1987;10:430–434.

26 Yamaya Y, Bogaard HJ, Wagner PD, Niizeki K, Hopkins SR: Validity of pulse oximetry during maximal exercise in normoxia, hypoxia, and hyperoxia. J Appl Physiol 2002;92:162–168.

27 Cooper DM: Rethinking exercise testing in children: A challenge. Am J Resp Crit Care 1995;152:1154–1157.

28 Reybrouck T, Weymans M, Stijns H, Knops J, van der HL: Ventilatory anaerobic threshold in healthy children: Age and sex differences. Eur J Appl Physiol 1985;54:278–284.

29 Baraldi E, Cooper DM, Zanconato S, Armon Y: Heart rate recovery from 1 minute of exercise in children and adults. Pediatr Res 1991;29:575–579.

30 Cooper DM, Berry C, Lamarra N, Wasserman K: Kinetics of oxygen uptake and heart rate at onset of exercise in children. J Appl Physiol 1985;59:211–217.

31 Cooper DM, Weiler Ravell D, Whipp BJ, Wasserman K. Growth-related changes in oxygen uptake and heart rate during progressive exercise in children. Pediatr Res 1984;18:845–851.

32 Troutman WB, Barstow TJ, Galindo AJ, Cooper DM: Abnormal dynamic cardiorespiratory responses to exercise in pediatric patients after Fontan procedure. J Am Coll Cardiol 1998;31:668–673.

33 Moser C, Tirakitsoontorn P, Nussbaum E, Newcomb R, Cooper D: Muscle size and cardiorespiratory response to exercise in cystic fibrosis. Am J Resp Crit Care Med 2000;162:1823–1827.

34 Cumming GR, Everatt D, Hastman L: Bruce treadmill test in children: Normal values in a clinic population. Am J Cardiol 1978;41:69–75.

35 James FW: Exercise testing in children and young adults: An overview. Cardiovasc Clin 1978;9:187–203.

36 Nagle F, Balke B, Baptista G, Alleyia J, Howley E: Compatibility of progressive treadmill, bicycle and step tests based on oxygen uptake responses. Med Sci Sports 1971;3:149–154.

37 Riopel DA, Taylor AB, Hohn AR: Blood pressure, heart rate, pressure-rate product and electrocardiographic changes in healthy children during treadmill exercise. Am J Cardiol 1979;44:697–704.

38 Godfrey S, Springer C, Noviski N, Maayan C, Avital A: Exercise but not methacholine differentiates asthma from chronic lung disease in children. Thorax 1991;46:488–492.

39 Speelberg B, Verhoeff NP, van den Brink WT: The prevalence of the early and late asthmatic reaction after exercise in patients with intrinsic and extrinsic asthma. Agents Actions Suppl 1989;28:375–378.

40 Bahous J, Cartier A, Pineau L, Bernard C, Ghezzo H, Martin RR, Malo JL: Pulmonary function tests and airway responsiveness to methacholine in chronic bronchiectasis of the adult. Bull Eur Physiopathol Resp 1984;20:375–380.

41 Crimi E, Balbo A, Milanese M, Miadonna A, Rossi GA, Brusasco V: Airway inflammation and occurrence of delayed bronchoconstriction in exercise-induced asthma. Am Rev Respir Dis 1992;146:507–512.

42 Avital A, Springer C, Bar-Yishay E, Godfrey S: Adenosine, methacholine, and exercise challenges in children with asthma or paediatric chronic obstructive pulmonary disease. Thorax 1995;50:511–516.

43 Cabral AL, Conceiecaao GM, Fonseca-Guedes CH, Martins MA: Exercise-induced bronchospasm in children: Effects of asthma severity. Am J Resp Crit Care Med 1999;159:1819–1823.

44 Mussaffi H, Springer C, Godfrey S: Increased bronchial responsiveness to exercise and histamine after allergen challenge in asthmatic children. J Allergy Clin Immunol 1986;77:48–52.
45 Bar-Yishay E, Gur I, Inbar O, Neuman I, Dlin RA, Godfrey S: Differences between swimming and running as stimuli for exercise-induced asthma. Eur J Appl Physiol Occup Physiol 1982;48:387–397.
46 Hofstra WB, Sterk PJ, Neijens HJ, Kouwenberg JM, Duiverman EJ: Prolonged recovery from exercise-induced asthma with increasing age in childhood. Pediatr Pulmonol 1995;20:177–183.
47 Theintz GE, Howald H, Weiss U, Sizonenko PC: Evidence for a reduction of growth potential in adolescent female gymnasts. J Pediatr 1993;122:306–313.
48 Eliakim A, Brasel JA, Mohan S, Cooper DM: Increased physical activity and the growth hormone insulin-like growth factor-I axis in adolescent males. Am J Physiol 1998;275:R308–314.
49 Eliakim A, Brasel JA, Mohan S, Barstow TJ, Berman N, Cooper DM: Physical fitness, endurance training, and the GH-IGF-I system in adolescent females. J Clin Endocrinol Metab 1996;81:3986–3992.
50 Anthony H, Bines J, Phelan P, Paxton S: Relation between dietary intake and nutritional status in cystic fibrosis. Arch Dis Child 1998;78:443–447.
51 Bell SC, Saunders MJ, Elborn JS, Shale DJ: Resting energy expenditure and oxygen cost of breathing in patients with cystic fibrosis. Thorax 1996;51:126–131.
52 Tirakitsoontorn P, Nussbaum E, Moser C, Hill M, Cooper DM: Fitness, acute exercise, and anabolic and catabolic mediators in cystic fibrosis. Am J Resp Crit Care Med 2001;164:1432–1437.
53 Moser C, Tirakitsoontorn P, Nussbaum E, Newcomb R, Cooper DM: Muscle size and cardiorespiratory response to exercise in cystic fibrosis. Am J Resp Crit Care Med 2000;162:1823–1827.
54 Nixon PA, Orenstein DM, Kelsey SF, Doershuk CF: The prognostic value of exercise testing in patients with cystic fibrosis. N Engl J Med 1992;327:1785–1788.
55 Shah AR, Gozal D, Keens TG: Determinants of aerobic and anaerobic exercise performance in cystic fibrosis. Am J Resp Crit Care Med 1998;157:1145–1150.
56 Pianosi P, Pelech A: Stroke volume during exercise in cystic fibrosis. Am J Resp Crit Care Med 1996;153:1105–1109.
57 Pianosi P, Wolstein R: Carbon dioxide chemosensitivity and exercise ventilation in healthy children and in children with cystic fibrosis. Pediatr Res 1996;40:508–513.
58 Coates AL, Canny G, Zinman R, Grisdale R, Desmond K, Roumeliotis D, Levison H: The effects of chronic airflow limitation, increased dead space, and the pattern of ventilation on gas exchange during maximal exercise in advanced cystic fibrosis. Am Rev Respir Dis 1988;138:1524–1531.
59 Hirsch JA, Zhang SP, Rudnick MP, Cerny FJ, Cropp GJ: Resting oxygen consumption and ventilation in cystic fibrosis. Pediatr Pulmonol 1989;6:19–26.
60 Jobe AH, Ikegami M: Prevention of bronchopulmonary dysplasia. Curr Opin Pediatr 2001;13:124–129.
61 Santuz P, Baraldi E, Zaramella P, Filippone M, Zacchello F: Factors limiting exercise performance in long-term survivors of bronchopulmonary dysplasia. Am J Resp Crit Care Med 1995;152:1284–1289.
62 Jacob SV, Lands LC, Coates AL, Davis GM, MacNeish CF, Hornby L, Riley SP, Outerbridge EW: Exercise ability in survivors of severe bronchopulmonary dysplasia. Am J Resp Crit Care Med 1997;155:1925–1929.
63 Pianosi PT, Fisk M: Cardiopulmonary exercise performance in prematurely born children. Pediatr Res 2000;47:653–658.
64 Smith RJ, Bauman NM, Bent JP, Kramer M, Smits WL, Ahrens RC: Exercise-induced laryngomalacia. Ann Otol Rhinol Laryngol 1995;104:537–541.
65 Bent JP, Miller DA, Kim JW, Bauman NM, Wilson JS, Smith RJ: Pediatric exercise-induced laryngomalacia. Ann Otol Rhinol Laryngol 1996;105:169–175.
66 Nussbaum E, Maggi JC: Laryngomalacia in children. Chest 1990;98:942–944.
67 Landwehr LP, Wood RP, Blager FB, Milgrom H: Vocal cord dysfunction mimicking exercise-induced bronchospasm in adolescents. Pediatrics 1996;98:971–974.
68 McFadden ER Jr, Zawadski DK: Vocal cord dysfunction masquerading as exercise-induced asthma: A physiologic cause for 'choking' during athletic activities. Am J Respir Crit Care Med 1996;153:942–947.
69 Kayani S, Shannon DC: Vocal cord dysfunction associated with exercise in adolescent girls. Chest 1998;113:540–542.
70 Lakin RC, Metzger WJ, Haughey BH: Upper airway obstruction presenting as exercise-induced asthma. Chest 1984;86:499–501.
71 Bittleman DB, Smith RJ, Weiler JM: Abnormal movement of the arytenoid region during exercise presenting as exercise-induced asthma in an adolescent athlete. Chest 1994;106:615–616.
72 Graham TP, Jr, Bricker JT, James FW, Strong WB: 26th Bethesda conference: Recommendations for determining eligibility for competition in athletes with cardiovascular abnormalities. Task Force 1: Congenital heart disease. Med Sci Sports Exerc 1994;26:S246–S253.
73 Graham TP Jr, Bricker JT, James FW, Strong WB: 26th Bethesda conference: Recommendations for determining eligibility for competition in athletes with cardiovascular abnormalities. Task Force 1: Congenital heart disease. J Am Coll Cardiol 1994;24:867–873.
74 Durongpisitkul K, Driscoll DJ, Mahoney DW, Wollan PC, Mottram CD, Puga FJ, Danielson GK: Cardiorespiratory response to exercise after modified Fontan operation: Determinants of performance. JACC 1997;29:785–790.
75 Perrault H, Drblik SP, Montigny M, Davignon A, Lamarre A, Chartrand C, Stanley P: Comparison of cardiovascular adjustments to exercise in adolescents 8 to 15 years of age after correction of tetralogy of fallot, ventricular septal defect or atrial septal defect. Am J Cardiol 1989;64:213–217.
76 Rhodes J, Garofano RP, Bowman FO, Grant GP, Bierman FZ, Gersony WM: Effect of right ventricular anatomy on the cardiopulmonary response to exercise: Implications for the fontan procedure. Circulation 1990;81:1811–1817.
77 Bink-Boelkens MT, Velvis H, van der Heide JJ, Eygelaar A, Hardjowijono RA: Dysrhythmias after atrial surgery in children. Am Heart J 1983;106:125–130.
78 Estes NA, III, Brockington G, Manolis AS, Salem D: Pacemakers and exercise: Current status, future developments and practical implications of physiological pacemakers. Sports Med 1989;8:1–8.
79 Bricker JT, Garson A, Jr, Traweek MS, Smith RT, Ward KA, Vargo TA, Gillette PC: The use of exercise testing in children to evaluate abnormalities of pacemaker function not apparent at rest. Pacing Clin Electrophysiol 1985;8:656–660.
80 Guenthard J, Wyler F: Exercise-induced hypertension in the arms due to impaired arterial reactivity after successful coarctation resection. Am J Cardiol 1995;75:814–817.
81 Sigurdardottir LY, Helgason H: Exercise-induced hypertension after corrective surgery for coarctation of the aorta. Pediatr Cardiol 1996;17:301–307.
82 Pelech AN, Kartodihardjo W, Balfe JA, Balfe JW, Olley PM, Leenen FH: Exercise in children before and after coarctectomy: Hemodynamic, echocardiographic, and biochemical assessment. Am Heart J 1986;112:1263–1270.
83 Hauser M, Bengel FM, Kuhn A, Sauer U, Zylla S, Braun SL, Nekolla SG, Oberhoffer R, Lange R, Schwaiger M, Hess J: Myocardial blood flow and flow reserve after coronary reimplantation in patients after arterial switch and ross operation. Circulation 2001;103:1875–1880.
84 Kato H, Ichinose E, Yoshioka F, Takechi T, Matsunaga S, Suzuki K, Rikitake N: Fate of coronary aneurysms in Kawasaki disease: Serial coronary angiography and long-term follow-up study. Am J Cardiol 1982;49:1758–1766.
85 Nakanishi T, Takao A, Kondoh C, Nakazawa M, Hiroe M, Matsumoto Y: ECG findings after myocardial infarction in children after Kawasaki disease. Am Heart J 1988;116:1028–1033.
86 Paridon SM, Galioto FM, Vincent JA, Tomassoni TL, Sullivan NM, Bricker JT: Exercise capacity and incidence of myocardial perfusion defects after Kawasaki disease in children and adolescents. J Am Coll Cardiol 1995;25:1420–1424.
87 Vetter VL, Tanner CS: Electrophysiologic consequences of the arterial switch repair of d-transposition of the great arteries. J Am Coll Cardiol 1988;12:229–237.

88 Perrault H, Coughlan M, Marcotte JE, Drblik SP, Lamarre A: Comparison of cardiac output determinants in response to upright and supine exercise in patients with cystic fibrosis. Chest 1992;101:42–51.
89 Gelatt M, Hamilton RM, McCrindle BW, Connelly M, Davis A, Harris L, Gow RM, Williams WG, Trusler GA, Freedom RM: Arrhythmia and mortality after the Mustard procedure: A 30-year single-center experience. J Am Coll Cardiol 1997;29:194–201.
90 Nollert G, Fischlein T, Bouterwek S, Bohmer C, Klinner W, Reichart B: Long-term survival in patients with repair of tetralogy of Fallot: 36-year follow-up of 490 survivors of the first year after surgical repair. J Am Coll Cardiol 1997; 30:1374–1383.
91 Gatzoulis MA, Balaji S, Webber SA, Siu SC, Hokanson JS, Poile C, Rosenthal M, Nakazawa M, Moller JH, Gillette PC, Webb GD, Redington AN: Risk factors for arrhythmia and sudden cardiac death late after repair of tetralogy of Fallot: A multicentre study. Lancet 2000; 356:975–981.
92 Therrien J, Siu SC, Harris L, Dore A, Niwa K, Janousek J, Williams WG, Webb G, Gatzoulis MA: Impact of pulmonary valve replacement on arrhythmia propensity late after repair of tetralogy of Fallot. Circulation 2001;103:2489–2494.
93 Reed FJ: Improving the preparticipation exam process. J SC Med Assoc 2001;97:342–346.
94 Metzl JD: The adolescent preparticipation physical examination: Is it helpful? Clin Sports Med 2000;19:577–592, v.
95 Drezner JA: Sudden cardiac death in young athletes. Causes, athlete's heart, and screening guidelines. [Comment in: Postgrad Med 2001; 109:18 UI: 21120625.] Postgrad Med 2000; 108:37–50.
96 Fuller CM, McNulty CM, Spring DA, Arger KM, Bruce SS, Chryssos BE, Drummer EM, Kelley FP, Newmark MJ, Whipple GH: Prospective screening of 5,615 high school athletes for risk of sudden cardiac death. Med Sci Sports Exer 1997;29:1131–1138.
97 Kurowski K, Chandran S: The preparticipation athletic evaluation (see comments). Am Fam Physician 2000;61:2683–2688.
98 Pinhas-Hamiel O, Zeitler P: Type 2 diabetes in adolescents, no longer rare. Pediatr Rev 1998;19:434–435.
99 Draznin MB, Patel DR: Diabetes mellitus and sports. Adolesc Med 1998;9:457–465.
100 Kiess W, Kapellen T, Siebler T, Deutscher J, Raile K, Dost A, Meyer K, Nietzchmann U: Practical aspects of managing preschool children with type 1 diabetes. Acta Paediatr Suppl 1998;425:67–71.
101 Galassetti P, Mann S, Tate D, Neill RA, Wasserman DH, Davis SN: Effect of morning exercise on counterregulatory responses to subsequent, afternoon exercise. J Appl Physiol 2001;91:91–99.
102 Galassetti P, Mann S, Tate D, Neill RA, Costa F, Wasserman DH, Davis SN: Effects of antecedent prolonged exercise on subsequent counterregulatory responses to hypoglycemia. Am J Physiol Endocrinol Metab 2001;280: E908–E917.
103 Sinaiko AR: Hypertension in children. N Engl J Med 1996;335:1968–1973.
104 Arar MY, Hogg RJ, Arant BS Jr, Seikaly MG: Etiology of sustained hypertension in children in the southwestern United States. Pediatr Nephrol 1994;8:186–189.
105 Flaherty KR, Wald J, Weisman IM, Zeballos RJ, Schork MA, Blaivas M, Rubenfire M, Martinez FJ: Unexplained exertional limitation: Characterization of patients with a mitochondrial myopathy. Am J Respir Crit Care Med 2001;164:425–432.
106 Selbst SM: Adolescent chest pain and cardiac emergencies. Adolesc Med 1993;4:23–34.
107 Selbst SM, Ruddy R, Clark BJ: Chest pain in children. Follow-up of patients previously reported. Clin Pediatr (Philadelphia) 1990;29: 374–377.
108 Selbst SM: Pediatric chest pain: A prospective study. Clin Pediatr (Philadelphia) 1990; 29:615.
109 Wiens L, Sabath R, Ewing L, Gowdamarajan R, Portnoy J, Scagliotti D: Chest pain in otherwise healthy children and adolescents is frequently caused by exercise-induced asthma. Pediatrics 1992;90:350–353.
110 Driscoll DJ, Jacobsen SJ, Porter CJ, Wollan PC: Syncope in children and adolescents. J Am Coll Cardiol 1997;29:1039–1045.
111 Alpert BS, Verrill DE, Flood NL, Boineau JP, Strong WB: Complications of ergometer testing in children. Pediatr Cardiol 1983;4:91–96.

Dan M. Cooper, MD
UCI College of Medicine
Clinical Research Center
Bldg. 25, ZOT 4094-03,101 The City Drive
Orange, CA 92868 (USA)
Tel. +1 714 456 2317
Fax +1 714 824 1595
E-Mail dcooper@uci.edu

Weisman IM, Zeballos RJ (eds): Clinical Exercise Testing.
Prog Respir Res. Basel, Karger, 2002, vol 32, pp 300–322

An Integrative Approach to the Interpretation of Cardiopulmonary Exercise Testing

Idelle M. Weisman[a] R. Jorge Zeballos[b]

[a]Human Performance Laboratory, Department of Clinical Investigation, Pulmonary-Critical Care Service, William Beaumont Army Medical Center, El Paso, Tex., and Department of Medicine, Pulmonary-Critical Care Division, University of Texas Health Science Center at San Antonio, San Antonio, Tex.;
[b]Human Performance Laboratory, Department of Clinical Investigation, William Beaumont Army Medical Center, and Department of Anesthesiology, Texas Tech University Health Sciences Center, El Paso, Tex., USA

Summary

Cardiopulmonary exercise testing (CPET) is currently being used in a wide spectrum of clinical applications because of the valuable information that it provides in patient diagnosis and management. The goals of this article are to provide an overview of our CPET interpretative strategy and to demonstrate how the information obtained during cardiopulmonary exercise testing can be appropriately presented, systematically approached, and meaningfully applied in the clinical decision-making process. A case study format will highlight this approach.

Introduction

Cardiopulmonary exercise testing (CPET) is currently being used in a wide spectrum of clinical applications because of the valuable information that it provides in patient diagnosis and management. Increasing use of CPET has been fueled by advances in technology, scientific advances in exercise physiology, and growing awareness of the importance of the integrative exercise response in clinical assessment [1–4].

In order to achieve optimal use of this modality in clinical practice, clarification of conceptual issues and stan-

The opinions or assertions contained herein are the private views of the authors and are not to be construed as official or as reflecting the views of the Department of the Army or the Department of Defense.

Glossary

AT	Anaerobic threshold
BP	Blood pressure
CPET	Cardiopulmonary exercise test
ECG	Electrocardiogram
EELV	End expiratory lung volume (TLC – IC = EELV)
extFVL/MFVL	Exercise tidal flow-volume loop referenced to resting maximal flow-volume loop
f	Breathing frequency
HCO_3^-	Bicarbonate
HR	Heart rate
HRR	Heart rate reserve
IC	Inspiratory capacity
IET	Incremental exercise test
LT	Lactate threshold
MVV	Maximal voluntary ventilation
O_2 pulse	Oxygen pulse
PaO_2	Arterial oxygen tension
$PaCO_2$	Arterial carbon dioxide tension
$P(A\text{-}a)O_2$	Alveolar-arterial oxygen pressure difference
P_{ETO_2}	End-tidal pressure of oxygen
P_{ETCO_2}	End-tidal pressure of carbon dioxide
pH	Hydrogen ion concentration
RER	Respiratory exchange ratio
SpO_2	Pulse oximetry
SaO_2	Arterial oxygen saturation
TI/TTOT	Ratio of inspiratory time to breath total time (duty cycle)
V_D/V_T	Physiologic dead space to tidal volume ratio
$\dot{V}_E$	Minute ventilation
$\dot{V}_E/\dot{V}_{O_2}$	Ventilatory equivalent for oxygen
$\dot{V}_E/\dot{V}_{CO_2}$	Ventilatory equivalent for carbon dioxide
$\dot{V}_E$/MVV	Ratio of indices of ventilatory demand to ventilatory capacity
$\dot{V}_{CO_2}$	Carbon dioxide output
V_T	Tidal volume
$\dot{V}_{O_2}$	Oxygen uptake
$\dot{V}/\dot{Q}$	Ventilation-perfusion ratio
VR	Ventilatory reserve

dardization of CPET practices are necessary [5]. Progress in this direction has begun with the publication of ERS guidelines [6] and the near completion of the joint ATS-ACCP statement on Cardiopulmonary Exercise Testing.

The goals of this article are to provide an overview of our CPET interpretative strategy and to demonstrate how the information obtained during cardiopulmonary exercise testing can be appropriately presented, systematically approached, and meaningfully applied in the clinical decision-making process. A case study format will highlight this approach. Exercise interpretation will emphasize cardiopulmonary results generated during maximal incremental cycle ergometry, which is currently the most popular approach. The complementary role of constant-work CPET in the interpretative and clinical decision-making processes will also be demonstrated.

Interpretative Strategies

An interpretative strategy that is scientifically based and sufficiently flexible to be applied to a variety of clinical entities/pathophysiologic conditions is required for the optimal utilization of CPET in clinical practice. Several approaches should be considered since there is no consensus on any one. Approaches that emphasize the mechanism for exercise limitation (i.e. ventilatory limitation to exercise) are limited by their lack of 'gold standard' definition and the realization that exercise limitation is often multifactorial [7–9]. Algorithms based on key measurements and conceptual framework [4, 10, 11] are limited by excessive reliance on single measurements. Interpretative error may result if that one measurement at a key branch point is wrong for whatever reason (i.e. anaerobic threshold). Standard algorithms are also inadequate for the evaluation of patients with early/mild disease, in patients with combined disease (heart-lung [see case study]), and when variable responses are borderline [3, 12]. The greatest diagnostic potential and impact of CPET on the clinical decision making process is best achieved by using an integrative approach to CPET interpretation, which emphasizes the interrelationships, trending phenomena, and patterns of key variable responses in a clinical setting framework [3, 6].

Integrative Approach

An integrative approach to the interpretation of CPET results includes consideration of the following: (1) reason(s) for CPET; (2) attention to pertinent clinical and laboratory information; (3) assessment of overall test quality, subject effort, and reason(s) for exercise cessation; (4) the identification of key measurements – initially $\dot{V}_{O_2}$, then HR, $\dot{V}_E$, and SaO_2 with other measurements evaluated subsequently based on the reasons for which CPET was obtained; (5) attention to trending phenomena (i.e. submaximal through maximal exercise results) using both tabular and graphic display formats; (6) determination of whether the measurements are normal or abnormal compared to appropriate (normal) reference values; (7) evaluation of limitations(s) to exercise including a determination of a physiologic vs. non-physiologic basis; (8) evaluation of patterns of exercise responses; (9) consideration of conditions/clinical entities which maybe associated with these patterns, and (10) correlation of exercise results with the patient's clinical information including results of other tests (i.e. PFTs, echocardiogram).

Additional salient comments for some of these considerations appear below although all are discussed subsequently.

Reason(s) for CPET: Should always be noted and addressed in the final report.

Clinical Status Evaluation: Results of history, physical examination, resting lab tests (i.e. PFTs, EKG), level of physical activity (most easily obtained using a health questionnaire), and medication history are all essential to accurate interpretation. A more meaningful physiologic-clinical correlation and, in turn, accurate interpretation of CPET is possible when a thorough clinical subject profile is available.

Assessment of Patient Effort: Knowledge of patient effort and motivation are necessary for the accurate interpretation of CPET. Several studies have shown that $\dot{V}_{O_2}$ peak is the same or similar to $\dot{V}_{O_2}$max when at least one of the following requirements occurs: (1) patient looks exhausted; (2) heart rate or $\dot{V}_E$ is close to predicted; (3) lactate is greater than 8 mEq/l, and/or (4) respiratory exchange ratio is greater than 1.15 [13–15]. A test may also be discontinued because of significant symptoms and/or serious ECG changes.

Reasons for Exercise Cessation: Should also be noted and quantitated (i.e. Borg scale for dyspnea/leg fatigue/chest pain) [16] (see chapter on Methodologic issues). Finally, as patients are often symptom rather than physiologically limited, a reduced $\dot{V}_{O_2}$peak may also reflect poor (or sub-maximal) effort with uncertainty persisting about exercise limitation and $\dot{V}_{O_2}$peak. The importance of assessing patient effort when $\dot{V}_{O_2}$peak is critical in clinical decision analysis has recently been underscored in a study involving patients for cardiac transplantation [17].

Reference Values: The selection of an appropriate set of reference values is a function of the patient population, age, height, weight, sex, and physical activity and may vary from lab to lab [4, 18, 19]. Knowledge of physical activity is important in accurately interpreting CPET results. For example, very fit individuals and athletes may experience significant reductions in their peak $\dot{V}_{O_2}$ as a result of pulmonary, cardiac or (peripheral) muscle illness and still be within the normal confidence interval for sedentary subjects. Different sets of maximal (or peak) reference values may have significant impact on the interpretation of CPET results as demonstrated in table 1. Therefore, for the future, standardization of normal reference values processes/practices for CPET is necessary to facilitate interpretation and optimize clinical application [3, 6].

Table 1. Impact of different reference values on interpretation of cardiopulmonary exercise testing results

59-year-old white female, nonsmoker, 160 cm, 83 kg
FVC = 100%; FEV_1 = 115%; FEV_1/FVC = 86%; TLC = 104%; DL_{CO} = 84%
Protocol: maximal, symptom-limited 10 W/min incremental exercise test

Variables	Peak	Hansen [80]	Jones [96]	Blackie [97, 98]
Work rate, W	70	95%	60%	50%
$\dot{V}_{O_2}$, liters/min	1.23	88%	79%	65%
$\dot{V}_E$, liters/min	61	74%	105%	102%
HR, beats/min	155	90%	97%	
O_2 pulse, ml/beat	8	100%	73%	

Measurements and Graphic Interrelationships

Computerized exercise systems permit an impressive number of variables to be measured during CPET (table 2). The number of variables to be measured will depend on the reasons for which CPET was requested. The graphic inter-relationships between these variables are discussed in the case studies. Also, in table 2, the measurements are represented as noninvasive or invasive (i.e. arterial sampling intervention). A listing of selected peak CPET measurements, including caveats and suggested normal guidelines for interpretation gleaned from the literature, appear in table 3.

$\dot{V}_{O_2}$max or $\dot{V}_{O_2}$peak

The measurement of $\dot{V}_{O_2}$max or $\dot{V}_{O_2}$peak remains the best index for the assessment of exercise capacity. $\dot{V}_{O_2}$peak should be directly measured since its estimation from resting indices, work rate, or exercise protocols is unreliable [20]. $\dot{V}_{O_2}$peak should be expressed in absolute values (liters/min) and as percent predicted. The optimal normalization for body mass remains controversial. The normalization could be done for body weight (ml/kg/min), body mass index (kg/m^2), or ideally for fat-free mass (ml/kg/min) [21]. Some prefer normalization by height ($\dot{V}_{O_2}$/ht) as it may prove to be a better correlate of lean body mass [4]. $\dot{V}_{O_2}$/kg is most commonly used (i.e. American Heart Association, American College of Sports Medicine) and is the easiest to calculate, but may produce deceptively low values in obese subjects [22]. $\dot{V}_{O_2}$max values have been regarded as most reliable when $\dot{V}_{O_2}$ does not increase (plateau) despite further increase in work rate [23, 24]. Such a plateau however, especially in patients is not often observed and the maximum $\dot{V}_{O_2}$

Table 2. Cardiopulmonary variables measured during cardiopulmonary exercise testing

Variables	Noninvasive	Invasive (ABGs)
Work	WR	
Metabolic	$\dot{V}_{O_2}$, $\dot{V}_{CO_2}$, R, AT	lactate
Cardiovascular	HR, ECG, BP, O_2 pulse	
Ventilatory	$\dot{V}_E$, V_T, f	
Pulmonary gas exchange	SpO_2, $\dot{V}_E/\dot{V}_{CO_2}$, $\dot{V}_E/\dot{V}_{O_2}$ P_{ETO_2}, P_{ETCO_2}	SaO_2, PaO_2, $P(A-a)O_2$, V_D/V_T
Acid, base		pH, $PaCO_2$, HCO_3^-
Symptoms	Dyspnea, leg fatigue, chest pain	

Abnormality of a variable does not necessarily define exercise limitation in that category.
Modified from Zeballos and Weisman [19], with permission.

Table 3. Selected peak cardiopulmonary exercise testing measurements

Variables	Measurement caveats	Comments	Suggested guidelines [3, 4, 80, 87, 91]
$\dot{V}_{O_2}$max or $\dot{V}_{O_2}$peak	max: When plateau is achieved peak: $\dot{V}_{O_2}$ at max exercise, but no plateau	global assessment of respiratory, cardiovascular, blood and muscle function	> 84 % predicted
Anaerobic threshold (a.k.a. lactate threshold)	direct: lactate in arterial blood; indirect: modified V-Slope ($\dot{V}_{CO_2}$ vs. $\dot{V}_{O_2}$) and conventional ($\dot{V}_E/\dot{V}_{O_2}$, $\dot{V}_E/\dot{V}_{CO_2}$, P_{ETO_2}, P_{ETCO_2}); no one noninvasive method is consistently superior	estimator of the onset of metabolic acidosis during exercise (AT); not an effective discriminator among different clinical entities; appears nonessential for exercise Rx in COPD; 50–60% $\dot{V}_{O_2}$max in average persons; higher in fit persons	>40% $\dot{V}_{O_2}$max predicted; wide range of normal: 35–80%; clinical validation is required
Heart rate (HR) Reserve (HRR)	predicted maximum HR: 210 – (age × 0.65) HRR: Age Predicted max HR – max HR achieved	age-related variability in max HR predicted; normals usually no HRR	max HR >90% age predicted HRR < 15 bpm
O_2 pulse ($\dot{V}_{O_2}$/HR)	determined at plateau, when max O_2 extraction and stroke volume have been reached	reflects stroke volume assuming that O_2 extraction is normal; its use in COPD/CHF remains unvalidated	>80%
$\Delta\dot{V}_{O_2}/\Delta WR$	measured during IET ($\dot{V}_{O_2}$peak – $\dot{V}_{O_2}$ min 3 unloading)/(W/min × duration test – 0.75)	used as index of O_2 delivery/utilization by the muscle; could be abnormal in patients with cardiovascular/pulm vascular disease; normal in patient with pulmonary disease	>8.3 ml/min/W
Ventilatory reserve (VR)	MVV – $\dot{V}_{Emax}$ or $\dot{V}_E$/MVV × 100 (widely used). MVV can be measured directly or calculated (FEV_1 × 40); extFVL/MFVL to visualize 'limitation'; quantitate: IC = TLC-EELV; EILV/TLC	potential ventilation in L that could be increased; percentage of the max breathing capacity used; no gold standard for its determination	MVV – $\dot{V}_{Emax}$: > 11 liters; $\dot{V}_E$/MVV × 100: <75% wide normal range: 72 ±15%
Breathing frequency (f)	different breathing strategies in COPD and ILD; erratic in malingers; high in psychogenic disorders	reflects abnormalities in the mechanics of breathing, control of breathing, and/or hypoxemia or psychological disorders	<60 brpm
$\dot{V}_E/\dot{V}_{CO_2}$ (at AT)	measured throughout but reported at AT (near nadir) when $PaCO_2$ is steady, to avoid the effect of hyperventilation acidosis, etc.	noninvasive measurement of efficiency of ventilation (L of $\dot{V}_E$ to eliminate 1 liter of $\dot{V}_{CO_2}$); reflects increase in V_D/V_T and or hyperventilation.	<34
V_D/V_T	$PaCO_2$ should be used in its determination; P_{ETCO_2} produces unreliable results	reflects efficiency of CO_2 exchange or lung units with proportionally higher $\dot{V}A$ than $\dot{Q}$ (increased VD); normally decreases with increased exercise intensity	<0.28
PaO_2	careful anaerobic collection at near maximal and peak exercise for consistency in the results	ability to exchange O_2 is best assessed by measurement of PaO_2 and not by pulse oximetry	>80 mm Hg
$P(A\text{-}a)O_2$	arterial blood should be collected slowly in the middle of the respective interval	evaluates gas transfer; abnormal high values may reflect $\dot{V}/\dot{Q}$ mismatching (shunt type), diffusion limitation, shunt and/or reduced PvO_2	< 35 mm Hg

Modified from Weisman and Zeballos [25], with permission.

achieved is called $\dot{V}_{O_2}$peak [13–14]. For practical purposes $\dot{V}_{O_2}$max and $\dot{V}_{O_2}$peak are used interchangeably.

A reduced $\dot{V}_{O_2}$peak response to exercise reflects problems with O_2 transport and/or peripheral abnormalities [1, 7–9]. A reduced $\dot{V}_{O_2}$peak may also reflect poor effort. $\dot{V}_{O_2}$peak is modulated by physical activity, and, consequently, is considered the gold standard for the evaluation of level of fitness. A normal $\dot{V}_{O_2}$peak reflects a normal aerobic power and exercise capacity and provides reassurance that no significant functional abnormality exists. Even though the $\dot{V}_{O_2}$peak is normal, CPET may reveal other abnormalities (i.e. abnormal breathing patterns [see case studies]) that may be of diagnostic value [25].

Anaerobic Threshold (AT)

Also known as lactate threshold (LT), is an estimator of the onset of metabolic acidosis caused predominantly by increases in lactic acid during exercise. After 30 years, the physiologic significance, clinical significance, and the methodology for the determination of the AT remain controversial [26–28]. Current knowledge would suggest that the AT may be considered to be affected by factors that impact both O_2 transport and O_2 utilization processes, pattern of muscle fiber recruitment, and possibly others [29]. The AT is usually 50–60% $\dot{V}_{O_2}$max in sedentary individuals and higher in fit individuals [4]. There is a wide range of normal predicted values (35–70%) [6].

The AT can be determined invasively by measurement of arterial lactate (gold standard) or, more often, noninvasively using ventilatory or gas exchange variables. Although there are several ways to determine the AT noninvasively, none appears consistently superior [30]. Currently, the modified V-slope method (change in the slope of the plot of $\dot{V}_{CO_2}$ vs. $\dot{V}_{O_2}$) is most popular [31]. The AT, using the ventilatory equivalents method, is defined as the lowest (nadir) for $\dot{V}_E/\dot{V}_{O_2}$ and P_{ETO_2} before beginning to consistently increase, while $\dot{V}_E/\dot{V}_{CO_2}$ and P_{ETCO_2} remain unchanged [4]. A 'dual methods' approach, which combines the modified V-slope and the ventilatory equivalents method, is recommended [19] (see case studies). $RER \approx 1$ is also useful [4]. False-positive noninvasive AT determinations have been reported in COPD and can be avoided by obtaining blood samples for standard bicarbonate or lactates [26]. The AT determination is helpful as an indicator of level of fitness and to monitor the effect of physical training [32]. The AT is reduced in a wide spectrum of clinical entities – i.e. heart disease, lung disease, deconditioning, post lung and heart transplantation, skeletal muscle abnormalities (metabolic myopathy, muscle dysfunction in chronic disease), etc., and, therefore, may be of limited discriminatory value in interpretative schemes [3].

Heart Rate

The best index for the evaluation of cardiac function during exercise would be the measurement of cardiac output. However, this is not routinely performed in the clinical exercise laboratory. Since it is well established that increase in cardiac output are initially accomplished by increases in stroke volume and HR, and then at higher work rates almost exclusively by increase in HR [24], the evaluation of HR yields an estimate of the level of cardiac output achieved during exercise.

It is important to remember that there is considerable variability (10–15 beats per minute) within an age group when these estimates of maximal HR are used. The difference between the age-predicted maximal HR and the maximum HR achieved during exercise is referred to as the HR reserve (HRR). Normally, at maximal exercise, there is little or no heart rate reserve. Peak heart rate achieved during exercise in patient populations, however, may vary considerably due to the disease itself or due to medications used in treatment. Finally, heart rate recovery has recently been reported to be important as an independent predictor of mortality in a cohort of patients referred for exercise electrocardiography [32a], see chapter Methods for Cardiopulmonary Exercise Testing, pp 43–59.

Ventilatory Reserve (VR)

This concept is used to denote if ventilatory limitation occurs during exercise. It expresses the relationship between the maximal ventilation achieved during exercise ($\dot{V}_Emax$) as an index of the ventilatory demand and the MVV as an estimator of the maximal ventilatory capacity. This relationship can be expressed as $\dot{V}_E$/MVV [4]. VR is dependent on many factors responsible for ventilatory demand including metabolic demand, body weight, mode of testing, dead space ventilation as well as neuroregulatory and behavioral considerations. Mechanical factors, ventilatory muscle function, genetic endowment, aging, and disease impact maximal ventilatory capacity [33]. Ventilatory capacity may also vary during exercise depending on bronchodilation or bronchoconstriction and operational lung volume [34].

A high $\dot{V}_E$/MVV is one of the criteria often used to indicate encroachment on the ventilatory reserve and possible ventilatory limitation to exercise. Although widely used and practical, MVV may not be a reliable indicator of maximal ventilatory capacity nor provide insight into breathing strategy (see chapter on methodology) [34]. Controversy has surrounded the assessment of VR and $\dot{V}_E$/MVV. Emerging methodologies compare aligned exercise tidal flow-volume loops to resting maximal flow-volume loops (extFVL/MFVL). The volume and the expiratory flow rate differences between the exercise tidal flow volume loops and MFVL curve maybe useful for the determination of ventilatory limitation and calculation of the theoretical maximal ventilatory capacity ($\dot{V}_{Ecap}$ [see chapter on Methodology]) [34]. Exercise tidal flow-volume loop analysis has been applied in several clinical settings [34–38]. Alternatively, the negative expiratory pressure (NEP) technique has been suggested as a means to determine expiratory flow limitation by applying negative pressure (5 cm) at the mouth during expiration and determining whether ventilation is able to increase [39]. However, unless NEP technique is combined with an assessment of exercise tidal flow volume loops, flow limitation is defined as 'all or none' without any quantitation of constraint.

Pulmonary Gas Exchange

The ventilatory equivalent for $\dot{V}_{CO_2}$ ($\dot{V}_E/\dot{V}_{CO_2}$) is a good noninvasive estimator of inefficient ventilation. This variable should be reported at the AT (near its nadir) when $PaCO_2$ is steady to avoid the effect of the lactic acidosis and other stimuli (anxiety) on ventilation. Higher values reflect hyperventilation and/or increased dead space (wasted) ventilation. Determination of P_{ETCO_2}, or preferably $PaCO_2$, is useful in distinguishing between these possibilities [3, 4, 18].

In clinical settings requiring accurate pulmonary gas exchange determinations, direct arterial blood gas (ABG) sampling during exercise should be considered for calculation of alveolar-arterial oxygen pressure difference ($PAO_2 - PaO_2$) and physiologic dead space to tidal volume ratio (V_D/V_T) [40]. V_D/V_T determined noninvasively using P_{ETCO_2} yields unreliable results [41]. PaO_2 and SaO_2 should be directly measured since pulse oximetry is only an estimator of SaO_2 [19]. Corroboration of incremental results may be achieved with ABG measurement during a 6-min constant work (CW) exercise test at 70% of the maximum work achieved, which is ≈ 90% $\dot{V}_{O_2}$peak (see case studies). Recently, validation of pulmonary gas exchange measurements during IET with CW testing above the AT has been reported [42]. Abnormal widening of $P(A\text{-}a)O_2$ with exercise usually reflects $\dot{V}/\dot{Q}$ mismatching, but also can be due to diffusion abnormalities, anatomical shunt and/or reduced O_2 saturation in mixed venous blood worsening the $\dot{V}/\dot{Q}$ mismatching (shunt effect) [43]. Normally, V_D/V_T decreases as exercise intensity increases [3, 4, 18, 43]. Failure of V_D/V_T to decrease normally with exercise is indicative of $\dot{V}/\dot{Q}$ abnormalities caused by increases in physiologic dead space (wasted ventilation) [3, 4, 18, 43]. V_D/V_T measurements can be impacted by exercise breathing patterns resulting in abnormally high values [44, 45]; both false-positive [46] and false-negative [47] results have been reported.

Clinical Signs and Symptoms

Ratings of perceived exertional symptoms (breathlessness, fatigue, chest pain) using the Borg Scale (0–10) [16] or other rating scores including visual analogue scales [48–49] should be noted with the physiologic measurements (table 2).

Exercise Limitation

Clinically, it is increasingly appreciated that exercise limitation or low $\dot{V}_{O_2}$max achieved is multifactorial and, as such, is not limited by any single component of the O_2 transport/utilization process, but rather by their collective quantitative interaction [7–9]. Although several factors may be involved, one factor often predominates with variable contributions to exercise intolerance from the other factors. Exercise in normal subjects is mainly limited by the cardiovascular system. Table 4 lists the most important categories and factors involved in exercise limitation resulting in reduced $\dot{V}_{O_2}$max. These include cardiovascular limitation (O_2 transport), ventilatory limitation, and peripheral limitation; the latter involves a broad spectrum of abnormalities that could impact tissue O_2 conductance, O_2 utilization and mechanisms of contraction [50–51].

Table 4. Mechanisms of exercise limitation

Pulmonary
Ventilatory (mechanical)
Respiratory muscle dysfunction (dynamic hyperinflation)
Gas exchange
Cardiovascular
Reduced stroke volume
Abnormal heart rate response
Abnormal systemic and pulmonary circulation
Hemodynamic consequences of dynamic hyperinflation
Abnormal blood (anemia, COHb)
Peripheral
Inactivity (disuse), loss of muscle mass (atrophy), neuromuscular dysfunction
Peripheral circulatory abnormalities
Reduced skeletal muscle oxidative capacity (metabolic myopathy, COPD)
Malnutrition
Perceptual
Motivational
Environmental
Exercise limitation is often multifactorial

Evaluation of Cardiopulmonary Exercise Testing Results

A reduced $\dot{V}_{O_2}$peak is the starting point in the evaluation of reduced exercise capacity. Typical CPET response patterns for several clinical conditions including chronic heart failure, COPD, ILD, pulmonary vascular disease, obesity, and deconditioning appear in table 5. This table is admittedly oversimplified and does not permit the wide range of responses that may be seen within a full spectrum (mild to severe) of patients with, for instance, COPD or heart disease. It must be clearly appreciated that significant overlap exists in the response patterns of patients with different cardiopulmonary diseases to exercise. Furthermore, coexisting conditions (obesity, deconditioning, etc.), often contribute to exercise intolerance and may confound CPET interpretation.

Cardiovascular Disease

Many factors contribute to exercise intolerance in patients with cardiovascular disease including inadequate

Table 5. Usual cardiopulmonary exercise response patterns

Measurements	Heart failure	COPD	ILD	Pulmonary vascular disease	Obesity	Deconditioned
$\dot{V}_{O_2}$max or peak	decreased	decreased	decreased	decreased	decreased for actual, normal for ideal weight	decreased
Anaerobic threshold	decreased	normal/decreased/ indeterminate	normal or decreased	decreased	normal	normal or decreased
Peak HR	variable, usually normal	decreased, normal in mild	decreased	normal/slightly decreased	normal/slightly decreased	normal/slightly decreased
O_2 pulse	decreased	normal or decreased	normal or decreased	decreased	normal	decreased
(Peak $\dot{V}_E$/MVV) × 100	normal or decreased	increased	normal or increased	normal	normal or increased	normal
$\dot{V}_E/\dot{V}_{CO_2}$ (at AT)	normal or increased	increased	increased	increased	normal	normal
V_D/V_T	increased	increased	increased	increased	normal	normal
PaO_2	normal	variable	decreased	decreased	normal/may increase	normal
$P_AO_2 - PaO_2$	normal	variable, usually increased	increased	increased	may decrease	normal

Decreased, normal, increased with respect to normal response.
Modified from multiple sources [4, 25, 67].

O_2 transport, abnormalities in the distribution of the peripheral circulation, skeletal muscle abnormalities (i.e. O_2 utilization, atrophy, etc.), deconditioning, and pulmonary abnormalities [52–55]. Consequently, these patients stop exercise prematurely with attainment of a lower $\dot{V}_{O_2}$. Early onset metabolic acidosis is manifested by a reduced AT. O_2 pulse, as an indirect measure of reduced stroke volume (assuming normal CaO_2-CvO_2), is reduced and cardiac output is maintained almost exclusively by increases in heart rate [56]. Usually, there is little or no heart rate reserve; however, this may be highly variable and is a function of the type and severity of the heart disease [56]. Patients with heart failure manifest an abnormal heart rate response with the likelihood of chronotropic dysfunction increasing as disease severity increases [56, 57]. The early exercise cessation is usually associated with a reduced $\dot{V}_E$max, a considerable ventilatory reserve and no arterial desaturation. Increases in V_D/V_T and $\dot{V}_E/\dot{V}_{CO_2}$ due to reduced pulmonary perfusion consequent to reduced cardiac output are also observed [58]. The presence of a reduced ventilatory reserve (high $\dot{V}_E$/MVV) in these patients may signal the presence of combined cardiovascular and respiratory limitation [12] (see case study 4).

Pulmonary Vascular Disease

Patients with pulmonary vascular disease are likewise usually cardiovascular limited, with a normal ventilatory reserve but with an abnormal breathing strategy consisting of rapid respiratory frequency and low tidal volumes. A spectrum of pulmonary gas exchange abnormalities including evidence of inefficient ventilation (increased $\dot{V}_E/\dot{V}_{CO_2}$) increased dead space ventilation (abnormal V_D/V_T responses), hypoxemia (↓ PaO_2), and arterial desaturation with abnormal widening of the $P(A\text{-}a)O_2$ are seen [4, 18, 56, 59, 60].

Deconditioning

Physical inactivity, for a variety of reasons. is the main cause of deconditioning or unfitness [61–63]. In deconditioning, early cessation of exercise is associated with low/low normal $\dot{V}_{O_2}$peak, normal or early onset of metabolic acidosis (normal/low AT), a reduced O_2 pulse, and little/no HRR but with increased HR at submaximal levels of $\dot{V}_{O_2}$. There is significant ventilatory reserve and no abnormal pulmonary gas exchange. Deconditioning is often difficult to distinguish form early or mild heart disease [3, 4, 18, 56]. Although occurring much less frequently, recent work has suggested that mitochondrial myopathy also be included within the differential diagnosis [64]. Deconditioning commonly co-exists in patients with chronic illness including those with heart and lung disease and in patients with mitochondrial myopathy. Response to an aerobic training regimen with monitoring of responses ($\dot{V}_{O_2}$, O_2 pulse, AT, HR) may help to distinguish between heart disease and deconditioning, but not necessarily between deconditioning and mitochondrial myopathy (see chapter on Mitochondrial Myopathy) [64].

Chronic Obstructive Pulmonary Disease

Depending on the stage of disease, a spectrum of exercise response patterns can be seen in patients with COPD. Whereas, patients with mild COPD have an essentially normal exercise response pattern with normal/near normal exercise capacity, patients with moderate-to-severe COPD will usually have reduced $\dot{V}_{O_2}$peak and work rate (see chapter on COPD) [65–67]. One of the distinguishing features of many patients with COPD is a reduced ventilatory reserve ($\dot{V}_E$/MVV approaching or exceeding 100%) suggesting ventilatory limitation to exercise [4]. There is usually significant heart rate reserve, a reflection that the cardiovascular system has been relatively unstressed. In a retrospective study of patients with COPD categorized as mild, moderate, or severe, as disease severity progressed, $\dot{V}_{O_2}$max and VR decreased and HRR increased [68]. Exercise limitation in COPD, however, is usually multifactorial [7–9].

In patients with COPD, the AT response may be normal, low or indeterminate. Early onset metabolic acidosis (low AT) usually reflects deconditioning due to physical inactivity and/or skeletal muscle dysfunction including alterations in exercise related substrate levels, especially glutamate [63, 69]. The O_2 pulse is usually (but not invariably) proportionately reduced to $\dot{V}_{O_2}$max due to ventilatory limitation, deconditioning and possibly hypoxemia. Reduction in O_2 pulse, as has been suggested, may also reflect the hemodynamic consequences of dynamic hyperinflation [70]. Other respiratory abnormalities include increasing dynamic hyperinflation (IC decreases with exercise), inefficiency of ventilation ($\dot{V}_E/\dot{V}_{CO_2}$) due to increased dead space ventilation with abnormal V_D/V_T responses, alveolar hypoventilation with $PaCO_2$ not changing or increasing compared to normals, and hypoxemia [3, 4, 18, 66, 67, 71]. PaO_2 may be variable but is more often reduced in patients with moderate-severe COPD; $PAO_2 - PaO_2$ usually increases abnormally, especially when PaO_2 decreases.

Interstitial Lung Disease (ILD)

$\dot{V}_{O_2}$peak and peak work rate are usually reduced. A spectrum of ventilatory and pulmonary gas exchange abnormalities are seen (see chapter on ILD). A reduced ventilatory reserve (high $\dot{V}_E$/MVV) and ventilatory limitation to exercise are often seen in patients with ILD. However, a recent retrospective analysis of patients with interstitial pulmonary fibrosis has suggested that the ventilatory reserve is normal and that cardiovascular/pulmonary circulatory limitation to exercise occurs [72]. The AT is usually normal, but pulmonary circulatory involvement may be suspected if the AT is low. A combined cardiovascular and respiratory limitation may exist [3]. Rapid, shallow breathing (high respiratory rate, low tidal volume) occurs commonly as does evidence of inefficient ventilation (↑ $\dot{V}_E/\dot{V}_{CO_2}$) in response to increases in V_D/V_T. Impressive arterial desaturation with abnormal widening of $PAO_2 - PaO_2$ is usually seen [73–76].

Obesity

$\dot{V}_{O_2}$ as percent of predicted can be normal or low in obese patients; however, when expressed as $\dot{V}_{O_2}$ per kg body weight is low and with increasing obesity; disproportionately lower. There is an excessive metabolic requirement manifested by an upwardly displaced $\dot{V}_{O_2}$-work rate relationship with a normal slope [77]. The $\dot{V}_E$ at a given external WR is higher as a reflection of increased mechanical work, but the ventilatory reserve ($\dot{V}_E$/MVV) can be normal or increased. A trend towards abnormally increased respiratory rate and reduced tidal volume is often seen [78]. Recent exercise tidal flow-volume loop analysis suggests that there is ventilatory constraint (flow limitation) during exercise as obese subjects breathe at low lung volumes [33–35]. HR is increased at submaximal work with attainment of normal or near normal peak HR with little or no heart rate reserve [79]. Resting PaO_2 and $P(A\text{-}a)O_2$ may improve with exercise, reflecting improved $\dot{V}/\dot{Q}$ relationships. Obesity is often associated with other conditions in negatively impacting exercise capacity.

Conclusions

The integrative approach to the interpretation of CPET results is evolving and requires attention to fundamental principles including a systematic analysis of factors discussed previously (see section on Integrative Approach, fig. 1, and tables 1–5). Inherent in this approach are 'operational' assumptions (precepts) that, although reasonable, require additional study. For instance, although a 'patterns based' approach is flexible and theoretically attractive, relatively few studies have evaluated the sensitivity, specificity, and positive predictive value of patterns of exercise responses in diagnosing and distinguishing different clinical entities. Moreover, the impact of this approach on clinical decision-making in well-estab-

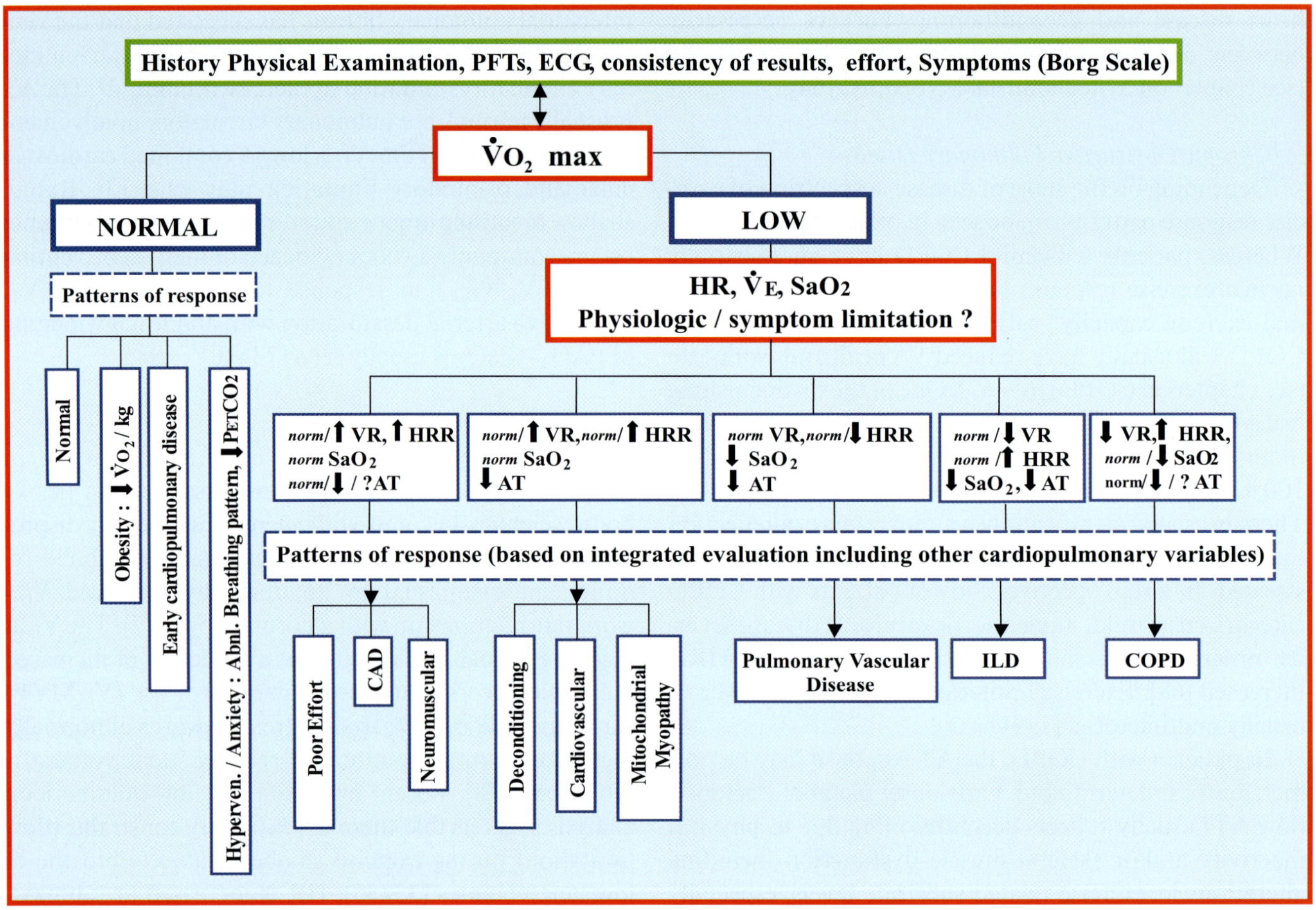

Fig. 1. Overview of a step approach to the interpretation of cardiopulmonary exercise testing results. Initial consideration of patient information, reason(s) for testing, and analysis of overall quality of the test are followed by determination of normality of $\dot{V}_{O_2}max/\dot{V}_{O_2}peak$. Subsequently, simultaneous assessment of three basic variables – HR, $\dot{V}_E$ and SaO_2. Determination of physiologic limitation is accomplished by analysis of ventilatory reserve ($\dot{V}_E$/MVV) and heart rate reserve (HRR). The AT may be helpful at this point in establishing generic diagnostic categories. Additional CPET measurements and patterns of response are established and (likely) associated clinical entities are considered resulting in more specific diagnostic pathways [99] (reprinted with permission).

lished clinical entities remains incompletely characterized. Fortunately, an increasing number of well-designed and executed clinical studies that fulfill evidence-based criteria are providing an expanded database of CPET results for systematic review that hopefully will provide answers to clinically relevant questions not immediately available.

Case Studies

The integrative approach to the interpretation of CPET results is highlighted in the following case studies. The 4 cases that will be presented reflect common clinical situations. In addition to the exercise response data, appropriate baseline clinical and laboratory data will be presented to enhance the physiologic-clinical correlation. The contribution of the exercise results in the clinical decision-making process is emphasized. For practical purposes, interpretation of these case studies was accomplished using information provided in tables 2–5 and figure 1.

The data are formatted for both tabular and graphic analysis. Maximal predicted values from Hansen et al. [80] were used. Multiple sources were used to provide the comparative normal responses for the graphic representation of the submaximal exercise [80–82]. Suggested criteria for normal maximal values for interpretation of CPET

Table 6. Maximal cardiopulmonary incremental exercise test with pre and post spirometry in a patient with exertional dyspnea (case 1)

20-year-old male, Hispanic, height: 173 cm, weight: 69 kg; clinical Dx: asthma
Medications: none
Reason for testing: unexplained exertional dyspnea

a Cardiopulmonary exercise test[1]

Variable	Peak	% pred
Work rate, W	200	83
$\dot{V}_{O_2}$, liters/min	2.92	98
$\dot{V}_{O_2}$, ml/kg/min	42.3	98
AT, liters/min	1.60	N (>1.19)
$\Delta\dot{V}_{O_2}/\Delta WR$	12.3	N (>8.3)
HR, bpm	181	91
O_2 pulse, ml/beat	16.1	108
BP, mm Hg		
$\dot{V}_E$, liters/min	106	63
f, br/min	96	H
$\dot{V}_E/\dot{V}_{CO_2}$, at AT	25	N

Stop: volitional exhaustion/fatigue 10/10.

b Spirometery before and after CPET (exercise-induced bronchoconstriction test)

	Baseline	5 min post	%[2]	15 min post	%[2]	30 min post	%[2]	Post BD	%[3]
FVC	5.06 (96%)	5.14	+2	4.51	−11	4.47	−12	4.58	+2
FEV_1	4.34 (97%)	4.25	−2	3.63	−16	3.34	−23	3.76	+13
FEV_1/FVC	86%	83%		80%		75%		82%	
FEF_{25-75}	5.09 (104%)	5.45	+7	3.82	−25	2.26	−49	4.60	+103

1 Protocol: maximal, symptom-limited incremental cycle ergometry, 25 W/min.
2 Percent change from baseline values.
3 Percent change post bronchodilator from 30-min values.

results obtained from several sources appears in table 3. These suggested guideline values are (at least for some variables) approximations of normality; evidence based criteria are necessary. Some of the data have been modified to enhance/focus the case relevant didactic message.

Exercise interpretation is limited to CPET results generated during maximal incremental cycle ergometry. In 2 cases, arterial blood gases were obtained at rest and then during minute 5 of constant work exercise testing which was used for an approximation of peak values for pulmonary gas exchange. Finally, the reader is reminded that for the interpretation of pulmonary gas exchange, our laboratory is at 1,270 m, mean barometric pressure 656 mm Hg (P_IO_2 = 128 mm Hg).

Case Study 1: Maximal CPET in a Subject with Exertional Dyspnea

Clinical History

A 20-year-old soldier, lifelong nonsmoker with a past medical history remarkable only for some poorly characterized childhood allergies was referred for evaluation of a 1-month history of exertional shortness of breath associated with chest tightness and inability to pass a required 2-mile run that he had successfully completed 3 months earlier. Physical examination, chest roentgenography, ECG, and screening laboratory tests, including pulmonary function tests, were all within normal limits. A methacholine challenge test was positive (PC_{20} = 4.2 mg/ml) and a diagnosis of exercise-induced bronchospasm (EIB) was established. After 6 weeks of an aggressive asth-

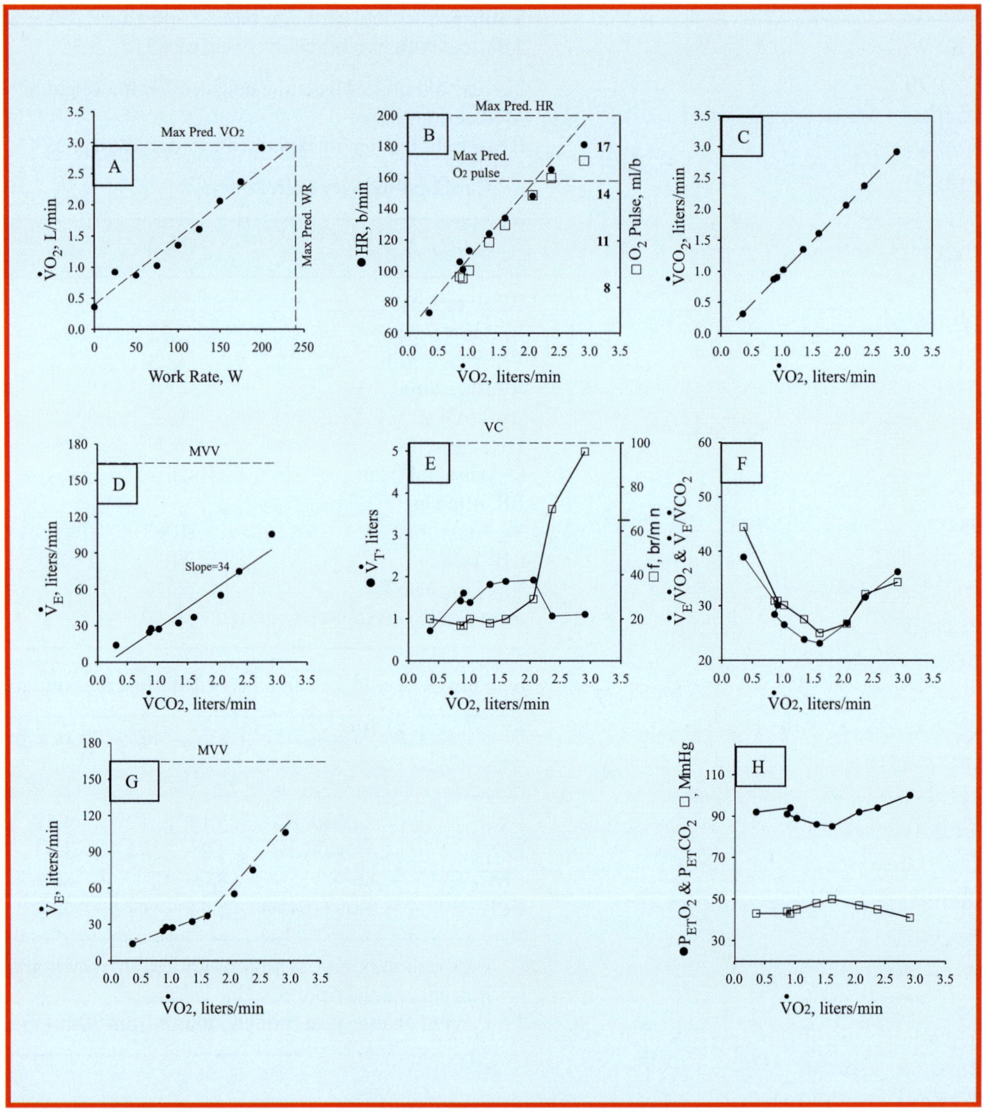

Fig. 2. Graphic representation of a maximal, incremental, cardiopulmonary exercise test in a subject with unexplained exertional dyspnea. These graphic data are 1-min interval averaged. The results are compared with calculated reference values obtained from several sources (dashed line). **A** Oxygen uptake ($\dot{V}_{O_2}$) vs. work rate. **B** Heart rate (HR) and O_2 pulse vs. $\dot{V}_{O_2}$. **C** Indirect determination of the anaerobic threshold (AT) using the modified V slope method in which the carbon dioxide production ($\dot{V}_{CO_2}$) is plotted vs. $\dot{V}_{O_2}$. **D** minute ventilation ($\dot{V}_E$) vs. carbon dioxide output ($\dot{V}_{CO_2}$). **E** Tidal volume (V_T) and respiratory frequency (f) vs. $\dot{V}_{O_2}$. **F** Ventilatory equivalent for O_2 ($\dot{V}_E/\dot{V}_{O_2}$), ventilatory equivalent for CO_2 ($\dot{V}_E/\dot{V}_{CO_2}$) vs. $\dot{V}_{O_2}$. **G** Minute ventilation ($\dot{V}_E$) vs. $\dot{V}_{O_2}$. **H** End-tidal pressure for O_2 (P_{ETO_2}) and end-tidal pressure for CO_2 (P_{ETCO_2}) vs. $\dot{V}_{O_2}$. Graphs **F** and **H** are also used for the determination of the AT using the ventilatory equivalents method.

ma treatment regimen, there was significant abatement of exertional chest tightness symptoms but shortness of breath persisted. While awaiting discharge from the Army for asthma, a CPET was performed to exclude the possibility of an additional etiology for his exertional shortness of breath. Anthropomorphic data, PFTs, and peak CPET results appear in table 6 and graphically in figure 2.

Interpretation of Exercise

Excellent effort was evidenced by near maximal predicted value for $\dot{V}_{O_2}$ (98%), greater than normal predicted O_2 Pulse (108% predicted), predicted HR = 91%, and the patient appearing exhausted. Exercise stopped because of leg fatigue (7/10). The aerobic capacity ($\dot{V}_{O_2}$ peak) was normal as was the $\dot{V}_{O_2}$-work rate relationship

(A). There was a normal cardiovascular response to exercise with a normal HR-$\dot{V}_{O_2}$ relationship (B) and O_2 pulse response (B). The AT was indeterminate using the V-slope method due to an abnormal breathing pattern (C [see below]). However, the AT was identified and within normal limits using the ventilatory equivalents method (F, H) thereby providing practical evidence that the 'dual methods' approach is preferable to using only 1 noninvasive methodology for AT determination [19]. There was plenty of ventilatory reserve at peak exercise (D, G) with a normal $\dot{V}_{O_2}$ vs. $\dot{V}_E$ relationship (G). An abnormal, atypical breathing pattern was noted with f dramatically increasing from 29 breaths per minute to 70 within 1 min and in the next minute achieving f = 96 at peak exercise (E)! This was associated with an increased but flattened V_T response, which actually decreased as f dramatically increased (E). Alveolar hypoventilation was noted as P_{ETCO_2} increased to 50 mm Hg during low-to-moderate intensity exercise and which decreased to only 42 mm Hg at peak exercise (H).

Spirometry performed before and after cycle exercise revealed a normal baseline study and significant reductions in FEV_1 at 15 and 30 min postexercise with significant improvement after inhaled bronchodilator (table 6). This is consistent with the diagnosis of EIB that was initially suggested by methacholine challenge [6, 83–85] (see chapters on Asthma and Exercise and Modalities of Clinical Exercise Testing – EIB).

Conclusion

Abnormal CPET with spirometry despite an aerobic capacity that was WNL. CPET was useful in establishing 2 coexisting diagnoses – EIB and psychogenic dysfunction.

Comment

This case underscores the value of noting both maximal and submaximal CPET responses especially in establishing a psychogenic etiology of unexplained exertional dyspnea [25]. The magnitude of the abnormal breathing response pattern is noteworthy and atypical for asthma. Furthermore, typically in asthma, the bronchoconstriction occurs postexercise [6, 84]. As 10% of patients with unexplained exertional dyspnea have 2 etiologies (see chapter on Unexplained Dyspnea), it is important to monitor response to treatment [25, 46]. A second CPET performed on another day while the patient was on an optimized asthma regimen elicited the same magnitude of abnormal breathing pattern but without significant changes in postexercise spirometry (negative test for EIB).

Table 7. Maximal cardiopulmonary incremental exercise test in a patient with non-ischemic, dilated, cardiomyopathy (case 2)

31-year-old female, Caucasian, height: 175 cm, weight: 94 kg; clinical Dx: cardiomyopathy

a Resting pulmonary function tests

Variable	Actual	% pred [100]
FVC, liters	4.23	96
FEV_1, liters	3.62	99
FEV_1/FVC	86%	
TLC, liters	5.81	100
RV, liters	1.43	99
DCO, ml/min/mm Hg	20.7	77

b Cardiopulmonary exercise test[1]

Variable	Peak	% pred
Work rate, W	135	76
$\dot{V}_{O_2}$, liters/min	1.51	76
$\dot{V}_{O_2}$, ml/kg/min	16.1	57
AT, liters/min	0.80	L (>1.24)
$\Delta\dot{V}_{O_2}/\Delta WR$	7.60	L (>8.3)
HR, bpm	170	90
O_2 Pulse, ml/beat	8.9	84
BP, mm Hg	125/75	
$\dot{V}_E$, liters/min	66	57
f, br/min	51	N
$\dot{V}_E/\dot{V}_{CO_2}$, at AT	32	N
SpO_2,% (rest 94%)	94%	
Stop: Leg fatigue 10/10; ideal weight = 71 kg.		

[1] Protocol: maximal, symptom-limited, incremental cycle ergometry, 15 W/min.

Postscript

The patient was referred for psychological evaluation and the diagnosis of separation anxiety (from family) was confirmed. The patient was discharged from the armed services.

Case Study 2: Maximal CPET in a Patient with Nonischemic Dilated Cardiomyopathy

Clinical History

A 31-year-old Caucasian female, lifelong nonsmoker with nonischemic dilated cardiomyopathy, with LVEF <30–35%, normal coronaries, increased filling pressures (LVEDP = 20 mm Hg, RV (systolic/diastolic) = 50/18 mm Hg, RA = 12 mm Hg), moderate pulmonary hyper-

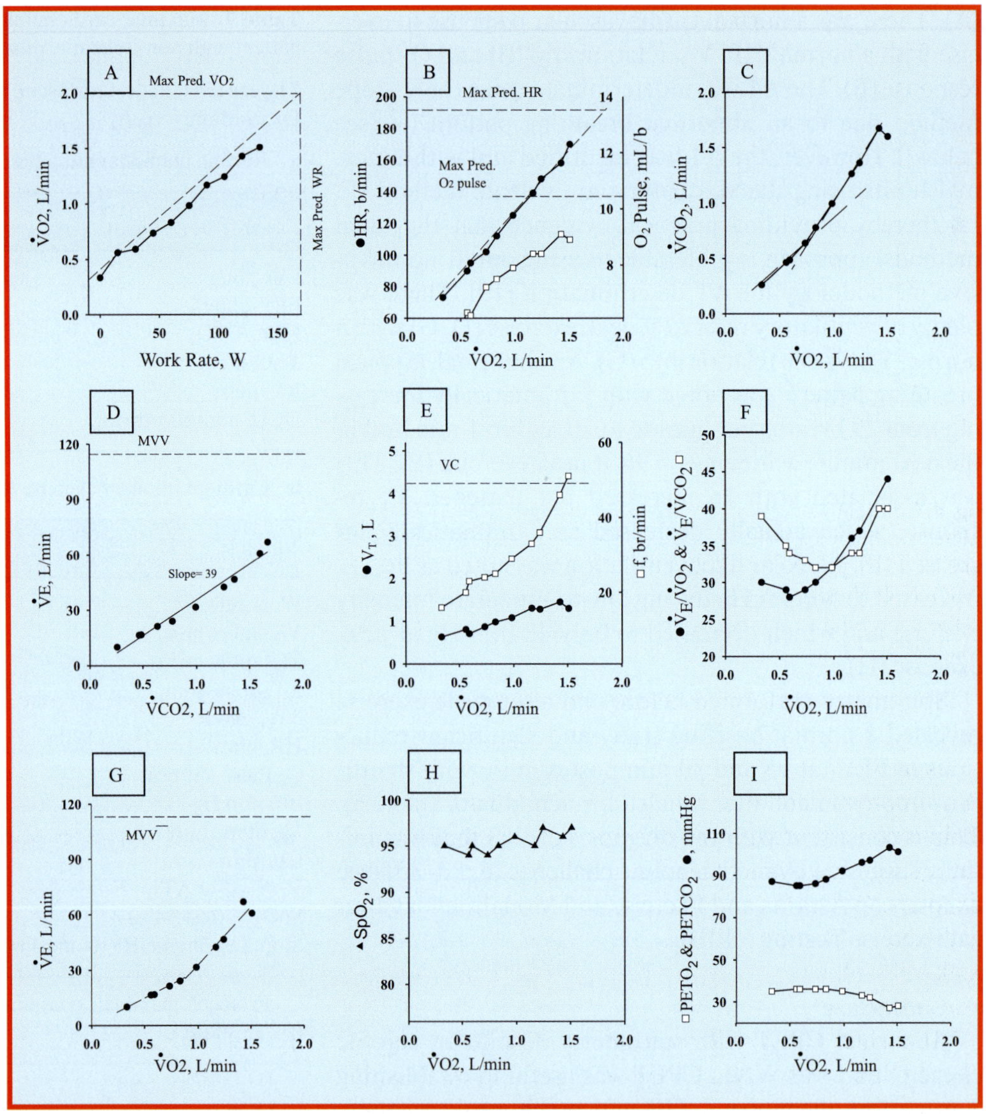

Fig. 3. Graphic representation of a maximal, incremental, cardiopulmonary exercise test in a patient with non-ischemic dilated cardiomyopathy. These graphic data are 1-min interval averaged. The results are compared with calculated reference values obtained from several sources (dashed line). **A** Oxygen uptake ($\dot{V}_{O_2}$) vs. work rate. **B** Heart rate (HR) and O_2 pulse vs. $\dot{V}_{O_2}$. **C** Indirect determination of the anaerobic threshold (AT) using the modified V slope method in which the carbon dioxide production ($\dot{V}_{CO_2}$) is plotted vs. $\dot{V}_{O_2}$. **D** Minute ventilation ($\dot{V}_E$) vs. carbon dioxide output ($\dot{V}_{CO_2}$). **E** Tidal volume (V_T) and respiratory frequency (f) vs. $\dot{V}_{O_2}$. **F** Ventilatory equivalent for O_2 ($\dot{V}_E/\dot{V}_{O_2}$), ventilatory equivalent for CO_2 ($\dot{V}_E/\dot{V}_{CO_2}$) vs. $\dot{V}_{O_2}$. **G** Minute ventilation ($\dot{V}_E$) vs. $\dot{V}_{O_2}$. **H** SpO_2 vs. $\dot{V}_{O_2}$. **I** End-tidal pressure for O_2 (P_{ETO_2}) and end-tidal pressure for CO_2 (P_{ETCO_2}) vs. $\dot{V}_{O_2}$. Graphs **F** and **I** are used for the determination of the AT using the ventilatory equivalents method.

tension PA (systolic/diastolic/ mean) = 45/20/28 mm Hg), and global hypokinesis was referred for CPET as part of a cardiac transplantation evaluation. Resting ECG revealed a left bundle branch pattern (LBBB). In the preceding 1 year she had progressive exertional dyspnea, generalized fatigue and had gained 12 kg. Prior to the onset of her illness, she was physically active running 3 × weekly. Current medications included carvedilol, lisinopril, furosemide, and paroxitene. Anthropomorphic data, PFTs, and peak incremental CPET results appear in table 7 and graphically in figure 3.

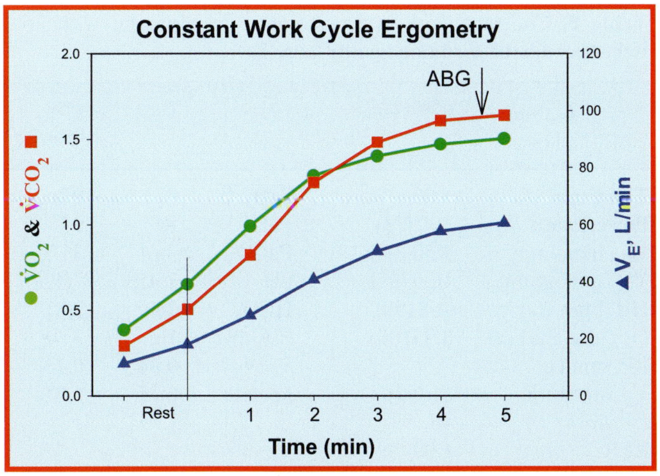

Fig. 4. Constant work cycle ergometry in a patient with nonischemic dilated cardiomyopathy. $\dot{V}_{O_2}$ (solid circle; green), $\dot{V}_{CO_2}$ (square; red), and $\dot{V}_E$ (triangle; blue) vs. time (min). An arterial blood sample (ABG) is obtained at minute 5 constant work exercise and referenced to the appropriate metabolic measurement interval for determination of $P(A\text{-}a)O_2$ and V_D/V_T (case 2).

Interpretation

Spirometry and lung volumes are WNL. DLCO is borderline reduced most probably reflecting reduced cardiac output and resultant $\dot{V}/\dot{Q}$ derangement and probable alveolar capillary loss.

Exercise: Maximal effort was evidenced by achieving a peak HR = 90% while on Carvedilol and clinically looking truly exhausted. Exercise stopped because of leg fatigue (10/10). There was a mild reduction in peak WR and peak $\dot{V}_{O_2}$ (A) that was associated with a low $\Delta\dot{V}_{O_2}/\Delta WR$, and a reduced O_2 pulse (B). When $\dot{V}_{O_2}$ is expressed per kg body weight, it is disproportionately reduced reflecting significant obesity (BMI = 33.2). The HR-$\dot{V}_{O_2}$ relationship was normal (A). The BP did not increase appropriately with exercise; there were no additional abnormal ECG changes (known LBBB pattern at rest noted). Exercise was cardiovascular limited as there was no heart rate reserve (15 bpm) at peak exercise (B). The AT was low using the 'dual methods' approach (C, F) [19]. This pattern of abnormalities is consistent with cardiovascular disease. Early onset metabolic acidosis (low AT) in this patient is consistent with cardiovascular disease but could also reflect deconditioning and/or skeletal muscle dysfunction.

There was plenty of ventilatory reserve at peak exercise ($\dot{V}_E$/MVV = 47%) (D, G). Abnormal ventilatory responses were observed including excessive ventilation for the metabolic rate requirement throughout exercise as manifested by an abnormal slope of the $\dot{V}_E$ vs. $\dot{V}_{CO_2}$ relationship (slope = 39, upper limit 95% CI <34) (D), which has been previously reported in heart failure patients [87] (D). There was a rapid, shallow breathing pattern (E); there were normal values for $\dot{V}_E/\dot{V}_{CO_2}$ and $\dot{V}_E/\dot{V}_{O_2}$ at near AT, which were slightly increased at peak exercise (F) with reduced values for P_{ETCO_2} at near peak exercise (I) likely reflecting mild alveolar hyperventilation. There was no desaturation with pulse oximetry (H).

To better characterize the abnormal ventilatory responses and to exclude a significant pulmonary gas exchange abnormality, a constant work rate exercise test approximating 75% of peak incremental WR was performed 1 h after the incremental CPET. An ABG obtained at minute 5 from a single radial arterial puncture approximates near maximal incremental exercise test values and may provide a clinically useful alternative to a radial arterial line (fig. 4) [42]. Resting and constant work ABG data appear in table 8 (note that at this level of CW, the patient achieved a $\dot{V}_{O_2}$ equal to the peak incremental CPET). The resting ABG revealed no hypoxemia and likely mixed metabolic and respiratory alkalosis at this altitude. There was no arterial desaturation during exercise. PaO_2 increased with exercise due to alveolar hyperventilation (decreased $PaCO_2$) and the $PAO_2 - PaO_2$ increased appropriately and was well within normal limits. V_D/V_T response decreased normally. Although not seen in this patient, abnormal V_D/V_T responses are often observed in patients with heart failure due to reduced cardiac output and resultant $\dot{V}/\dot{Q}$ derangement [58]. The CW exercise ABG revealed a combined metabolic acidosis and respiratory alkalosis with ↑ in arterial lactate and appropriate reciprocal ↓ in serum HCO_3^-.

Conclusion

Abnormal exercise test. There was a mild reduction in aerobic capacity ($\dot{V}_{O_2}$peak) with an abnormal exercise response pattern consistent with cardiovascular disease and a predominantly O_2 transport limitation to exercise. The abnormal ventilatory responses do not appear exercise limiting; this is consistent with the heart failure literature as is the normal SaO_2, PaO_2, and $PAO_2 - PaO_2$ obtained during CW exercise. As exercise limitation is usually multifactorial, the variable contribution of deconditioning, skeletal muscle dysfunction, and obesity to this patient's exercise intolerance should be considered.

Comments

A $\dot{V}_{O_2}$peak = 76% on a cycle ergometer (≈80–84% on a treadmill) is well above the 50% level of $\dot{V}_{O_2}$max associated with poor survival in patients with chronic heart failure [54, 88]. Consequently, emergent cardiac transplantation was not necessary and the patient continued to receive optimized medical management. Importantly, this patient had only a mildly reduced $\dot{V}_{O_2}$peak when reference values for sedentary subjects were used demonstrating that physically fit individuals such as this patient may experience significant reductions in their peak $\dot{V}_{O_2}$ as a result of illness and still either be within the normal confidence interval for sedentary subjects, borderline, or only mildly abnormal.

The addition of CW exercise testing permitted the evaluation of pulmonary gas exchange at (near) maximal $\dot{V}_{O_2}$ (tables 7, 8) [42]. Increasingly, CW exercise testing is being utilized in clinical decision-making [89, 90]. Finally, the patient's CPET results provided the basis for an individualized cardiac rehabilitation prescription and an objective measure of interval evaluation.

Table 8. Constant work cycle ergometry in a patient with non-ischemic, dilated cardiomyopathy (case 2)

	CW (%)[1]		Rest	CW (5 min)[2]
Time, min	5:00	SaO_2, %	97	97
Power, watts	100 (75)	PaO_2	84	95
$\dot{V}_{O_2}$, liters/min	1.50 (99)	$PaCO_2$	36.1	31.3
$\dot{V}_{O_2}$, ml/kg/min	16.0 (99)	pH	7.453	7.422
HR, bpm	168 (99)	HCO_3^-	24.9	20.1
O_2 pulse, ml/beat	8.9 (100)	$P(A-a)O_2$	1	3
BP, mm Hg		V_D/V_T	0.34	0.23
$\dot{V}_E$, liters/min	61 (92)	Lactate	0.75	5.01
f, br/min	46			
RER	1.09			

1 % max incremental CPET.
2 Single stick ABG.

Postscript

After 1 year of an optimized medical regimen and cardiac rehabilitation, repeat CPET revealed significant improvement in aerobic capacity – $\dot{V}_{O_2}$peak (↑ 10%), O_2 pulse, AT, and exertional symptoms while ventilatory abnormalities were reduced. This was consistent with improvements in cardiac echocardiography and quality of life. Although improving, the etiology of the non-ischemic dilated cardiomyopathy remains uncertain.

Case Study 3: Maximal CPET in a Patient with COPD

Clinical History

A 63-year-old Caucasian male with moderate-severe COPD was referred for CPET because of increasing exertional dyspnea over the last 1 year with stable PFTs and ECG. He was considering relocating to a New Mexico ski resort (altitude ≈ 3,000 m). The patient had a >50 pack year smoking history but had stopped when the diagnosis of COPD was established 10 years earlier. His present medications included ipratropium bromide, triamcinalone acetate, and albuterol metered dose inhalers. His weight had been stable for the past 5 years. He had become a self-declared 'couch potatoe' as a result of his increasing exertional dyspnea. His chest radiograph showed hyperinflation and routine labs were within normal limits. Anthropomorphic data, PFTs, and peak CPET responses appear in table 9 and graphically in figure 5.

Table 9. Maximal cardiopulmonary incremental exercise test in a patient with COPD (case 3)

63-year old male, Caucasian, height: 180 cm, weight: 88.9 kg; clinical Dx: COPD.

a Resting pulmonary function tests

Variable	Actual	% pred [100]
FVC, liters	4.28	89
FEV_1, liters	1.80	48
FEV_1/FVC, %	42%	
TLC, liters	8.83	123
DCO, ml/min/mm Hg	17.9	52

b Cardiopulmonary exercise test[1]

Variable	Peak	% pred
Work rate, W	120	78
$\dot{V}_{O_2}$, liters/min	1.43	64
$\dot{V}_{O_2}$, ml/kg/min	16.0	59
AT, liters/min	0.87	L (>0.89)
HR, bpm	152	90
O_2 pulse, ml/beat	9.4	71
$\dot{V}_E$, liters/min	82	115
f, br/min	42	N
$\dot{V}_E/\dot{V}_{CO_2}$, at AT	48	H

Stop: dyspnea 9/10. Ideal weight = 82 kg.

1 Protocol: maximal, symptom-limited, incremental cycle ergometry, 20 W/min.

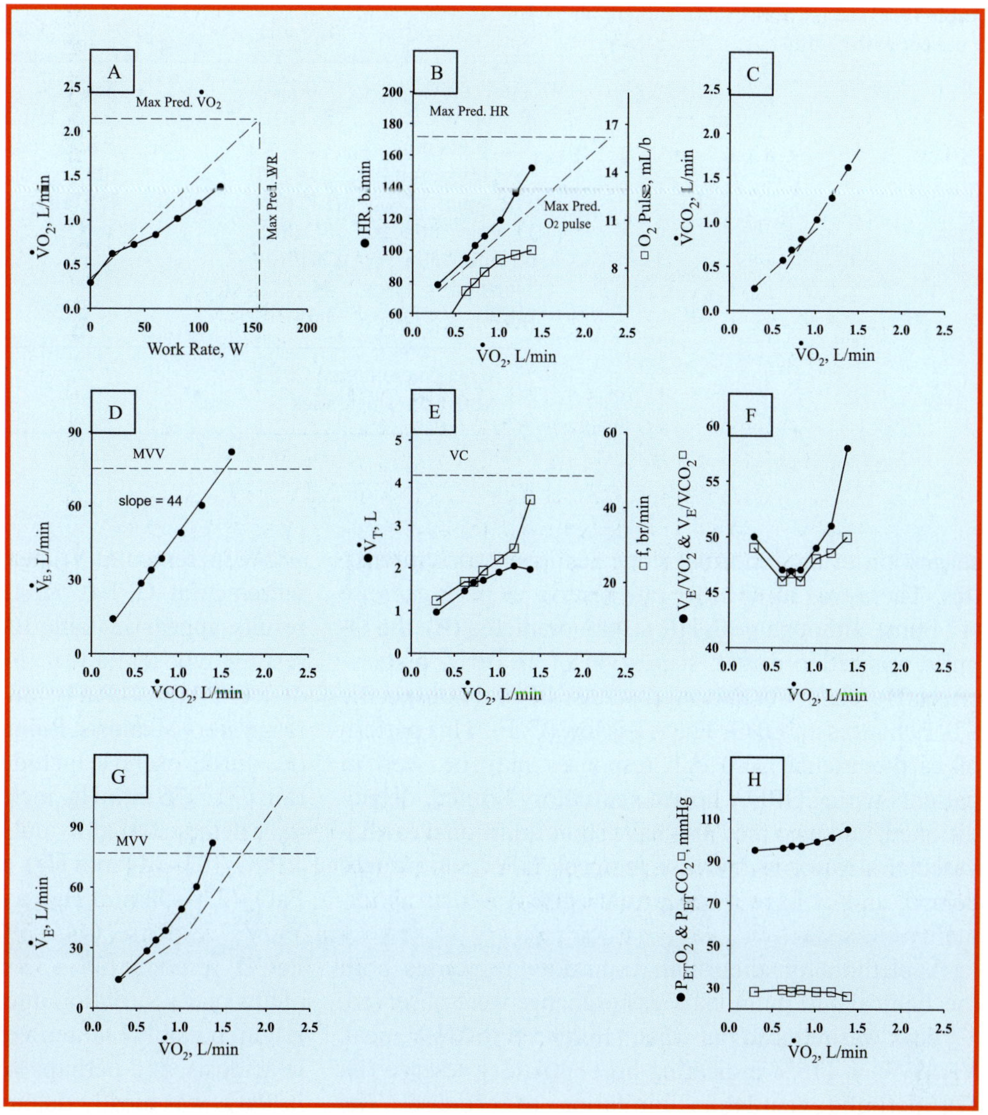

Fig. 5. Graphic representation of a maximal, incremental, cardiopulmonary exercise test in a patient with COPD. These graphic data are 1-min interval averaged. The results are compared with calculated reference values obtained from several sources (dashed line). **A** Oxygen uptake ($\dot{V}_{O_2}$) vs. work rate. **B** Heart rate (HR) and O_2 pulse vs. $\dot{V}_{O_2}$. **C** Indirect determination of the anaerobic threshold (AT) using the modified V slope method in which the carbon dioxide production ($\dot{V}_{CO_2}$) is plotted vs. $\dot{V}_{O_2}$. **D** Minute ventilation ($\dot{V}_E$) vs. carbon dioxide output ($\dot{V}_{CO_2}$). **E** Tidal volume (V_T) and respiratory frequency (f) vs. $\dot{V}_{O_2}$. **F** Ventilatory equivalent for O_2 ($\dot{V}_E/\dot{V}_{O_2}$), ventilatory equivalent for CO_2 ($\dot{V}_E/\dot{V}_{CO_2}$) vs. $\dot{V}_{O_2}$. **G** Minute ventilation ($\dot{V}_E$) vs. $\dot{V}_{O_2}$. **H** Illustrates end-tidal pressure for O_2 (P_{ETO_2}) and end-tidal pressure for CO_2 (P_{ETCO_2}) vs. $\dot{V}_{O_2}$. Graphs **F** and **H** are also used for the determination of the AT using the ventilatory equivalents method.

Interpretation

PFTs: Moderate-to-severe obstructive ventilatory impairment. Lung volumes are consistent with air trapping. A moderate-severe reduction in DLCO is observed.

Exercise: Outstanding effort as reflected by patient achieving physiologic (ventilatory) limitation, HR = 90% predicted, RER = 1.16, and patient appearing truly exhausted; exercise stopped due to dyspnea (9/10). Moderate reduction in $\dot{V}_{O_2}$peak was noted (A). There was a mild reduction in peak WR with the $\dot{V}_{O_2}$-WR relationship appearing somewhat right-shifted (A). The HR-$\dot{V}_{O_2}$ relationship was left-shifted (↑ HR at submaximal $\dot{V}_{O_2}$) with

Table 10. Constant work cycle ergomerty in a patient with COPD

	CW (%)[1]		Rest	CW (5 min)[2]
Time, min	5:00	SaO_2, %	93	76
Power, W	85 (70)	PaO_2, mm Hg	63	42
$\dot{V}_{O_2}$, liters/min	1.22 (85)	$PaCO_2$, mm Hg	34	33
$\dot{V}_{O_2}$, ml/kg/min	13.6 (85)	pH	7.445	7.362
HR, bpm	148 (97)	$P(A\text{-}a)O_2$, mm Hg	23	58
O_2 Pulse ml/beat	8.3 (88)	V_D/V_T	0.44	0.39
$\dot{V}_E$, liters/min	79 (96)			
f, br/min	44			
RER	1.18			

[1] % max incremental CPET.
[2] ABG from single stick.

suggestion of an abnormal slope at higher work intensities. There was mild heart rate reserve at peak exercise (17 bpm), although peak HR = 90% predicted (B); the O_2 pulse was reduced with suggestion of an early 'plateau' effect (B). There were normal exercise BP and nonspecific ST-T changes on ECG. The AT is low (C, F). This pattern of cardiovascular and AT responses may be seen in patients with COPD who are ventilatory limited, deconditioned, and who may also have some additional cardiovascular stressor to increase the peak HR response (see below), and/or have a concurrent cardiovascular abnormality.

A plethora of abnormal respiratory responses both mechanical and pulmonary gas exchange were observed. $\dot{V}_E$ peak was reduced but when referenced to MVV, peak $\dot{V}_E$/MVV = 115% indicating no ventilatory reserve (D, G), defining ventilatory limitation to exercise. The breathing strategy reflected that the increase in V_T was limited (possibly related to dynamic hyperinflation) with increases in $\dot{V}_E$ achieved mostly through increases in f (E). Other abnormal ventilatory responses included excessive ventilation for the metabolic requirement throughout exercise as manifested by an abnormal slope of the $\dot{V}_E$ vs. $\dot{V}_{CO_2}$ relationship (slope = 44 using linear regression) (D), an abnormal $\dot{V}_E$ vs. $\dot{V}_{O_2}$ relationship (G), and increased values for $\dot{V}_E/\dot{V}_{CO_2}$ and $\dot{V}_E/\dot{V}_{O_2}$ throughout exercise (F). P_{ETCO_2} did not change significantly with exercise (H). There was a significant decrease in exercise SpO_2 (93%→85%), but with poor correlation to arterial pulsation.

To better characterize the abnormal pulmonary gas exchange responses and in view of DLCO = 51%, a constant work rate exercise test approximating 70% of peak incremental WR (achieving during min 5 CW exercise ≈85% incremental $\dot{V}_{O_2}$peak) was performed 1 h after the incremental CPET. Resting and minute 5 CW ABG results appear in table 10. Resting ABG revealed mild resting hypoxemia (for this altitude) with borderline widened $PAO_2 - PaO_2$, an abnormal V_D/V_T, and acute respiratory alkalosis. Pulmonary gas exchange abnormalities during exercise included impressive arterial desaturation (93→76 mm Hg, including a greater magnitude drop than demonstrated by pulse oximetry), hypoxemia with a ↓ PaO_2 (63→42 mm Hg), an abnormally widened $PAO_2 - PaO_2$ (23→58 mm Hg), a minimally changed (abnormal) V_D/V_T response (44→39). The essentially unchanged $PaCO_2$ response (34→33 mm Hg) reflects a reduced level of alveolar ventilation due to increased dead space ventilation, possibly blunted ventilatory responses to metabolic acidosis, and perhaps ventilatory limitation. The drop in PaO_2 was mostly due to $\dot{V}/\dot{Q}$ mismatching and also to alveolar hypoventilation. The acid-base status at near peak exercise is consistent with a metabolic (lactic) acidosis.

Conclusion

Abnormal exercise test. Moderate reduction in aerobic capacity. Abnormal respiratory factors were exercise limiting. Ventilatory limitation due to mechanical derangement was associated with a spectrum of pulmonary gas exchange abnormalities including inefficient ventilation (↑ $\dot{V}_E/\dot{V}_{CO_2}$), increased dead space ventilation (V_D/V_T), arterial desaturation (↓ SaO_2), hypoxemia (↓ PaO_2), and a possible blunted ventilatory response to metabolic acidosis. These factors contributed to this patient's ventilatory demand exceeding capacity and consequent ventilatory limitation and overall exercise intolerance. The HR response most probably reflects the additional cardiovascu-

Table 11. Maximal cardiopulmonary incremental exercise test in a patient with non-ischemic dilated cardiomyopathy and COPD (case 4)

56-year-old, male, black, height: 180 cm, weight: 71 kg, Hb 9.6; clinical Dx: dilated cardiomyopathy.

a Resting pulmonary function tests

Variable	Actual	% pred [100]
FVC, liters	2.80	66
FEV_1, liters	1.33	40
FEV_1/FVC	48%	
MVV, liters/min	54	
TLC, liters	3.73	104
RV, liters	2.60	138
DCO, ml/min/mm Hg	12.1	43

b Cardiopulmonary exercise test[1]

Variable	Peak	% pred	Variable	Rest	Peak
Work Rate, W	80	52	SaO_2, %	89%	78%
$\dot{V}_{O_2}$, liters/min	1.13	53	SpO_2, %	90%	86%
$\dot{V}_{O_2}$, ml/kg/min	16.0	53	PaO_2, mm Hg	65	54
AT, liters/min	0.75	L (>0.85)	$PaCO_2$, mm Hg	40	39
HR, bpm	168	97	pH	7.39	7.31
O_2 Pulse, ml/beat	7.0	55	HCO_3^-, mEq/l	24	20
$\Delta\dot{V}_{O_2}/\Delta WR$	7.2	L (>8.3)	$P(A\text{-}a)O_2$, mm Hg	19	39
$\dot{V}_E$, liters/min	61	112	V_D/V_T	0.48	0.42
f, br/min	44	N	Lactate, mEq/l	1.0	5.3
$\dot{V}_E/\dot{V}_{CO_2}$, at AT	50	H			
RER	1.12	H			

Stop: dyspnea and fatigue 10/10. Ideal weight = 81 kg.

[1] Protocol: maximal, symptom limited, incremental cycle ergometry, 10 W/min.

lar stress of severe hypoxemia. The O_2 pulse could have been reduced due to the early termination of exercise (ventilatory limitation), hypoxemia, deconditioning and/or skeletal muscle dysfunction, and theoretically, also to the hemodynamic consequences of dynamic hyperinflation. The multifactorial etiology of exercise limitation is nicely demonstrated in this patient.

Postscript

The patient was started on supplemental O_2 for activities requiring exertion. It was recommended that he not relocate to 3,000 m. Maximal CPET and subsequent CW exercise testing were valuable in establishing the need for and titration of supplemental O_2 during exercise. CPET results were also used to exclude clinically significant coronary artery disease and for writing an individualized exercise prescription for pulmonary rehabilitation.

Case Study 4: Maximal CPET in a Patient with Combined Heart and Lung Disease

Clinical History

A 56-year-old black man with a 5-year history of non-ischemic dilated cardiomyopathy (NIDCM) (class 111-NYHA) and COPD with a greater than 60 pack years smoking history (recently stopped) was referred for CPET because of progressive increase in dyspnea on exertion and fatigue associated with reduced exercise tolerance over the preceding 12 months. He had noted a decrease in muscle mass/strength in the last 1–2 years. The patient was referred for CPET for cardiac transplantation evaluation and determination of exercise limitation in this patient with both heart and lung disease. A recent cardiac echocardiogram revealed global chamber enlargement, depressed left ventricular function (LVEF ≈ 15%), apical

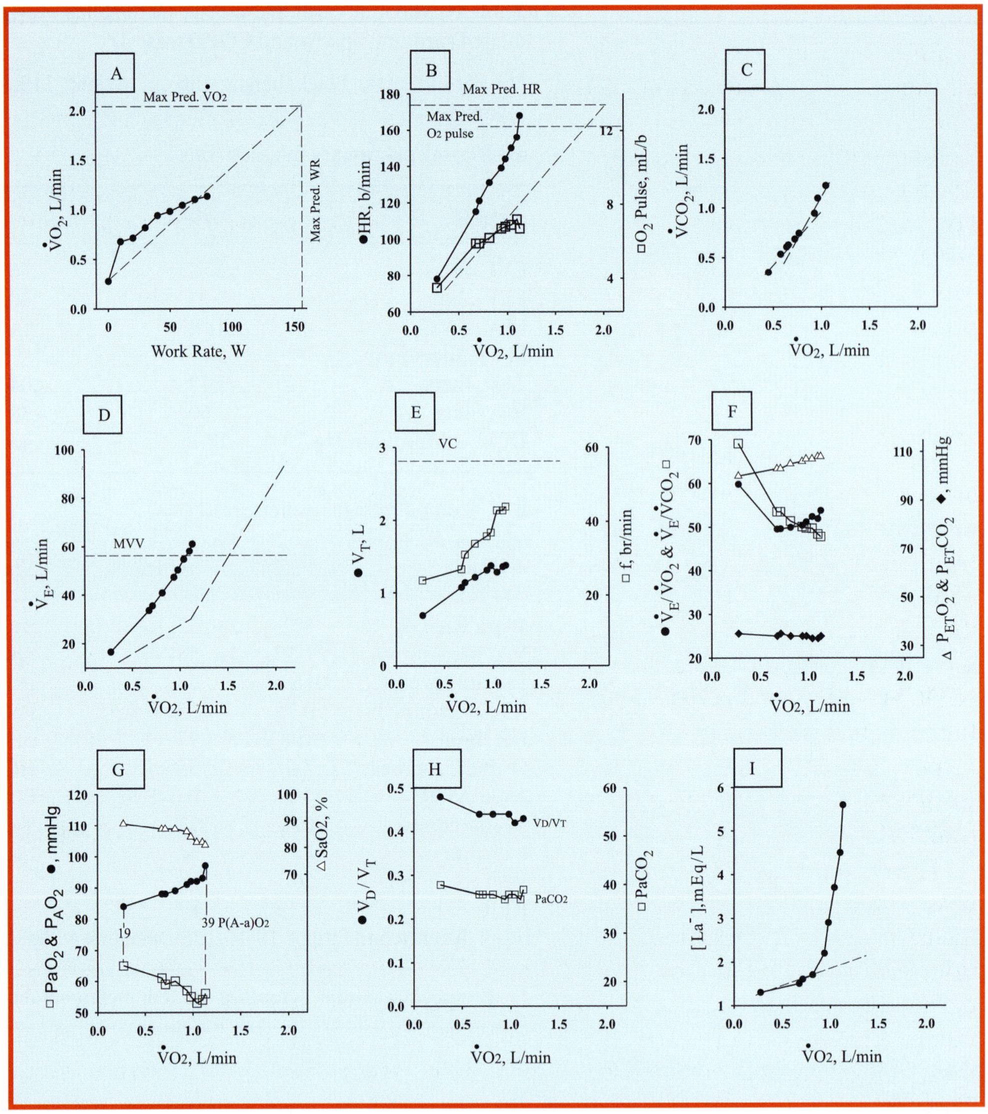

Fig. 6. Graphic representation of a maximal, incremental, cardiopulmonary exercise test in a patient with nonischemic dilated cardiomyopathy and COPD. These graphic data are 1-min interval averaged. The results are compared with calculated reference values obtained from several sources (dashed line). **A** Oxygen uptake ($\dot{V}_{O_2}$) vs. work rate. **B** Heart rate (HR) and O_2 pulse vs. $\dot{V}_{O_2}$. **C** Indirect determination of the anaerobic threshold (AT) using the modified V slope method in which the carbon dioxide production ($\dot{V}_{CO_2}$) is plotted vs. $\dot{V}_{O_2}$. **D** Minute ventilation ($\dot{V}_E$) vs. oxygen uptake ($\dot{V}_{O_2}$). **E** Tidal volume (V_T) and respiratory frequency (f) vs. $\dot{V}_{O_2}$. **F** Ventilatory equivalent for O_2 ($\dot{V}_E/\dot{V}_{O_2}$), ventilatory equivalent for CO_2 ($\dot{V}_E/\dot{V}_{CO_2}$), end-tidal pressure for O_2 (P_{ETO_2}) and end-tidal pressure for CO_2 (P_{ETCO_2}) vs. $\dot{V}_{O_2}$. This graph is also used for the determination of the AT using the ventilatory equivalents method. **G** Alveolar O_2 pressure (P_AO_2), arterial O_2 tension (PaO_2), alveolar-arterial O_2 pressure difference ($P_AO_2 - PaO_2$), and arterial O_2 saturation (SaO_2) vs. $\dot{V}_{O_2}$. **H** Physiologic dead space to tidal volume ratio (V_D/V_T) and arterial CO_2 tension vs. $\dot{V}_{O_2}$. **I** Determination of AT using the plot of arterial lactate vs. $\dot{V}_{O_2}$.

LV thrombus, intact valves and moderate pulmonary hypertension (PA systolic/diastolic = 49/20 mm Hg). Resting ECG revealed nonspecific ST-T changes, occasional PVCS, and an abnormal P wave axis in AVL. Medications included: ipratropium MDI, albuterol MDI, digoxin, lisinopril, furosemide, and Coumadin. Labs: hemoglobin/hematocrit = 9.6/34.8. Anthropomorphic data, PFTs, and peak CPET results appear in table 11 and graphically in figure 6, respectively.

Interpretation

PFTs: Severe obstructive ventilatory impairment with air trapping. Severe reduction in DLCO.

Exercise: Because of this patient's severe COPD and likelihood for desaturation and the fact that pulse oximetry may potentially be unreliable in patients with heart failure [92] and in black subjects [19, 93], CPET with radial arterial line was performed. Outstanding effort was evidenced by patient achieving $\dot{V}_E$/MVV = 112% predicted, HR = 97% predicted, R = 1.12, and patient appearing exhausted. Exercise stopped because of dyspnea (10/10) and fatigue (9/10). There was a moderate reduction in aerobic capacity ($\dot{V}_{O_2}$peak) and peak WR achieved (A). The $\dot{V}_{O_2}$-WR relationship appears to reach an early plateau with a low$\Delta\dot{V}_{O_2}/\Delta$WR (A), reflecting reduced O_2 transport and/or O_2 utilization. The $\dot{V}_{O_2}$-HR relationship was left-shifted (↑ HR at submaximal levels of $\dot{V}_{O_2}$ with an abnormal slope) (B). Also, noteworthy is the achieved peak HR = 97% predicted in a patient who is ventilatory limited and who has moderate-to-severe NIDCM and more likely to manifest chronotropic dysfunction (see section on Cardiovascular Disease) [56]. Hypoxemia and anemia [94, 95] provided additional cardiovascular stresses responsible for achieving that peak HR.

The O_2 pulse was markedly reduced (B). This patient possessed a number of factors known to impact O_2 pulse including reduced stroke volume due to systolic dysfunction, hypoxemia with progressive arterial desaturation during exercise, anemia, deconditioning, ventilatory limitation to exercise and possibly even dynamic hyperinflation and its potential for hemodynamic consequences. There were no abnormal BP or ECG responses. Interestingly, ventricular premature contractions decreased during exercise despite ↓SaO_2 and ↓PaO_2. The AT was low using the noninvasive 'dual methods' approach (C, F) [19] and confirmed through direct lactate measurements (I). Clearly, a cardiovascular (O_2 transport) abnormality is evidenced.

Respiratory Responses: Abnormal ventilatory responses were observed including excessive ventilation for the metabolic requirement throughout exercise as manifested by an abnormal $\dot{V}_E$ vs. $\dot{V}_{O_2}$ relationship (D), an abnormal slope of the $\dot{V}_E$ vs. $\dot{V}_{CO_2}$ relationship (slope = 45, 95% CI <34 [not shown]), and increased values for $\dot{V}_E/\dot{V}_{CO_2}$ and $\dot{V}_E/\dot{V}_{O_2}$ throughout exercise (F). A rapid shallow breathing pattern was observed (E).

$\dot{V}_E/\dot{V}_{CO_2}$, a noninvasive estimator of ventilation efficiency is often abnormal in patients with lung disease due to increased contribution of high $\dot{V}/\dot{Q}$ regions or more often due to increased dead space ventilation. In turn, patients with heart failure can also have abnormal $\dot{V}_E/\dot{V}_{CO_2}$ responses, especially patients with more severe disease. Recent work has suggested that the slope of $\dot{V}_E$ vs. $\dot{V}_{CO_2}$ relationship is a valuable supplemental prognostic indicator for survival ($\dot{V}_{O_2}$max was still better) in patients with chronic heart failure [87]. However, in this patient with co-existing severe heart and lung disease, $\dot{V}_E/\dot{V}_{CO_2}$ has limited discriminatory value and is most probably, primarily abnormal due to severe COPD.

Importantly, there was no ventilatory reserve as $\dot{V}_E$/MVV = 112% predicted (D). $\dot{V}_E$/MVV is usually <75% in patients with heart failure. In patients with severe COPD, the $\dot{V}_E$/MVV often approaches or exceeds the ventilatory ceiling ($\dot{V}_E$/MVV ≥ 100%).

Abnormal pulmonary gas exchange responses in this patient including significant arterial desaturation (↓ Δ 11%) (G), hypoxemia (↓ PaO_2) with widened $PAO_2 - PaO_2$ (normal <35) (G), and abnormal (essentially unchanged) V_D/V_T responses (H) with no real change in $PaCO_2$ (40→39) (H) were observed. The lack of change in $PaCO_2$ reflects a reduced level of alveolar ventilation due to a mechanical limitation and a blunted ventilatory response to metabolic acidosis. These pulmonary gas exchange abnormalities are most likely due to COPD. V_D/V_T abnormalities occurring in patients with heart failure are explained by the same pathophysiology noted above for abnormal $\dot{V}_E/\dot{V}_{CO_2}$ responses [58, 87].

Importantly, patients with heart failure usually do not develop arterial desaturation and maintain relatively normal PaO_2 during exercise. Therefore, a primary respiratory etiology of these pulmonary gas exchange abnormalities due to COPD is more likely in this patient. The ↓ in PaO_2 and in SaO_2 are consistent with DLCO = 39% predicted. Pulmonary hypertension may also have contributed to these pulmonary gas exchange abnormalities. The acid-base status at peak exercise is consistent with a metabolic acidosis without the appropriate respiratory compensation due to COPD. The increase in serum lactate with exercise was paralleled by a reciprocal decrease in serum bicarbonate.

Conclusion

Abnormal exercise test, moderate-to-severe reduction in aerobic capacity but above the 50% level associated with poor outcome in patients being evaluated for cardiac transplantation [54, 88]. Exercise limitation in this patient is multifactorial: (1) ventilatory (mechanical) and pulmonary gas exchange derangements (hypoxemia, arterial desaturation, ↑ dead space ventilation) due to

COPD appear to be the predominant cause (s) of exercise limitation; (2) O_2 transport abnormalities due to cardiovascular dysfunction and compensated nonischemic dilated cardiomyopathy certainly contributed, as did pulmonary hypertension; (3) deconditioning with skeletal muscle dysfunction and attendant O_2 utilization abnormalities were also likely, and (4) anemia may also have contributed to reduction in O_2 carrying capacity [94, 95].

Comment

Standard algorithms are inadequate in interpreting CPET results in patients with both heart and lung disease. $\dot{V}_E$/MVV exceeding 100% predicted in patients with heart failure may signal the presence of combined heart and lung disease. Currently, the exercise variables most helpful in distinguishing between heart failure and COPD include $\dot{V}_E$/MVV, SaO_2 and PaO_2 responses, and BP and ECG responses. CPET was able to identify, prioritize, and (relatively) quantitate exercise-limiting factors contributing to this patient's exercise intolerance so that an effective clinical management scheme could be initiated. Based on the results of the CPET, the following recommendations were made: (1) supplemental O_2 especially during exercise; (2) aggressive treatment to optimize respiratory function; (3) consider adding carvedilol to cardiac regimen; (4) anemia work-up, including GI evaluation; (5) cardiopulmonary rehabilitation with an individualized exercise program based on CPET results, and (6) interval evaluation after above recommendations.

Postscript

A GI work-up revealed a guiac-positive stool; subsequent colonoscopy revealed 2 polyps, which were removed. Iron supplementation was initiated with improvement in hemogram. Exertional oxygen supplementation was prescribed, respiratory, and cardiac medications were optimized, and cardiopulmonary rehabilitation was begun.

Acknowledgements

The authors wish to acknowledge Mr. Raul Hernandez, Ms. Luz B. Torres and Mr. Sean Connery for their diligence in preparation of the manuscript.

References

1 Hamilton AL, Killian KJ, Summers E, Jones NL: Muscle strength, symptom intensity, and exercise capacity in patients with cardiorespiratory disorders. Am J Respir Crit Care Med 1995;152:2021–2031.
2 Sue DY, Wasserman K: Impact of integrative cardiopulmonary exercise testing on clinical decision making. Chest 1991;99:981–992.
3 Weisman IM, Zeballos RJ: An integrated approach to the interpretation of cardiopulmonary exercise testing. Clin Chest Med 1994;15:421–445.
4 Wasserman K, Hansen JE, Sue DY, Casaburi R, Whipp BJ: Principles of Exercise Testing and Interpretation, ed 3. Philadelphia, Lippincot Williams & Wilkins, 1999.
5 Weisman IM, Zeballos RJ: Cardiopulmonary exercise testing-the need for standardization. Pulmon Persp 1992;9:5–8.
6 ERS Task Force on Standardization of Clinical Exercise Testing: Clinical exercise testing with reference to lung diseases: Indications, standardization, and interpretation strategies. Eur Respir J 1997;10:2662–2689.
7 Dempsey JA, Babcock MA: An integrative view of limitations to muscular performance. Adv Exp Med Biol 1995;384:393–399.
8 Jones NL, Killian KJ: Exercise limitation in health and disease. N Engl J Med 2000;343:632–641.
9 Wagner PD: Determinants of maximal oxygen transport and utilization. Annu Rev Physiol 1996;58:21–50.
10 Eschenbacher WL, Mannina A: An algorithm for the interpretation of cardiopulmonary exercise tests. Chest 1990;97:263–267.
11 Neuberg GW, Friedman SH, Weiss MB, Herman MV: Cardiopulmonary exercise testing: The clinical value of gas exchange data. Arch Intern Med 1988;148:2221–2226.
12 Weisman IM, Connery SM, Belbel RJ, Zeballos RJ: The role of cardiopulmonary exercise testing in the selection of patients for cardiac transplantation. Chest 1992;102:1871–1874.
13 Cumming GR, Borysyk LM: Criteria for maximum oxygen uptake in men over 40 in a population survey. Med Sci Sports Exerc 1972;14:18–22.
14 Myers J, Walsh D, Buchanan N, Foelicher VF: Can maximal cardiopulmonary capacity be recognized by a plateau in oxygen uptake? Chest 1989;96:1312–1316.
15 Lange-Andersen K, Shepard RJ, Denolin H, Varnauskas E, Masironi R: Fundamentals of Exercise Testing. Geneva, World Health Organization, 1971.
16 Borg GAV: Psychophysical bases of perceived exertion. Med Sci Sports Exerc 1982;14:377–381.
17 Ramos-Barbon D, Fitchett D, Gibbons WJ, Latter DA, Levy RD: Maximal exercise testing for the selection of heart transplantation candidates: Limitation of peak oxygen consumption. Chest 1999;115:410–417.
18 Jones NL: Clinical Exercise Testing, ed 4. Philadelphia, Saunders, 1997.
19 Zeballos RJ, Weisman IM: Behind the scenes of cardiopulmonary exercise testing. Clin Chest Med 1994;15:193–213.
20 ACC/AHA guidelines for exercise testing: A report of the American College of Cardiology/ American Heart Association Task Force on Practice Guidelines (Committee on Exercise Testing). J Am Coll Cardiol 1997;30:260–315.
21 Cotes JE: Lung Function: Assessment and Application in Medicine, ed 5. Oxford, Blackwell Scientific Publications 1993, pp 54–58.
22 American College of Sports Medicine: ACSM's Guidelines for Exercise Testing and Prescription, ed 6. Philadelphia, Lippincott Williams & Wilkins, 2000
23 Shephard RJ: Tests of maximum oxygen intake: A critical review. Sports Med 1984;1:99–124.
24 Astrand PO, Rodahl K: Textbook of Work Physiology: Physiological Bases of Exercise, ed 3. New York, McGraw-Hill, 1986.
25 Weisman IM, Zeballos RJ: Clinical evaluation of unexplained dyspnea. Cardiologia 1996;41:621–634.

26 Belman MJ, Epstein LJ, Doornbos D, Elashoff JD, Koerner SK, Mohsenifar Z: Noninvasive determinations of the anaerobic threshold: Reliability and validity in patients with COPD. Chest 1992;102:1028–1034.
27 Brooks GA: Current concepts in lactate exchange. Med Sci Sports Exerc 1991;23:895–906.
28 Wasserman K, Beaver WL, Whipp BJ: Gas exchange theory and the lactic acidosis (anaerobic) threshold. Circulation 1990;81:II.14–II.30.
29 Myers J, Ashley E: Dangerous curves: A perspective on exercise, lactate, and the anaerobic threshold. Chest 1997;111:787–795.
30 Dickstein K, Barvik S, Aarsland T, Sanpinn S, Karlsson J: A comparison of methodologies in detection of the anaerobic threshold. Circulation 1990;81:II-38–II-46.
31 Sue DY, Wasserman K, Moricca RB, Casaburi R: Metabolic acidosis during exercise in patients with chronic obstructive pulmonary disease: Use of v-slope method for anaerobic threshold determination. Chest 1988;94:931–938.
32 Casaburi R, Patessio A, Loli F, Zanaboni S, Donner CF, Wasserman K: Reductions in exercise lactic acidosis and ventilation as a result of exercise training in patients with obstructive lung disease. Am Rev Respir Dis 1991;143:9–18.
32a Nishime EO, Cole CR, Blackstone EH, Pashkow FJ, Lauer MS: Heart rate recovery and treadmill exercise score as predictors of mortality in patients referred for exercise ECG. JAMA 2000;284:1392–1398.
33 Babb TG: Mechanical ventilatory constraints in aging, lung disease, and obesity: Perspective and brief review. Med Sci Sports Exerc 1999; 31(suppl):S12–S22.
34 Johnson BD, Weisman IM, Zeballos RJ, Beck KC: Emerging concepts in the evaluation of ventilatory limitation during exercise: The exercise tidal flow-volume loop. Chest 1999;116: 488–503.
35 Johnson BD, Beck KC, Zeballos RJ, Weisman IM: Advances in pulmonary laboratory testing. Chest 1999;116:1377–1387.
36 Marciniuk DD, Sridhar G, Clemens RE, Zintel TA, Gallagher CG: Lung volumes and expiratory flow limitation during exercise in interstitial lung disease. J Appl Physiol 1994;77:963–973.
37 Belman M, Botnick W, Shin J: Inhaled bronchodilators reduce dynamic hyperinflation during exercise in patients with chronic obstructive pulmonary disease. Am J Respir Crit Care Med 1996;153:967–975.
38 Martinez FJ, Montes de Oca M, Whyte RI, Stetz J, Gay SE, Celli BR: Lung-volume reduction improves dyspnea, dynamic hyperinflation, and respiratory muscle function. Am J Respir Crit Care Med 1997;155:1984–1990.
39 Koulouris NG, Dimopoulou I, Valta P, Finkelstein R, Cosio MG, Milic-Emili J: Detection of expiratory flow limitation during exercise in COPD patients. J Appl Physiol 1997;82:723–731.
40 Anthonisen NR, Fleetham JA: Ventilation: Total, alveolar, and dead space; in Fishman AP (ed): Handbook of Physiology: The Respiratory System: Gas Exchange. Bethesda, American Physiological Society, sect 3, vol IV, chap 7, 1987, pp 113–117.
41 Lewis DA, Sietsema KE, Casaburi R, Wasserman K: Inaccuracy of non-invasive estimates of VD/VT in clinical exercise testing. Chest 1994;106:1476–1480.
42 Zeballos RJ, Weisman IM, Connery SM: Comparison of pulmonary gas exchange measurements between incremental and constant work exercise above the anaerobic threshold. Chest 1998;113:602–611.
43 Wagner PD: Ventilation-perfusion matching during exercise. Chest 1992;101:S192–S198.
44 Jones NL, McHardy GJR, Naimark A, Campbell EJM: Physiological dead space and alveolar-arterial gas pressure differences during exercise. Clin Sci 1966;31:19–29.
45 Mohsenifar Z, Brown HV, Koerner SK: Effect of breathing pattern on dead space ventilation VD/VT during exercise. Respiration 1985;47: 232–236.
46 Martinez FJ, Stanopoulos I, Acero R, Becker FS, Pickering R, Beamis JF: Graded comprehensive cardiopulmonary exercise testing in the evaluation of dyspnea unexplained by routine evaluation. Chest 1994;105:168–174.
47 Mohsenifar ZAB, Tashkin DP, Levy SE, Bjerke RD, Clements PJ, Furst D: Lack of sensitivity of measurements of VD/VT at rest and during exercise in detection of hemodynamically significant pulmonary vascular abnormalities in collagen vascular disease. Am Rev Respir Dis 1981;123:508–512.
48 Mahler DA, Guyatt GH, Jones PW: Clinical measurement of dyspnea; in Mahler DA (ed): Dyspnea. Lung Biology in Health and Disease Series, vol 111. New York, Marcel Dekker, 1998, pp 149–198.
49 Aitken RCB: Measurement of feelings using visual analogue scales. Proc R Soc Med 1969; 62:989–993.
50 Evans AB, Al-Himyary AJ, Hrovat MI, Pappagianopoulos P, Wain JC, et al: Abnormal skeletal muscle oxidative capacity after lung transplantation by ^{31}P-MRS. Am J Respir Crit Care Med 1997;155:615–621.
51 Richardson RS, Sheldon J, Poole DC, Hopkins SR, Ries AL, Wagner PD: Evidence of skeletal muscle metabolic reserve during whole body exercise in patients with chronic obstructive pulmonary disease. Am J Respir Crit Care Med 1999;159:881–885.
52 Johnson BD, Beck KC, Olson LJ, O'Malley KA, Allison TG, Squires RW, Gau GT: Ventilatory constraints during exercise in patients with chronic heart failure. Chest 2000;117: 321–332.
53 Mancini DM: Pulmonary factors limiting exercise capacity in patients with heart failure. Prog Cardiovasc Dis 1995;37:347–370.
54 Mancini DM, Eisen H, Kussmaul W, et al: Value of peak oxygen consumption for optimal timing of cardiac transplantation in ambulatory patients with heart failure. Circulation 1991; 83:778–786.
55 Mancini D, Reichek N, Chance B, Lenkinski R, Mullen J, Wilson JR: Contribution of skeletal muscle atrophy to exercise intolerance and altered muscle metabolism in heart failure. Circulation 1992;85:1364–1373.
56 Weber KT, Janicki JS: Cardiopulmonary Exercise Testing: Physiologic Principles and Clinical Application. Philadelphia, Saunders, 1986.
57 Francis GS, Goldsmith SR, Ziesche S: Nakajma H, Cohn JN, et al: Relative attention of sympathetic drive during exercise in patients with congestive heart failure. J Am Coll Cardiol 1985;5:832–839.
58 Myers J, Froelicher VF: Hemodynamic determinants of exercise capacity in chronic heart failure. Ann Intern Med 1991;115:377–386.
59 Janicki JS, Weber KT, Likoff MJ, Fishman AP: Exercise testing to evaluate patients with pulmonary vascular disease. Am Rev Respir Dis 1984;129:S93–S95.
60 D'Alonzo GE, Gianotti LA, Pohil RL, Reagle RR, Du Ree SL, Fuentes F, et al: Comparison of progressive exercise performance of normal subjects and patients with primary pulmonary hypertension. Chest 1987;92:57–62.
61 Saltin B, Blomquist G, Mitchell JH, Johnson RL, Wildenthal K, Chapman CB: Response to exercise after bed rest and after training. Circulation 1968;38(suppl 7):1–78.
62 Gosselink R, Troosters T, Decramer M: Peripheral muscle weakness contributes to exercise limitation in COPD. Am J Respir Crit Care Med 1996;153:976–980.
63 Engelen MPKJ, Schols AMWJ, Does JD, Gosker HR, Deutz NEP, Wouters EFM: Exercise-induced lactate increase in relation to muscle substrates in patients with chronic obstructive pulmonary disease. Am J Respir Crit Care Med 2000;162:1697–1704.
64 Flaherty KR, Wald J, Weisman IM, Zeballos RJ, Schork MA, Blaivas M, Rubenfire M, Martinez FJ: Unexplained exertional limitation: Characterization of patients with a mitochondrial myopathy. Am J Respir Crit Care Med 2001;164:425–432.
65 Babb TG, Viggiano R, Hurley B, Staats B, Rodarte JR: Effect of mild-to-moderate airflow limitation on exercise capacity. J Appl Physiol 1991;70:223–230.
66 Gallagher CG: Exercise limitation and clinical exercise testing in chronic obstructive pulmonary disease. Clin Chest Med 1994;15:305–326.
67 Marciniuk DD, Gallagher CG: Clinical exercise testing in chronic airflow limitation. Med Clin North Am 1996;80:565–587.
68 LoRusso TJ, Belman MJ, Elashoff JD, Koerner SK: Prediction of maximal exercise capacity in obstructive and restrictive pulmonary disease. Chest 1993;104:1748–1754.
69 Maltais F, Simard AA, Simard C, et al: Oxidative capacity of the skeletal muscle and lactic acid kinetics during exercise in normal subjects and in patients with COPD. Am J Respir Crit Care Med 1996;153:288–293.
70 Montes de Oca M, Rassulo J, Celli BR: Respiratory muscle and cardiopulmonary function during exercise in very severe COPD. Am J Respir Crit Care Med 1996;154:1284–1289.

71 O'Donnell DE, Lam M, Webb KA: Measurement of symptoms, lung hyperinflation, and endurance during exercise in chronic obstructive pulmonary disease. Am J Respir Crit Care Med 1998;158:1557–1565.
72 Hansen JE, Wasserman K: Pathophysiology of activity limitation in patients with interstitial lung disease. Chest 1996;109:1566–1576.
73 Keogh BA, Lakatos E, Price D, Crystal RG: Importance of the lower respiratory tract in oxygen transfer: Exercise testing in patients with interstitial and destructive lung disease. Am Rev Respir Dis 1984;129:S76–S80.
74 Marciniuk DD, Gallagher CG: Clinical exercise testing in interstitial lung disease. Clin Chest Med 1994;15:287–303.
75 Risk C, Epler GR, Gaensler EA: Exercise alveolar-arterial oxygen pressure difference in interstitial lung disease. Chest 1984;85:69–74.
76 Watters LC, King TE, Schwarz MI, Waldron JA, Stanfrod RE, et al: A clinical, radiographic, and physiologic scoring system for the longitudinal assessment of patients with idiopathic pulmonary fibrosis. Am Rev Respir Dis 1986; 133:97–103.
77 Whipp BJ, Davis JA: The ventilatory stress of exercise in obesity. Am Rev Respir Dis 1992; 145:101–105.
78 Sakamoto S, Ishikawa K, Senda S, Nakajima S, Matsuo H: The effect of obesity on ventilatory response and anaerobic threshold during exercise. J Med Syst 1993;17:227–231.
79 Salvadori A, Fanari P, Fontana M, Buontempi L, Saezza A, Baudo S, Miserocchi G, Longhini E: Oxygen uptake and cardiac performance in obese and normal subjects during exercise. Respiration 1999;66:25–33.
80 Hansen JE, Sue DY, Wasserman K: Predicted values for clinical exercise testing. Am Rev Respir Dis 1984;129(Suppl):S49–S55.
81 Riddle W, Younes M, Remmers J: Graphical analysis of patient performance in the pulmonary function laboratory. Fourth Annual Symposium on Computer Applications in Medical Care. IEEE 1980;282–290.
82 Wasserman K, Whipp BJ: Exercise physiology in health an disease. Am Rev Respir Dis 1975; 112:219–249.
83 American Thoracic Society: Guidelines for methacholine and exercise challenge testing – 1999. Am J Respir Crit Care Med 2000;161: 309–329.
84 National Heart, Lung and Blood Institute: National Asthma Education and Prevention Program. Expert Panel Report 2: Guidelines for the Diagnosis and Management of Asthma. Bethesda, National Institutes of Health, 1997, publ 97-4051.
85 European Respiratory Society: Airway responsiveness. Standardized challenge testing with pharmacological, physical and sensitizing stimuli in adults. Eur Respir J 1993;16(suppl):53–83.
86 Zeballos RJ, Weisman IM, Connery SM, Bradley JP: Standard treadmill (STE) vs. incremental cycle ergometry (IET) in the evaluation of airway hyperreactivity in unexplained dyspnea. Am J Respir Crit Care Med 1999;159: A419.
87 Chua TP, Ponikowski P, Harrington D, Anker SD, Webb-Peploe K, et al: Clinical correlates and prognostic significance of the ventilatory response to exercise in chronic heart failure. J Am Coll Cardiol 1997;29:1585–1590.
88 Stelken AM, Younis LT, Jennison SH, et al: Prognostic value of cardiopulmonary exercise testing using percent achieved of predicted peak oxygen uptake for patients with ischemic and dilated cardiomyopathy. J Am Coll Cardiol 1996;27:345–352.
89 Oga T, Nishimura K, Mitsushiro T, Hajiro T, Ikeda A, Izumi T: The effect of oxitropium bromide on exercise performance in patients with stable chonic obstructive pulmonary disease. Am J Respir Crit Care Med 2000;161:1897–1901.
90 O'Donnell DE, Lam M, Webb KA: Spirometric correlates of improvement in exercise performance after anticholinergic therapy in chronic obstructive pulmonary disease. Am J Respir Crit Care Med 1999;160:542–549.
91 American Association Respiratory Care (AARC): Clinical practice guideline: Exercise testing for evaluation of hypoxemia and/or desaturation. Respir Care 1992;37:907–912.
92 Hansen JE, Casaburi R: Validity of ear oximetry in clinical exercise testing. Chest 1987; 91:333–337.
93 Zeballos RJ, Weisman IM: Reliability of noninvasive oximetry in black subjects during exercise and hypoxia. Am Rev Respir Dis 1991;144:1240–1244.
94 Schaffartzik WE, Barton D, Poole K, Tsukimoto M, Hogan D, Bebut J, Wagner P: Expectations of reduced [Hb] on leg VO_2 during maximal exercise in humans. J Appl Phys 93; 75:491–498.
95 Warren GL, Cureton KJ: Modeling the effects of alternations in hemoglobin concentration on VO_2max. Med Sci Sports Exerc 1989;21: 256–231.
96 Jones NL, Makrides L, Hitchcock C, Chypchar T, McCartney N: Normal standards for an incremental progressive cycle ergometer test. Am Rev Respir Dis 1985;131:700–708.
97 Blackie SP, Fairbarn MS, McElvaney GN, Morrison NJ, Wilcox PG, Pardy RL: Prediction of maximal oxygen uptake and power during cycle ergometry in subjects older than 55 years of age. Am Rev Respir Dis 1989;139: 1424–1429.
98 Blackie SP, Fairbarn MS, McElvaney NG, Wilcox PG, Morrison NJ, Pardy RL: Normal values and ranges for ventilation and breathing pattern at maximal exercise. Chest 1991; 100:136–142.
99 Weisman IM, Zeballos RJ: Clinical exercise testing. Clin Chest Med 2001;22:679–701.
100 Morris AH, Kanner RE, Crapo RO, et al: Clinical Pulmonary Function Testing, ed 2. Salt Lake City, Utah Intermountain Thoracic Society, 1984.

Idelle M. Weisman, MD
Human Performance Laboratory
Department of Clinical Investigation
Pulmonary-Critical Care Service
William Beaumont Army Medical Center
5005 N. Piedras Street
El Paso, TX 79920-5001 (USA)
Tel. +1 915 569 2664/2296
Fax +1 915 569 2554
E-Mail iweisman@aol.com or
Idelle.weisman@amedd.army.mil

Author Index

Subject Index